OXFORD MEDICAL PUBLICATIONS

CLINICAL DIETETICS AND NUTRITION

CLINICAL DIETETICS AND NUTRITION

SECOND EDITION

F. P. ANTIA

M.D. (Bom.), F.R.C.P. (Lond.)
M.S. (Ill.)

Honorary Physician in Charge, Department of Gastro-enterology, B. Y. L. Nair Charitable Hospital, Bombay. Consulting Physician and Gastroenterologist, Tata Memorial Hospital, Bombay. Consulting Honorary Physician, Radiation Medical Centre, Bhabha Atomic Research Centre, Bombay. Consulting Physician, B. D. Petit Parsi General Hospital, Bai Jerbai Wadia Hospital for Children and Habib Hospital, Bombay

DELHI
OXFORD UNIVERSITY PRESS
LONDON   NEW YORK
1973

Oxford University Press, Ely House, London W. 1

GLASGOW   NEW YORK   TORONTO   MELBOURNE   WELLINGTON
CAPE TOWN   IBADAN   NAIROBI   DAR ES SALAAM   LUSAKA   ADDIS ABABA
DELHI   BOMBAY   CALCUTTA   MADRAS   KARACHI   LAHORE   DACCA
KUALA LUMPUR   SINGAPORE   HONG KONG   TOKYO

2/11 *Ansari Road, Daryaganj, Delhi 110006*

Framroz Pirojshaw ANTIA 1916

First Published 1966
Second Edition 1973

Printed in India by Aroon Purie at Thomson Press (India) Limited, Faridabad, Haryana, and published by John Brown, Oxford University Press, 2/11, Ansari Road, Daryaganj, Delhi 110006.

CONTENTS

Part III CLINICAL DIETETICS

Part IV TABLES OF FOOD VALUES, ETC.

PREFACE

TO THE SECOND EDITION

The knowledge of human nutrition no longer entails merely prevention of deficiency diseases like pellagra, beriberi or scurvy. Nutrition now plays a major role in the prevention and management of many diseases. Indeed, one of the most important advances in modern medicine is not the discovery of antibiotics, but the better understanding of basic requirements of fluids and electrolytes. This helps in the management of seriously ill medical cases and is very vital in the successful outcome of surgery. For, ill-conceived notions may even lead to over-enthusiasm, whereby an acutely ill medical or surgical patient is literally drowned with excess fluids or electrolytes.

Human diseases are mostly the result of heredity, environment or food. It is not possible to change heredity, it is difficult to change environment, but it is relatively easy to change food habits. The lower the income, the higher the proportion of money spent on food. Knowledge of proper nutrition, therefore, is essential for economy and health. It is therefore surprising that nutrition does not form a part of the regular medical curriculum, to bring about better management of patients.

The aim of this second edition is to acquaint clinicians, as well as undergraduate and postgraduate students, with recent trends in the practice of nutrition for better management of patients. It will also help dietitians in understanding the reasoning behind the diet prescriptions for patients. No attempt is made to describe nutrition for a particular community or nation.

I thank Dr R. H. Dastur for contributing chapters on Lipids, Vitamin B_{12}, Calcium, and Atherosclerosis and Coronary Heart Disease. My thanks are also due to Dr H. G. Desai who has contributed the chapter on Folic Acid and has rendered considerable help in preparing the manuscript.

Dr Himmatlal N. Maniar has corrected the manuscript and offered criticism. I thank him for his most valuable help.

It was possible to complete the second edition of this book through the kind help of my colleagues, Dr C. K. Deshpande, Dr F. P. Soonawalla, Dr R. D. Ganatra, Dr S. M. Sharma, Dr (Mrs) A. M. Samuel, Dr Rusi Colah and Mr N. Deshikachar.

My thanks are also due to Librarians Mr V. M. Matkar, Mr J. P. Fernandes and Mr S. A. Sawant.

I thank Mr Marian A. D'Souza for his very valuable secretarial help in preparation of the manuscript.

I am indebted to P. A. for ably helping me in my work.

F. P. A.

534, Sandhurst Bridge
Bombay 400007
April 1972

FOREWORD

TO THE FIRST EDITION

This book is written by a physician who has had an exceptionally wide experience of clinical medicine particularly gastroenterology and its title 'Clinical Dietetics and Nutrition' indicates that the book is written for the benefit of men and women in clinical practice and in training.

It is clear, straightforward, accurate and extremely practical. The many interesting points added give the book a character of its own and stimulate the interest of the readers.

There is always a gap between knowledge and practice and this is particularly true in nutrition and dietetics. Great attention to nutritional disturbances is particularly needed in countries where intestinal disorders are common and where nutritional needs may be impaired by feeding customs or by population problems.

Dr Antia has done a splendid service for his country by producing this book and it will be of particular value in many other parts of the world where there are important nutritional problems and elsewhere it will constitute a very useful reference book.

I feel proud to have had my name associated with this publication which I regard as a real contribution to world medicine.

F. AVERY JONES

London
June 1966

PREFACE

TO THE FIRST EDITION

My interest in nutrition and dietetics was stimulated when working at the Central Middlesex Hospital, London, as clinical assistant to Dr F. Avery Jones. It is his subsequent help and encouragement that has made this work possible. When teaching clinical nutrition and dietetics the need was felt for a simple book for students and that has prompted me to undertake this task.

The first part of the book consisting of chapters on Calories, Proteins, Fats, Carbohydrates, Vitamins and Minerals may help the pre-clinical students of physiology. The book as a whole is meant for senior students, medical practitioners and dietitians. References are given to stimulate interest in those seeking detailed information.

The tables of food values were derived from the following sources: (1) *Bowes and Church's Food Values of Portions Commonly Used*, 9th ed., revised by Church, C. F., and Church, C. N. (1963), J. B. Lippincott Company, Philadelphia; (2) McCance, R. A., and Widdowson, E. M. (1960) *The Composition of Foods*, Medical Research Council Special Report Series No. 297, Her Majesty's Stationery Office, London; (3) Aykroyd, W. R. *The Nutritive Value of Indian Foods and Planning of Satisfactory Diets*, 6th ed., revised by Gopalan, C., and Balasubramanian, S. C. (1963), Indian Council of Medical Research, New Delhi. I am thankful to Dr Charles F. Church for material from the ninth edition of *Food Values of Portions Commonly Used* and to Mrs Anna de Planter Bowes, Her Majesty's Stationery Office and the Indian Council of Medical Research for permission to draw from their material.

The work was started in collaboration with Dr R. H. Dastur, but due to a very busy schedule he could not spare time to continue. I am thankful to him for contributing the following chapters: Fat and Cholesterol, Vitamin B_{12}, Calcium, Atherosclerosis and Coronary Heart Disease.

I am deeply thankful to Dr J. E. Lennard-Jones for most painstakingly correcting the manuscript and offering valuable criticisms. His help has made this book easy to read.

It is with pleasure that I acknowledge help by my colleagues: Prof. T. H. Rindani, Dr M. M. Desai, Dr K. N. Jeejeebhoy, Prof. S. N.

Narayanrao, Dr L. R. Patel, Dr Aubrey Kail, Dr Jamshed Pohowala, Prof. P. M. Dalal, Dr Noshir Wadia, Dr Darab Dastur, Dr G. A. Dhopeshwarker, Dr P. E. Billimoria, Dr Rusi Colah, Dr Hiralal G. Desai, Dr Pragna Rindani and Mrs Rashmi G. Desai. Dr N. N. Dastur, Principal, Dairy Science College, has helped in the chapter on Milk. Dr N. Desikachar supplied information on Fats.

Mr Y. P. Antia rendered considerable help in preparing the tables. My thanks are also due to Mr V. M. Matkar, Librarian to Tata Memorial Hospital, and to Messrs Prem Nath, K. N. Mistry, M. Sundareswaran and R. Natarajan for secretarial help. Thanks are also due to the staff of the Oxford University Press in London and Bombay for their cordial co-operation.

I am indebted to my wife Pilloo who induced me to complete this work. My apologies to Leaela and Minoo for the inability to give them company at the time of life they needed me most.

F. P. A.

534, Sandhurst Bridge
Bombay-7
1 October 1965

PART I

NUTRITION

1. CALORIES

Energy is necessary to meet the needs of body basal metabolism, building and replacement of body tissue, excretory losses and physical activity. Man derives all the energy from plants. Even the origin of animal or fish flesh is plants. Simple substances from the soil and air with the aid of solar energy are converted by plants into proteins, fats and carbohydrates that are used as a source of energy.

Food requirements are estimated in terms of heat units known as the large Calorie or physiological Calorie. It is defined as the amount of heat required to raise the temperature of a litre of water from 15° to 16°C. The available energy from food is usually calculated as 4 Cal/g protein or carbohydrate and 7 Cal/g alcohol. The available energy from fat is 9 Cal/g. For short chain fatty acids (e.g. butyric) the available energy is calculated as 6·7 Cal/g.

Calorie Requirement

The Food and Agriculture Organization (FAO) of the United Nations in 1957 issued a Report on Calorie Requirements. The FAO mentioned the 'Reference Man' and 'Reference Woman' as healthy, doing average physical work and taking adequate rest, living in a climate with a mean annual temperature of 10°C with 65 kg weight for 'Reference Man' and 55kg for 'Reference Woman'. The recommendations of FAO for Calorie requirements are shown in TABLES 1 and 2. The requirements, however, have to be modified as follows:

Age. With increasing age there is: (1) a decline in physical activity and less strenuous employment; (2) decrease in the basal metabolic rate. It is therefore recommended that beyond 25 years there should be decrease in calories by 3 per cent per decade up to 45 years and 7·5 per cent thereafter up to 65 years.

Climate. For every 10°C rise in the mean annual temperature over reference temperature of 10°C a decrease in calories by 5 per cent is recommended.

For every 10°C fall of mean external temperature below the reference temperature of 10°C only 3 per cent increase in calories is

3

recommended because it is assumed that man takes more protection against cold than heat.

Physical Activity. Physical activity is an important factor in determining the calorie requirement. With average physical activity about 15 per cent additional calories are necessary, while with heavy manual work 25–50 per cent increase may be required.

Capacity to do physical work does not necessarily depend upon the state of nutrition as laid down by Western standards. It is possible that long-standing inadequacy of diet elicits available mechanisms of adaptation, and the official figures given for 'practical allowances' or 'minimum requirement' of various nutrients are perhaps somewhat high [1].

TABLE 1

ENERGY EXPENDITURE OF A 'REFERENCE MAN'

Age 25 years.   Weight 65 kg.
Mean Annual Temperature 10°C.

				CAL/DAY
A	8 hours	WORKING ACTIVITIES: mostly standing (over-all rate, 2·5 Cal/min)		1200
B	8 hours	NON-OCCUPATIONAL ACTIVITIES:	Cal/day	
		1 hour washing, dressing etc. at 3 Cal/min	180	
		1½ hours walking at about 6 km/hr at 5·3 Cal/min	480	
		4 hours sitting activities at 1·54 Cal/min	370	
		1½ hours active recreation and/or domestic work at 5·3 Cal/min	470	1500
C	8 hours	REST IN BED at basal metabolic rate		500
				3200

Children. Newborn infants require 110–120 Cal/kg up to 6 months and 100 Cal/kg up to 1 year. Thereafter up to the age of 12 the requirements are identical for boys and girls.

Between 13 and 15 years 3100 Calories are recommended for boys and 2600 for girls.

In the *adolescent period* between 16 and 19 years the calorie requirement may vary considerably with the physical activity. The requirements are about 113 and 104 per cent respectively of requirements of males and females at 25 years.

TABLE 2

ENERGY EXPENDITURE OF A 'REFERENCE WOMAN'

Age 25 years.   Weight 55 kg.
Mean Annual Temperature 10°C.

				CAL/DAY
A	8 hours	WORKING ACTIVITIES: in the home or in industry; mostly standing (over-all rate, 1·83 Cal/min)		880
B	8 hours	NON-OCCUPATIONAL ACTIVITIES:	Cal/day	
		1 hour washing, dressing etc. at 2·5 Cal/min	150	
		1 hour walking at about 5 km/hr at 3·6 Cal/min	220	
		5 hours sitting activities at 1·41 Cal/min	420	
		1 hour active recreation and/or heavier domestic work at 3·5 Cal/min	210	1000
C	8 hours	REST IN BED at basal metabolic rate		420
				2300

Pregnancy and Lactation

During pregnancy additional calories are required for the formation of the foetus, placenta, increased metabolic rate and increased work load associated with the movement of the mother. For this purpose an additional 40,000–80,000 Calories are necessary. Daily increase of about 300 Calories for the mother is recommended during the second and third trimester. A total average weight increase by 10 kg (22 lb) occurs during pregnancy. Observing the body weight of the mother can indicate whether an increase or decrease in calorie intake is necessary.

Lactation. Lactating mothers require 600 additional calories over and above their usual intake.

Calorie Requirement of an Individual

The recommendations of FAO can be used as a general guide for assessing the requirements of a large group of people, for example an army or a nation. Since the calorie requirement varies not only with the environment but also with the metabolism of an individual, the best guide to the actual calorie requirement is periodic observation of body weight. In a normal weight healthy individual, maintenance of body weight presumes adequate calorie intake.

Calorie Requirement of Indians. Based on FAO report of 1957, the recommendations for the calorie allowance for Indians is revised, taking 55 kg 'Reference Man' and 45 kg 'Reference Woman'.

Calorie Requirement in Great Britain. The recommendations of the Committee on Nutrition of the British Medical Association (1950) are given in a later table.

Calorie Requirement in North America. The North American recommendations for calorie requirement consider 70 kg 'Reference Man' and 58 kg 'Reference Woman' at a mean temperature of 20°C. The recommendation of the Food and Nutrition Board is given in TABLE 57.

REFERENCE

[1] ARESKOG, N.H., SELINUS, R., and VAHLQUIST, B. (1969) Physical work capacity and nutritional status in Ethiopian male children and young adults, *Amer. J. clin. Nutr.*, **22**, 471.

2. PROTEINS

The word 'protein' is derived from the Greek word *protos* meaning 'first'. Protein is the basic chemical unit of the living organism essential for nutrition, growth and repair. Proteins contain nitrogen but the nutritive value of protein-rich foods does not depend upon the total nitrogen content but on the constituent amino acids. Gelatin is rich in nitrogen but does not contain all the essential amino acids and is of little nutritive value. The total body proteins constitute about 15 per cent of the body weight [1].

Origin of all Proteins

Amino acids, which contain nitrogen, are the building stones from which proteins are synthesized. Plants synthesize amino acids from: (1) the soil, which supplies the necessary nitrogen and sulphur; (2) water which provides oxygen and hydrogen; and (3) atmospheric carbon dioxide which supplies carbon and oxygen. With the help of symbiotic bacteria and fungi these elements are synthesized by plants into amino acids. Animals cannot synthesize amino acids from basic elements but derive them from food and synthesize them from pre-formed products of metabolism. Thus the primary source of all foods containing protein, including meat and fish, is the vegetable kingdom.

CHEMISTRY

Protein molecules are made up of amino acids in various proportions and arrangements. Nitrogen as an amino group is the characteristic component of all amino acids.

Nitrogen. Carbon, hydrogen and oxygen are utilized in the metabolic pool for the formation of carbohydrates or fats required by the body, but for the formation of proteins nitrogen has to be supplied either from the intake of food containing proteins or from the endogenous breakdown of proteins.

The nitrogen content of proteins varies from 14 to 20 per cent, the average being 16 per cent. It is, therefore, assumed that when 100 g of protein is broken down in the body 16 g of nitrogen is excreted, thus $\frac{100}{16} = 6 \cdot 25$ is the factor used to calculate the protein breakdown in the body from nitrogen excretion. The nitrogen excretion on a protein-free diet depends upon the metabolic rate and amounts to 2 mg per Calorie of metabolism. An average man metabolizing 1500 Calories per day excretes about 3g nitrogen daily on a protein-free diet.

NITROGEN EQUILIBRIUM. The proteins of the body are in a state of dynamic equilibrium, there being continuous breakdown and synthesis. An individual is said to be in nitrogen equilibrium when the intake over a known period equals the loss through urine, faeces and perspiration. When the intake of nitrogen is greater than the output a person is said to be in *positive* nitrogen balance. An output of nitrogen greater than the intake, as seen in starvation or disease states, is referred to as *negative* nitrogen balance.

The other elements always present in proteins are carbon, hydrogen and oxygen. Sulphur, phosphorus, iron, copper and zinc may also be present in some proteins.

Plasma Albumin and Globulin

The human plasma protein concentration depends upon the state of nutrition, condition of the liver and associated diseases. The values also differ according to whether: (1) chemical fractionation; (2) electrophoresis; (3) immunological; or (4) dye binding method is employed for its estimation. In clinical practice chemical and electrophoretic methods are generally employed. No single method of protein estimation is superior to another.

Chemical Method. It consists of precipitating globulin by half saturation with salts such as sodium or ammonium sulphate and estimating the albumin in the supernatant fluid.

Electrophoretic Method. Proteins differ in their isoelectric points. They generally carry net charges of different magnitude at a given pH. As a result the individual components in a mixture of proteins migrate at different velocities in an electrical field. Electrophoretic analysis of plasma gives more accurate and detailed information about the various fractions. The albumin value is higher by the chemical method because with ammonium sulphate, part of the globulin fraction remains in solution with albumin. The approximate percentage of proteins by the chemical and electrophoretic methods is given in TABLE 3.

ALBUMIN. The molecular weight of serum albumin is about 67,000.

TABLE 3

HUMAN PLASMA PROTEINS

PROTEIN	MOLECULAR WEIGHT	CHEMICAL ANALYSIS, GRAMMES PER CENT	ELECTROPHORESIS	
			Grammes per cent	Percentage of total protein fraction
Albumin	67,000 to 70,000	4·0 to 5·5	3·5 to 5·0	50
Globulins		1·5 to 2·5	2·5 to 4·0	46
Alpha	200,000 to 300,000	—	1·0	14
Beta	150,000 to 1,300,000	—	1·2	20
Gamma	156,000 to 300,000	—	1·0	12
Fibrinogen	400,000	0·3	0·3	4

There are several fractions of *alpha, beta* and *gamma* globulins which have a wide range of molecular weight.

In the clinical assessment of nutritional status the albumin level alone is of significance. Albumin is formed in the liver and hence in chronic liver damage the serum albumin level is low. Whenever there is a loss of proteins from the body as in proteinuria, albumin is lost in greater quantity because the low molecular weight permits easy permeation through the damaged capillaries. Paracentesis, employed for the treatment of ascites, causes a loss of albumin from the body but the use of diuretics helps to conserve it. When there is a marked albumin depletion, as in cirrhosis of the liver, nephrotic syndrome and kala-azar, the globulin value may be high. In these patients estimation of total plasma proteins alone without estimation of various fractions provides incorrect inference in respect to the nutritional status.

Synthesis of albumin occurs only in the liver, at a rate of about 200 mg/kg daily (daily 14 g in 70 kg man) [2]. Synthesis increases in a cold climate and decreases with heat acclimatization and raised *gamma* globulin levels. *Total extravascular* albumin is 4 g/kg body weight. Albumin binds bilirubin, cortisol and other hormones and aids their transport.

Degradation site of albumin is not known. *Loss* of albumin occurs in urine, stool, exudates or burns.

ANALBUMINAEMIA. This is a rare disorder which is characterized by a congenital absence of serum albumin due to a genetic defect resulting in an inability to synthesize it. Such patients have little oedema and are clinically remarkably well.

GLOBULIN. The molecular weights of various fractions of globulin vary from 90,000 to 1,300,000. The gamma globulin fraction contains antibodies and is credited with the resistance mechanism to body infection.

HYPOGAMMAGLOBULINAEMIA. This is rather a rare condition with susceptibility to recurrent infection with Gram-positive organisms, but does not predispose to viral infections except viral hepatitis. Hypogammaglobulinaemia occurs in three forms. (1) *Congenital inherited* as a sex-linked recessive and confined to boys. In such patients the lymph nodes are devoid of follicles and plasma cells. (2) *Primary acquired* in which it occurs in adult male and female patients. The relatives have hypergammaglobulinaemia. In these cases there is lymph follicular hyperplasia. (3) *Secondary acquired* hypogamma-globulinaemia in obvious cases of multiple myeloma, Hodgkin's disease, lymphatic leukaemia and lymphoma.

The term *albumin-globulin ratio* is extensively used in medicine but does not help in clinical evaluation as the albumin fraction in the blood is independent of globulin. A patient with cirrhosis of the liver may have a serum albumin of 1·6 g per cent, and a globulin of 3·2 g per cent, a ratio of 1 : 2. Another patient may have an albumin of 3·5 g per cent with globulin of 7 g per cent, again a ratio of 1 : 2. Despite the same ratio the former indicates poor synthesis or albumin loss, while in the latter albumin metabolism is probably normal.

IMMUNOGLOBULINS [3]. Gamma globulin fraction of the plasma has the ability to react specifically in a detectable fashion with some foreign substances. The term *immunoglobulin* is now applied to any constituent of this fraction that can be shown to possess either specific antibody properties, or the structure now known to be characteristic of them. Five major immunoglobulins that take part in the defence mechanism are recognized: G (IgG), A (IgA), M (IgM), D (IgD), and E (IgE).

IgG is the most abundant immunoglobulin, containing antibodies that react with soluble antigens such as toxins. *IgA* in serum does not reach adult levels until the age of 4. Its plasma concentration is only 20 per cent that of *IgG*. It originates in the plasma cells of the secreting glands and is found in the body secretions such as tears, saliva, milk, and in the respiratory and alimentary tracts. *IgM* (macroglobulin) causes lysis of micro-organisms in the presence of complement, and contains cold agglutinins, rheumatoid factor and Wassermann antibodies. *IgD* is found to contain insulin antibody [4]. *IgE* has the capacity to fix mast cells and is associated with body sensitivity, but its utility is not clear.

IMMUNOLOGICAL SPECIFICITY. Every species of animal has its own characteristic protein which can be easily distinguished by immunological studies although the present methods of chemical analysis may not reveal any differences.

Fibrinogen is the soluble precursor of the protein fibrin that forms a solid clot. The body contains 10–20 g fibrinogen, mostly in the plasma. The plasma half life is 80 hours in man. Fibrin clot can be broken down by the action of *plasmin* (fibrinolysin). Fibrinogen level may be low due to : (1) Increased plasma volume. (2) Decreased synthesis due to inherited anomaly or liver disease. (3) Increased catabolism with bleeding or intravascular clotting due to coagulants entering the blood following trauma, surgery or complications of obstetrics.

DIGESTION OF PROTEINS

Proteins are digested to form proteoses, peptones, polypeptides and amino acids. Digestion of proteins in fried food is slower because of delayed gastric emptying and the fat envelope requires digestion in the small intestine, before the proteolytic enzymes act.

Stomach. The enzyme *pepsin* secreted by the stomach breaks down proteins into proteoses and peptones. The enzyme *rennin* converts the milk protein caseinogen into casein. The latter, in combination with calcium is converted into an insoluble clot of calcium caseinate, which is digested to peptones.

Duodenum. *Trypsin* and *chymotrypsin* are pancreatic enzymes. They act in an alkaline medium on partially digested proteoses and peptones and hydrolyse them into simpler polypeptides. A few amino acids are also liberated.

Intestinal Peptidases [5]. The intestinal peptidases (like disaccharidases) are located in the intestinal mucosa. The pancreatic proteases have also been shown to bind to the brush border [6]. The gastric and pancreatic digestion releases 3–6 linked amino acids that are then broken down by peptidases to single amino acids. There are apparently several peptidases acting on different digested proteins.

PEPTIDASE DEFICIENCY. At least two specific *peptidase deficiency* states are known: (1) Congenital deficiency of *peptide hydrolase,* that hydrolyses *gluten,* produces coeliac disease [7]. (2) Deficiency of *pteroyl polyglutamate hydrolase* (PPH or folate conjugase) results in failure to break down dietary folates (pteroyl moieties linked to series of glutamic acid by peptide bonds). Since monoglutamates for absorption are not formed, there is malabsorption of folates.

Protein Putrefaction. When unabsorbed proteins enter the large intestine as a result of intestinal malabsorption, massive intestinal resection or pancreatic disease, bacterial protein putrefaction occurs producing foul-smelling flatus. A stool examination may reveal undigested meat fibres. In the clinical condition of Hartnup's disease tryptophan is not absorbed and is passed into the colon where it is broken down into indole which when absorbed may cause neurological disorders.

ABSORPTION OF PROTEINS

Only in the newborn is there direct protein absorption of colostrum and antibodies. *The main form of absorption is of amino acids.* There is also some peptide absorption. *The essential amino acids* as a group are more rapidly absorbed, probably by a dual mechanism of mucosal uptake of free amino acids as well as oligopeptides [8]. Absorption of amino acids is decreased after calorie or protein starvation [9] that may further aggravate protein deficiency, as in kwashiorkor. The amino acids reach the liver via the portal vein. Some amino acids are removed by the liver cells, while others pass into the systemic circulation and reach the tissues, where they replace the corresponding amino acids of the protoplasmic proteins.

Absorption of Bacterial Decomposed Products of Proteins in Portacaval Shunt. The absorbed products of bacterial decomposition of proteins in the intestine like indoles, ammonia, phenols, etc. impair cerebral functions. A surgical portacaval shunt is sometimes performed for portal hypertension. The absorbed products enter the systemic circulation directly and reach the brain with consequent neurological disturbances leading to coma. This condition occurs especially on a high protein diet and can be treated by withholding proteins and inhibiting intestinal bacterial flora by the administration of non-absorbable antibiotics neomycin or streptomycin.

STORAGE OF PROTEINS

In an average healthy person about 15 per cent of body weight is constituted by proteins. Unlike fats, proteins in excess of the body requirements are not stored. When adequate amounts of proteins are not available in the diet, stores from vital organs, especially the liver, are utilized. Animals kept on a low protein diet show a reduction in the protein content of the liver, kidney, heart and skeletal muscles, the maximum fall being in the liver. Proteins of one tissue can be converted to meet the needs of another. A foetus can grow and develop from the protein stores of the mother even if she is protein deficient. In protein malnutrition, the serum albumin level could be used as a rough guide to the degree of protein deficiency.

Labile Protein. The body contains some form of readily available protein, which is utilized in emergencies and is known as labile protein. It does not exceed 5 per cent of the total body protein.

The effect of albumin infusions on the circulating albumin is worthy of special mention. Such infusions will not increase the circulating albumin to a level which would be expected if all the infused material remained in the circulation, because a part of the infused albumin is diverted to extravascular stores. For example, if the serum albumin is 2 g per 100 ml and the plasma volume 2000 ml, then the total circulating albumin would be $\frac{2}{100} \times 2000 = 40$ g. In such a patient, infusion of another 40 g of albumin would be expected to increase the total circulating albumin to 80 g but in practice this does not occur due to diversion to extravascular stores.

AMINO ACIDS

Chemistry

Amino acids are so called because they have an amino group (NH_2) attached to an organic acid (COOH). The basic amino group (NH_2) and the acidic carboxyl group (COOH) are attached to the same carbon atom. An amino acid thus has the following structural formula:

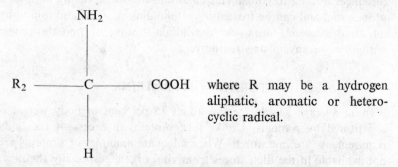

where R may be a hydrogen aliphatic, aromatic or hetero-cyclic radical.

The amino acids in a protein molecule are joined by peptide linkages in which the carboxyl group of one amino acid is linked with the amino group of another, with the elimination of one molecule of water.

$$
\begin{array}{ccccc}
NH_2 & & & & COOH \\
| & & & & | \\
R_1 \text{——} & C & \text{——CONH——} & C & \text{——} R_2 \\
& | & \text{(peptide bond)} & | & \\
& H & & H &
\end{array}
$$

The molecular weight of a simple amino acid like glycine is 75, while more complex ones have a molecular weight of several hundreds.

Essential Amino Acids

Certain amino acids are not synthesized in the body but are indispensable for growth and well-being. These are referred to as *essential amino acids* and are supplied from the diet. Other amino acids are termed *non-essential amino acids* as these can be synthesized by the body when required, from metabolic precursors.

Twenty-three amino acids have been identified of which eight are essential to man [TABLES 4 and 5]. The amino acids arginine and histidine are essential for the growing child but not for adults. Exclusion of any one of the eight essential amino acids from the diet leads to loss of appetite, nervous irritability and a negative nitrogen balance. Nitrogen balance and health are restored when the missing amino acid is added to the diet. It should not, however, be construed that if only essential amino acids are supplied the protein intake is adequate. The quantities of essential amino acids as recommended in TABLES 4 and 5 are sufficient only if other non-essential amino acids are also taken. In rats fed on essential amino acids alone, the rate of growth is only 70-75 per cent of their mates fed on 19 amino acids.

TABLE 4

AMINO ACID REQUIREMENTS OF MAN*

All values were determined with diets containing the
eight essential amino acids and sufficient extra nitrogen
to permit the synthesis of the non-essentials.

AMINO ACID	VALUE PROPOSED TENTATIVELY AS MINIMUM; G PER DAY	VALUE WHICH IS DEFINITELY A SAFE INTAKE; G PER DAY
L—Tryptophan	0·25	0·50
L—Phenylalanine	1·10	2·20
L—Lysine	0·80	1·60
L—Threonine	0·50	1·00
L—Methionine	1·10	2·20
L—Leucine	1·10	2·20
L—Isoleucine	0·70	1·40
L—Valine	0·80	1·60

* Rose *et al.* (1955).

TABLE 5

AMINO ACID REQUIREMENTS OF INFANTS*

AMINO ACID	MINIMUM REQUIRE-MENT MG/KG/ DAY	HUMAN MILK (153 ML/KG)	COW'S MILK FED AT LEVEL PROVIDING 2 G PRO-TEINS/KG	SOYA FORMULA
Histidine	34	32	45	33–57
Isoleucine	119	123	128	67–117
Leucine	150	230	216	91–159
Lysine	103	112	156	73–127
Methionine (in presence of cystine)	45	73	52	31–55
Phenylalanine (in presence of tyrosine)	90	92	104	65–115
Threonine	87	89	92	51–89
Tryptophan	22	31	30	11–20
Valine	105	128	138	67–117

* Holt, L. E., and Snyderman, S.E. (1961) The amino acid requirements of infants, *J. Amer. med. Ass.*, **175**, 100.

Laevo (*l*) and Dextro (*d*) Amino Acids. Amino acids exist, as seen by polarized light, as *laevo* (*l*) and *dextro* (*d*) forms. The *naturally* occurring amino acids are *l*-forms. The body utilizes only *l*-forms of the amino acids for protein synthesis. The only exceptions known are *d*-methionine and *d*-phenylalanine which the body can convert to the *l*-forms to synthesize protein. The *d*-forms of amino acids are *chemically synthesized* and rarely exist in nature. They are metabolized by amino acid oxidase to form carbohydrate for energy, while ammonia and urea are produced from the nitrogen component.

Properties of Some Amino Acids

Glycine. This is the simplest amino acid. It is derived from glucose and is sweet to taste. Glycine detoxicates aromatic compounds like benzene or benzoic acid to form hippuric acid which is excreted in the urine. This is the basis of the hippuric acid test of liver function. Glycine is necessary for the formation of the bile acid, glycocholic acid and glutathionine. It can be utilized to form ribose, glucose, fatty acid, aspartic acid, purines, pyrimidines and porphyrin structure of haemes for the formation of haemoglobin. Although from a dietetic standpoint it is not an essential amino acid, glycine is indispensable for many biological activities.

Tyrosine. The thyroid gland utilizes tyrosine and iodine for the formation of the mono-iodotyrosine, di-iodotyrosine and the hormone thyroxine. The hormone adrenaline and the pigment melanin are also synthesized from tyrosine. Transient tyrosinaemia may occur in premature infants. However, *tyrosinosis* (tyrosinaemia) is characterized by hepatic cirrhosis, vitamin D resistant rickets, and serum tyrosine about 10 mg (normal 3 mg) 100 ml.

Lysine. Lysine is necessary for growth. A diet consisting mainly of rice or wheat is deficient in lysine and has to be supplemented by milk and soya bean, both of which are rich in lysine. Congenital lysine intolerance produces ammonia intoxication and coma.

Tryptophan. Tryptophan is partly converted to nicotinamide in the body. The ability of tryptophan to substitute for nicotinamide in the prevention of pellagra is known as the 'niacin equivalent'. About 60 mg tryptophan is equivalent to 1 mg of nicotinamide. A congenital defect in the absorption of tryptophan from the bowel produces hereditary pellagra or Hartnup's disease. Tryptophan has an antidepressive activity. *Blue diaper syndrome* occurs with tryptophan malabsorption and indigo blue formation.

Methionine. Methionine contains a methyl group and sulphur. The methyl group helps to form choline which is a lipotropic factor because it removes fat from the liver. Demethylation of methionine results in the formation of the sulphur-containing amino acid cystine which prevents necrosis of liver cells. Methionine, therefore, is a parent substance which protects the liver from fatty changes as well as necrosis. It is abundant in casein, the protein of milk. The methionine content of cereals and pulses is low. Many Indians who obtain their protein from cereals and pulses have a deficient intake of methionine.

Cystine and Cysteine. Cystine and cysteine are other sulphur-containing amino acids. Cysteine is converted to cystine by oxidation and condensation of two molecules of the former. Hepatotoxic drugs produce necrosis of the liver cells more readily in the presence of a deficiency of sulphur-containing amino acids; on the other hand excess of cystine predisposes to a fatty liver. Cystine is present in nails and hair. Insulin is rich in cystine. Cystinuria occurs as an inborn error of metabolism. Rarely cystine renal calculi occur.

Phenylalanine. It is a precursor of the amino acid tyrosine and thus aids in the formation of the hormones adrenaline and thyroxine and the pigment melanin. *Phenylketonuria* and mental retardation in childhood occur as an inborn error of metabolism due to an enzyme defect *phenylalanine dehydrogenase,* and phenylalanine is not converted to tyrosine.

Histidine. It is essential for growth and repair of human tissues. Histidine can be converted to histamine which when released in the skin produces urticarial rash.

Leucine. Leucine *depresses blood sugar* in most individuals. It inhibits hepatic output of glucose [10] and stimulates pancreatic insulin secretion. Some people are more sensitive to leucine, and develop hypoglycaemia and even convulsions with dietary leucine [11]. In such cases protein restriction and high carbohydrate diet help.

Arginine. This amino acid, essential to children but not to adults, is a constituent of many proteins including albumin. In addition it is concerned with the formation of urea in the liver from ammonia and carbon dioxide.

Amino Acid Metabolism
The amino acid 'pool' represents the stores available for protein synthesis. The amino acids of the body pool are derived from proteins

in the diet and constant breakdown of tissue proteins. All amino acids
undergo one or other of the following changes:
  1. *Conversion into another amino acid* through a metabolic cycle. For
example: (a) glycine can form serine and N-free precursors; (b) arginine can be synthesized from carbon dioxide and ammonia derived
from the metabolism of amino acid; or (c) by direct transamination
where an amino group of one amino acid is shifted to a keto acid in
the presence of the enzyme transaminase as alpha-ketoglutaric acid
and alanine giving pyruvic acid and glutamic acid.
  2. When all the necessary amino acids are present they may be
condensed into protein. This is shown by the finding that an essential
amino acid tagged with radioactive carbon is converted into protein
only if all the constituent amino acids for the required protein are simultaneously present. Otherwise, the tagged amino acid is degraded and
excreted within a few hours. As long as the protein intake is mixed
there is a pool of amino acids for the synthesis of proteins. This is of
practical importance. A mixture of protein-containing foods taken at
one meal is better utilized for tissue growth than a single protein-rich
food which may not contain all the required amino acids.
  3. Amino acids may be deaminated to form alpha-keto acids and
ammonia. Alpha-keto acids may be oxidized further to yield *energy*
or are utilized for *synthesis of carbohydrates and fats.*

Storage
  Normally the rate of supply of amino acids approximately equals
the needs of tissues for growth and repair. Limited amounts of amino
acids are stored in the body in a 'pool' which is largely intracellular.

Excretion
  Average normal excretion of amino acids is about 150 mg of free
acid or between 400 mg and 1 g of total acid in 24 hours.

Aminoaciduria. When amino acids appear in excess in the blood
due to abnormal metabolism or when renal tubular damage prevents
their reabsorption, the amino acids are excreted in the urine. Examples
are severe liver damage, congenital metabolic defects as in Fanconi's
syndrome and hepatolenticular degeneration (Wilson's disease),
cystinuria, heavy metal poisoning and Hartnup's disease which is a
defect in the tubular reabsorption of tryptophan.

Biosynthesis of Proteins from Amino Acids

This complex problem has received a lot of attention recently and in brief the concept currently held is that the amino acids necessary for protein synthesis are placed in their correct sequence on a template of RNA which therefore acts like a 'mould' in which the amino acids are 'poured' and condensed into a protein molecule. The order and types of amino acids for a particular protein are determined by the sequence of bases in the RNA template. It is thought that certain sequences of bases represent the code for a particular amino acid.

Nutrition after Partial Gastrectomy

After partial or subtotal gastrectomy patients may exhibit symptoms of the so called 'dumping syndrome' so that small frequent meals in place of the usual three meals a day are necessary. Hypoproteinaemia is not uncommon after such operations and these patients can be helped by providing, even in small feeds, a mixture of proteins rather than a single protein-rich food. Small frequent feeds such as milk shakes containing eggs, milk with biscuit or *dal* (pulses) with bread, are more helpful than any one of them given individually. In this way, a mixture of amino acids can be provided simultaneously for the formation of proteins. Indians may suffer from hypoproteinaemia after partial gastrectomy because their diet is comparatively poor in protein-rich foods and they probably are unable to eat sufficient food at a time to derive all the required amino acids for the formation of proteins.

Oral and Intravenous Protein Hydrolysates and Amino Acids : Intravenous Amino Acids. *See* Intravenous Feeding.

Amino Acids in Hepatic Failure. The knowledge that methionine is helpful in the prevention and treatment of fatty liver and that cystine can prevent necrosis of the liver, has induced some clinicians to administer a high protein diet or intravenous amino acids in severe hepatic disease. A high protein diet or supplements of amino acids are positively harmful during severe liver damage because the products of bacterial decomposition of proteins are not detoxicated by the liver and depress cerebral functions.

Functions of Amino Acids

Amino acids are utilized for the formation of proteins, hormones, vitamins and enzymes.

EFFECT OF TOTAL CALORIES AND CARBOHYDRATES ON PROTEIN METABOLISM

Total Calories

The amino acids absorbed from food are not utilized for the formation of proteins unless adequate calories are provided from fats or carbohydrates. However, despite deficient supply of calories in a malnourished pregnant woman the foetus continues to grow, or in tumours, growth can continue despite an inadequate intake of calories.

Specific Dynamic Action of Proteins

More calories are 'burnt' than expected from the amount of ingested food because food stimulates metabolism resulting in an increased production of heat. To furnish this extra energy the food stores of the body are drawn upon. This increase in metabolism is less with carbohydrates and fat than with proteins. On a protein-rich diet the metabolism is stimulated by 10–30 per cent; this effect is known as the 'specific dynamic action' (S.D.A.) of proteins. S.D.A. is believed to be due to the stimulation of cellular metabolism by the remnants of amino acid molecules after the amino group has been removed. A diet containing 60 g of protein supplies 240 Calories, but about 72 extra Calories are derived from the S.D.A. and these are utilized in maintaining the body temperature. Clinically, this effect of increasing caloric expenditure is sometimes utilized by giving a high protein deit for weight reduction.

Protein Sparing Effect of Carbohydrates

The requirement for proteins is markedly influenced by the amount of carbohydrates in the diet. Withholding proteins, but giving carbohydrates to provide calories, reduces the total body metabolism of proteins and reduces the excretion of nitrogen in the urine to a minimum is called the 'protein sparing effect'. The protein sparing effect of carbohydrates is greatest when proteins and carbohydrates are ingested together. When a single feed of extra carbohydrate is given the nitrogen sparing action lasts 12 hours. Repeated daily supplements of extra carbohydrates results in nitrogen retention. This retained nitrogen is excreted within a few days if extra carbohydrate is stopped.

Clinically, the protein sparing effect of carbohydrates is utilized in severe liver and kidney disease when the endogenous breakdown products of protein metabolism have to be kept at a minimum. Administration of small frequent feeds containing carbohydrates, or a slow continuous intravenous drip of 5–10 per cent glucose or a continuous nasogastric drip of 20 per cent glucose or maltose, helps to minimize tissue protein breakdown. The administration of concentrated glucose over a short period once a day is not as effective in its protein sparing effect as small repeated administrations.

Nitrogen Excretion
Nitrogen loss occurs through urine, faeces, skin, hair and nails.

The amount of *endogenous* urinary loss is 2 mg nitrogen per 1 basal calorie. The *faecal* nitrogen is lost through digestive juices and desquamation of the intestinal epithelium. In a protein-free diet this amounts to 1 g nitrogen daily. Total protein loss from the whole *small intestine* in man is 84 g per day, about 10 g coming from within exfoliated cells and the rest from plasma, mucoprotein and interstitial fluid. The normal intestine must reabsorb most of the material [12].

Cutaneous loss through minimal sweat amounts to 0.36 g nitrogen daily, which may increase 10 times with profuse sweating. With acclimatization less nitrogen is lost. With minimal sweating, epithelial debris, hair, and nail nitrogen loss is estimated to be between 0.5–1.4 g daily. The total daily nitrogen loss × 6.25 is also calculated to be the amount of protein requirement.

FUNCTIONS OF PROTEINS

1. Proteins are necessary for growth. Fats and carbohydrates cannot be substituted for proteins as they do not contain nitrogen.

2. The human body is constantly undergoing 'wear and tear' which is repaired by proteins.

3. Dietary proteins supply raw materials for the formation of digestive juices, hormones, plasma proteins, haemoglobin, vitamins and enzymes.

4. Each gramme of protein supplies 4 calories.

5. Proteins function as buffers, thus helping to maintain the reaction (pH) of various media such as plasma, cerebrospinal fluid, intestinal secretions, etc. at a constant level.

6. Proteins aid *transport of nutrients* (e.g. lipoproteins) and *drugs*. Drugs bind to specific sites of the protein molecule. When combinations of drugs are administered their effects or reactions depend upon

whether the protein binding site is already utilized or free.

PROTEIN REQUIREMENTS

The daily requirement of proteins is a complex problem because:

1. Protein requirements depend upon the *composition of the amino acids*. Food should supply not only the full quota of essential amino acids but also the non-essential amino acids should be supplied [13] for the optimum results.

2. The mere administration of protein-rich foods does not mean that the proteins are adequately digested and utilized. Unless all the *component amino acids are present simultaneously* the protein molecule will not be formed. The unutilized amino acids are not stored but deaminated and metabolized within a few hours. Thus it is the mixture of proteins in the diet which determines utilization.

3. Most studies on protein requirements are based on 'nitrogen balance' studies which are influenced by the body stores of protein in an individual.

4. If *calories supplied by carbohydrates and fats* are adequate, then there is less tissue protein breakdown (protein sparing effect) and less proteins are required.

5. *Protein requirements increase with the calorie intake.* Kwashiorkor does not develop when both the caloric and the protein intake are low but manifestations occur when calorie intake is high relative to protein intake. Therefore, an important consideration for protein requirement is the total intake of calories.

6. *Stress* increases protein metabolism due to greater secretion of glucocorticoids [14].

7. The nitrogen of raised serum ammonia in kidney failure is also utilized to form non-essential amino acids.

The concept of protein requirement has undergone a drastic reorientation by nutritionists during the last decade. The nutritive value of protein varies according to the amino acid content, and protein requirements are now termed *reference protein*.

Reference protein is 100 per cent utilized. Egg protein, which is almost completely utilized, is the usually mentioned reference protein. Since all the dietary proteins are not first class, on a mixed *British diet an* 80 *per cent conversion ratio* utilization is assumed. A *vegetarian Indian diet* has a conversion ratio of 65 per cent of reference protein that approximates to 1 g of preponderantly vegetable protein per kg adult body weight [15]. The recommended protein requirement is stated in TABLE 6.

TABLE 6

MINIMUM PROTEIN REQUIREMENT

	BRITISH RECOMMENDATION* BIOLOGICAL VALUE OF BRITISH DIET 80%	INDIAN RECOMMENDA- TION** BIOLOGICAL VALUE OF VEGETARIAN INDIAN DIET 65%
0—6 months	2 g/kg (human milk protein)	2·3—1·8 g/kg (human milk)
6—12 months	2 g/kg	1·8—1·5 g/kg (human milk protein)
4 years	30 g	20 g
12 years	50 g	41 g
ADULT (male)	50 g	55 g
ADULT (female)	40 g	45 g
Pregnancy (2nd half)	55 g	55 g
Lactation	65 g	65 g

* *Modified from: Requirement of Man for Protein* (1964) Reports of Public Health and Medical Subjects, No. 111, London, H.M.S.O.
** *Modified from:* Rao, B.S.N. (1969) Studies on nutrient requirements of Indians, *Indian J. med. Res.,* **57,** 16. (Recommendation of I.C.M.R., 1968.)

FIRST AND SECOND CLASS DIETARY PROTEINS

Foods vary in their amino acid content. Protein-rich foods like meat, fish, poultry, eggs and milk contain essential amino acids and are called 'first class' proteins. The vegetable proteins derived from pulses, wheat, millet and vegetables, are individually termed 'second class' proteins as they do not contain all the essential amino acids in adequate amounts.

The distinction between 'first class' and 'second class' protein foods is not rigid. Though second class proteins may be individually deficient in supplying all the amino acids, yet, if ingested collectively, they may supplement to some extent. The biological values of vegetable proteins are higher when derived from mixed cereals and pulses rather than from a single cereal such as wheat [16]. Even a first class protein like milk is better utilized when fed with the second class vegetable proteins of bread or potato [17]. If protein-containing foods of low biological value are ingested simultaneously and the essential amino acids supplied by them have adequate proportions, this combination can be of high biological value. Cows, subsisting solely on vegetable proteins of low biological value synthesize them into beef which is of high biological value but this is not true of man who cannot synthesize essential amino acids.

Biological Value of Proteins

Nutritionists use the term 'biological value of proteins' to indicate the percentage of nitrogen that is retained. Biological value therefore is a comprehensive term which includes the composition of amino acids of proteins in food, their digestion, absorption and reconversion into proteins in the body. Thus proteins of egg, milk, meat, fish and poultry have a high biological value. Vegetable proteins of cereals and pulses have varying biological values according to the combinations in which they are eaten.

Family Budget and Protein Intake

People of moderate means who cannot afford expensive first class protein-rich foods would do well if they took a combination of second class proteins at considerably less cost. Money spent on a liberal quantity of wheat, rice, pulses, potatoes and a little milk gives better nourishment on a limited budget than the same amount spent on meat or eggs.

PROTEIN DEFICIENCY

Proteins are necessary for the growth and repair of tissues. The intestinal epithelium is shed at regular intervals and proteins are required for its regeneration. Unless the mucous membrane of the intestine is healthy impairment of digestion and absorption occurs.

Protein deficiency occurs in: (1) *low intake* due to poverty or loss of appetite; (2) *poor digestion and absorption* as after partial gastrectomy, in pancreatic deficiency and malabsorption syndrome; (3) *reduced synthesis* when the absorbed amino acids are not converted to albumin; and (4) *excessive loss* in diseases like nephritis, cirrhosis of the liver with ascites, chronic dysentery, ulcerative colitis, protein-losing gastro-enteropathy and profuse expectoration in bronchiectasis or lung abscess.

When protein deficiency occurs in disease states it is usually a deficiency in the albumin fraction. The globulin fraction does not reflect protein deficiency as in cirrhosis of the liver, nephrotic syndrome and kala-azar as mentioned before.

Clinically, protein deficiency manifests itself as weakness, anaemia, oedema, delayed wound healing and decreased resistance to infection as antibody formation is decreased. A deficient protein intake has also been associated with a high incidence of toxaemia of pregnancy. Serum albumin of less than 3 g per 100 ml is indicated by myoedema. It is elicited by striking a percussion hammer on the biceps, deltoid or pectoralis muscle when a muscle ridge is noted [18]. Serum albumin lower than 2·2 g per 100 ml may manifest as transverse bands on the fingernails [19].

Adaptation to low protein occurs as follows:

There is diminished nitrogen excretion, increased protein synthesis in the liver and re-utilization of the broken down amino acids in the cells. These changes are regulated by increased enzymatic and hormonal activities [20]. During protein starvation the organs that have a greater protein turnover lose proportionally more protein. The highest losses occur in the liver, small intestine, pancreas and subsequently the skeletal muscles. This results in fatty liver, small intestinal mucosal atrophy, and pancreatic exocrine enzyme deficiency.

Sprue Syndrome. Deficient protein *intake* produces clinical and histological changes that resemble sprue [22, 23]. This is not surprising as the intestinal mucosal turnover is very rapid (3–5 days) and protein is required for regeneration. These patients also have fatty livers. The pancreatic enzyme formation is deficient, leading to pancreatic steatorrhoea and fat-soluble vitamin deficiency. With adequate protein intake there is marked clinical as well as histological improvement in the liver and small intestine [23] and the exocrine pancreatic secretions [24].

Protein-calorie Malnutrition. *See* Kwashiorkor.

Protein-losing Gastro-enteropathy

Hypo-albuminaemia in gastro-intestinal disorders was until recently thought to be due to malnutrition. However, in hypertrophic gastritis a diminished serum albumin may be associated with exudation of albumin into the stomach. The albumin thus exuded would be digested like any other protein entering the bowel and even through the digested products are normally reabsorbed they are not available to the body as 'albumin' which is not re-synthesized by the liver completely. For some obscure reason the rate of synthesis of albumin by the liver does not compensate for the loss. Thus this process of gastro-intestinal loss would deplete the serum of albumin although there is no over-all loss of other proteins from the body. Later, a similar process was found to be a cause of hypo-albuminaemia in other gastro-intestinal disorders like sprue, colitis and regional enteritis, carcinoma of the stomach, blind loop syndrome and in idiopathic hypo-albuminaemia. Protine loss has also been reported in cardiac disease.

Gastro-intestinal Protein Allergy. Patients suffering from this condition have oedema, anaemia, hypo-albuminaemia, hypogammaglobulinaemia, eosinophilia, growth retardation, excessive faecal protein loss, and shortened albumin survival time (3–4 days). Those with milk allergy show marked amelioration of symptoms on withholding milk, with recurrence on resumption. Precipitating antibodies to milk can be demonstrated [25] in the serum.

Protein Intake and Urea Clearance

The urea clearance test performed in normal healthy Indians on low protein intake was found to be low, but when the daily protein intake was raised the urea clearance was comparable to the normal Western standards. This increased clearance was due to increased urea excretion with a higher protein intake [26].

HIGH PROTEIN DIET

A diet of high protein content of over 1·5 g per kg body weight is indicated in pregnancy, lactation, fatty liver, kwashiorkor and cirrhosis of the liver without liver failure. High protein intake is not associated with harmful effects if the kidney function and fluid intake are adequate.

Skimmed milk powder helps to enhance the intake of proteins. It is less expensive, easily digestible and many palatable preparations can be made with it. In a vegetarian diet skimmed milk powder is a useful supplement to increase the protein intake. Pulses (*dal*), including *chana* (Bengal gram) and groundnuts, are inexpensive protein-rich foods.

Salt poor human albumin for intravenous use is expensive. However, it is directly utilized by the body without being first broken down into its component amino acids, and thus the metabolic load on the liver is also reduced. It can be administered 25–50 g per day by slow intravenous drip. *Intravenous amino acid mixture* is useful for people who cannot be fed orally (*see* Parenteral Feeding).

Fortification with Amino Acids. It has been repeatedly proposed that in an undernourished population cereals should be fortified with amino acids. Diets vary, however, in different parts of the world and adequate information about the benefits of amino acid supplement is not yet available. Large-scale supplementation of cereals is therefore an expensive gamble [27].

Leaf Proteins [21, 28]

It has been pointed out that the origin of all proteins is the vegetable kingdom. Leaves contain proteins which can be extracted and utilized for human consumption. The leaves of pea, sugar cane, potato, banana, pumpkin, groundnut and even wild leaves are utilized.

The plant protein machine squeezes out the juice with pressure and this juice is then heated to coagulate proteins. The by-product of cellulose is used for cattle feeds. The machine costs £8000 with an annual operating cost of £10,000 [29].

The domestic process consists in macerating crushed green leaves with 2 per cent sodium bicarbonate solution, straining the extract through cloth and slightly acidifying with lemon or tamarind juice. The proteins are precipitated by warming and the liquid filtered through a cloth, yielding a green protein-rich material.

Rubber tree seeds contain 32 per cent fat, 27 per cent protein, and a high content of lysine and tryptophan. Proper processing to remove toxic products is suggested in order to make it suitable as a protein supplement in South-East Asia [30].

Such a source of protein is likely to be deficient in certain essential amino acids. Leaf protein appears to be a cheap potential source of protein to feed our starving millions or to supplement their inadequate intake. It can be added for the preparation of soups, curries or *chappatis*.

Synthesis of proteins by unicellular bacteria and yeast can produce cheap and abundant protein by assimilating hydrocarbons from paraffin of oil refinery type, nitrogen from ammonium salts, and atmospheric oxygen.

LOW PROTEIN DIET

The products of protein metabolism and decomposition by bacteria in the bowel are detoxicated by the liver and excreted by the kidneys. With marked damage to the liver or kidneys there is an accumulation of the products of protein breakdown which produce toxic symptoms. With incipient hepatic failure as in fulminating viral hepatitis and advanced cirrhosis of the liver, or during suppression of urine as in severe nephritis, it is advisable to withhold proteins till the patient is tided over the crisis.

In hepatic failure carbohydrates should be the only source of calories as neither proteins nor probably fats are metabolized by the liver. *During suppression of urine* fats as well as carbohydrates are allowed.

REFERENCES

[1] WIDDOWSON, E.M., McCANCE, R.A., and SPRAY, C.M. (1951) Chemical composition of human body, *Clin. Sci.,* **10,** 113.

[2] ROTHSCHILD, M.A., ORATZ, M., and SCHREIBER, S.S. (1970) Current concepts of albumin metabolism, *Gastroenterology,* **58,** 402.

[3] BRITISH MEDICAL JOURNAL (1970) The immunoglobulins, *Brit. med. J.,* **4,** 445.

[4] DAVEY, M., CARTER, D., SANDERSON, C.J., and COOMBS, R.R.A. (1970) IgD antibody to insulin, *Lancet,* **ii,** 1280.

[5] PETERS, T.J. (1970) Intestinal peptidases, *Gut,* **11,** 720.

[6] GOLDBERG, D.M., CAMPBELL, R., and ROY, A.D. (1969) Studies on binding of trypsin and chymotrypsin by human intestinal mucosa, *Scand. J. Gastroent.,* **4,** 217.

[7] DOUGLAS, A.P., and PETERS, T.J. (1970) Peptide hydrolase activity of human intestinal mucosa in adult coeliac disease, *Gut,* **11,** 15.

[8] ASATOOR, A.M., *et al.* (1970) Intestinal absorption of two dipeptides in Hartnup disease, *Gut,* **11,** 380.

[9] ADIBI, S.A., and ALLEN, E.R. (1970) Impaired jejunal absorption rates of essential amino acids induced by either dietary caloric or protein deprivation in man, *Gastroenterology,* **59,** 404.

[10] GREENBERG, R., and REAVEN, G. (1966) The effect of L-leucine on hepatic glucose formation, *Pediatrics,* **37,** 934.

[11] GRUMBACH, M.M., and KAPLAN, S.L. (1970) Amino acid and alpha-keto acid induced hyperinsulinism in leucine sensitive type of infantile and childhood hypoglycaemia, *J. Pediat.,* **57,** 346.

[12] DA COSTA, L.R., CROFT, D.N., and CREAMER, B. (1971) Protein loss and cell loss from the small-intestinal mucosa, *Gut,* **12,** 179.

[13] ROSE, W.C., WIXOM, R.L., LOCKHART, H.B., and LAMBERT, G.F. (1955) The amino acid requirements of man, XV. The valine requirement; summary and final observations, *J. biol. Chem.,* **217,** 987.

[14] SCRIMSHAW, N.S., *et al.* (1966) Protein metabolism of young men during University examinations, *Amer. J. clin. Nutr.,* **18,** 321.

[15] GOPALAN, C. (1970) Some recent studies in the Nutrition Research Laboratories, Hyderabad, *Amer. J. clin. Nutr.*, **23**, 35.

[16] PHANSALKAR, S.V., and PATWARDHAN, V.N. (1956) Utilization of animal and vegetable proteins, *Indian J. med. Res.*, **44**, 1.

[17] HENRY, K.M., and KON, S.K. (1942) The effect of the method of feeding on the supplementary relationships between the proteins of dairy products and those of bread or potato, *Chem. and Ind.*, **61**, 97.

[18] CONN, R.D., and SMITH, R.H. (1965) Malnutrition myoedema and Muehrcke's lines, *Arch. intern. Med.*, **116**, 875.

[19] MUEHRCKE, R.C. (1956) The fingernails in chronic hypoalbuminaemia, *Brit. med. J.*, **1**, 1327.

[20] WATERLOW, J.C. (1968) Observations on the mechanism of adaptation to low protein intakes, *Lancet*, **ii**, 1091.

[21] GUHA, B.C. (1960) Leaf protein as human food, Letter to the Editor, *Lancet*, **i**, 704.

[22] CHUTTANI, H.K., MEHRA, M.L., and MISRA, R.C. (1968) Small bowel in hypoproteinaemic states, *Scand. J. Gastroent.*, **3**, 529.

[23] TANDON, B.N., MAGOTRA, M.L., SARAYA, A.K., and RAMALINGASWAMI, V. (1968) Small intestine in protein malnutrition, *Amer. J. clin., Nutr.*, **21**, 813.

[24] TANDON, B.N., *et al.* (1970) Recovery of exocrine pancreatic function in adult protein-calorie malnutrition, *Gastroenterology*, **58**, 358.

[25] WALDMANN, T.A., WOCHNER, R.D., LASTER, L., and GORDON, R.S. (1967) Allergic gastroenteropathy. A cause of excessive gastrointestinal protein loss, *New Engl. J. Med.*, **276**, 761.

[26] CHITRE, R.G., NADKARNI, D.S., and MONTEIRO, L. (1955) The effect of protein nutrition on the 'urea clearance' in human subjects, *J. postgrad. Med.*, **1**, 79.

[27] HEGSTED, D.M. (1968) Amino acid fortification and protein problem, *Amer. J. clin. Nutr.*, **21**, 688.

[28] PIRIE, N.W. (1969) The production and use of leaf protein, *Proc. Nutr. Soc.*, **28**, 85.

[29] BRITISH MEDICAL JOURNAL (1968) Protein concentrates from vegetables, *Brit. med. J.*, **3**, 246.

[30] GOIK, L.T., SAMSUDIN, H., and TARWOTIJO, (1967) Nutritional value of rubber seed protein, *Amer. J. clin. Nutr.*, **20**, 1300.

3. LIPIDS

(FATS AND CHOLESTEROL)

Contributed by R.H. Dastur

Lipids are organic substances which are soluble in fat solvents such as alcohol, ether and chloroform but insoluble in water. The term embraces fatty acids, soaps, neutral fats, phospholipids, steroids and waxes.

Fats are the reserve fuel of the animal kingdom supplying 9 Calories per gramme, which is more than twice the calories supplied per gramme by proteins or carbohydrates. A high fat diet is suitable for manual workers who require food with a high calorie content but of reasonable bulk. Fats also provide fat-soluble vitamins A, D, E and K, impart flavour to the food and remain longer in the stomach than other foods, thus producing a sense of satiety. Foods rich in fats are more expensive than carbohydrates because the cost of production per acre is greater.

CHEMISTRY

Fats contain carbon, hydrogen and oxygen. They supply more energy than carbohydrates because they contain proportionately more combustible carbon and hydrogen. The *body depot fats* (adipose fat) are mainly composed of triglycerides which are esters of glycerol and fatty acids. The most commonly encountered fatty acids in such glycerides are oleic, palmitic and stearic acids. *Most oils* are liquid at 20°C, are usually derived from vegetable products and have glycerol in combination with unsaturated fatty acids like oleic, linoleic and linolenic acid. Oils or *ghee* are pure fats without the admixture of proteins, carbohydrates or water.

The neutral fats, or triglycerides, are formed from one molecule of glycerol and three molecules of fatty acids.

CH_2	OH	HOOC	R_1	CH_2O	OC R_1	
CHO	H	HOOC	R_2	CHO	OC R_2	
CH_2	OH	HOOC	R_3	CH_2O	OC R_3	
Glycerol		Fatty acids		Neutral fat		$+H_2O$

R_1, R_2 and R_3 represent fatty acid chains which may or may not all be the same.

Physical and Chemical Properties

Melting Point. Each fat has its own melting point which is different from its solidification point. Fats which contain a high proportion of saturated fatty acids, like stearic and palmitic acids, are usually solid at room temperature.

Emulsification. Fats and oils are lighter than water. They are insoluble, but form a homogeneous mixture with water when emulsified as very small globules. In the small intestine, bile salts emulsify triglycerides and fatty acids, and in the blood, phospholipids and proteins maintain an emulsion.

Saponification. Neutral fats are largely composed of fatty acids esterified with glycerol which is chemically a triglyceride alcohol (an ester is a compound formed by interaction of an alcohol and an acid with the elimination of water). Such glycerol esters are termed *glycerides*. Thus fats are glycerides having two components, one being the fatty acid and the other being glycerol. If neutral fats are heated with sodium or potassium hydroxide they readily undergo hydrolysis at the ester linkage into glycerol and the sodium or potassium salts of the fatty acids. Salts of fatty acids such as sodium oleate, potassium stearate or potassium palmitate are known as *soaps*. This hydrolysis of fats with heat and alkali into soap is known as saponification.

Saturated and Unsaturated. Saturated fatty acids have all the carbon atoms in the chain completely saturated with hydrogen atoms. Fatty acids are termed unsaturated when some of the hydrogen atoms attached to the carbon atoms have been removed and replaced by a double bond. The degree of unsaturation (conveniently measured by the ability to take up iodine or hydrogen) depends on the number of double bonds.

Double Bonds. A fatty acid which contains one or more double bonds is termed an unsaturated fatty acid. If the fatty acid contains more than one double bond it is termed a *poly-unsaturated* fatty acid. The double bonds can occur between any two consecutive carbon atoms along the fatty acid chain. It is at the unsaturated linkages that the fatty acids combine with hydrogen.

Saturated fatty acids have no double bonds. The degree of unsaturation depends on the number of double bonds, for example arachidonic acid with four double bonds, is more unsaturated (iodine value 334) than oleic acid with a single double bond (iodine value 90) [TABLE 7].

TABLE 7

FATTY ACIDS IN FOODS

NAME OF ACID	FORMULA	IODINE VALUE	NO. OF DOUBLE BONDS	OCCURRENCE
SATURATED				
Palmitic	$C_{15}H_{31}COOH$	0	0	All fats and oils
Stearic	$C_{17}H_{35}COOH$	0	0	Lard, tallow
Butyric	C_3H_7COOH	0	0	Butter
UNSATURATED				
Oleic	$C_{17}H_{33}COOH$	90	1	All fats and oils
Linoleic	$C_{17}H_{31}COOH$	181	2	Mostly in vegetable oils like sunflower, saf-flower, soya-bean, corn and cotton-seed, walnut.
Linolenic	$C_{17}H_{29}COOH$	274	3	Mainly in linseed oil
Arachidonic	$C_{19}H_{31}COOH$	334	4	Fish oils and animal fats

Iodine Number (Value). The iodine number (value) is defined as the number of grammes of iodine which can combine with 100 g of fat. Since iodine combines at the site of double bonds, the greater the number of double bonds in an unsaturated fatty acid, the higher is its iodine number. Many factors such as soil, climate, feeding and season, affect the fatty acid composition of fats and oils, and for this reason samples may show a considerable variation. The iodine numbers of common cooking fats are given in TABLE 8.

TABLE 8*

IODINE NUMBER OF FATS

OIL OR FAT	IODINE NUMBER	OIL OR FAT	IODINE NUMBER
Coconut	7·5 — 10·5	Peanut (groundnut)	84 — 100
Corn	103 — 128	Sardine	170 — 190
Cotton-seed	106 — 113	Sesame (sweet, gingelly, *till*)	103 — 116
Herring	130 — 144	Soya-bean	120 — 141
Lard	50 — 70	Sunflower	125 — 136
Linseed	170 — 204	Tallow (beef)	40 — 50
Olive	74 — 94	Walnut	154 — 162
Palm	44 — 58		

* Average fatty acid composition and constants of fats and oils; Armour and Company, Chemical Division, revised September 1944.

Hydrogenation (Margarine, Vegetable Ghee, Vanaspati). An unsaturated fat becomes saturated if it combines with hydrogen at the site of double bonds. This occurs during the process of hydrogenation when the unsaturated fat is exposed to hydrogen at high temperature in the presence of a catalyst like nickel or cobalt. Hydrogenation makes vegetable fats easily marketable because it converts oils, which are liquid at room temperature, into odourless solids which are easy to transport, have an attractive white colour and do not turn rancid. Rancidity is developed due to the chemical changes like oxidation or degradation at unsaturated linkages giving rise to foul-smelling products. Hence saturated or hydrogenated fats do not usually turn rancid. Groundnut, coconut, cotton-seed and other oils are usually used for hydrogenation. The melting point of hydrogenated oils should be between 35° and 37°C.

Vegetable oils, unlike animal fats such as butter and *ghee*, are deficient in vitamin A. Whatever *beta* carotene (provitamin A) is originally present in the vegetable oil is lost due to chemical changes brought about by the process of hydrogenation. It is compulsory in India for the manufacturers of *vanaspati* (hydrogenated vegetable oil, vegetable *ghee*) to add not less than 700 IU of synthetic vitamin A per 30 g of hydrogenated oil product.

Margarine is extensively used as a cheap substitute for butter. Margarine was originally prepared by a French scientist in 1870. The word margarine is derived from the Greek *margaron* (pearl), as fat when churned with milk produces globules resembling pearls. Margarine is prepared from vegetable oils such as coconut, groundnut or soya-bean, the heated oil being churned with skimmed milk. Yellow colouring material is added to make the margarine look like butter. Vitamins A and D are usually added to equal the amounts present in butter.

Argemone oil derived from the common plant in India *Argemone mixicana* (prickly poppy: Dhotra) may be adulterated with edible oils, *vanaspati* or *ghee* that may result in *epidemic dropsy* and *glaucoma* [1].

Fatty Acids

The animal and vegetable fats eaten by man are mixed triglycerides since they contain different fatty acids. There are over forty fatty acids found in nature, most of them having an *even number* of carbon atoms. Fatty acids may be saturated or unsaturated. The fats found in the animal body are composed of palmitic, stearic and oleic acids, with small amounts of linoleic, myristic and other acids.

Saturated Fatty Acids

The empirical formula for fatty acids is $C_nH_{2n}O_2$ where n is an even number of carbon atoms varying from 2 to 24. The common saturated fatty acids are palmitic, stearic, lauric and myristic. *Palmitic* acid $(C_{16}H_{32}O_2)$ is the most widely distributed, and constitutes about 25–30 per cent of the depot fat of animals like lambs and sheep. *Stearic* acid $(C_{18}H_{36}O_2)$ is present in higher proportion in beef, tallow and lard. *Lauric* acid $(C_{12}H_{24}O_2)$ and *myristic* acid $(C_{14}H_{28}O_2)$ are present in vegetable oils, particularly coconut and palm oils. The saturated fats are usually solid at room temperature. They do not have any double bonds and hence cannot combine with halogens or hydrogen.

Unsaturated Fatty Acids

These can be classified according to the number of double bonds, for example:

One double bond—Oleic acid: $O_nH_{2n}\text{-}2O_2 = (C_{18}H_{34}O_2)$
Two double bonds—Linoleic acid: $C_nH_{2n}\text{-}4O_2 = (C_{18}H_{32}O_2)$
Three double bonds—Linolenic acid: $C_nH_{2n}\text{-}6O_2 = (C_{18}H_{30}O_2)$
Four double bonds—Arachidonic acid: $C_nH_{2n}\text{-}8O_2 = (C_{20}H_{32}O_2)$

The unsaturated fatty acids are present in marine oils (whale, shark, etc.) and vegetable oils (except coconut and palm oils which have a preponderance of saturated fatty acids). The unsaturated fatty acids are usually liquid at room temperature.

Multiple sclerosis (disseminated sclerosis) tends to occur in areas where the diet is rich in saturated fats. In cases of this disease the serum linoleate is lower than in normal subjects and supplements of sunflower seed oil or corn oil to the usual diet augment linoleate intake and raise the serum linoleate level. Whether higher linoleate intake benefits patients with multiple sclerosis is not known [2].

Essential Fatty Acids (EFA)

Fatty acids which are nutritionally important and necessary for growth are known as essential fatty acids. These are *linoleic, linolenic* and *arachidonic* acids. Like the non-essential amino acids, they cannot be synthesized by the body and have to be supplied in the diet. *Linoleic and linolenic acids* are of vegetable origin and are present in cottonseed, groundnut and linseed oils, while *arachidonic* acid is synthesized from linolenic acid in fish and animals. *Deficiency* of EFA in animals results in skin changes and malabsorption due to defective intestinal epithelial regeneration [3].

Cholesterol [*see also* Heart Disease]

The publicity given to blood cholesterol and heart disease has left the impression that cholesterol is an unnecessary substance which must be eliminated if a heart attack is to be avoided. This is not the case. Man cannot live without cholesterol since it is an important raw material for the manufacture of steroid hormones and bile salts.

Source. The sources of cholesterol are: (1) *exogenous* from food [TABLE 9]; (2) *endogenous synthesis* from acetate by the *liver* and the *intestines,* particularly the ileum.

TABLE 9

CHOLESTEROL IN FOODS

FOOD	CHOLESTEROL mg per 100 g	FOOD	CHOLESTEROL mg per 100 g
Egg yolk, dried	2950	Lard and other animal fat	95
Brains, raw	2000	Veal	90
Egg yolk, fresh	1500	Cheese (25 to 30 per cent fat)	85
Egg yolk, frozen	1280	Milk, dried, whole	85
Egg, whole	550	Beef, raw	70
Kidney, raw	375	Fish, steak	70
Caviar or fish roe	300	Fish, fillet	70
Liver, raw	300	Lamb, raw	70
Butter	250	Pork	70
Sweetbreads (thymus)	250	Cheese spread	65
Oysters	200	Margarine, (2/3 animal fat, 1/3 vegetable)	65
Lobster	200	Mutton	65
Heart, raw	150	Chicken, flesh only, raw	60
Crab meat	125	Ice-cream	45
Shrimp	125	Cottage cheese, creamed	15
Cheese, cream	120	Milk, fluid, whole	11
Cheese, cheddar	100	Milk, fluid, skim	3
		Egg white	0

Absorption. Cholesterol present in the intestinal lumen is obtained from food, intestinal secretions, and bile. Cholesterol is solubilized with bile acids and phospholipids to form mixed micelles, and is then absorbed. *Chylomicrons* are formed of cholesterol, triglycerides and proteins. The asorbed chylomicrons enter the lymphatics. Higher fat intake enhances cholesterol absorption by increasing bile flow and chylomicron formation. *Crystalline* cholesterol is poorly absorbed, and cholesterol absorption capacity is limited to only 300–500 mg a day [4]. Despite high cholesterol diet a major part of serum cholesterol is derived from *endogenous synthesis* [5], mainly from carbohydrate.

Plasma Cholesterol. The plasma cholesterol is *raised* in pregnancy, diabetes, nephrosis, obstructive jaundice, primary biliary cirrhosis, hypothyroidism and cholecystitis. It is *diminished* in hyperthyroidism, anaemia and acute infections.

EXCRETION. *Unabsorbed* cholesterol is reduced to coprosterol by the intestinal bacteria and excreted. *Intestinal excretion* consists of dietary cholesterol, derived from bile and from desquamation of the intestinal epithelial cells. Cholesterol is also *catabolized* to bile acids and excreted in the intestine. Increased bile acid destruction by intestinal bacteria, or diversion of bile by drainage or ileostomy, enhances bile formation from cholesterol catabolism. *Urinary excretion occurs* through the catabolic products of steroid hormones.

FUNCTIONS. Cholesterol is the precursor of steroid hormones and bile salts. Progesterone, possibly oestrogen, and the adrenal corticoids are derived from cholesterol. Similarly, cholic acid, derived from cholesterol, combines with glycine and taurine to produce the bile salts sodium glycocholate and sodium taurocholate. Cholesterol in the blood plays an important role in the transport of fatty acids.

Cholesterol exists as both free cholesterol and cholesterol esters. The cholesterol esters are formed by the liver and are markedly diminished in severe hepatocellular damage.

DIGESTION AND ABSORPTION OF FATS

Emptying the stomach of fats may not be a complex mechanism, but a simple physical phenomenon may also have a role. Fat floats in the stomach. In the erect posture fat emptying is considerably delayed but is rapid when lying on the left side.

Lipid absorption consists of emulsification, hydrolysis, solubilization,

absorption, triglyceride resynthesis, chylomicron formation, and chylomicron transport [6]. Dietary triglyceride is *emulsified* by bile salts and
is *hydrolysed* by the pancreatic (and intestinal mucosal) lipase into
monoglycerides and fatty acids prior to absorption.

Bile Salts

The *conjugated bile salts* act as detergent to form a mixed micelle in
which fatty acids and monoglycerides are *solubilized* to form a clear
aqueous solution for absorption. Concentration of bile salts of 4–10 m
Mol per litre allows fat absorption while below 4 mMol per litre
results in malabsorption of fats. Conjugated bile salts: (1) emulsify fats;
(2) provide optimum pH for the pancreatic lipase; (3) activate lipase
to split fat into monoglycerides and fatty acids; and (4) form *micelles*
which are suspensions in water of small globules of fat for absorption.

In the absence of bile salts, fat absorption occurs to a lesser extent
as a result of intestinal mucosal hydrolysis of triglycerides and absorption of resulting free fatty acid. With bile salt deficiency, instead of the
normal duodenal and jejunal absorption, absorption also occurs from
the distal small intestine [7].

Lipase

Gastric lipase probably digests milk triglycerides in *infants* and
hydrolyses medium-chain triglycerides in *children,* but has no significant
role in adults [8]. *Pancreatic lipase,* in the presence of bile salts at pH
6–7, splits fats into monoglycerides, diglycerides, free fatty acids and
glycerol. The mono- and diglycerides, which are water soluble, are
absorbed by the portal vein. The *lipase in the intestinal mucosal cells*
acts on the medium-chain but not on long-chain fatty acids.

Absorption

Absorption of short- and medium-chain fatty acids is different from
that of long-chain fatty acids.

The *short- and medium-chain fatty acids* (up to 10 carbon atoms)
are rapidly broken down by the pancreatic, and to an extent by the
intestinal mucosal, lipase. These fatty acids do not require bile salts
for their absorption and do not form chylomicrons. As they are water
soluble they are absorbed in the *portal system.* Thus, despite small
intestinal mucosal damage in coeliac disease, the medium-chain fatty
acids are absorbed.

The *long-chain* fatty acids (over 14 carbon chain) require bile salts for their digestion and absorption. Healthy small intestinal mucosal cells reconvert fatty acids and monoglycerides into triglycerides. The triglycerides are then surrounded by protein (*lipoprotein* synthesized by the intestinal cells) to form *chylomicrons* that are carried by the *lymphatics* into the thoracic duct. In the liver the chylomicrons are converted into free fatty acids and bound to albumin for transport to the adipose tissues. The absorption of triglycerides is also regulated by adrenals as their removal produces fat malabsorption [9].

Malabsorption of Fats : (Steatorrhoea)

The normal human intestine can absorb up to 300 g fat. In a healthy person on a diet of 50–150 g fat the daily faecal fat excretion is less than 6 g. Most people take between 50–150 g fat daily and therefore on a *normal diet* faecal fatty acid excretion is less than 6 g a day. Increase in daily faecal content over 6 g is called steatorrhoea.

Steatorrhoea may be due to defective fat breakdown (lipolysis) or defective absorption. The causes of malabsorption stated elsewhere also produce steatorrhoea (see Malabsorption Syndrome).

BLOOD LIPIDS

The plasma contains about 500 mg of lipids per 100 ml during the post-absorptive phase. The value tends to rise with increasing age.

Average lipid content of blood plasma

	mg per 100 ml
Neutral fat (triglycerides)	140–225
Free cholesterol	40– 60
Cholesterol esters	110–190
Phospholipids	160–200

Triglycerides

Chemically, fats are fatty acid esters of alcohol and glycerol. Glycerol has 3 carbon atoms and when 3 fatty acids are attached to it, *triglyceride* is formed. The dietary fats, triglycerides, are broken down in the intestine into fatty acids and glycerol. Fatty acids, on absorption, are reconverted to triglycerides by the intestinal cell, and with the addition of protein form chylomicron. The circulating lipoproteins and most of the body fat depot contain triglycerides.

Phospholipids

Phospholipids are those lipids which, on hydrolysis, yield one molecule of phosphoric acid in addition to a molecule of glycerol, and two molecules of fatty acids with or without a molecule of nitrogenous base. The blood contains phospholipids such as lecithin, cephalin, etc. Phospholipids, because of their detergent or surface active properties, help to *disperse* lipids into the cells and back from the cells into the plasma. Lecithin, the bile secretion, helps to keep cholesterol in solution.

LIPID TRANSPORT

Plasma transport of lipids occurs by means of the *chylomicrons, free fatty acids* and *lipoproteins* [10].

Chylomicrons

Chylomicrons are covered with a small layer of protein and are also classed as lipoprotein. The chylomicron core contains triglycerides and cholesterol, while the membrane consists of phospholipid and some lipoprotein [11]. Chylomicrons are absorbed by the intestinal lymphatics for transport to various sites for deposition. On dark-field microscopic examination of the blood, chylomicrons are visible for a few hours after food ingestion. Blood withdrawn within an hour or two after a fatty meal and kept standing overnight displays chylomicrons as a creamy layer on top of the plasma.

Free Fatty Acids (FFA)

Depot fat triglycerides are released for energy requirement as: (1) glycerol, which is metabolized as carbohydrate; and (2) fatty acids which are known as *free fatty acids* (FFA) bound to albumin, and circulate in the blood in small amounts. FFA are either broken down for energy by the muscle cell enzymes and produce carbon dioxide and water, or are resynthesized to form body triglycerides. For resynthesis in the cell, the glycerol required is newly formed from glycerose-phosphate derived from glucose. Normal carbohydrate metabolism is therefore essential for resynthesis of body triglycerides. In the absence of adequate carbohydrate metabolism, as in starvation, excess FFA circulate in the blood. The release of FFA from fat depots is considerably reduced on administration of glucose or insulin. Many hormones, particularly adrenaline, release fat from depots and raise plasma FFA while insulin prevents release.

Lipoproteins

Lipids are insoluble, but their attachment to proteins of different densities makes them *soluble* for transport as lipoproteins. Parts of the cholesterol, neutral fat and phospholipids are bound with protein to form lipoproteins. The various lipoproteins can be separated by:

1. *Ultracentrifugation.* Variations *in densities* separate the lipoproteins as high (*alpha*), low (*beta*) and very low (*pre-beta*) density lipoproteins; and chylomicrons that contain very little lipoprotein.

2. *Electrophoresis.* Due to variations in migrating properties of these proteins, electrophoresis is the commoner and easier method for indentification of *alpha, beta* and *pre-beta* lipoproteins.

The *lipoproteins* consist of (1) the specific lipoprotein, mentioned above; (2) cholesterol; (3) and phospholipid. *Beta* lipoproteins contain more cholesterol than other lipoproteins. In coronary heart disease the *pre-beta* and *beta* lipoproteins are increased.

OXIDATION AND STORAGE OF FAT

After absorption, fats may be oxidized to carbon dioxide and water or stored in the fat depots. *Lipoprotein lipase* present in the fat cells hydrolyses circulating triglycerides prior to deposition in the cells. Glycerol from hydrolysed triglyceride returns to the liver, while glucose in the cell is converted to glycerol that combines with fatty acids to form triglycerides for deposition in the cells, Insulin is *lipogenic* (aids body storage of fat).

After the energy requirements of the body have been met, excess fat is stored in fat depots under the skin, in the peritoneal cavity, between the muscles and around the kidneys and ovaries. In a normal individual fats consitute about 15–18 per cent of the body weight. A man weighing 60 kg has about 9 kg (9000 g) of fat, enough to supply his calorie requirements for well over 4 weeks. This is in sharp contrast to the negligible amount of energy available from the body stores of carbohydrates. Fats are thus ideally constituted as the reserve fuel of the body.

Composition of Depot Fat

The *intracellular lipid pool* is composed of triglycerides and phospholipids. *For energy requirements* during exercise or fasting states the storage fat is released as free fatty acids (FFA) and utilized by the tissues.

In the newborn, adipose tissues contain 40 per cent lipid which increases in old age to as much as 75 per cent, while the water and nitrogen contents are decreased [12]. The composition of depot fat depends upon the type of dietary fat. In animals fed on unsaturated vegetable fats, depot fat tends to be unsaturated with a high iodine value and a low melting point. If fed on saturated fats the animal's depot fat has a higher proportion of saturated fatty acids with a higher melting point and a lower iodine value. In aquatic life, changes in the composition of body fat with the change in water temperature have been observed [13]. In humans too, administration of vegetable fats only reduces serum cholesterol and the adipose tissues contain more unsaturated fatty acids than do controls [14]. The composition of dietary fats such as eggs and animal fats can therefore be changed by feeding different diets to animals. It may be possible to employ such animal foods in the future with special therapeutic values.

Obesity is excessive store of depot fat, and is usually due to consumption of excess fat and carbohydrates that are converted into fatty acids.

Functions

1. The most important function of fats is to provide an energy reserve, a bank balance which can be drawn upon when necessary. Fats supply about 9 Calories per gramme which is more than double the energy yield of protein or carbohydrate. The short-chain fatty acids like butyric acid from tributyrin of butter yield only 6.7 Calories per gramme.

2. Fats serve as a vehicle for the absorption of the fat-soluble vitamins A, D, E and K.

3. Fats supply the essential fatty acids which are necessary for growth and nutrition. The exact role of the essential fatty acids in the prevention of atherosclerosis and ischaemic heart disease has been the subject of extensive research.

4. If fats and carbohydrates are utilized as energy sources, proteins are spared for tissue growth and repair. This is known as the protein sparing effect of fats and carbohydrates.

5. Fats help in producing a sense of satiety as they retard the emptying of the stomach.

Fat Content of Diets

The fat content of diets varies with the food habits as well as with the economic prosperity of a nation. In the United States of America fats supply over 40 per cent of the total calories. In England fats supply 35 per cent of the calories, whilst in Japan fats supply only 8–10 per cent. In the tropics, the vast majority of the population derives barely 10–15 per cent of the daily calorie intake from fats. The chief sources of fat amongst the poorer classes are vegetable oils like groundnut, coconut, mustard or gingelly oil. Amongst the middle classes, who cannot afford the high price of *ghee,* hydrogenated vegetable oils (*vanaspati*) are used extensively for cooking. The richer classes consume butter and *ghee.* Non-vegetarians may also consume fats from meat, fish, poultry and eggs.

Requirements

The most important function of fats is to supply calories. If the calorie requirements can be largely met from carbohydrate and protein then the demand for fats is proportionately reduced. In tropical countries, like India, the fat requirements are less than in colder countries; about 50–60 g would be an adequate intake for a normal person.

FRIED FOODS

The temperature of fat during frying is 180°–200°C. Frying causes a big increase in the calorie value of food. A boiled potato weighing 100 g supplies only 87 calories, whilst the same weight of fried potato has twice the calorie value. The amount of fat absorbed during frying, and hence the calorie increase, depends on: (1) the foodstuff; (2) the surface area in contact with fat; (3) mode of cooking; and (4) temperature of the cooking medium.

(1) Porous foods, like *brinjals* (egg plant), when sliced and fried, absorb so much fat that the calorie value is increased by over 600 per cent. In contrast, frying of eggs increases their calorie value by only 50 per cent. (2) A whole potato when fried absorbs less fat than chipped potato because the area in contact with the cooking fat is larger. (3) Covering cutlets or fish with eggs and bread crumbs reduces the amount of fat during frying. (4) Food fried at a low temperature absorbs much fat and has a greasy taste. When fried at higher temperatures, the food is coated with fat but less is absorbed. These factors are

of importance in considering the calorie value of fried foods.

The common cooking fats and oils are:

1. *Vegetable oils.* Groundnut oil and sweet oil (also known as gingelly oil or *till* oil or sesame oil) are extensively used in the Maharashtra State. Coconut oil is used on the west coast of India, Kerala and Goa. Mustard oil is used in Bengal, Bihar and Uttar Pradesh.

2. *Hydrogenated oils.* Vegetable *ghee* or *vanaspati* is made by hydrogenating vegetable oils.

3. *Ghee* is butter from which moisture has been expelled by boiling, a process which improves its keeping qualities.

4. *Butter* is the most expensive fat and is used only by the richer classes.

5. *Margarine* is extensively used as a cheap substitute for butter.

Frying fat should not contain any moisture or it will splutter as the water forms steam. Food should not be added until frying fat is hot, otherwise excess fat absorbed by the foods makes it unpalatable.

Contra-indications. Fried food is difficult to digest. As fats are not digested in the stomach, the digestion of proteins and carbohydrates is delayed. Fried foods are contra-indicated in acute illness, gastritis, cholecystitis, dysentery, sprue, steatorrhoea, obesity and atherosclerosis.

Indications. Food is fried to make it more appetizing and to increase its calorie content. Fried foods are thus specially indicated for people who need to gain weight.

REFERENCES

[1] HAKIM, S.A.E. (1966) Argemone oil, epidemic dropsy, glaucoma and cancer, *Bombay Hosp. J.,* **8**, 137.

[2] BRITISH MEDICAL JOURNAL (1971) Fats and multiple sclerosis, *Brit. med. J.,* **2**, 545.

[3] SNIPES, R.L. (1968) The effect of essential fatty acid deficiency on the ultrastructure and functional capacity of the jejunal epithelium, *Lab. Invest.,* **18**, 179.

[4] KAPLAN, J.A., COX, G.E., and TAYLOR, C.B. (1963) Cholesterol metabolism in man, *Arch. Path.,* **76**, 359.

[5] WILSON, J.A., and LINDSEY, C.A. (1965) Studies on the influence of dietary cholesterol on cholesterol metabolism in the isotopic steady state in man, *J. clin. Invest.,* **44**, 1805.

[6] ISSELBACHER, K.J. (1966) Biochemical aspects of fat absorption, *Gastroenterology,* **50**, 78.

[7] PORTER, H.P., *et al.* (1971) Fat absorption in bile fistula in man, *Gastroen-terology,* **60,** 1008.

[8] COHEN, M., MORGAN, R.G.H., and HOFFMAN, A.F. (1971) Lipolytic activity of human gastric and duodenal juice against medium and long chain triglycerides, *Gastroenterology,* **60,** 1.

[9] RODGERS, J.B., RILEY, E.M., DRUMMEY, G.D., and ISSELBACHER, K.J. (1967) Lipid absorption in adrenalectomised rats: the role of altered enzyme activity in the intestinal mucosa, *Gastroenterology,* **53,** 547.

[10] CARLSON, L.A. (1967) Lipid metabolism and muscle work, *Fed. Proc.,* **26,** 1755.

[11] ZILVERSMIT, D.B. (1967) Formation and transport of chylomicrons, *Fed. Proc.,* **26,** 1599.

[12] BAKER, G.L. (1969) Human adipose tissue composition and age, *Amer. J. clin. Nutr.,* **22,** 829.

[13] MEAD, A.F. (1963) Lipid metabolism, *Ann. Rev. Biochem.,* **32,** 262.

[14] TURPEINEN, O., *et al.* (1968) Dietary prevention of coronary heart disease. Long term experiment, *Amer. J. clin. Nutr.,* **21,** 255.

4. CARBOHYDRATES

Carbohydrates are so called because they ordinarily contain carbon, with oxygen and hydrogen in the same proportion as in water. They are utilized as fuel by the human body and constitute the only source of energy for nervous tissues. Carbohydrates are the cheapest and most important source of calories for the vast majority of people in the tropics.

CHEMISTRY

Carbon, hydrogen and oxygen are formed into units known as saccharide groups. Carbohydrates are classified according to the number of saccharide groups present, monosaccharides have one, disaccharides two, whilst starches and glycogen are examples of polysaccharides which have more than two saccharide groups linked together.

Monosaccharides

Monosaccharides are the simplest form of carbohydrates. All carbo-hydrates are reduced to this state before absorption and utilization.

Monosaccharides may contain from 3 to 6 carbon atoms and are as such termed triose, tetrose, pentose or hexose according to the number of carbon atoms. Hexoses have 6 carbon atoms with the formula $C_6H_{12}O_6$. Glucose, fructose and galactose are hexoses, important for human nutrition.

1. *D-Glucose* (dextrose or grape sugar) rotates polarized light to the right (*dextro*=right). It is a white crystalline substance, freely soluble in water with a sweet taste. Glucose is not as sweet as the household sugar, sucrose.

Relative sweetness in water of some compounds [1]:

LESS SWEET THAN SUCROSE		MORE SWEET THAN SUCROSE	
Lactose	0·16	Fructose	1·1
Liquid glucose	0·23	Cyclamate	30
Sorbitol	0·54	Saccharin	350
Glucose (dextrose)	0·67		

SUCROSE (Household sugar)=1

The ability of glucose to reduce copper compounds from the cupric to the cuprous state is utilized to detect glucose in the urine (Benedict's test), but other reducing substances also give positive results. The *glucose oxidase* method detects glucose specifically. Glucose is readily ingested as a drink, does not require digestion, can be absorbed from the stomach and easily utilized. Fruits may contain free glucose with laevulose and sucrose.

2. *Fructose* (laevulose or fruit sugar) rotates polarized light to the left (*laevo*=left). It is present in honey, fruits and vegetables. *Sucrose* (household sugar) breakdown releases glucose and fructose. The latter is converted to glucose mainly by the liver cells and also by the mucosal cells of the intestine. Fructose enters the cells *without* the aid of insulin, and is hence sometimes recommended for diabetes.

Fructosuria. (1) *Essential fructosuria* is a benign condition, found mostly in Jews, and is due to hepatic deficiency of enzyme fructokinase that aids conversion of fructose to glucose. Fructose appears in the urine. (2) *Hereditary fructose intolerance* is due to deficiency of enzyme fructose-1-phosphate aldolase in the liver resulting in fructosaemia, fructosuria, vomiting and hypoglycaemia, subsequent development of hepatomegaly, and even death. The mechanism of hypoglycaemia is not known. The symptoms appear when the child is started with household sugar sucrose (glucose+fructose). The *treatment* is exclusion of sugar and fruits.

3. *Galactose.* Lactose is milk sugar which breaks down into glucose and galactose during digestion. Galactose is not present in fruits or vegetables.

Galactosaemia. The enzyme galactose-1-phosphate uridyl transferase is essential for the conversion of galactose (from milk sugar lactose) to glucose [2]. This results in the accumulation of galactose-1-phosphate in the tissues. The clinical features are jaundice, cirrhosis, cataract and mental retardation. The urine shows reducing substances which by means of glucose oxidase testing are found to be negative for glucose. Treatment consists of eliminating milk and substituting carbohydrate by dextrimaltose.

Sorbitol and mannitol. Reduction of glucose to alcohol forms *sorbitol,* while fructose when reduced to alcohol produces a mixture of *sorbitol* and *mannitol. Oral sorbitol* is absorbed slowly and is first converted to fructose before being utilized for energy. *Intravenous mannitol* is not metabolized and is excreted in the urine as such; it is therefore used for producing osmotic diuresis to forestall renal shutdown.

Disaccharides

Disaccharides contain 2 saccharide groups per molecule and have the formula $C_{12}H_{22}O_{11}$. The disaccharides sucrose, maltose and lactose are broken up into the corresponding monosaccharides by the action of enzymes or acids.

1. *Sucrose (cane sugar)* is the table or household sugar. In the tropics it is made from sugar cane and in Western countries from sugar beet. Sugar is a comparatively cheap source of energy. In the intestine, sucrose is broken down into the monosaccharides, *glucose* and *fructose,* which are then absorbed.

2. *Maltose* is an intermediate product formed in the process of conversion of starch into glucose. One molecule of maltose yields *two molecules of glucose.* It is formed during the breakdown of starch in the process of malting barley.

3. *Lactose (milk sugar)* is the sugar of human and animal milk. It is a white powder which does not readily dissolve in cold water but is

more soluble in hot water. It is easily digestible but not as sweet as cane sugar, hence it can be added to foods to increase calories without making them too sweet. Excess of lactose, however, produces diarrhoea. Lactose is broken down by the intestinal enzyme *lactase* into *glucose* and *galactose*. In late pregnancy and during lactation, lactose may be passed in the urine and the detection of a reducing substance in the urine during this period requires to be distinguished from true diabetes mellitus. Infants suffering from enteritis may also show lactosuria.

Polysaccharides

Polysaccharides are composed of many molecules of monosac-charides linked together and have the formula $(C_6H_{10}O_5)n$. The important polysaccharides in human nutrition are: (1) starch; (2) glycogen; and (3) cellulose.

1. *Starch* is the stored carbohydrate found in the vegetable kingdom and is the counterpart to glycogen of the animal kingdom. Starch is found in cereals, pulses, potatoes and sweet potatoes. Starch granules are seen within the thin-walled cells. Starches derived from different sources have granules of different appearance, for instance the microscopic appearances of rice and potato starch differ. Cooking facilitates the digestion of starch. Boiling causes swelling of the starch granules and rupture of the cell walls.

The enzyme amylase, present in salivary and pancreatic juices, converts starch into maltose which is subsequently broken down into glucose and absorbed. Starch present in some unripe fruits is converted on maturing into sucrose, glucose and fructose (laevulose), which then impart a sweet taste.

2. *Glycogen* is a complex molecule consisting of many glucose units. Monosaccharides, in whatever form they are absorbed, whether as glucose, fructose or galactose, are ultimately converted into glycogen which represents the storage or reserve form of carbohydrate fuel for animals. The total glycogen reserve of the body is capable of supplying energy for just over half a day but whatever amount utilized is replenished.

3. *Cellulose* is a long chain-like molecule composed of many glucose units. It forms the cell wall of vegetables, fruits and cereals. Cattle can digest and utilize cellulose but the human intestinal juices cannot digest it. If the cell of a nutrient like rice is covered with cellulose, the digestive juices cannot act unless the cellulose barrier is broken down. This is accomplished by cooking or by mastication, which mechanically

breaks down the cellulose barrier, thereby allowing the digestion of starch by the amylase of the saliva and the intestinal juices.

Constipated persons can be helped by cellulose which provides an unabsorbable bulk and distends the intestine and stimulates peristalsis. A liberal intake of cellulose-containing foods, like wheat bran, leafy vegetables and fruits is helpful. Flour from which bran has been removed contains little cellulose and provides less bulk in the intestines. Brown bread made from whole wheat flour is more helpful in cases of constipation than white bread prepared from white flour, devoid of bran. The colour of brown bread sold in the market may be due to the addition of molasses which is easily distinguished from bread made with bran by taking a piece and rolling it between the fingers for a few minutes when the bran particles can be easily recognized.

Isphgul (*Isogel*) is cellulose with a capacity to absorb over 25 times its weight of water. It is extensively used for treating constipation because the absorbed water forms a huge bulk which stimulates intestinal peristalsis. Administration of *isphgul* is a physiological way of treating constipation rather than irritating the bowel with purgatives.

Agar-agar, which is obtained from sea-weed, has properties similar to *isphgul.*

Liquid Glucose

Liquid glucose[1] [TABLE 10] is a complex carbohydrate *predigested*

TABLE 10

CARBOHYDRATE COMPOSITION OF LIQUID GLUCOSE BPC

CARBOHYDRATE COMPONENT	GRAMMES PER 100 g CARBOHYDRATE
Glucose (dextrose)	19·3
Maltose, including isomaltose	14·3
Trisaccharides	11·8
Tetrasaccharides	10·0
Pentasaccharides	8·4
Hexasaccharides	6·6
Heptasaccharides	5·6
Octa-and high saccharides	24·0
Total carbohydrate	100·0

by hydrolysis of starch into tri-, tetra-, penta- or higher saccharides as desired. *Its composition of viscosity and sweetness can be changed* by varying the hydrolysis to greater or lesser extent with acids or specific enzymes. It has one-fifth the sweetness of fructose and one-third that of dextrose. It can be dried, powdered or demineralized to suit any requirement. Liquid glucose and dextrose are absorbed twice as fast as sucrose and ten times as fast as fructose. In animals, liquid glucose causes less increase in serum lipids than sucrose. Since liquid glucose can be made up into various forms and compositions it is widely used in the United Kingdom for the preparation of various foods.

DIGESTION

Mouth. Digestion of carbohydrates begins in the mouth. Chewing breaks down the cellulose envelope and makes starch and sugar readily available for subsequent digestion. Saliva contains a starch-splitting enzyme, ptyalin or salivary amylase which acts best between a pH of 4 and 9. Ptyalin converts starch into dextrines of decreasing complexity and liberates some maltose.

Stomach. The digestive action of ptyalin is continued in the stomach until acidity of the gastric juice rises and stops its action.

Small Intestine. Carbohydrates are mainly digested in the small intestine. Amylase, of the pancreatic juice, acting in an alkaline medium, rapidly converts starch into maltose. It was believed until recently that the intestinal juice or succus entericus contained enzymes called invertase (sucrase), maltase and lactase which convert disaccharides into monosaccharides. The reactions being

Sucrose ——————— Invertase ——————— glucose and fructose

Maltose ——————— Maltase ——————— glucose and glucose

Lactose ——————— Lactase ——————— glucose and galactose

It is now known that these reactions occur inside the intestinal mucosal cells where these enzymes reside [3].

The end product of carbohydrate digestion is mainly glucose together with some fructose and galactose. Human digestive enzymes do not act on polysaccharides like cellulose, which pass unchanged to the large bowel where they constitute the bulk of the faeces. Improper digestion of carbohydrate produces carbohydrate dyspepsia.

Intestinal Disaccharidase Deficiency

Specific deficiency of disaccharidase, *lactase* and sometimes *sucrase* and *maltase* may cause severe diarrhoea with the passage of pale frothy stools and malnutrition. The age of onset of this condition varies. In lactose intolerance the symptoms appear during the first few days of life and in adult life when there is diarrhoea with the intake of milk. With intolerance for sucrose or maltose, the symptoms appear when mixed feeding is started for infants. The diarrhoea is due to osmotic water retention in the intestine, and the action of micro-organisms on unabsorbed carbohydrates causes the formation of acids that irritate the bowel. Treatment consists of avoiding milk, sucrose or starches, according to the deficiency, and substituting monosaccharides.

Carbohydrate Dyspepsia (Intestinal Carbohydrate Dyspepsia)

It is characterized by abnormal fermentation of carbohydrates in the intestines producing excessive gas. Carbohydrates are well absorbed from the small intestine, except in the presence of intestinal hurry, chronic pancreatic disease, or intestinal disaccharidase deficiency.

Undigested and unabsorbed carbohydrates pass into the large bowel where they are fermented by bacteria. Predominantly vegetarian diets containing cereals, potatoes, pulses and vegetables have a high content of carbohydrates and cellulose which may ferment and may also form short-chain fatty acids. The symptoms are abdominal distension, colic and unformed stools with froth (gas bubbles). The flatus is relatively odourless compared to the offensive smell of protein putrefaction in the intestine . The stool examination may reveal excess of vegetable fibres and starch granules.

Reducing the intake of carbohydrates and avoiding indigestible pulses improves the condition. Spices are reduced to a minimum as their excess produces intestinal hurry and the increased amount of unabsorbed carbohydrates passes into the colon.

ABSORPTION

Carbohydrates are reduced to monosaccharides (glucose, fructose and galactose) before absorption, which takes place mainly in the small intestine. A small amount of glucose can be absorbed from the stomach and the large bowel.

During absorption, concentrated sugar solutions in the intestine are rapidly diluted. *Fructose* diffuses from the brush border of the intestine into the blood. *Glucose* (and ? *galactose*), with sodium ion, is absorbed from the brush border. Sodium is then dissociated from glucose, and free sodium returns to the brush border. Thus, in Addison's disease with low sodium glucose absorption is poor. The same glucose/sodium link operates for glucose reabsorption in the kidney tubules.

The rate of absorption of carbohydrates from the small intestine is regulated by:

1. *Condition of the intestinal tract.* The motility of the stomach and the tone of the pyloric sphincter determine the rapidity with which food enters the small intestine. The quicker the carbohydrates enter the small intestine the more rapid is the absorption.

In thin subjects with a lower border of the stomach in the pelvis (*gastroptosis*) in the erect posture, the glucose tolerance test done in the sitting position shows lower values due to gradual emptying. Repetition of the test with the patient lying on the right side shows a higher value due to rapid stomach emptying [4]. The *oral* glucose tolerance test shows lower blood values during the period of *menstrual flow* and worsens as the cycle progresses, while the intravenous glucose tolerance does not vary. The rapid gastric emptying during the mid-cycle may be responsible for decreased tolerance[5]. When the intestinal mucous membrane is atrophied, as in idiopathic steatorrhoea, absorption is diminished.

2. *Endocrine glands.* Endocrine glands, particularly the anterior pituitary, thyroid and adrenal cortex influence the rate of absorption. Deficiency of the *anterior pituitary* diminishes the rate of absorption, giving a 'flat' glucose tolerance curve. This effect is probably due to secondary hypofunction of the thyroid. In *hypothyroidism,* glucose absorption is depressed. In *hyperthyroidism,* the rate of absorption is enhanced and the glucose tolerance test shows a diabetic type of curve. Glucose absorption is diminished in *suprarenal deficiency,* but can be restored to normal by the administration of sodium chloride. *Insulin* has no effect on the rate of absorption of sugar, but a rise in blood sugar stimulates insulin secretion and facilitates glycogen deposition.

Vitamin B increases the absorption of carbohydrates. *Intravenous glucose* 5 per cent solution is commonly used, while 10 per cent solution produces venous thrombosis. Intravenous glucose can be oxidized, stored as liver or muscle glycogen, converted to fat or excreted in the urine.

Carbohydrate Absorption after Partial Gastrectomy (Dumping Syndrome)

The sudden influx of ingested carbohydrates into the jejunum produces symptoms known as the 'dumping syndrome'. This occurs in mild to moderate form in about 10–12 per cent of cases after partial gastrectomy and gastro-enterostomy. The dumping syndrome may be due to: (1) withdrawal of circulating fluid; (2) intestinal distension; or (3) hypoglycaemia.

1. *Withdrawal of circulating fluid* (*early dumping syndrome*). *In a normal person* the pylorus regulates the flow of food into the jejunum and the food passed into the intestine is gradually digested and absorbed, but symptoms of dumping syndrome are produced by infusing glucose rapidly into the duodenum or jejunum through a tube. After partial gastrectomy, food rapidly enters the jejunum in a hypertonic form which causes a rapid transfer of fluid from the vascular compartment of the body into the intestines. This results in intestinal distension and an abrupt fall in the circulating plasma volume [6] the symptoms being abdominal distension, borborygmi, palpitation, exhaustion, faintness and sweating. If insulin is given to these patients sugar is more rapidly stored in the liver, and a high concentration in the intestine which withdraws fluid from the circulation is prevented [7]. The symptoms of dumping syndrome can be *reproduced* by orally feeding 175 ml of 50 per cent glucose.

2. *Intestinal distension.* A hypertonic solution of glucose in the intestine withdraws circulating fluid and causes intestinal distension. This releases *serotonin* from the intestinal chromaffin cells, which stimulates intestinal peristalsis and produces vasomotor changes. Experimentally, distension of the small intestine with a balloon may also reproduce some of the symptoms of the dumping syndrome.

3. *Hypoglycaemia* (*late dumping syndrome*). In some patients with partial gastrectomy, about 2–3 hours after a meal there may be symptoms of weakness, faintness, palpitation, tremors, hunger or nausea. These symptoms resemble those of hypoglycaemia. The diagnosis is established by examining during symptoms the blood sugar level, which will be well below 60 mg per cent. The mechanism in these cases appears to be quick transit of carbohydrates into the

intestine where there is a rapid breakdown into glucose. The sudden absorption of glucose stimulates over-secretion of insulin which may be responsible for the subsequent low blood sugar and symptoms of hypoglycaemia. Treatment is with small and more frequent meals, consisting mainly of protein-rich foods which during absorption do not produce sudden rise in blood sugar but maintain the blood sugar level by gluconeogenesis. *Lactase deficiency* after gastric surgery also contributes to dumping syndrome and avoiding milk is helpful.

Surgical treatment in an intractable case of dumping syndrome consists of inserting a 6 cm segment of jejunum (either iso- or antiperistaltic) between the stomach and duodenum. (The segment is taken from 12–24 cm beyond duodenal jejunal flexure.) Vagotomy is necessary for an iso- but not for antiperistaltic segment [8].

BLOOD SUGAR

The normal fasting level of reducing substances in blood is 80–120 mg per 100 ml which includes besides sugar other substances which reduce copper such as glutathione, ergothionine, creatinine and cysteine. The concentration of these non-sugar substances is about 20 mg per 100 ml of blood. When these substances are eliminated, the 'true glucose value' in a normal fasting person is 60–100 mg per 100 ml of blood, as determined by the glucose oxidase method. Blood sugar normally does not exceed this level because excess sugar is stored and released as required. The kidneys usually excrete some sugar when the blood level rises over about 180 mg per cent.

Hormonal Control of Blood Sugar

The blood sugar level is regulated by hormones of the anterior pituitary and suprarenals, insulin and also by the state of the intestine and liver.

The anterior pituitary growth hormone increases the blood glucose level and prevents the entry of glucose into the tissues. The action of the anterior pituitary is opposite to that of insulin.

Insulin is secreted by the beta cells of the islets of Langerhans in the pancreas. Insulin makes the cell membrane permeable to glucose and reduces the blood sugar level by increasing the deposition of glycogen in the liver and by helping the oxidation of glucose to carbon dioxide in the tissues.

Adrenaline raises the blood sugar and may be injected to counteract the hypoglycaemic effect of an overdose of insulin by mobilizing glycogen from the liver. *Cortisone,* secreted by the suprarenal cortex, also raises the blood sugar.

Arterial and Venous Blood

In a normal person there is little difference between the peripheral venous blood drawn from the cubital vein and arterial blood taken from capillaries by pricking the finger tip. After the administration of 50–100 g of glucose the arterial blood level is higher than the venous blood level by 20 mg. This difference is due to the utilization of sugar by the tissues, hence the values for venous blood are lower.

Total sugar in the blood. An average adult having 5 litres of circulatory blood with 100 mg per cent sugar, the total blood sugar is less than 5 g which is a mere teaspoonful supplying 20 Calories, just enough to provide calories for the body for about 15 minutes; but there is, however, a constant conversion of liver glycogen to maintain blood sugar level.

Hyperglycaemia (High Blood Sugar)

Hyperglycaemia occurs in diabetes mellitus.

Hypoglycaemia (Low Blood Sugar)

Lowered blood sugar produces clinical symptoms. There is no fixed level at which these symptoms occur but they are usually noted when the level is below 60 mg per 100 ml. Diabetics, who are used to a high sugar level, may have symptoms of hypoglycaemia even when the level is over 100 mg per 100 ml.

Functional hypoglycaemia is the commonest cause of low blood sugar in which, after a preponderantly carbohydrate meal, there is over-stimulation of the islets of Langerhans and the excess insulin produces symptoms about 3–4 hours after breakfast or lunch giving rise to a feeling of weakness, palpitation, sweating, tremulousness and a feeling of hunger and nausea. The symptoms may automatically disappear in a short time probably due to the release of adrenaline which converts liver glycogen into glucose. These symptoms are subjectively distressing to the patient but as no physical signs are noted on subsequent examination by the physician the patient may be diagnosed as 'neurotic'. If hypoglycaemia is suspected the blood sugar should be examined during an attack. *The treatment* consists of advising snacks of biscuits, sandwiches or milk drinks about two and a half hours after breakfast or lunch. If the patient is seen during a mild attack, the administration of fruit juice, sweet lemon squash, tea or coffee with sugar is helpful. Intravenous administration of glucose gives prompt relief if the symptoms are severe.

Tumours of the islets of Langerhans of the pancreas produce bizarre neuropsychiatric symptoms or more severe symptoms of hypoglycaemia as coma and convulsions. The diagnostic features of an islet cell tumour are a triad of symptoms called Whipple's triad consisting of: (1) attacks induced by starving for 12–24 hours; (2) blood sugar less than 50 mg per cent during the height of attack; (3) rapid relief of symptoms with intravenous glucose. Subsequently the patient should be surgically explored.

Hypoglycaemia also occurs with hepatic diseases, Addison's disease, pituitary deficiency and antidiabetic drugs. Alcoholic hypoglycaemia results from diminished glucose formation by the liver (decreased gluconeogenesis).

Migraine attacks in some susceptible individuals are precipitated by low blood sugar which probably affects the autonomic system [9].

STORAGE

Monosaccharides are stored in the liver and muscles as *glycogen* which, when required for energy, is converted to glucose.

Glycogen Storage Disease

This is a rare metabolic disease due to six different types of enzyme deficiency, which reconverts glycogen into glucose. *Von Gierke's disease* is due to glucose-6-phosphate deficiency. The liver, heart, and kidneys are grossly enlarged by excessive accumulation of glycogen. The fasting blood sugar is low, acetone may be present in the urine and hypoglycaemic convulsions may occur.

McArdle's syndrome is the result of deficiency of muscle phosphorylase activity, and muscle glycogen is not broken down when required for muscle exercise. This results in pain in exercised muscles.

Diet for Athletes

An athlete taking normal combinations of foods and consuming 4000–5000 Calories naturally ingests twice the amount of protein. Thus, the advocated high protein diet for athletes has only a psychological effect [10]. With a sufficient oxygen supply, muscles utilize up to

66 per cent fat for energy, but with heavy muscular exercise, involving anaerobic processes, a major energy source is carbohydrates that increase the duration and efficiency of work. An individual whose one limb is rested and the other put to heavy exercise has glycogen depletion in the exercised limb. If a high carbohydrate diet is taken for 3 days, the exercised limb shows marked glycogen increase, while the other limb shows no such variations.

On exhausting muscle glycogen with exercise and feeding a *protein-fat* diet, the glycogen content of the muscle is reduced to 0.6 per cent, which is subsequently raised to 4.7 per cent on a high *carbohydrate* diet. This increased muscle glycogen enhances the work period [11]. In order to augment muscle glycogen for a competition lasting over 30–60 minutes, it is suggested that the preparations start a week before. For the first 3 days the muscles should be exercised on a *protein-fat* diet, while thereafter a high carbohydrate diet enhances the muscle glycogen store on the day of the competition.

FUNCTIONS

Energy. Carbohydrates supply energy for immediate use by the body. One gramme of carbohydrate provides approximately four Calories. The total body store of carbohydrates is about 300–400 g and assuming that this amount is converted to energy, then only 1200–1600 Calories could be derived from carbohydrates, enough to last for less than a day. The carbohydrates stores are negligible compared to the stores of fats which may last for a month. Though the store of carbohydrates is very low, yet it is being continuously replenished from fats and proteins. Brain and erythrocytes require glucose for metabolism, while other tissues can utilize free fatty acids and ketones.

The sources of carbohydrates in the body are: (1) the total sugar content of extracellular fluids; (2) liver glycogen—about 5 per cent of the total weight of the liver is glycogen, but this amount is reduced in starvation; (3) muscle glycogen—about 0.7 to 1 per cent of the weight of the muscle is glycogen which cannot be easily released for energy even in the presence of severe hypoglycaemia.

Apart from supplying ready fuel, carbohydrates also play a vital role in the proper function of the liver, the central nervous system, the heart and muscle contraction.

Liver. Glycogen protects the liver against bacterial toxins and poisonous substances. Glycuronic acid produced by the liver from carbohydrates converts harmful substances containing alcoholic or phenolic groups into harmless compounds which are excreted. The liver also produces the acetyl group, mainly from carbohydrates, which combines with substances like sulphonamides producing harmless acetylated forms which are excreted by the kidneys.

Central Nervous System. Glucose is the food required by the brain for its metabolism. Brain tissue is very sensitive to lack of glucose and deficiency can lead to semipermanent or permanent alterations in the cells in a few minutes. If a very low blood sugar is allowed to persist for long periods, then permanent changes may occur in the brain resulting in porencephaly (cysts or cavities in the brain).

Heart. The efficiency of the heart as a pump depends upon carbohydrates as a fuel. The carbohydrate supply is derived from the blood sugar and glycogen stored in the heart muscle. Unlike the brain tissue, the heart has a reserve store of glycogen which can be utilized in an emergency. When there is a temporary reduction in the blood sugar, a healthy heart is not damaged because of the reserve muscle glycogen. When a damaged heart, containing little reserve of glycogen is subjected to low blood sugar, anginal pain may be experienced, and in extreme cases, death may follow. Insulin increases the irritability of ectopic foci in a damaged heart [12]. When treating a diabetic with a damaged heart, care should be taken to avoid insulin over-dosage.

Muscle Contraction. Every movement of a muscle requires energy for which carbohydrate is the most efficient and economical fuel; this is derived from glycogen in the muscles. All muscle glycogen is not converted to energy. Anaerobic glycolysis produces *lactate* that diffuses into the blood, and the liver reconverts it to glucose or glycogen.

Protein Sparing Effect. When carbohydrates and fats are supplied to a person to meet the demand for energy, proteins are spared for growth and repair which is known as the 'protein sparing effect'. When carbohydrates are insufficient to meet the requirements of an individual, amino acids are deaminated to form fatty acids used for gluconeogenesis. The deaminated products are converted into urea by the liver and excreted by the kidneys. In severe liver or kidney damage these products may accumulate and produce toxic symptoms. The endogenous breakdown of proteins is reduced if the patient is given a minimum of 150 g (600 Calories) of carbohydrate for energy. Even in a comatose patient carbohydrate can be given by nasogastric tube feeding or by intravenous infusion of glucose.

The mechanism of the protein sparing effect is not clear. Insulin also has the action of depositing amino acids in the cells for protein synthesis. Secretion of insulin with a carbohydrate diet probably aids amino acid deposition.

Ketosis and Carbohydrate Metabolism. Ketone bodies are not abnormal products of fat metabolism as was presumed. During normal metabolism, fat is broken down by the liver into beta hydroxybutyric acid, aceto-acetic acid and acetone. They are collectively known as ketone (acetone) bodies. Ketone bodies are used by the peripheral tissues as a source of energy but only to a limited extent. When carbohydrates are not readily available, as in starvation, or cannot be utilized as in severe deficiency of insulin, fats are broken down in greater quantities for energy and an increased amount of ketone bodies are produced. These being in excess of the limited capacity of the tissue utilization, accumulate in the blood (ketonaemia) and are excreted in the urine (ketonuria).

In clinical practice, urine examination of an unconscious starving patient may show absence of sugar but excess of ketone bodies. An inexperienced physician may be tempted to give insulin mistaking this condition for diabetic ketosis. Ketone bodies, without sugar in the urine, are due to starvation and require glucose to supply energy and reduce the breakdown of fats.

Conversion of Carbohydrates into Fats. After fulfilling the energy demands and replenishing the stores in the liver and muscles an excess of ingested carbohydrates is converted into fats and stored in the fat depots which can be expanded to an unlimited capacity producing obesity.

SOURCES

Carbohydrates form the staple food in the tropics. Rice, wheat, *bajra, jowar,* pulses (*mung dal, tuver dal,* etc.), fruits, vegetables, tubers (potato, sweet potato), sugar, honey and jaggery are the main sources.

Oral Glucose. Glucose is given orally to supply immediate energy. It is also given during prolonged fevers to enhance the caloric intake. An excessive amount of glucose given orally produces distension of the abdomen which is detrimental to an ill patient.

Intravenous Glucose. An acutely ill patient requires intravenous administration of a 5–10 per cent solution of glucose in order to reduce the abnormal breakdown of his body proteins. Administration of 25–50 per cent glucose is irritating to the veins and may produce thrombosis. Moreover, it is rapidly excreted in the urine. Such high concentrations of glucose are given only to reduce pulmonary or cerebral oedema or when many calories are needed with little fluid as in anuria when a central vein may be cannulated and used.

REQUIREMENTS

Carbohydrates are interchangeable with fats for the necessary caloric requirements. There is no minimum necessary requirement for carbohydrates provided adequate calories are supplied. The usual daily intake of carbohydrates by an adult male is approximately 4–6 g per kg body weight. The optimal intake of carbohydrates is calculated by first determining the total calories needed by a person according to his height, weight and occupation. Total caloric requirements are then supplied as: (1) proteins, 11 per cent (14 per cent in children, pregnant and lactating mothers) of the total calories; (2) fat, 1 g per kg body weight; and (3) carbohydrates make up the rest of the calories. *For example,* an adult male weighing 60 kg, height 175 cm, with a sedentary occupation, requires 30 Calories per kg, i.e. $60 \times 30 = 1800$ Calories. Proteins should provide 200 Calories (11 per cent of calories $= 50$ g), fats should provide 540 Calories (1 g per kg$=60$ g); therefore the remaining 1060 Calories will be provided by 265 g carbohydrates.

Vitamin B Complex and Carbohydrate Metabolism

Vitamins of the B group take part in the metabolism of carbohydrates at various stages. Carbohydrates increase the demand for vitamin B complex. Nature has combined vitamin B with carbohydrates in most grains and plants. Modern methods of food refining, such as polishing rice in which vitamin B is lost, lead to vitamin B deficiency and impaired metabolism of carbohydrates. It is advisable to administer vitamin B complex whenever glucose is given parenterally.

REFERENCES

[1] ALLEN, R.J.L., and BROOK, M. (1967) Carbohydrate and the United Kingdom food manufacturer, *Amer. J. clin. Nutr.*, **20**, 163.

[2] ISSELBACHER, K.J., ANDERSON, E.P., KURAHASKI, K., and KALCKAR, H.M. (1956) Congenital galactosemia, a single enzymatic block in galactose metabolism, *Science*, **123**, 635.

[3] DAHLQVIST, A., and BORGSTROM, B. (1961) Digestion and absorption of disaccharides in man, *Biochem. J.*, **81**, 411.

[4] DESAI, H.G., and ANTIA, F.P. (1968) Effect of posture on glucose tolerance curve, in *Diabetes in the Tropics. Proceedings of the World Congress on Diabetes in the Tropics, 20–22 January*, Diabetic Association of India, Bombay, p. 191.

[5] MACDONALD, I., and CROSSLEY, J.N. (1970) Glucose tolerance during the menstrual cycle, *Diabetes*, **19**, 450.

[6] LE QUESNE, L.P., HOBSLEY, M., and HAND, B.H. (1960) The dumping syndrome. I. Factors responsible for the symptoms, *Brit. med. J.*, **1**, 141.

[7] HOBSLEY, M., and LE QUESNE, L.P. (1960) The dumping syndrome. II. Cause of the syndrome and the rationale of its treatment, *Brit. med. J.*, **1**, 147.

[8] BOUCHALD, H. (1968) Dumping syndrome and its treatment, *Amer. J. Surg.*, **116**, 81.

[9] BLAU, J.N., and PYKE, D.A. (1970) Effect of diabetes on migraine, *Lancet*, **ii**, 241.

[10] ASTRAND, P.O. (1970) Diet and athletic performance, *Fed. Proc.*, **26**, 1772.

[11] BERGSTROM, J., HERMANSEN, L., HULTMAN, E., and SALTIN, B. (1967) Diet, muscle glycogen and physical performance, *Acta physiol. scand.*, **71**, 140.

[12] SOSKIN, S., KATZ, L.N., STROUSE, S., and RUBINFELD, S.H. (1933) Treatment of elderly diabetic patients with cardiovascular disease, *Arch. intern. Med.*, **51**, 122.

5. VITAMIN B₁ (Thiamine, Aneurine)

Vitamin B₁ is historically very important. It was deficiency of this vitamin which proved conclusively for the first time that a disease syndrome could be produced by an inadequate supply of minute amounts of certain factors in food. Casimir Funk in 1911 obtained vitamin B₁ as a crystalline substance from rice polishings. He called it 'vitalamine' (now called vitamin) because it contained nitrogen as an amine. Some food factors active in minute amounts, and discovered since then, are not 'amines', yet the term vitamin is still used to describe them. Just as the discovery of microbes as a cause of disease opened a new era in medicine, so the discovery that deficiency of vitamins in food can produce debilitating and even fatal diseases, has helped millions especially in the East, where the diet is generally poor.

Takaki, a physician in the Japanese Navy, first demonstrated that a grossly debilitating and fatal disease like beriberi could not only be treated but also eradicated from the Japanese Navy by adding vegetables, fish and meat, to the rice diet. Though the disease could be successfully prevented by a change in the diet, the exact factor which prevented beriberi was not known. Later, Eijkman, a Dutch physician in Java, noted that a diet consisting mainly of polished rice was responsible for beriberi; hence, as a corollary, rice polishings were extensively investigated in an attempt to extract the antineuritic principle.

The word 'thiamine', originally used in the United States, has been adopted internationally as the standard name for vitamin B$_1$. Aneurine is the British pharmacopoeial word derived from '*anti-neur*itic vitam*in*'.

Chemistry

Thiamine hydrochloride has a thiazole and a pyrimidine nucleus. Its empirical formula is $C_{12}H_{17}N_4$ OSCI.HCl. It is a white crystalline substance soluble in water and stable at 100°C in acid solution. It is unstable in an alkaline medium and for this reason the practice of adding sodium bicarbonate (soda) during cooking, to render meat and pulses tender or to retain the green colour of vegetables, results in considerable loss of this vitamin.

Thiamine was *synthesized* in 1936.

Unit. Three micrograms of thiamine hydrochloride are equivalent to one International Unit. One milligram of commercially available vitamin B$_1$ represents 333 International Units. It is customary to express amounts of vitamin B$_1$ in terms of milligrams rather than in International Units.

Absorption

Vitamin B$_1$ is readily absorbed from the small and large intestine. It can be administered parenterally.

Storage

Little vitamin B_1 is stored in the body. It is mainly concentrated in the liver, muscles, heart, kidneys and brain. The body stores can be considerably reduced in a few days and so vitamin B_1 should be administered during an acute illness when the food intake is poor.

Excretion

Vitamin B_1 is excreted in the *urine* and a little is present in the faeces, though how much of this is the result of bacterial synthesis in the intestine is not known. *Breast milk* also contains vitamin B_1.

Action

Thiamine pyrophosphate (diphosphothiamine) is the physiologically active form of thiamine. Thiamine pyrophosphate also functions as a co-enzyme in the 'transketolase system' associated with the direct oxidative pathway of glucose metabolism. In its absence, the inter-mediate products of carbohydrate metabolism, lactic acid and pyruvic acid, accumulate in the body.

Nervous tissue in particular derives all its energy from carbohydrate. If carbohydrates cannot be properly metabolized the peripheral nerves degenerate, giving rise to peripheral neuropathy.

Source

Vitamin B complex consists of several factors and none of them is found in abundance in any food. In order to supply the daily require-ments of any vitamin of the B group, food has to be taken in con-siderable quantities. This is unlike vitamin C, such large amounts of which are concentrated in certain fruits that the daily needs can be supplied, for instance, by one orange. Usually the food-stuffs which provide most of the caloric intake also provide enough of the vitamin B complex. Cereals provide the major part of the caloric intake in Eastern countries; hence the source of B_1 depends upon: (1) the staple cereal eaten in the area; and (2) the mode of processing the cereal.

Rice contains adequate amounts of vitamin B complex but a large proportion of the vitamin B_1 is lost when it is polished. If polished rice is cooked with too much water which is then thrown away, a further loss of the vitamin occurs. Parboiled rice or home pounded rice preserves the vitamins better than polished rice.

Wheat milled with 70 per cent or less extraction, to produce white flour for baking bread or cake, is poor in vitamin B$_1$. In India baked bread is eaten in large cities by relatively wealthy people who supplement their diet with other foodstuffs containing vitamin B$_1$. In the villages, wheat is usually eaten as unleavened bread (*chappatis*) made from wheat flour ground at home. This is passed through a sieve which removes only about 5 per cent of the coarse bran; flour of 95 per cent extraction is thus used for preparing *chappatis* and vitamin B$_1$ is preserved.

Millets like *bajra* (*Pennisetum typhoides*) or *jowar* (*Sorghum vulgare*) eaten by the villagers are similarly about 95 per cent extracted and the loss of natural vitamins is not great.

There is no convincing evidence that intestinal bacteria are a source of vitamin B$_1$ in humans.

Commercial preparations of vitamin B$_1$ are either extracted from a natural source like rice, or are synthesized.

Requirements

The minimum thiamine requirements are studied from: the urinary excretion, dose retention, or appearance and disappearance of deficiency symptoms. Erythrocyte analysis for transketolase activity and tests for thiamine pyrophosphate have also been employed for estimating thiamine requirement.

Various factors influence the daily requirement of vitamin B$_1$. (1) An *increased metabolic rate* as occurs with exercise and fever increases the requirement. Children have a higher metabolic rate than adults and thus require more vitamin B$_1$ per kg of body weight. (2) *Pregnancy and lactation* increase the demand for vitamin B$_1$. (3) Vitamin B$_1$ is necessary for the *metabolism of carbohydrates* and thus the needs depend on the carbohydrate intake. As carbohydrates supply the bulk of calories, vitamin B$_1$ requirements are usually related to the calories consumed.

Vitamin B$_1$ deficiency produced experimentally in men by restricting its intake showed the 'minimal' requirement to be between 0·22 and 0·5 mg per 1000 Calories and 'optimal' requirement between 0·5 and 1·5 mg per 1000 Calories of diet [1].

The British Medical Association [2] recommends 0·4 mg per 1000 Calories for *infants, children* and *adults*. As vitamin B$_1$ is present in human milk, more vitamin B$_1$ is required by *nursing mothers*. The total daily vitamin B$_1$ requirement for an average adult can be taken as about 1 mg while for a nursing mother it can be taken as 1·4 mg.

The FAO/WHO Expert Group (1967) also recommend 0·4 mg thiamine per 1000 Calories. The minimum requirement of thiamine in Indian females is 0·26 mg/1000 Calories and for men 0·36 mg/1000 Calories [3].

DEFICIENCY

Deficiency of vitamin B_1 is frequently associated with a low calorie intake and deficiency of other factors of the vitamin B complex that are found in the same foods. In clinical practice, therefore, pure vitamin B_1 deficiency is not usually seen. Those who live on cereals alone may take just enough vitamin B_1 to supply their minimum requirements and any reduction in their intake, because of a change to refined flour or due to loss during cooking, may precipitate a deficiency. Deficiency of vitamin B_1 can be caused by: (1) low intake; (2) poor absorption; or (3) excessive demand.

1. *Low intake.* Deficiency of vitamin B_1 occurs in areas where refined cereals are the major source of calories, either as polished rice, or as highly refined flour for baking bread. Alcoholics suffer from vitamin B_1 deficiency because their food intake is usually low and because alcohol increases the metabolism and demand for the vitamin.

2. *Poor absorption.* Patients suffering from various diseases of the gastro-intestinal tract absorb vitamin B_1 poorly.

3. *Excessive demand.* The demand for vitamin B_1 is increased during pregnancy and lactation, when the basal metabolic rate is high as in hyperthyroidism or fever, and when large amounts of refined carbohydrate, like sugar, are taken.

Severe deficiency of vitamin B_1 produces the disease *beriberi*. The exact causative mechanisms producing beriberi are not known, but the accumulation of partial breakdown products of carbohydrate metabolism such as lactic and pyruvic acids, play an important role.

Clinically, vitamin B_1 deficiency manifests as: (1) subclinical deficiency; (2) infantile beriberi; (3) dry beriberi; (4) polyneuropathy associated with alcohol, diabetes or prolonged fever; (5) wet beriberi; and (6) Wernicke-Korsakoff syndrome.

Subclinical Deficiency

Subclinical forms are more common in females because of the reducing diets of the high income group and the inadequate diets of the low income group cannot cope with the large demands for vitamin

B$_1$ during pregnancy and lactation. Vitamin B$_1$ deficiency may also be associated with anaemia, deficiency of proteins and other vitamins.

The symptoms and signs of early vitamin B$_1$ deficiency are indefinite. Typical *symptoms* are anorexia, weakness, evening tiredness and constipation. On *examination,* there may be slight tenderness on pressing the calf muscles and sluggish ankle jerks. Vitamin B$_1$ deficiency is suspected when the history suggests a poor intake or excessive loss. If the symptoms are due to deficiency of vitamin B$_1$, administration of the vitamin produces rapid relief.

Infantile Beriberi

Infantile beriberi occurs in the first few months of life if the diet of the mother is deficient in vitamin B$_1$. The infant is constipated and may even appear well nourished and plump due to oedema. The heart is enlarged and the heart sounds muffled. Oedema of the glottis manifests itself as a peculiar cry, and later, as aphonia. Ultimately, there may be cardiac failure, twitchings, coma and death.

Dry Beriberi

In dry beriberi there is a polyneuropathy (polyneuritis) with involvement of the peripheral nerves, first of the legs and later of the arms. Degeneration of the myelin sheath of the nerves is followed by degeneration of the axis cylinder.

The symptoms described in the subclinical form may progress to frank manifestations of peripheral neuropathy. *Subjective symptoms* are bilateral and symmetrical tingling, numbness, and burning in the feet and hands. *Examination* shows tenderness of the calf muscles and hypo-aesthesia at the periphery of the limbs. Hypo-aesthesia is best appreciated when a pin is drawn up the lower limbs starting at the toes. In the toes there is little sensation but as the pin is drawn towards the calf sensation becomes more distinct. The knee and ankle jerks are sluggish. With progress of the disease there is marked wasting of the muscles of the feet and hands resulting in foot-drop and wrist-drop; loss of knee and ankle jerks; and complete loss of sensation at the periphery with 'glove' and 'stocking' anaesthesia.

Polyneuropathy

The *polyneuropathy* associated with alcohol, diabetes and prolonged fever resembles dry beriberi and is probably due to deficiency of vitamin B$_1$. In alcoholics thiamine intake is reduced, and the absorption is also diminished. It returns to normal with abstinence.

Experimentally-produced vitamin B_1 deficiency in man resembles dry beriberi.

Wet Beriberi

What determines whether a patient will get the dry or the wet type of beriberi is not known. If a man with vitamin B_1 deficiency does not get bedridden with polyneuropathy he is likely to continue his activities and thus precipitate cardiac failure.

Pathologically, there is enlargement of the heart, the right side being more affected than the left. Microscopically, the cardiac muscle fibres are separated by oedema. *Clinically,* pitting oedema of the extremities develops, possibly with ascites and hydrothorax. Heart failure is manifested by oliguria, dyspnoea, palpitations, tachycardia, engorged neck veins and cardiac enlargement. The electrocardiogram shows a rapid heart rate but there are no diagnostic electrocardiographic changes in wet beriberi.

Beriberi heart disease is sometimes seen among alcoholics in Western countries.

Wernicke-Korsakoff Syndrome (see Alcohol)

Treatment

1. *Prophylactic.* Those whose staple diet is refined cereals should be advised to eat the whole grain flour. This knowledge, spread by Government propaganda, will not only prevent vitamin B_1 deficiency but also other deficiencies. Enrichment of wheat flour with vitamin B_1 is practised in Western countries but as most people grind their own cereals in India, the enrichment of flour would not solve the problem.

Supplements of oral vitamin B_1, about 5 mg per day, are indicated in diabetes, alcoholism, pregnancy, lactation, and prolonged fever.

2. *Subclinical vitamin B_1 deficiency.* Therapy for subclinical states requires 5 mg of vitamin B_1 orally three times a day. It is desirable to prescribe a multivitamin preparation as well and to educate the patient about a proper diet.

3. *Manifest deficiency of vitamin B_1.* Therapy for dry or wet beriberi consists in daily parenteral administration of 10 mg of vitamin B_1. This may also be supplemented by oral supplements, 5 mg three times a day. It is best to give multivitamin preparations both parenterally and orally because manifest deficiency seldom occurs unless the

diet has been poor for a long time. In cases where there is cardiac involvement it is advisable to give 10–20 mg vitamin B$_1$ diluted with glucose by slow intravenous drip.

Wet beriberi responds to therapy rapidly and the patient improves within a few days. It may be several weeks before polyneuropathy improves.

Intravenous Feeding. Patients who are maintained on intravenous fluids with glucose, for example during acute vomiting or after surgical operations, require a vitamin B supplement because: (1) vitamin B$_1$ is not stored in the body and the food intake may have been low for several days; and (2) a large glucose intake increases the need for vitamin B complex.

Unnecessary Use. Some years ago, vitamin B$_1$ was claimed to be a panacea for all unknown diseases, and in this respect is now being replaced by vitamin B$_{12}$. Vitamin B$_1$ has been prescribed for neurological disorders of known aetiology, like prolapsed intervertebral disc, and for others where the cause is not obvious such as Bell's palsy. Even during marked vitamin B$_1$ deficiency, facial nerve paralysis does not occur, and thus it is apparent that thiamine will not be of any use in such cases. A careful and detailed assessment of the food intake and symptomatology will exclude the possibility of any deficiency state and avoid unnecessary vitamin therapy when it is not indicated.

Toxicity

Toxicity has not been reported due to excessive administration of vitamin B$_1$. However, allergic manifestations like urticaria, sensations of burning or warmth, nausea, sweating, and tachycardia may occur, and rarely, anaphylactic shock with collapse and death have been reported after parenteral therapy.

REFERENCES

[1] WILLIAMS, R.D., MASON, H.L., SMITH, B.F., and WILDER, R.M. (1942) Induced thiamine (vitamin B$_1$) deficiency and the thiamine requirement of man, *Arch. intern. Med.,* **69**, 721.
[2] BRITISH MEDICAL ASSOCIATION (1950) *Report of the Committee on Nutrition,* London.
[3] BAMJI, M.S. (1970) Transketolase activity and urinary excretion of thiamine in

the assessment of thiamine-nutrition status in Indians, *Amer. J. clin. Nutr.*, **23**, 52.

6. RIBOFLAVINE

The isolation of vitamin B_1 as a heat labile component from natural sources left a heat stable component which was originally known as vitamin B_2. Later it was discovered that the heat stable B_2 was not a single factor but contained, besides riboflavine, other vitamins such as pyridoxine, niacin and pantothenic acid. Riboflavine derives its name from its yellow colour (flavus=yellow) and is found in many substances. The suffix 'flavine' was added to the name of the source from which it was obtained, for instance, lactoflavine from milk, ovoflavine from egg, hepatoflavine from liver and uroflavine from urine. Ultimately it was established that all these were the same compound. When it was discovered that the molecule contained a group similar to the sugar ribose, the name 'riboflavine' was coined. Riboflavin is the accepted name in the *Pharmacopeia of the United States* while the *British Pharmacopoeia* adds an 'e' as riboflavine.

Chemistry

Riboflavine is dimethyl iso-alloxazine attached to d-ribitol, which is sugar pentose. The empirical formula is $C_{17}H_{20}N_4O_6$. In nature it may occur as the *free pigment,* as riboflavine phosphate or as *flavoproteins.* The latter are a combination of riboflavine with phosphoric acid and adenine to form riboflavine-adenine-dinucleotide, and the whole joined with a protein [1].

Riboflavine was *isolated* in 1933 and *synthesized* in 1935.

Stability. Riboflavine is relatively stable to heat. Ordinary cooking does not destroy it by more than 20 per cent. Cooking in an excess of water which is later thrown away entails a considerable loss. Milk exposed to sunlight in a transparent glass bottle loses riboflavine.

Absorption

Riboflavine is absorbed from the intestine. It is also absorbed when given parenterally.

Excretion

Riboflavine is excreted in the urine and milk. Excess in the body is rapidly excreted in the urine to which it imparts a yellow colour.

Action

Flavoproteins act as enzymes and take part in cell respiration. There are several flavoproteins, each one having its own specific activity. For example, xanthine oxidase acts on hypoxanthine.

Source

1. *Food.* Riboflavine is found in milk, meat, cereals and pulses. There is little in fruits, vegetables, nuts and tubers.

2. *Bacterial synthesis.* Human intestinal bacterial flora [2] probably synthesize riboflavine. Thus, men on a vitamin-free diet with supplements of pure vitamins excreted twice the daily intake of riboflavine in the urine, and five to six times the intake in the faeces.

Requirement

Experimental restriction of riboflavine in men showed that the daily requirement was 1·1–1·6 mg. A reserve of riboflavine cannot be maintained on an intake below 1·1 mg per day [3]. A well balanced diet supplies 1–2 mg of riboflavine daily.

DEFICIENCY

Riboflavine deficiency is usually associated with deficiency of other factors of the vitamin B group. Manifestations of riboflavine deficiency may be overshadowed by the more prominent manifestations of pellagra or beriberi. Deficiency can be precipitated by: (1) inadequate intake, particularly of milk which is a good source of riboflavine; (2) poor absorption as in diseases associated with chronic diarrhoea; and (3) excessive demands, as with the raised metabolic rate in thyrotoxicosis, fevers or pregnancy. During lactation, 30 micrograms per 100 ml is excreted in milk.

Observations with Restricted Riboflavine Intake

The effect of diet deficient in riboflavine but otherwise adequate was studied in 15 male subjects with 14 controls. A diet containing 2200 Calories and 0·55 mg riboflavine was maintained for 9–17 months, during which period angular stomatitis, seborrhoeic dermatitis, scrotal skin lesions and diminished ability to perceive a flicker were noted [3].

Subclinical Deficiency. Subclinical riboflavine deficiency may be suggested by general 'run down condition' with anorexia, weakness, apathy and burning at the angles of mouth, in the eyes and over the skin. A therapeutic response to riboflavine proves the diagnosis.

Manifest Deficiency. The manifestations of riboflavine deficiency are: (1) angular stomatitis and cheilosis; (2) changes in the tongue; (3) changes in the skin; and (4) corneal vascularization.

1. *Angular stomatitis.* The angles of the mouth appear pale and moist with a yellow crust and formation of fissures. *Cheilosis.* The parts of the lips which touch one another are crusted and removal of the crust leaves a red margin known as cheilosis. Changes occurring on the lips and at the angle of the mouth have been ascribed to local trauma which is not repaired.

2. *Tongue.* The tongue has been described as 'magenta' coloured with a peculiar reddish hue.

3. *Skin.* There is a fine scaly desquamation of the skin which is particularly well seen on the nasolabial folds, ears, the vulva in the female and scrotum in the male.

4. *Corneal vascularization.* Vascularization of the cornea may be due to the low riboflavine content of lachrymal secretions. The earliest changes in the eyes are seen by slit lamp examination. There is proliferation and engorgement of the limbic plexus which progresses to superficial vascularization of the cornea and finally to interstitial keratitis. Congestion of the sclera, vascularization, opacities of the cornea and abnormal pigmentation of the iris respond rapidly to the administration of riboflavine [4].

Riboflavine, 5 mg three times a day by mouth or parenterally, is necessary for the treatment of the acute deficiency state.

Despite well described manifestations ascribed to riboflavine deficiency the following remarks by Meiklejohn [5] are of interest. 'Riboflavine is one of those embarrassing vitamins which has been offered to us by the chemical industry before we felt the need for it...attempts have been made in the past to identify certain clinical signs as specific indications of riboflavine deficiency and to dignify them with the diagnosis of "ariboflavinosis" but this, like the sign of Jonas the prophet, is best forgotten'.

Toxicity

Toxicity has not been noted following the therapeutic use of riboflavine because of its rapid excretion by the kidney.

REFERENCES

[1] HARRIS, L.J. (1955) *Vitamins in Theory and Practice,* 4th ed., Cambridge, p. 263.
[2] NAJJAR, V.A., JOHNS, G.A., MEDAIRY, G.C., FLEISCHMANN, G., and HOLT, L.E. (1944) The biosynthesis of riboflavin in man, *J. Amer. med. Ass.,* **126,** 357.
[3] HORWITT, M.K., HILLS, O.W., HARVEY, C.C., LIEBERT, E., and STEINBERG, D.L. (1949) Effects of dietary depletion of riboflavin, *J. Nutr.,* **39,** 357.
[4] SYDENSTRICKER, V.P., SEBRELL, W.H., CLECKLEY, H.M., and KRUSE, H.D. (1940) The ocular manifestations of ariboflavinosis, *J. Amer. med. Ass.,* **114,** 2437.
[5] MEIKLEJOHN, A.P. (1959) Riboflavine, *Practitioner,* **182,** 35.

7. VITAMIN B$_6$ (Pyridoxine, Adermin)

Vitamin B$_6$ is not a single factor but consists of three compounds with similar activity. They are pyridoxine, its aldehyde pyridoxal and its amine pyridoxamine. All three are found in foods in varying proportions. The word pyridoxine is derived from the fact that it is a PYRIDine hydrOXyl and vitamIN. It was also known as adermin which originally signified A(nti)-DERM (atitis)-(vitam)IN [1].

Chemistry

Pyridoxine is a white crystalline substance soluble in water and alcohol. It was *isolated* in 1938 and subsequently *synthesized*. Its empirical formula is $C_8H_{11}O_3N$.

Absorption

The absorption of vitamin B$_6$ from the intestine is rapid, and occurs by diffusion mainly from the jejunum. It is also absorbed from the skin. If applied over a large area of skin, enough is absorbed to relieve all clinical and chemical signs of vitamin B$_6$ deficiency.

Excretion

All three compounds are found in urine after ingestion but

4-pyridoxic acid is quantitatively the most important excretion product. On a vitamin B_6-deficient diet the excretion can be higher than the intake. In rats on a dextrin diet the intestinal flora synthesize vitamin B_6 which is utilized. Similar synthesis is postulated in man.

Storage

The storage of vitamin B_6 in the body is usually sufficient to last for about eight weeks.

Action

Pyridoxine is necessary for the tissue metabolism. As an enzyme it aids in decarboxylation and transamination of the amino acids.

Amino Acids. During normal metabolic activity the amino group of amino acids is either utilized to form other amino acids (transamination) or converted into ammonia which is subsequently excreted as urea. In pyridoxine deficiency, the transamination activity decreases and more nitrogen is lost from the body as urea.

Tryptophan. Normally trytophan is converted to kynurenine, which with the aid of vitamin B_6, is metabolized through hydroxy-kynurenine to nicotinic acid. If there is a deficiency of vitamin B_6 this conversion is blocked and kynurenine accumulates, being excreted by the kidneys after conversion to xanthurenic acid. Estimation of xanthurenic acid in urine can thus be a measure of vitamin B_6 deficiency.

Lipid Metabolism. Vitamin B_6 aids in lipid metabolism.

Maturation of Red Blood Cells. Vitamin B_6 plays a role in iron utilization.

Source [TABLE 11]

The foods richest in pyridoxine are egg yolk, meat, fish and milk among animal sources. The vegetable sources are whole grains, cabbage and other green vegetables. Vitamin B_6 is probably also synthesized by the intestinal bacteria.

Requirement

Infants require 0·2–0·3 mg and adults about 2–3 mg vitamin B_6 per day. The requirement increases with a high protein diet. An average

TABLE 11*

VITAMIN B$_6$ IN FOODS

	Microgram/g		Microgram/g
CEREALS			
Cambu	10·7	Rice, raw highly milled	3·3
Cholam	8·0	Wheat, whole	8·1
Maize (whole, yellow)	7·9	Wheat flour	3·3
Rice, raw husked	6·9		
PULSES			
Bengal gram	10·9	Red gram	10·0
Black gram	9·9	Soya-bean	8·6
Green gram	10·1		
VEGETABLES			
Beetroot	1·1	Carrots	1·9
Cabbage	2·9	Potato	1·6
FLESH FOOD			
Liver, sheep	13·6	Muscle, sheep	4·6
MISCELLANEOUS			
Milk, cow's	1·8	Yeast, dried brewer's	51·8
Rice polishings	19·0	Yeast, dried brewer's (autoclaved at pH 9·4)	52·1

* Swaminathan, M. (1940) A chemical test for vitamin B$_6$ in foods, *Indian J. med. Res.*, **28**, 427.

mixed diet supplies the necessary amount of pyridoxine. The average Indian diet supplies 3·5–5 mg of vitamin B$_6$ daily.

DEFICIENCY

A well defined clinical syndrome due to isolated deficiency of vitamin B$_6$ is not recognized. It is usually part of a general deficiency of vitamin B complex and is, therefore, seen in association with pellagra or beriberi. No specific picture of deficiency could be produced experimentally by depriving a normal adult of vitamin B$_6$ for 54 days [2]. A specific deficiency of vitamin B$_6$ has been produced in 34 of 50 normal subjects, without a deficiency of other factors of vitamin B group, by giving them 4-desoxypyridoxine, an antagonist to pyridoxine. Symptoms appeared quicker if 4-desoxypyridoxine was given with a pyridoxine-deficient diet than with a normal diet. There was: (1) anorexia, nausea, restlessness and lethargy; (2) seborrhoea; (3) hyperpigmentation and pellagra-like dermatitis which resembled nicotinic acid deficiency; (4) cheilosis, glossitis and stomatitis which resembled that due to deficiency of the other factors of vitamin B group; (5) changes in the peripheral nerves with first sensory impairment and later motor abnormalities; (6) lymphocytopenia and eosinophilia; (7) a large amount of xanthurenic acid was excreted in the urine after a dose of tryptophan. Daily administration of pyridoxine, pyridoxal or pyridoxamine, parenterally or as an ointment, alleviated the clinical and chemical manifestations of vitamin B_6 deficiency.

Convulsions in Infants. During the manufacture of milk powder vitamin B_6 is destroyed. Infants fed on artificial feeds of powdered milk develop convulsions which are easily controlled by the administration of vitamin B_6. Convulsions soon after birth due to pyridoxine deficiency are also reported.

Anaemia. Pyridoxine appears to be essential for erythrocyte formation. There is elevated serum iron concentration, saturation of iron binding protein and increased haemosiderin deposits in the bone marrow and the liver, suggesting failure of iron utilization in haemoglobin synthesis. The serum iron level drops with pyridoxine therapy. *Familial pyridoxine-responsive anaemia* requires 100–1000 mg daily for the correction of anaemia and maintenance therapy [3].

Xanthurenic Aciduria. This is associated with *mental retardation*. Pyridoxine deficiency does not allow conversion of tryptophan to nicotinic acid [4].

Isoniazid Therapy. This treatment for tuberculosis may produce neuritic symptoms that respond to vitiamin B_6 therapy. Isoniazid inhibits the physiological action of this vitamin.

Kidney stone formation in humans is decreased with daily oral magnesium oxide 200 mg and pyridoxine 10 mg [5]. In *homocystinuria* daily 150–450 mg oral pyridoxine helps restore normal plasma amino acid level [6].

Nausea, Vomiting and Radiation Sickness. Whether pyridoxine prevents nausea and vomiting, particularly that occurring during pregnancy and radiation sickness, has not been proved. Double blind trials are needed to establish its efficacy.

Treatment

For therapy 10 mg vitamin B$_6$ per day is given orally, intramuscularly or intravenously.

Local Application in Seborrhoeic Dermatitis. Seborrhoeic dermatitis of the dry type is probably due to defective fat metabolism in the skin which increases the local requirement of pyridoxine. Local application of pyridoxine-containing ointment has helped when oral or parenteral vitamin B$_6$ had no effect [7].

REFERENCES

[1] HARRIS, L.J. (1955) *Vitamins in Theory and Practice,* 4th ed., Cambridge, p. 266.
[2] HAWKINS, W.W., and BARSKY, J. (1948) An experiment on human vitamin B$_6$ deprivation, *Science,* **108**, 284.
[3] BOURNE, M.S., ELVES, M.W., and ISRAELS, M.C.G. (1965) Familial pyridoxine-responsive anaemia, *Brit. J. Haemat.,* **11**, 1.
[4] O'BRIEN, D., and JENSEN, C.B. (1963) Pyridoxine dependency in two mentally retarded subjects, *Clin. Sci.,* **24**, 179.
[5] GERSHOFF, S.N., and PRIEN, E.L. (1967) Effect of daily MgO and vitamin B$_6$ administration to patients with recurring calcium oxalate kidney stone, *Amer. J. clin. Nutr.,* **20**, 393.
[6] CARSON, N.A.J., and CARRIE, I.J. (1969) Treatment of homocystinuria with pyridoxine. A preliminary study, *Arch. Dis. Childh.,* **44**, 387.
[7] SCHREINER, A.W., SLINGER, W.N., HAWKINGS, V.R., and VILTER, R.W. (1952) Seborrheic dermatitis: a local metabolic defect involving pyridoxine, *J. Lab. clin. Med.,* **40**, 121.

8. NICOTINIC ACID (Niacin)

Pellagra, a clinical condition due to deficiency of nicotinic acid occurs sporadically in India. However, it used to assume epidemic proportions amongst the Negroes in the Southern United States. Since pellagra is seen amongst poor patients, its skin manifestations were considered at first to be due to dirt and bad hygiene but Goldberger cured and prevented pellagra in the inmates of asylums by adding meat, vegetables, fruits and eggs to their diet. He thus demonstrated a pellagra-preventing factor (P-P factor) in food and showed that pellagra is a deficiency disease. Ultimately, Elvehjem *et al.* [1] in 1937 found nicotinic acid and nicotinamide effective in curing black tongue in dogs (a condition similar to human pellagra) and suggested a clinical trial with these compounds in human pellagra.

Nicotinic acid had been synthesized as early as 1867 by oxidation of nicotine, which is a well-known alkaloid of tobacco. The physiological activity of nicotinic acid bears no resemblance to the activity of nicotine. That a poison-like nicotine could be changed into a life-preserving vitamin was surprising. In order to remove doubts in the public mind that the vitamin might have some of the bad effects of tobacco, it was renamed 'niacin', derived from the words '*Ni*-cotinic-*acid*-vitam*in*' [2].

Chemistry

Nicotinic acid was isolated in 1911 from rice polishings by Funk but its significance was not apparent at the time. It is pyridine beta carboxylic acid, with an empirical formula of $C_6H_5O_2N$. It is a white crystalline compound soluble in water.

Nicotinamide is formed by the addition of an NH_2 radical to nicotinic acid. In the animal tissues nicotinic acid exists as nicotinamide only. Taken orally, nicotinic acid is rapidly converted into nicotinamide.

Cooking. Nicotinamide in food is not destroyed by cooking but can be lost if excessive water used is drained off.

Absorption

Nicotinic acid or nicotinamide is rapidly absorbed from the stomach, the small and the large bowel.

Storage

As an essential tissue co-enzyme, nicotinamide is distributed in cells throughout the body.

Excretion

The excretion of nicotinic acid is mainly through the kidneys, partly as N-methyl nicotinamide and its glycine conjugate. The estimation of N-methyl nicotinamide in the urine is, therefore, used as a test of nicotinic acid deficiency. There are other end products of excretion which are not yet identified. After an intravenous injection the urinary excretion is rapid, hence frequent small oral doses are therapeutically the most effective.

Action

Like other members of the vitamin B group, nicotinic acid is essential for tissue metabolism. It forms a part of co-enzyme I diphosphoridine nucleotide (DPN) and co-enzyme II triphosphopyridine nucleotide (TPN) and thus aids in tissue respiration.

Source

As the co-enzymes DPN and TPN are found in every cell, nicotinamide is found in the cells of all food-stuffs, mainly in cereals and flesh foods. Processing cereals in order to make white flour or polished rice reduces the nicotinamide content.

Tryptophan. Tryptophan is an essential amino acid which can also prevent and cure pellagra. Tryptophan is a precursor of nicotinic acid and the administration of the former also increases the urinary excretion of N-methyl nicotinamide. The conversion of tryptophan to nicotinamide requires the presence of other factors of vitamin B, thiamine, riboflavine and pyridoxine. The interrelationship of the various factors of the B group is thus apparent. Animal foods rich in proteins also contain a fair quantity of tryptophan. Milk is relatively poor in nicotinamide but rich in tryptophan, hence milk is a good pellagra-preventing food. Food analysis should thus indicate the nicotinic acid as well as the tryptophan content, just as the vitamin A content of food is determined in terms of vitamin A as well as carotenes. Approximately 60 mg (range 31–87 mg) of tryptophan is equivalent to 1 mg of nicotinic acid [3].

Leucine. With the same intake of niacin and tryptophan pellagra could be produced more easily in humans on a 'corn diet' than on a 'wheat diet' [4]. It was, therefore, postulated that an imbalance of amino acids could be a factor in the production of pellagra. This finds support as the higher content of the amino acid leucine is responsible for the pellagra seen in people of Southern India eating jowar (*Sorghum vulgare*), while rice consumption with a lower leucine content does not produce pellagra. Maize (corn) eaten in the Southern United States, where epidemics of pellagra used to occur, also has a high leucine content [TABLE 12]. How leucine interferes with nicotinic acid in producing pellagra is not understood. Probably leucine increases the metabolism of nicotinamide, for administration of 5 g of leucine metabolizes 3·5 mg of additional nicotinic acid as estimated by urinary excretion of N-methyl nicotinamide.

TABLE 12

TRYPTOPHAN, LEUCINE AND NICOTINIC ACID CONTENT OF MAIZE, JOWAR AND RICE*

	Tryptophan G PER 100 G PROTEIN	Leucine G PER 100 G PROTEIN	Nicotinic acid MG PER 100 G
Maize (corn)	0·8	14·9	1·4
Jowar (Sorghum vulgare)	1·2	12·9	1·8
Rice	1·2	8·0	1·2

* Gopalan, C., and Srikantia, S.G. (1960) Leucine and pellagra, Lancet, i, 954.

Requirements [TABLE 13]

The daily requirements of nicotinic acid vary with: (1) physical exertion and the metabolic rate; and (2) the tryptophan content of the diet. The Food and Nutrition Board of the United States defines the nicotinic acid requirement as the *niacin equivalent* which means: (1) the nicotinic acid content of the food-stuff in mg; and (2) the tryptophan content of the diet, 60 mg of tryptophan being equivalent to 1 mg of nicotinic acid. The recommended allowance is about 6·6 mg niacin equivalent per 1000 Calories. The British Medical Association recommends 4 mg nicotinic acid per 1000 Calories, with an additional 2 mg during lactation. There is general agreement between the American and British recommendations as in the latter tryptophan intake is not considered. Niacin deficiency does not occur when 15 per cent of the calories are supplied by milk casein which contains tryptophan. The average milk diet of infants supplies this amount.

TABLE 13

	B.M.A. RECOMMENDATION NIACIN PER DAY mg	FOOD AND NUTRITION BOARD, U.S.A. NIACIN EQUIVALENT mg
Men	17 – 20	18 – 21
Women	6 – 15	17
Pregnancy, 2nd half	11	20
Lactation	14	19
Boys	11 – 14	21 – 25
Girls	10	17
Children	6 – 8	8 – 14
Infants	4	7

DEFICIENCY

Deficiency of nicotinic acid is caused by: (1) deficient intake of nicotinic acid as well as tryptophan; (2) defective digestion as in diarrhoea. Lack of absorption can possibly occur, but once the food is digested absorption is rapid; (3) Excessive demand during pregnancy, rapid growth or during increased metabolic rate as in thyrotoxicosis and fevers. During lactation there is extra excretion of niacin in the milk.

A deficiency of nicotinic acid in certain clinical conditions is of interest:

1. *Carcinoid tumours.* Normally a small amount of tryptophan is converted by the argentaffin cells of the gut into serotonin (5-hydroxytryptamine). With a carcinoid tumour argentaffinoma of the small intestine or appendix, or with widespread secondary deposits most of the available tryptophan is converted into serotonin and a clinical state resembling nicotinic acid deficiency is produced.

2. *Isoniazid therapy.* Isonicotinic acid hydrazide (isoniazid), a

derivative of nicotinic acid, is extensively used in the treatment of tuberculosis. If the diet is not adequate during isoniazid administration a nicotinamide deficiency can be precipitated.

3. *High leucine diet.* Pellagra is more common in communities eating maize (corn) and *jowar* (*Sorghum vulgare*) than among those eating foods less rich in leucine. There is a temporary deterioration in the mental state of pellagrins when 20-30 g of leucine is added to their diet [4].

CLINICAL MANIFESTATIONS OF DEFICIENCY

A deficiency of nicotinic acid may occur as: (1) subclinical deficiency; (2) pellagra.

Subclinical Deficiency

Subclinical nicotinic acid deficiency manifests itself as weakness, lassitude, irritability, burning tongue and constipation. The diagnosis can be established by the dietetic history and confirmed by clinical improvement noted within a fortnight after therapeutic administration of the vitamin.

Pellagra

Pellagra is classically characterized by three Ds: (1) dermatitis: (2) diarrhoea; and (3) dementia. The full-blown picture is not always seen.

1. *Dermatitis.* Pellagra derives its name from the skin manifestations, *pelle* = skin and *agra* = rough. Changes are marked on the skin exposed to the sun and friction. The parts exposed to the sun are the back of the hands, the wrists, feet, ankles, and neck; on the face, the nose and either side of the cheeks, the so-called butterfly distribution. The friction areas are the elbows, extensor surface of the arms, knees, scrotum and perineal region. The affected parts are usually symmetrically distributed and are well demarcated from the surrounding skin. Erythema, thickening and pigmentation is followed by exfoliation, leaving a parchment-like skin. To an untrained eye the thickening of the skin on the knuckles with pigmentation looks like dirt.

2. *Diarrhoea.* The word diarrhoea is symbolic of changes in the gastro-intestinal tract. The papillae are lost; the tongue appears raw and the mucous membrane of the mouth is inflamed. Spiced or hot

food cannot be tolerated. Involvement of the stomach is shown by achlorhydria in the majority. Diarrhoea accentuates the deficiency state. No description of gastroscopic or sigmoidoscopic appearances are available but a few cases having nutritional deficiency observed by me showed a reddish dry colonic mucous membrane, probably due to nicotinic acid deficiency.

3. *Dementia.* The word dementia is symbolic of involvement of the nervous system. There is irritability, depression, poor concentration and loss of memory. Cases of pellagra with dementia may be admitted to lunatic asylums, the mental symptoms being interpreted as a primary psychosis and the skin pigmentation being ascribed to poor hygiene. Involvement of the lateral columns of the spinal cord (pyramidal tracts) is manifested as paraplegia, exaggerated jerks and extensor plantar responses. Involvement of the posterior columns (Goll and Burdach) leads to ataxia. Peripheral neuropathy may be associated due to deficiency of other vitamins of the B group.

Anaemia of the macrocytic type may occur in pellagra.

Encephalopathy due to nicotinic acid deficiency responding dramatically to intravenous nicotinamide may occur [6].

Treatment. Pellagra in humans is always associated with other nutritional deficiencies; thus a well-balanced diet is of the utmost importance. Milk and fresh meat are particularly needed.

VITAMINS. Pellagrins are usually deficient in other vitamins of the B group. Yeast tablets provide a cheap and effective supplement. Oral nicotinic acid or nicotinamide is also advised, the former being converted by the body into nicotinamide.

Nicotinic acid is quickly absorbed from the stomach. When 50–100 mg is administered on an empty stomach it produces within a few minutes symptoms of burning under the skin, itching, a rise in temperature and throbbing of the head. The symptoms start from the head and spread downwards, lasting for about 15 minutes. If given soon after food, absorption is gradual, and these symptoms may not occur.

Nicotinamide, though well absorbed, does not produce these symptoms and so is a preferable form of treatment.

DOSAGE. For the treatment of pellagra, 25–50 mg of nicotinamide is administered four to six times a day. It is necessary to give frequent small doses, rather than a single large dose, which is rapidly excreted.

Intravenous administration of nicotinamide is not warranted if the patient can take it by mouth. With severe diarrhoea, 25 mg may be given intravenously three times a day.

RESULTS OF TREATMENT. The skin changes and diarrhoea improve within a week of therapy. Nervous symptoms improve gradually and even a deranged mental state can be restored to normal.

Nikethamide (*Coramine*), a diethyl amide of nicotinic acid, can also alleviate the symptoms of pellagra. It is commonly used as a cardiovascular stimulant.

Hartnup's Disease (Hereditary Pellagra)

It is a hereditary disease characterized by intermittent attacks, rough scaly reddened skin on moderate exposure to sunlight, more severe exposure produces severe rash similar to pellagra. The disease gets its name from a study of a family with the surname of Hartnup. The primary defect is of amino acid transport and malabsorption of free amino acids while oligopeptides may be partly absorbed [5]. Amino acids, tryptophan, phenylalanine, arginine and lysine are not absorbed and are passed into the colon where tryptophan is acted upon by the normal intestinal flora to form indole compounds which are absorbed and excreted in the urine. Such excretion of indole can be stopped by sterilizing the gut with antibiotics. A corresponding defect in the amino acid reabsorption in the renal tubules produces amino-aciduria.

Clinically there are intermittent attacks of scaly reddened skin on moderate exposure to light but with more severe exposure the appearance is like clinical pellagra. The absorption of indole compounds produces attacks of cerebellar ataxia from which the patient may recover.

Other Uses of Nicotinic Acid

Vascular Disease. The vasodilator effect of nicotinic acid (not nicotinamide) has prompted physicians to use it in cases of angina pectoris and cerebral thrombosis with a view to improving the circulation. The dosage is 100 mg of nicotinic acid three times a day one hour before meals, but no beneficial effect has been proved.

Pain of Coronary Thrombosis. During an attack of coronary thrombosis, nicotinic acid, 50 mg given subcutaneously, or 100 mg sublingually, has helped in the relief of pain and shock.

High Serum Cholesterol. High doses of nicotinic acid have been reported to reduce the serum cholesterol level in cases of atherosclerosis. The side-reactions to such high doses are the same as with 50–100 mg of nicotinic acid. Sodium or potassium salts of nicotinic acid also reduce the serum cholesterol without side-effects.

Toxicity

Prolonged administration of nicotinic acid for hypercholesterolaemia has produced alterations in liver function and raised serum uric acid values [7]. A physician who took 6 g nicotinic acid for a year to reduce his serum cholesterol level developed bilateral amblyopia with paracentral scotomas [8].

REFERENCES

[1] ELVEHJEM, C.A., MADDEN, R.J., STRONG, F.M., and WOOLLEY, D.W. (1937) Relation of nicotinic acid and nicotinic acid amide to canine black tongue, Letter to the Editor, *J. Amer. chem. Soc.*, **59**, 1767.

[2] HARRIS, L.J. (1955) *Vitamins in Theory and Practice*, 4th ed., Cambridge, p. 89.

[3] GOLDSMITH, G.A. (1956) Experimental niacin deficiency, *J. Amer. diet. Ass.*, **32**, 312.

[4] GOPALAN, C., and SRIKANTIA, S.G. (1960) Leucine and pellagra, *Lancet*, i, 954.

[5] ASATOOR, A.M., *et al.* (1970) Intestinal absorption of two dipeptides in Hartnup disease, *Gut*, **11**, 380.

[6] TABAQCHALI, S., and PALLIS, C. (1970) Reversible nicotinamide-deficiency encephalopathy in a patient with jejunal diverticulosis, *Gut*, **11**, 1024.

[7] PARSONS, W.B. (1961) Studies of nicotinic acid use in hypercholesterolemia, *Arch. intern. Med.*, **107**, 653.

[8] HARRIS, J.L. (1963) Toxic amblyopia associated with administration of nicotinic acid, *Amer. J. Ophthal.*, **55**, 133.

9. FOLIC ACID (Pteroylglutamic Acid)

Contributed by H.G. Desai

The word folic acid is derived from the Latin *folium* (leaf), because folic acid is found extensively in green vegetables. Many bacteria synthesize folic acid but *Lactobacillus casei* grows well only if folic acid is supplied. Folic acid was therefore named the *Lactobacillus casei* factor. Thus, both the anti-anaemia vitamins, folic acid and vitamin B_{12}, were originally discovered as essential factors for the growth of organisms, folic acid as *Lactobacillus casei* factor and vitamin B_{12} as a factor for the growth of *Lactobacillus lactis*.

Chemistry

The phrase *folic acid* indicates monoglutamate, while the word *folate* denotes mono- as well as polyglutamates. Folic acid contains a pteridyl group and glumatic acid and is therefore called *pteroylglutamic acid*. There is also an additional para-aminobenzoic acid molecule. Naturally occurring dietary folates exist, about a quarter as *monoglutamates* and three-quarters as polyglutamates (6–7 pteroylglutamic acid molecules linked together).

The simpler folate compounds, containing one, two or three such residues, are also known as 'free' folates and can be assayed microbiologically using *Lactobacillus casei,* whereas the higher polyglutamates cannot be so assayed without previous enzymatic digestion with folate conjugase [1]. Folates are sensitive to light, aerobic conditions, extremes of pH, and boiling. From 50–95 per cent of food folate can be destroyed by cooking, canning and other processing methods. Anti-oxidant agents such as ascorbic acid (vitamin C) in food prevents folate destruction during cooking. Ascorbic acid is now used in analytical procedures to prevent loss due to oxygen-labile folates. In the *body* folic acid exists as tetrahydrofolic acid.

Folic acid was *synthesized* in 1954 and only synthetic preparations are now marketed.

Folinic Acid (Citrovorum Factor).

Folinic acid is a formyl derivative of tetrahydrofolic acid. *Dihydroreductase* is an enzyme that converts folic acid into a *metabolically active reduced form* of folinic acid. Folic acid is partly excreted in the urine as folinic acid.

Absorption

Crystalline folic acid is primarily absorbed from the jejunum, unlike vitamin B_{12} which is primarily absorbed from the ileum. The absorption probably takes place by active transport and also by diffusion when administered in large amounts. Monoglutamates are absorbed in the ileum even in the absence of the jejunum. Alkaline intestinal pH or simultaneous administration of sodium bicarbonate decreases folic acid absorption [2]. On absorption, conversion to methyltetrahydrofolate occurs in the gut wall [3].

Polyglutamates are predominant (about 75 per cent) in dietary folates. They are hydrolysed for absorption to monoglutamates by the enzyme *pteroylglutamate hydrolase (folate conjugase)* which is abundant in the upper small intestinal mucosa. If the intestine does not deconjugate the dietary folate, most of it is not absorbed.

Serum Level

The normal level of serum *folate* assayed by its effect on the growth of *Lactobacillus casei* varies between 6 and 15 millimicrograms per ml. In folic acid deficiency the serum level falls below 5 millimicrograms per ml.

Cerebrospinal folate levels are about three times higher than the serum level and reflect concentration in the central nervous system.

Excretion

Folic acid is excreted in the urine as: (1) substances which have folic acid activity and hence promote the growth of *Lactobacillus casei* and *Streptococcus faecalis;* (2) *inactive* degradation products. The amount excreted depends upon the serum level. When the serum level is less than 10 millimicrograms per ml only 6 per cent is excreted, but when it rises to 70 millimicrograms per ml over 30 per cent is excreted [4].

Action

Folic acid is itself inactive. It is converted in the body to a biologically active form, folinic acid.

Folic acid is essential for nucleoprotein synthesis and is therefore required for the cell division and also for the maturation of erythrocytes.

Folic acid acts as a co-enzyme and is necessary for the transfer of one carbon atom moiety to amino SH groups. An example of the former is the *formimino glutamic acid* (FIGLU), a product of histidine breakdown. FIGLU is further converted to glutamic acid and folinic acid is essential for this step. In folic acid deficiency this step is retarded, consequently FIGLU accumulates and is excreted in the urine.

Storage

The body store of 5–10 mg is adequate for 3–4 months' requirements. Storage occurs mainly in the liver as 5-methyltetrahydrofolate.

TABLE 14

FOLATE CONTENT OF COOKED FOODS*

COOKED FOOD	FOLATE µg / g	COOKED FOOD	FOLATE µg / g
MEAT AND FISH			
Bacon (fried)	0·02	Lamb kidney (in pie, stewed)	0·31
Beef (minced, boiled)	0·03	Lamb liver (boiled)	6·37
Chicken (roast)	0·07	Mutton (roast)	0·03
Cod (fried)	0·16	Sardines (tinned in oil)	0·32
DAIRY PRODUCTS			
Cheese (cheddar)	0·06	Ovaltine (powder)	0·86
Milk (pasteurized)	0·085	Egg (hen's, boiled)	0·3
VEGETABLES			
Beans (baked)	0·1	Onions (boiled)	0·25
Beetroot (boiled)	0·2	Peas (tinned)	0·08
Cabbage (boiled)	0·11	Potato (boiled)	0·12
Carrots (boiled)	0·03	Spaghetti (tinned, in tomato sauce)	0·06
Cauliflower (boiled)	0·04	Spinach (boiled)	0·29
Cucumber (fresh)	0·14	Tomato (fresh)	0·18
Lettuce (fresh)	2·0	Vegetable soup	0·04
FRUIT			
Apple (fresh)	0·02	Orange (fresh)	0·45
Apricots (tinned)	0·04	Pineapple (tinned)	0·02
Banana (fresh)	0·27	Plums (tinned)	0·02
CEREALS			
Bread (white)	0·17	Cornflakes	0·05
Biscuit (plain)	0·08	Porridge (boiled)	0·02
MISCELLANEOUS			
Walnuts	0·58	Peanuts	0·25
Chocolate	0·12	Marmite	3·05

*Adapted from: Hurdle, A.D.F., Barton, D., and Searles, I.H. (1968) A method for measuring folate in food and its application to a hospital diet, Amer. J. clin. Nutr., **21**, 1202.

Source

Folates are derived from cereals, vegetables, meat and liver. Dietary folates exist as monoglutamates (about one-quarter) and polyglutamates (about three-quarters). The variation in the microbiological assay values reported by various authors are due to whether: (1) the food is treated with conjugase to get the *total* (mono and polyglutamates) activity or whether (2) ascorbic acid is added to the culture medium to prevent folate destruction. Folate destruction also occurs during cooking. TABLE 14 gives folate values of *cooked* foods. Folates synthesized by the colonic bacteria are not absorbed.

Requirement

Depriving volunteers of dietary folic acid, the *minimum* supplement required to maintain normal blood level was 50–100 micrograms a day [5]. The FAO/WHO recommendations for *absorbable* folates are as follows:

TABLE 15

RECOMMENDED DAILY INTAKE
OF 'FREE' (ABSORBABLE) FOLATE*

0 – 6 months	40 µg	13 years and over	200 µg
7 – 12 months	60 µg	Lactation	300 µg
1 – 12 years	100 µg	Pregnancy	400 µg

* *Wld Hlth Org. techn. Rep. Ser.*, No. 452 (1970), p. 46.

The normal human total daily intake varies from 700–1500 micrograms but may not be absorbed without being converted to monoglutamate.

DEFICIENCY [6, 7]

Folic acid deficiency occurs as follows :

DEFICIENT INTAKE	INCREASED DEMAND	MALABSORPTION	INHIBITION OF FOLATE METABOLISM
Poor diet	Pregnancy	Tropical sprue	Folic acid antagonists (antifols)
Lengthy cooking	Infancy	Coeliac syndrome	Alcoholism
Alcoholism	Hyper-thyroidism	Stagnant loop syndrome	Vitamin B deficiency
	Haemolytic anaemias	Small intestinal diseases	Liver disease
	Leukaemia	Jejunal resection	
	Carcinoma Loss in dialysis		
		Drugs: Phenytoin (anti-epileptic) Contraceptives	
		Congenital folate malabsorption	

Deficient Intake. Folic acid, being both heat-labile and water-soluble, is easily destroyed and lost by repeatedly boiling food or by using excess water during cooking that is discarded. Indeed, this method

is used to produce experimental folate deficiency in humans [8]. *The major cause of folic acid deficiency is its destruction during cooking.*
Increased demand is created by rapidly proliferative tissue.

Malabsorption is due mainly to deficiency of polyglutamate hydrolase (conjugase) following diseases of the jejunum. The dietary folates which are essentially polyglutamates are not absorbed. On the other hand, folic acid (monoglutamate) are absorbed throughout the small intestine, and the folic acid absorption test may be normal in less severe intestinal damage.

Stagnant loop syndrome may sometimes be associated with raised serum folate due to the absorption of folates synthesized in the jejunum by the proliferative bacteria [9]. On the other hand, bacterial deconjugation of bile salt may decrease the intestinal folate conjugase activity and decrease the absorption.

Congenital isolated defect of folic acid absorption is rare [10].

Clinical Manifestations

Clinically, folate deficiency results in: (1) megaloblastic anaemia; (2) tropical sprue.

The symptoms of folic acid deficiency are fatigue, pallor, diarrhoea and and glossitis. The buccal, vaginal and intestinal mucosal biopsies show large immature nuclei. The peripheral smear exhibits large oval erythrocytes and hypersegmented nuclei in polymorphs. The bone marrow is hypercellular and megaloblastic. In some cases of tropical sprue arising from primary folic acid deficiency, fatty diarrhoea is marked.

Folic acid deprivation for 1 month shows low serum folate. In the second month there is an increase in lobes of polymorphonuclear leucocytes, while megaloblastic anaemia occurs after 3 months [11].

Diagnosis of Deficiency

(1) *Serum* folate levels are low (normal 6–15 millimicrograms/ml. (2) *Packed erythrocyte folate* estimation reflects tissue folates[12] (normal values 160–640 millimicrograms/ml). (3) *Absorption test* with titrium-labelled folic acid should be carried out. (4) *FIGLU excretion test* should be done. Demonstration of FIGLU in the urine is a *test* of folic acid deficiency. As FIGLU is a metabolite in the pathway of the breakdown of the amino acid histidine to glutamic acid, the urinary excretion of FIGLU is measured after an oral dose of 15 g of histidine hydrochloride. A normal subject excretes on an average 9 mg of FIGLU per hour between the third and eighth hour after administration of

histidine. In megaloblastic anaemia requiring folic acid therapy, more than 17 mg of FIGLU per hour is excreted. However, during pregnancy the test is not reliable as the oral dose of histidine may be utilized by the foetus for protein synthesis and therefore, despite folic acid deficiency, FIGLU excretion may be low. (5) A *therapeutic test* to prove folate deficiency is the easiest test to conduct in any clinical laboratory. Along with the usual diet, 200 micrograms of folic acid is administered daily. A reticulocyte peak in 7–10 days confirms folate deficiency.

Treatment

An *expectant mother* should eat more vegetables and meat products than usual. An oral supplement of 5 mg folic acid may be given. An adequate folic acid intake prevents macrocytic anaemia in both the mother and child.

Some cases of *tropical sprue* from Puerto Rico are reported to show dramatic response to folic acid therapy. A reticulocyte crisis occurs within a week and the diarrhoea and appetite improve. This suggests that such cases of sprue are primarily due to deficient folate intake or deficient absorption. However, such favourable response in tropical sprue is not noted from other regions.

When it is established that macrocytic anaemia in an adult is due to folic acid (and not due to vitamin B_{12} deficiency), 5 mg folic acid is administered orally three times a day until the haemoglobin level is normal. There is a drop in serum iron in 24 hours, and peak reticulocyte response appears in 7–10 days. Thereafter, 2–5 mg of folic acid should be given daily as a maintenance dose.

Folic acid is usually effective when given orally, but parenteral injection may be necessary when there is intestinal malabsorption.

Epilepsy

Diphenylhydantoin (phenytoin, *Dilantin*), and also phenobarbitone and primidone, used over prolonged periods as anticonvulsant therapy for epilepsy produce macrocytic anaemia, megaloblastic bone marrow, reduced serum folate and deteriorating mental condition. Phenytoin probably inhibits the action of enzyme folate conjugase since the malabsorption is of dietary polyglutamates but not of folic acid. Administration of folate may improve the mental state but there is also a falling serum vitamin B_{12} level and sometimes an increase in the number of fits. The fits can then be reduced by the administration of vitamin B_{12}. The *therapy* consists of initial administration of folic acid 10–15 mg daily with 1000 micrograms vitamin B_{12} weekly. *Preventive therapy* recommended for children treated with anticonvulsant drugs is 5 mg folic acid once a week and 250 micrograms vitamin B_{12} once a month [13].

FOLIC ACID ANTAGONISTS

Folic acid analogues, which biologically counteract the effect of folic acid as a growth factor, are known as folic acid antagonists (*antifols*). Notable among them is an amino derivative known as *aminopterin*. This compound depresses *dihydrofolate reductase,* the enzyme necessary for normal folate metabolism. Advantage is taken of this fact in the treatment of leukaemia, where temporary remission may occur with aminopterin. If the bone marrow becomes dangerously depressed during aminopterin therapy, its effect may be counteracted by folinic acid but not by folic acid.

Pyrimethamine (antimalarial) also induces folic acid deficiency by depressing dihydrofolate reductase. However, malaria itself may cause folate deficiency, which may be prevented by folic acid supplements [14].

Caution

Folic acid-vitamin B_{12} *antagonism* is seen in: (1) pernicious anaemia, where administration of folic acid alone improves the blood picture but may precipitate subacute combined degeneration of the cord; (2) *anticonvulsant therapy,* that requires supplements of both folic acid and vitamin B_{12}.

Folic acid also provides fuel to malignant cells of *leukaemia, myeloma,* and *Hodgkin's disease,* and therefore in such cases folic acid should not be administered except to correct anaemia or leucopenia.

Toxicity

A daily 15 mg dose of folic acid is reported to produce mental changes, sleep disturbances and gastro-intestinal upset [15]. This observation requires confirmation.

REFERENCES

[1] WORLD HEALTH ORGANIZATION (1970) *Wld Hlth Org. techn. Rep. Ser.,* No. 452, p. 17.
[2] BENN, A., *et al.* (1971) Effect of intraluminal pH on the absorption of pteroyl-monoglutamic acid, *Brit. med. J.,* **1,** 148.

[3] CHANARIN, I., and PERRY, J., (1969) Evidence for reduction and methylation of folate in the intestine during normal absorption, *Lancet,* **ii,** 776.

[4] CHANARIN, I., and BENNETT, M. (1962) The disposal of small doses of intravenously injected folic acid, *Brit. J. Haemat.,* **8,** 28.

[5] HERBERT, V. (1962) Minimal daily adult folate requirement, *Arch. intern. Med.,* **110,** 649.

[6] SHAW, M.T., and HOFFBRAND, A.V. (1970) Use and abuse of folic acid, *Practitioner,* **204,** 795.

[7] STREIFF, R.R. (1970) Folic acid deficiency anaemia, *Seminars in Haematology,* **7,** 23.

[8] HERBERT, V. (1963) A palatable diet for producing experimental folate deficiency in man, *Amer. J. clin. Nutr.,* **12,** 17.

[9] HOFFBRAND, A.V., TABAQCHALI, S., and MOLLIN, D.L. (1966) High serum folate levels in intestinal blind-loop syndrome, *Lancet,* **i,** 1339.

[10] LANZKOWSKY, P. (1970) Congenital malabsorption of folate, *Amer. J. Med.,* **48,** 580.

[11] HERBERT, V. (1967) Biochemical and hematologic lesions in folic acid deficiency, *Amer. J. clin. Nutr.,* **20,** 562.

[12] HOFFBRAND, A.V., NEWCOMBE, B.F.A., and MOLLIN, D.L. (1966) Method of assay of red cell folate activity and the value of the assay as a test for folate deficiency, *J. clin. Path.,* **19,** 17.

[13] NEUBAUER, C. (1970) Mental deterioration in epilepsy due to folate deficiency, *Brit. med. J.,* **2,** 759.

[14] TONG, M.J., STRICKLAND, G.T. VOTTERI, B.A., and GUNNING, J. (1970) Supplemental folates in the therapy of *Plasmodium falciparum* malaria, *J. Amer. med. Ass.,* **214,** 2330.

[15] HUNTER, R., BARNES, J., OAKELEY, H.F., and MATHEWS, D.M. (1970) Toxicity to folic acid given in pharmacological doses to healthy volunteers, *Lancet,* **i,** 61.

10. VITAMIN B_{12} (Cyanocobalamin)

Contributed by R. H. Dastur

Vitamin B_{12} is interesting because:

1. Its presence was discovered in 1948 almost simultaneously in the United States and England by employing different methods of approach.

2. This vitamin is extensively produced by fungi and bacteria.

3. It is active even in a millionth part of a gramme (there is no drug in clinical medicine which has a purity and potency in such a small amount).

4. It is unusual for a marked deficiency to occur from a deficient intake, such a state being usually due to malabsorption.

5. It is the only vitamin containing the element cobalt.

The discovery of this vitamin in the United States started with the work of Mary Shrob who found that *Lactobacillus lactis Dorner* bacteria required for their growth a factor from the liver and this factor was proportional to the antipernicious anaemia activity of the liver extract. This knowledge led others to isolate a crystalline factor in the liver which was effective in microgram quantities against pernicious anaemia.

Almost simultaneously in England, Lester Smith was conducting clinical trials with purer extracts of the liver exhibiting antipernicious anaemia activity. He finally isolated a highly concentrated red substance, vitamin B$_{12}$ which had specific activity against pernicious anaemia.

Chemistry

The name cyanocobalamin is given because vitamin B$_{12}$ contains a cyanide group and cobalt. The empirical formula is $C_{63}H_{90}O_{14}N_{14}PCo$. It is a red crystalline substance, the red colour being due to cobalt. It is slightly soluble in water and is stable to ordinary heat. It is destroyed by prolonged exposure to sunlight.

Vitamin B$_{12}a$ is aquacobalamin where H_2O replaces cyanide (CN). *Vitamin B$_{12}b$* (*hydroxocobalamin*) is the anhydrous form of B$_{12}$. Hydroxocobalamin can be retained in the body for longer periods than cyanocobalamin [14].

Vitamin B$_{12}$ is produced by micro-organisms only. Many bacteria produce it for their own growth even with an infinitely small supply of cobalt. Some organisms which produce vitamin B$_{12}$ far in excess of their requirement are used for the commercial production of vitamin B$_{12}$. *Streptomyces griseus* is used for the production of streptomycin and from it vitamin B$_{12}$ is produced as a by-product. Similarly, *Streptomyces aureofaciens* which is used for the production of aureomycin yields vitamin B$_{12}$ as a by-product. The intestinal bacteria also produce appreciable amounts of vitamin B$_{12}$ which is excreted in the faeces and its further activation enhances the content of vitamin B$_{12}$. Fertilizers made from dried sludge may contain as much as 7 micrograms of vitamin B$_{12}$ per gramme.

Absorption

Castle's Observations. In pernicious anaemia, feeding liver together with human gastric juice produced a remarkable improvement while feeding of liver alone was not effective. This led Castle to postulate that two factors: (1) intrinsic and (2) extrinsic were necessary for the relief of pernicious anaemia.

1. *Intrinsic factor.* Purified intrinsic factor is a glycoprotein with a molecular weight of 50,000. It is produced in humans by the gastric parietal cells. Intrinsic factor combines with an extrinsic factor of food (vitamin B_{12}). In pernicious anaemia the stomach wall is atrophied, a little neutral or alkaline juice and very scanty intrinsic factor are produced. Intrinsic factor has no other role than that of aiding ileal mucous membrane to *absorb* vitamin B_{12} and transfer it into the blood stream, because parenteral injection of vitamin B_{12} alone produces a specific anti-anaemia effect.

2. *Extrinsic factor* (vitamin B_{12}). It is now known that when liver is fed along with normal gastric juice it is the vitamin B_{12} (extrinsic factor) in the liver that produces remission in pernicious anaemia.

Absorption from the Intestine. (1) *Active absorption* of vitamin B_{12} from food (bound by intrinsic factor), occurs from the brush border of mucosal cells of *ileum* in alkaline pH in the presence of calcium. Patients with ileal inflammation, resection or ileal bypass, have poor vitamin B_{12} absorption [1]. After penetrating the ileal mucosa the intrinsic factor is detached, and vitamin B_{12} attaches to transport-protein *transcobalamin II*. In pernicious anaemia, administration of 50–100 ml of gastric juice from a healthy person (which supplies intrinsic factor), together with oral vitamin B_{12}, is effective in producing a remission. (2) *Passive absorption* occurs by means of diffusion throughout the length of the small intestine when *large therapeutic oral doses* (100 micrograms) of vitamin B_{12} are administered. *Iron* deficient patients may have deficient vitamin B_{12} absorption that improves with iron administration alone [2]. Free *calcium ion* probably takes part in the absorption of vitamin B_{12}. In malabsorption syndromes, free calcium ion may not be available and the administration of calcium lactate improves vitamin B_{12} absorption [3].

Parenteral Injection. Parenteral therapy is necessary in pernicious anaemia, as oral vitamin B_{12} is not absorbed in the absence of intrinsic factor secretion by the stomach.

Gastric Atrophy. Gastric atrophy in pernicious anaemia is mostly complete with total loss of gastric secretion. *Genetic* defect is the most likely cause of achlorhydria as gastric atrophy is also noted in the relatives of patients with pernicious anaemia. In pernicious anaemia, gastric parietal cell antibodies and intrinsic factor antibodies are detected, hence gastric atrophy is also ascribed to *auto-immune* disease.

The *intrinsic factor antibodies* may be demonstrated either in the *serum* or *gastric juice,* or both [4]. *Gastric parietal cell antibodies* are detected in the serum and in the gastric juice. Whether the antibodies are the primary cause of gastric mucosal injury or are secondary to gastric mucosal cell damage is not settled. However, the gastric atrophy may be temporarily *reversed.* With corticosteroid therapy there is recovery in vitamin B$_{12}$ absorption, mucosal cell regeneration, secretion of hydrochloric acid and intrinsic factor [5] but the effect stops on withholding corticosteroids.

Serum Vitamin B$_{12}$

Transcobalamin is the protein that binds vitamin B$_{12}$. *Transcobalamin II* is a *beta* globulin, concerned with binding *intestinal absorbed* vitamin B$_{12}$ and delivering it to storage sites in the liver and bone marrow. *Transcobalamin I* is an *alpha* globulin, binds the *stored* vitamin B$_{12}$, and transports it for the body's needs.

The normal serum vitamin B$_{12}$ level is 200–1000 micromicrograms per ml. In *pernicious anaemia* values are always below 170 and frequently below 100 micromicrograms per ml [6]. *Low serum levels* are also found in *pregnancy* and in strict *vegetarians.* Some patients with megaloblastic anaemia due to *folic acid deficiency* have low serum vitamin B$_{12}$ levels that return to normal with folic acid therapy only. *Iron deficiency anaemia,* after administration of iron therapy, shows low serum vitamin B$_{12}$ levels.

High serum levels of vitamin B$_{12}$ are observed in diseases of the liver, and the highest serum level occurs in hepatic necrosis, possibly due to the *release* of stored vitamin B$_{12}$ from the liver and also an increased vitamin B$_{12}$ binding capacity of the serum. With hepatic disease, vitamin B$_{12}$ uptake from the portal circulation by the liver is diminished, which may again account for the high serum levels.

Storage

The bulk of body stores of vitamin B$_{12}$ is in the form of coenzyme B$_{12}$. The total body store is 3000–5000 micrograms and the main storage in the *liver* is about 1500 micrograms. This supply is adequate for years. A healthy liver stores more vitamin B_{12} than a diseased liver. Storage of vitamin B_{12} in the liver is estimated as 1·0 (0·70–1·2) micrograms per g of wet liver in the normal person. The storage in cirrhosis of the liver and pernicious anaemia is 0·25 micrograms and 0·10 micrograms per g of wet liver respectively. The liver store becomes depleted in conditions where vitamin B_{12} is not absorbed, as after gastrectomy, sprue and ileitis.

Excretion
Urine. A normal person excretes in the urine about 30 micromicrograms of vitamin B_{12} per day. A small dose of vitamin B_{12} in a normal subject is retained but a dose over 50 micrograms is quickly excreted in the urine. When 1000 micrograms is injected in a normal person well over 95 per cent is excreted but in a person whose store of vitamin B_{12} in the liver is depleted, more is retained and the excretion is lower.

Faeces. The faecal vitamin B_{12} in the human represents mostly that produced by bacteria in the colon. As the colon does not absorb vitamin B_{12}, it is excreted.

Bile. Vitamin B_{12} excreted in bile is largely reabsorbed in enterohepatic circulation.

Milk. Vitamin B_{12} is secreted in human milk, the concentration being nearly equal to that in blood. Patients with deficiency of vitamin B_{12} may secrete very little in the milk and breast-fed infants may develop vitamin B_{12} deficiency.

Action
Vitamin B_{12} plays a role in DNA synthesis. Therefore deficiency manifests early in rapidly dividing cells, as in the bone marrow and the gastro-intestinal tract. In deficiency of vitamin B_{12} the maturation of red blood cells in the bone marrow is disturbed. The nuclear chromatin of the maturing red blood cell appears abnormal, and the cell is known as a megaloblast, a characteristic finding in vitamin B_{12} deficiency anaemias.

Source [TABLE 16]
Daily dietary intake is 3–30 micrograms from milk, cheese, eggs, etc. Vitamin B_{12} is *not* synthesized by mammalian cells. It is synthesized

by bacteria of the soil, water, human or animal intestine.

The human source of vitamin B$_{12}$ is mainly from the animal food-stuffs. Those who live on a pure vegetarian diet in which even milk is excluded (vegans), are in danger of developing deficiency. The production of vitamin B$_{12}$ by the intestinal bacteria does not contribute to nutrition because these bacteria thrive in the colon from which vitamin B$_{12}$ is not absorbed. Thus the excretion of vitamin B$_{12}$ in the faeces may be high despite marked deficiency in the body.

Requirement

The daily requirement of vitamin B$_{12}$ is difficult to assess and appears to vary from person to person. The drawbacks in experimental human studies are the huge stores in the liver sufficient to last for years. Even a parenteral dose as low as 1 or 2 micrograms a day can be adequate to maintain remission in a case of pernicious anaemia.

One microgram is needed to maintain haemopoiesis while as little as 0·1 microgram is effective in producing haematological improvement in pernicious anaemia [7].

The WHO recommendations on requirements are as follows:

RECOMMENDED DAILY INTAKE OF VITAMIN B$_{12}$*

	RECOMMENDED DAILY INTAKE IN MICROGRAMS
0–12 months	0·3
1–3 years	0·9
4–9 years	1·5
10–years and over	2·0
Pregnancy	3·0
Lactation	2·5

* *Wld Hlth Org. techn. Rep. Ser.*, No. 452 (1970), p. 40.

TABLE 16

VITAMIN B₁₂ IN ANIMAL PRODUCTS*

	Micrograms per 100 g fresh weight		Micrograms per 100 g fresh weight
Beef muscle	2–8	Egg yolk	1·2 (per yolk)
Beef kidney	20–50	Egg white	0
Beef heart	25	Herring (whole)	11
Beef liver	50–130	,, (fillet)	13
Pork	0·1–5	,, (liver)	34
Veal	2	Fish meal	10–25
Leg of lamb	8	Fish solubles	15–40
Milk (cow)	0·2–0·6	Meat scrap	3·5
Milk (goat)	0·01	Pasture soil	1
Cheese	1·4–3.6	Silage	0·1–2
Chicken liver	8		

* Smith, E.L. (1960) *Vitamin B₁₂*, London, p. 20.

DEFICIENCY

INTAKE DEFICIENCY	INTRINSIC FACTOR DEFICIENCY	ABSORPTION DEFECTS	EXCESSIVE DEMAND
Lack of animal protein	Congenital *Pernicious anaemia* Gastrectomy	Coeliac syndrome Sprue *Diphyllobothrium latum* infestation Stagnant loop syndrome Ileal defects Congenital malabsorption Inflammation Resection Drugs	Pregnancy

1. *Lack of intake.* Pure vegetarians who refuse to take even milk or milk products (vegans) are likely to get deficiency of vitamin B$_{12}$. Mothers with deficient intake of animal protein and vitamin B$_{12}$ may deliver babies with poor hepatic vitamin B$_{12}$ stores, and when these infants are breast-fed they may develop vitamin B$_{12}$ deficiency and megaloblastic anaemia. *Therapy* is with vitamin B$_{12}$ but folic acid alone should not be administered [8].

2. *In pernicious anaemia* vitamin B$_{12}$ is not absorbed from the gut due to the absence of gastric intrinsic factor. After total or partial *gastrectomy* the absence of intrinsic factor leads to vitamin B$_{12}$ deficiency when the liver store is exhausted. This occurs many years after operation since even 1 per cent of the stomach capacity can produce intrinsic factor for vitamin B$_{12}$ absorption. *Bacterial overgrowth* in the intestine following gastric surgery also contributes to vitamin B$_{12}$ malabsorption. *Congenital intrinsic factor deficiency* occurs as an isolated defect in infants and children, resulting in vitamin B$_{12}$ malabsorption. Their gastric mucosa and acid secretion are normal.

3. *Deficiency of intestinal absorption.* The ileum is the site of absorption of B$_{12}$ intrinsic factor complex. Diseases of the ileum such as *regional enteritis, intestinal tuberculosis, coeliac syndrome* and *sprue* result in lack of absorption of vitamin B$_{12}$. *Diphyllobothrium latum* infestation is common in Finland where 20 per cent of the population is affected. These parasites utilize ingested vitamin B$_{12}$ causing deficiency in the host. Analysis of the parasites shows a high concentration of vitamin B$_{12}$. *Stagnant loop syndrome* occurs after intestinal surgery or is due to multiple small intestinal diverticula, which promote the growth of bacteria. These bacteria bind vitamin B$_{12}$ and prevent its absorption [9]. Administration of broad-spectrum antibiotics inhibits the growth of these bacteria in the stagnant area, and the anaemia improves.

Congenital vitamin B$_{12}$ malabsorption. Despite normal intrinsic factor secretion by the stomach, there may be a deficiency of receptors in the ileum in absorbing vitamin B$_{12}$ intrinsic factor complex [10]. On biopsy the small intestinal mucosa is normal.

Vitamin B$_{12}$ deficiency itself decreases ileal capacity for B$_{12}$ absorption. With vitamin B$_{12}$ therapy normal absorption occurs. The absorption is also impaired with *drugs*—neomycine, colchicine, para-amino-salicylic acid and alcohol.

4. *Excessive demand,* particularly with low intake, shows manifestation of vitamin B$_{12}$ deficiency in pregnancy.

Vitamin B$_{12}$ Deficiency in Childhood [6]. (1) Congenital intrinsic factor deficiency, and (2) congenital vitamin B$_{12}$ malabsorption have been described above. These disorders are not associated with antibodies against gastric juice. *Treatment* is with parenteral vitamin B$_{12}$ for life.

Diagnosis of Vitamin B$_{12}$ Deficiency

Clinical. The example of extreme degree of vitamin B$_{12}$ deficiency is *pernicious anaemia* which actually is not due to deficiency of vitamin B$_{12}$ but of the intrinsic factor of the stomach leading to malabsorption of orally-taken vitamin B$_{12}$. The specific manifestations of vitamin B$_{12}$ deficiency are: (1) haematological, and (2) neurological.

1. *The haematological changes* are: (a) macrocytic anaemia in which the blood smear shows variation in the size and shape of the red blood cells; (b) the bone marrow shows megaloblasts; (c) the average survival time of the red blood cells, which normally is 120 days, is reduced to about 60 days. When a patient is undergoing treatment for vitamin B$_{12}$ deficiency the characteristic blood changes are not noted.

In pernicious anaemia there is yellowish pallor of the skin. The tongue may be sore, particularly on eating spiced food, it may be red and denuded of papillae. In patients with Addisonian pernicious anaemia gastric secretion is markedly reduced and there is histamine-fast achlorhydria. Gastroscopy shows atrophic changes of the stomach mucosa.

2. The *neurological changes* are characteristically manifest as *subacute combined degeneration of the spinal cord*. The neurological involvement is generally seen in neglected cases of pernicious anaemia or when pernicious anaemia is treated with folic acid alone, but some authorities maintain that occasionally neurological manifestations may occur even before the anaemia becomes manifest. The exact mechanism by which vitamin B$_{12}$ deficiency produces neurological changes is not known. There is: (a) degeneration of the lateral and posterior columns of the spinal cord; (b) peripheral neuropathy; and (c) occasionally mental changes.

(a) Changes in the lateral columns produce weakness, spasticity and extensor plantar response while involvement of the posterior columns gives loss of joint and vibration sense.

(b) Changes in the peripheral nerves give bilateral and symmetrical tingling, numbness, paraesthesiae and diminished or absent sensation involving the distal parts of the limbs. The combination of lateral column involvement and peripheral nerves gives exaggerated knee jerks but absent ankle jerks.

(c) Mental changes may manifest as loss of mental energy, depression, paranoia and psychosis. The mental changes respond to therapy with vitamin B$_{12}$.

Special Laboratory Investigations

Serum Vitamin B$_{12}$. Vitamin B$_{12}$ is less than 170 micromicrograms per ml of serum, but even less than 100 micromicrograms per ml commonly occurs with gross deficiency.

Methylmalonic Acid in Urine. Methylmalonic acid is converted to succinate in the presence of vitamin B$_{12}$. The estimation of serum vitamin B$_{12}$ so far has been made by *bacterial assay,* but urinary methylmalonic acid estimation is a useful *chemical method.* In the absence of vitamin B$_{12}$, daily urinary excretion of methylmalonic acid is over 5 mg. After 10 g valine load the urinary excretion of methylmalonic acid is over 40 mg in 24 hours in vitamin B$_{12}$ deficient patients. This method of rapid demonstration of vitamin B$_{12}$ deficiency is suitable even for debilitated patients [11].

Intrinsic Factor Deficiency. This can be demonstrated by:

(1) *Gastric secretion.* After histamine or pentagastrin injection, an absence of gastric hydrochloric acid and alkaline gastric pH of between 7 and 8 is noted in pernicious anaemia. (2) *Intrinsic factor deficiency.* Absence or marked diminution of intrinsic factor is demonstrable by radioimmunoassay. (3) *Radioactive vitamin B$_{12}$ absorption studies* can be done to confirm the diagnosis of pernicious anaemia. Radioactive cobalt-labelled vitamin B$_{12}$ is administered orally and the absorption is noted by estimating the excretion in the (a) *stool*, (b) *urine*, or (c) by estimating the vitamin B$_{12}$ level in the *blood. Hepatic uptake of* vitamin B$_{12}$ is not usually carried out in practice.

(a) *Unabsorbed faecal excretion.* In pernicious anaemia oral administration of radioactive vitamin B$_{12}$ results in high faecal excretion. Repeating the test with simultaneous administration of hog's stomach or 25 to 100 ml gastric juice from a normal person (intrinsic factor), the intestinal absorption of vitamin B$_{12}$ is increased and faecal excretion is considerably reduced. This cumbersome method of stool collection is not usually followed in practice, but is a useful method when patients are in remission due to treatment.

(b) *Excretion in the urine* (Schilling test) [12]. The modified method now generally adopted consists of an *oral* dose of 1 microgram of radioactive vitamin B_{12} and one hour later 1000 micrograms (1 mg) B_{12} (non-radioactive) is given *subcutaneously*. The injected inactive vitamin B_{12} helps to flush out the absorbed circulating radioactive vitamin B_{12} that is not incorporated in tissues. Four to six hours after the oral dose in a normal person radioactive B_{12} appears in the urine and persists for 24 hours. The amount excreted in 24 hours in normal people is about 20 per cent of the dose, but with malabsorption it is reduced to below 10 per cent. Repeating the test with oral 25–100 ml of neutralized gastric juice from normal persons, together with 1 microgram of radioactive vitamin B_{12} and the 'flushing' injection of non-radioactive vitamin B_{12} 1000 micrograms, the absorption is increased and the urinary excretion is also enhanced. Collecting urine specimens in older confused patients is difficult and the test is fallacious in patients with renal disease. The high flushing dose of non-radioactive vitamin B_{12} may produce haematological improvement even in folate deficient patients.

(c) *Plasma radioactivity* may also be measured in blood drawn 8 hours after the oral dose of radioactive vitamin B_{12} for Schilling test. The average radioactivity in a litre of plasma is 0·66 per cent of the oral dose, while in pernicious anaemia it is less than 0·15 per cent [13].

(d) *A therapeutic test* is a daily injection of a small dose of 2–5 micrograms vitamin B_{12}. This results in a reticulocyte peak by the end of the week. This test is most practical and devoid of fallacies where there are limited laboratory facilities.

Treatment of Pernicious Anaemia

The dosage schedule of vitamin B_{12} for pernicious anaemia varies from clinic to clinic. Three factors which guide the schedule are: (1) a vitamin B_{12} deficient person can accumulate a store in the liver sufficient to last for a long time if given a sufficiently large dose; (2) very high doses lead to a considerable loss in the urine; and (3) the individual requirements for producing a remission as well as for maintenance are variable.

Parenteral Therapy. *Hydroxocobalamin* is retained more efficiently and is preferred for parenteral therapy [14] in pernicious anaemia. In a moderately severe case the dosage schedule would be 100 micrograms of vitamin B$_{12}$ intramuscularly three times a week for about 2–3 weeks. Thereafter, the *maintenance dose* of 100 micrograms once every 3–5 weeks appears to be the most economical. Alternatively, maintenance therapy of 1000 micrograms of hydroxocobalamin every 4 months, or cyanocobalamin every 2 months, and an even more frequent dose in patients with associated liver or kidney diseases is advocated [14]. However, the progress of the patient should determine any necessary alteration in the dosage. When vitamin B$_{12}$ was first discovered the administration of even 1 microgram a day was found sufficient to produce remission in pernicious anaemia.

Oral Therapy. For pernicious anaemia oral therapy of vitamin B$_{12}$ is not advised but can be given. The usual method is to administer vitamin B$_{12}$ with intrinsic factor in the form of hog's stomach extract or even 50–100 ml of normal gastric juice to facilitate absorption. Pernicious anaemia can sometimes be shown to respond to as little as 1 microgram of vitamin B$_{12}$ together with 10 ml of human gastric juice. If the intrinsic factor as normal gastric juice is not given then oral administration of vitamin B$_{12}$ alone can also be helpful provided a larger dose is given when it is absorbed by a mass action effect. Oral vitamin B$_{12}$ in a dose of 100 micrograms daily can be an effective therapy for maintenance.

Treatment of Subacute Combined Degeneration of the Cord

For the treatment of subacute combined degeneration of the cord parenteral vitamin B$_{12}$, 100 micrograms, should be given on alternate days and continued till the neurological signs and symptoms improve.

Folic Acid Contra-indicated. Folic acid, though it improves the blood picture in pernicious anaemia, may actually precipitate neurological complications; it is therefore a dangerous treatment. On the other hand in cases of sprue and idiopathic steatorrhoea, though the blood picture improves with vitamin B$_{12}$, steatorrhoea responds only to parenteral administration of folic acid.

Nutritional Vitamin B$_{12}$ Deficiency

Those with dietary deficiency of vitamin B$_{12}$ (without pernicious anaemia, in vegetarians) respond even to *oral* 1 microgram vitamin B$_{12}$ [15].

Prophylactic Vitamin B_{12} Therapy

Deficiency of vitamin B_{12} has been described after partial gastrectomy and after resection of ileum, and therefore prophylactic monthly injections of 100 micrograms vitamin B_{12} are advised.

Tobacco Amblyopia

Hydroxocobalamin is the physiologically active form of vitamin B_{12} and is safe to administer in preference to cyanocobalamin [16]. Tobacco amblyopia is related to cyanide metabolism, and hydroxocobalamin is a powerful cyanide antagonist. In patients with tobacco amblyopia only hydroxocobalamin should be administered [17].

Unnecessary Use

Innumerable claims are made about the utility of vitamin B_{12} in conditions like alcoholic neuritis, trigeminal neuralgia, herpes zoster, migraine, asthma, eczema, dermatitis, infectious hepatitis and as a 'general tonic'. In fact it is claimed to be panacea for all ills but without a double blind study the therapeutic utility of vitamin B_{12} in these diseases should be considered doubtful.

Toxicity

Even with a high dose of vitamin B_{12} no toxicity is noted, but anaphylactic reaction may occur [18].

REFERENCES

[1] BOOTH, C.C., and MOLLIN, D.L. (1959) The site of absorption of vitamin B_{12} in man, *Lancet*, **i**, 18.

[2] COX, E.V., MEYNELL, M.J., GADDIE, R., and COOKE, W.T. (1959) Inter-relation of vitamin B_{12} and iron, *Lancet*, **ii**, 998.

[3] GRASBECK, R., KANTERO, I., and SIURALA, M. (1959) Influence of calcium ions on vitamin B_{12} absorption in steatorrhoea and pernicious anaemia, *Lancet*, **i**, 234.

[4] ROSE, M.S., and CHANARIN, I. (1971) Intrinsic factor antibody and absorption of vitamin B_{12} in pernicious anaemia, *Brit. med. J.*, **1**, 25.

[5] ARDEMAN, S., and CHANARIN, I. (1965) Steroids in Addisonian pernicious anaemia, *New Engl. J. Med.*, **273**, 1352.

[6] CHANARIN, I. (1970) Pernicious anaemia and other vitamin B_{12} deficiency states, *Abstr. Wld Med.*, **44**, 73.

[7] SULLIVAN, L.W. (1970) Vitamin B_{12} metabolism and megaloblastic anaemia, *Seminars in Haematology*, **7**, 6.

[8] JADHAV, M., WEBB, J.K.G., VAISHNAVA, S., and BAKER, S.J. (1962) Vitamin B_{12} deficiency in Indian infants. A clinical syndrome, *Lancet*, **ii**, 903.

[9] SCHJONSBY, H., PETERS, T.J., HOFFBRAND, A.V., and TABAQCHALI, S. (1970) The mechanism of vitamin B$_{12}$ malabsorption in the blind loop syndrome, *Gut,* **11,** 371.

[10] GRASBECK, R., GORDIN, R., KANTERO, I., and KUHLBACK, B. (1960) Selective vitamin B$_{12}$ malabsorption and proteinuria in young people. A syndrome, *Acta med. scand.,* **167,** 289.

[11] GREEN, A.E., and PEGRUM, G.D. (1968) Value of estimating methylmalonic acid excretion in anaemia, *Brit. med. J.,* **3,** 591.

[12] SCHILLING, R.F. (1953) A new test for intrinsic factor activity, *J. Lab. clin. Med.,* **42,** 946.

[13] COINER, D., and WALSH, J.R. (1971) Comparison of Schilling test and plasma level of cyanocobalamin Co[57], *J. Amer. med. Ass.,* **215,** 1642.

[14] BODDY, K., *et al.* (1968) Retention of cyanocobalamin, hydroxocobalamin and coenzyme B$_{12}$ after parenteral administration, *Lancet,* **ii,** 710.

[15] STEWART, J.S., ROBERTS, P.D., and HOFFBRAND, A.V. (1970) Response of dietary vitamin B$_{12}$ deficiency to physiological oral doses of cyanocobalamin, *Lancet,* **ii,** 542.

[16] FOULDS, W.S., FREEMAN, A.G., PHILLIPS, C.I., and WILSON, J. (1970) Cyanocobalamin. A case for withdrawal, *Lancet,* **i,** 35.

[17] CHISHOLM, I.A., BRONTE-STEWART, J., and FOULDS, W.S. (1967) Hydroxocobalamin versus cyanocobalamin in the treatment of tobacco amblyopia, *Lancet,* **ii,** 450.

[18] HOVDING, G. (1968) Anaphylactic reaction after injection of vitamin B$_{12}$, *Brit. med. J.,* **3,** 102.

11. PANTOTHENIC ACID (Filtrate Factor)

Pantothenic acid derives its name from its distribution in all foodstuffs (*pantothen* = everywhere). It was also known as *filtrate factor* because originally the term vitamin B$_2$ was applied to the heat resistant combination of riboflavine, niacin and vitamin B$_6$ which were all adsorbed on fuller's earth; pantothenic acid was not adsorbed but passed into the filtrate. Interest in this factor was aroused by the observation that it prevented greying of fur in rats. The absence of this factor was also known to produce changes in the skin of chicks which superficially resembled human pellagra, hence it was also known as chick *pellagra factor.*

Chemistry

Pantothenic acid is a peptide derivative. d-Pantothenic acid is a viscous oil but its calcium salt, calcium pantothenate is a crystalline substance soluble in water. Commercially pantothenic acid is available as soluble calcium pantothenate. Pantothenic acid was *isolated* in 1938 and *synthesized* in 1940 [1].

Absorption and Excretion
Pantothenic acid is absorbed from the alimentary tract and excreted in the urine and also in milk.

Blood Level
The normal value of pantothenic acid in the blood is 0·225 micrograms per ml [2].

Action
Pantothenic acid is concerned with acetylation reactions within living cells; for this reason it is known as co-enzyme A (A for acetylation) [3]. Pantothenic acid also plays a part in: (1) metabolism of amino acids; (2) synthesis of fatty acids and cholesterol; (3) formation of steroids.

Pantothenic Acid Antagonist
Omega-methyl-pantothenic acid acts antagonistically to pantothenic acid.

Source
This co-enzyme is distributed throughout all animal tissues, the highest concentration being found in the liver, kidneys, spleen, heart and adrenals.

Requirement
No clear data exist to show the daily requirement. An average diet contains 6–10 mg of pantothenic acid and this is evidently adequate. Cow's milk yields 10·5 mg per 2500 Calories and human milk yields 10·9 mg per 2500 Calories [4].

DEFICIENCY

Test for Pantothenic Acid Deficiency
Pantothenic acid aids in acetylation, hence the ability of the body to acetylate 100–200 mg of para-aminobenzoic acid has been used as a test of deficiency. In pantothenic acid deficiency, as in the burning

feet syndrome, the excretion of acetylated para-aminobenzoic acid in the urine was diminished [5].

Experimental deficiency in human volunteers produced by administering the pantothenic acid antagonist omega-methyl-pantothenic acid, together with a purified diet devoid of pantothenic acid produced the following manifestations [6, 7]: apathy, depression, vasomotor instability most marked when standing, paraesthesia, burning pains, muscle weakness, abdominal pain and disturbed bowel function. Laboratory investigations showed histamine-fast achlorhydria, altered glucose tolerance and increased sensitivity to insulin. Administration of ACTH did not produce eosinopenia. Whether these manifestations were due to the pantothenic acid deficiency alone or whether due to poisoning by omega-methyl-pantothenic acid is not known.

Burning Feet Syndrome

It is a syndrome characterized by sensation of pins-and-needles, tingling, numbness and burning in the feet, seen amongst poor patients in South India [8]. Administration of nicotinic acid, thiamine and riboflavine, improved the general state of nutrition but no relief was obtained from paraesthesia. The symptoms improved on daily intramuscular administration of 20–40 mg of calcium pantothenate. The burning disappeared first, the sensation of pins-and-needles disappeared last in 2 to 4 weeks. These results have not been confirmed. In an organized trial among 60 patients with burning feet syndrome no benefit was noted when treated with pantothenic acid [9].

Grey Hair

Fame and fortune awaits any person who can prevent greying of hair. The anti-grey fur factor for the rat was pantothenic acid but even large doses over a prolonged period have failed to affect human hair. It is not certain that greying in adult humans is even caused by dietary deficiency [10].

Burns

Encouraging results from topical application of pantothenic acid for burns have been reported [11].

Paralytic Ileus

Pantothenic acid is also advocated in the treatment of paralytic ileus but it is probable that most cases of paralytic ileus are due to low grade peritonitis or deficiency of potassium.

REFERENCES

[1] WILLIAMS, R.J., and MAJOR, R.T. (1940) The structure of pantothenic acid, *Science,* **91**, 246.

[2] STANBERY, S.R., SNELL, E.E., and SPIES, T.D. (1940) A note on an assay method for pantothenic acid in human blood, *J. biol. Chem.,* **135**, 353.

[3] HARRIS, L.J. (1955) *Vitamins in Theory and Practice,* 4th ed., p. 271, Cambridge.

[4] WILLIAMS, R.J. (1942) The approximate vitamin requirements of human beings, *J. Amer. med. Ass.,* **119**, 1.

[5] SARMA, P.S., MENON, P.S., and VENKATACHALAM, P.S. (1949) Acetylation in the laboratory diagnosis of 'burning feet syndrome' (pantothenic acid deficiency), *Curr. Sci.,* **18**, 367.

[6] Bean, W.B., and HODGES, R.E. (1954) Pantothenic acid deficiency induced in human subjects, *Proc. Soc. exp. Biol. (N.Y.),* **86**, 693.

[7] BEAN, W.B., HODGES, R.E., and DAUM, K. (1955) Pantothenic acid deficiency induced in human subjects, *J. clin. Invest.,* **34**, 1073.

[8] GOPALAN, C. (1946). The 'burning feet' syndrome, *Indian med. Gaz.,* **81**, 22.

[9] BIBILE, S.W., LIONEL, N.D.W., DUNUWILLE, R., and PERERA, G. (1957) Pantothenic acid and the burning feet syndrome, *Brit. J. Nutr.,* **11**, 434.

[10] FROST, D.V. (1948) The relation of nutritional deficiencies to greying, *Physiol. Rev.,* **28**, 368.

[11] MATANIC, V. (1958) Pantothenic acid and burns, *Practitioner,* **180**, 771.

12. CHOLINE, BIOTIN, INOSITOL AND PARA-AMINOBENZOIC ACID

Choline, biotin, inositol and para-aminobenzoic acid have been raised to the status of vitamins and so will be reviewed in brief. All vitamins so far discussed have been effective in small doses but these substances have to be given in bigger quantities to produce a clinical effect.

CHOLINE

Choline was identified in the last century. It is a component of the phospholipid lecithin and in combination with alcohol it forms acetylcholine and supplies a labile methyl group for transmethylation.

Fatty Liver and Choline

Phospholipids are concerned with the mobilization of fat in the body. In the absence of choline, neutral fat and to some extent cholesterol esters accumulate in the liver producing fatty liver. As choline prevents fatty liver it is called *lipotropic factor* [1]. Choline is of no help in hepatic cirrhosis without fatty changes.

The mode of action of choline is not understood. It either : (1) enhances the oxidation of fatty acids in the liver; or (2) promotes the formation of some lecithin-containing-lipoproteins in the liver which are essential for oxidation of fatty acids.

Source

Egg-yolk, wheat germ, liver, brain, kidney, heart, lean meat, yeast, soya-beans, peanut and skimmed milk are good sources of choline. The amino acid methionine can act as a donor of labile methyl groups to convert ethanolamine to choline by transmethylation so proteins with a high methionine content such as casein, can act as a source of choline. For this reason the requirement of choline cannot be assessed.

REFERENCE

[1] BEST, C.H., CHANNON, H.J., and RIDOUT, J.H. (1934) Choline and dietary production of fatty livers, *J. Physiol. (Lond.)*, **81**, 409.

BIOTIN

Biotin was originally called vitamin H or Haut (from the German word *Haut*=skin) [1] because it protected rats from dermatitis. Biotin is a component of human tissues and is necessary for bacterial growth in culture media.

DEFICIENCY OF BIOTIN

'Egg White Injury' (Avidin). The study of biotin was stimulated by the 'egg white injury' produced in chicks [2] and rats [3]. Rats kept on a diet which contained uncooked egg white, developed dermatitis and spasticity of the hind legs preventable by giving either cooked eggs or biotin. The damage is not due to any toxic substance acting directly on the body but to the presence of a protein substance in egg white called *avidin*, the term meaning avid (hungry) albumin. Avidin combined with biotin and the avidin-biotin complex is excreted in the stool. Hence excess avidin prevents the absorption of biotin. Heat destroys avidin and so cooked eggs do not produce biotin deficiency.

Biotin has also been shown to act as a co-enzyme for carboxylation of acetyl Co-A to form malonyl Co-A, which is an important step in the fatty acid synthesis and fat metabolism.

Biotin Deficiency in Humans. Sydenstricker [4] has produced biotin deficiency in man by giving 30 per cent of the calories as desiccated egg white. The diet was poor in all vitamins of the B group, except riboflavine and was supplemented with adequate amounts of available synthetic vitamins. The subjects developed dermatitis, lassitude, somnolence, muscle pains and hyperaesthesia. The symptoms disappeared with the parenteral administration of 150–300 micrograms of biotin daily.

REFERENCES

[1] HARRIS, L.J. (1955) *Vitamins in Theory and Practice,* 4th ed., p. 283, Cambridge.
[2] EAKIN, R.E., McKINLEY, W.A., and WILLIAMS, R.J. (1940) Egg-white injury in chicks and its relationship to a deficiency of vitamin H (Biotin), *Science,* **92,** 224.
[3] GYÖRGY, P., ROSE, C.S., EAKIN, R.E., SNELL, E.E., and WILLIAMS, R.J. (1941) Egg-white injury as the result of nonabsorption or inactivation of Biotin, *Science,* **93,** 477.
[4] SYDENSTRICKER, V.P., SINGAL, S.A., BRIGGS, A.P., DeVAUGHN, N.N., and ISBELL, H. (1942) Observations on 'egg-white injury' in man and its cure with biotin concentrate, *J. Amer. med. Ass.,* **118,** 1199.

INOSITOL

Inositol has been found to cure alopecia in the mouse. It is plentiful in human tissues but its significance is not clear. Inositol is a component of phospholipids, e.g. inositol phosphatide or lipositol. In tissue culture experiments, 18 different human cell strains required addition of meso-inositol for normal growth. In human diabetics the excretion of inositol is increased and the excretion rate falls after treatment with insulin.

An inositol derivative, known to nutritionists as *phytin* (inositol hexaphosphate), is present in cereals and prevents the absorption of calcium from the gut.

Source

Inositol is widely distributed and is found in fruits, meat, milk, nuts, vegetables, whole grain, yeast and bacteria.

PARA-AMINOBENZOIC ACID

Para-aminobenzoic acid is a growth factor for chicks. Bacteria also require para-aminobenzoic acid for their growth. If a sulphonamide is added to the culture medium, bacteria take it up instead of para-aminobenzoic acid because both have a similar chemical structure. Sulphonamides thus act as competitors for the vitamin and so inhibit bacterial growth. Para-aminobenzoic acid is a component of the folic acid molecule.

13. VITAMIN C (Ascorbic Acid)

James Lind, a British Naval surgeon, by the first clinical trial ever performed, demonstrated in the eighteenth century that citrus fruit juices prevented and cured scurvy which was the scourge amongst sailors. The experimental study of vitamin C started with the production of scurvy in guinea-pigs by Holst and Frölich. It was fortunate that they worked on guinea-pigs because it has now been shown that guinea-pigs and primates do not synthesize their own vitamin C, while other animals and plants are able to do so. Szent-Györgyi isolated a substance from orange juice, cabbage and the suprarenal glands which was identified as hexuronic acid, but its antiscorbutic properties were not apparent till Waugh and King showed that hexuronic acid was identical with vitamin C which they had isolated from lemon juice.

Chemistry

Ascorbic acid is a white crystalline substance readily soluble in water. Its empirical formula is $C_6H_8O_6$. Laevo-ascorbic acid is an active antiscorbutic substance, while dextro-ascorbic acid is not. Ascorbic acid is destroyed by oxidation, heat and strong alkalies, all of which are important considerations in the destruction of vitamin C during cooking. Ascorbic acid was *synthesized* in 1933 by Reichstein *et al.*

Synthesis of Ascorbic Acid in Animals and Plants. Ascorbic acid is synthesized both by animals (except guinea-pigs and primates) and plants, from simple sugars. There is experimental evidence to show that the biosynthesis of ascorbic acid occurs from dextrose (D-glucose) and D-galactose. The probable steps simply stated are:

D-glucose — D-glucuronic acid — L-gulonic acid — L-ascorbic acid

D-galactose — D-galacturonic acid — L-galactonic acid — L-ascorbic acid.

The failure of guinea-pigs and primates to synthesize their own ascorbic acid from glucose is due to a deficiency of the enzymes in the liver which convert L-gulonic acid to ascorbic acid.

TEST FOR ASCORBIC ACID. There are many tests for the detection of ascorbic acid but as it is a powerful reducing substance, the most commonly employed is reduction with 2–6 dichlorophenol indophenol.

Destruction of Ascorbic Acid. *Ascorbic oxidase.* Vegetable cells contain an enzyme called ascorbic oxidase. When vegetables are finely cut a greater quantity of the enzyme is released and more vitamin C is destroyed. The rate of enzymic oxidation increases as the temperature is raised and so gradual heating of vegetables destroys vitamin C. Ascorbic oxidase is destroyed on boiling. If vegetables are immersed directly in boiling water then ascorbic oxidase is destroyed immediately and the loss of vitamin C due to ascorbic oxidase does not occur.

Vitamin C is more easily destroyed than other vitamins. During cooking, loss of vitamin C occurs due to: (1) cutting the vegetables finely; (2) using an excess of water which is later thrown away; (3) gradually heating the vegetables rather than putting them in boiling water; (4) overcooking; (5) keeping vegetables hot for a long time before being served; (6) adding sodium bicarbonate in order to preserve the colour of vegetables as alkalinity destroys vitamin C.

Tablets of ascorbic acid do not deteriorate at room temperature. Aqueous solutions for injections, however, are less stable.

PRESERVED FOOD. Modern methods of dehydration, freezing and canning preserve the vitamin C content of food to a considerable extent.

Absorption

Ascorbic acid is absorbed from the intestines. It is also easily absorbed when given parenterally.

Plasma Level

The plasma level of ascorbic acid in normal persons is over 1 mg per 100 ml, with lower values found in deficiency states. The level falls to zero several months before clinical manifestations of scurvy appear. Ascorbic acid levels in leucocytes reflect the tissue levels. Normal values are about 25 micrograms per 10^8 leucocytes. Smoking lowers plasma and leucocyte vitamin C levels.

Storage

The concentration of ascorbic acid in the tissues appears to be related to metabolic activity. It is present in descending order of concentration in the adrenal glands (55 mg per 100 g), brain, pancreas, thymus (in infants and children), kidneys, lungs, spleen and heart muscle. The total body pool is about 2–3 g. When the body content exceeds 4 g, extra amounts are quickly excreted. The half life of isotopically labelled ascorbic acid is 20 days.

Excretion

Ascorbic acid is excreted by the *kidneys* when the plasma level exceeds 1·4 mg per 100 ml. Large amounts given intravenously are mostly excreted. Excretion is diminished or absent when the tissues are depleted of vitamin C. This observation forms the basis of the 'saturation test' for the diagnosis of vitamin C deficiency, in which a large loading dose is given. If the tissues are saturated most of it is excreted, but if the tissues are deficient a large part is retained.

Normally, very little ascorbic acid is excreted in the *faeces*, but the loss is appreciable in diarrhoea. *Expired air* is also shown to contain isotopically labelled ascorbic acid.

Action

Ascorbic acid is a reducing substance and forms part of the tissue enzyme system concerned with oxidation and reduction It is concerned in the formation of collagen present between cells. If collagen is defective, the cells are not bound together so that the proper formation of tissues such as bone matrix, teeth and the lining of blood vessels does not occur. Ascorbic acid is also necessary for the formation of osteoblasts and for haemopoiesis.

Source

The main sources of vitamin C are green vegetables and fruits.

Cereals and pulses do not contain vitamin C in the dry state, but if soaked in water for about 48 hours and allowed to germinate, they form a good source of vitamin C. Thus vitamin C can be made available even in the absence of fresh fruits and vegetables.

Requirement

The recommended requirements vary from 30 to 100 mg a day. A British study on 20 human volunteers [1] showed that a dose of 10 mg per day would prevent clinical scurvy in adults. The committee, allowing a margin of safety, recommended 30 mg as the total requirements.

The FAO/WHO recommendations are as follows:

RECOMMENDED DAILY INTAKES OF ASCORBIC ACID*

A G E	RECOMMENDED DAILY INTAKE IN MG
Birth—12 years**	20
13 years and over	30
Pregnant women (second and third trimesters)	50
Lactating women	50

* *Wld Hlth Org. techn. Rep. Ser.,* No. 452 (1970), p. 28.
** For infants aged 0–6 months it is accepted that breast-feeding by a well-nourished mother is the best way to satisfy requirements for ascorbic acid.

DEFICIENCY

Scurvy

Scurvy is produced by prolonged deficiency of vitamin C. Human volunteers deprived of vitamin C showed no clinical manifestations for 17 weeks. The first signs noted were hyperkeratotic hair follicles from 17 to 21 weeks, followed by perifollicular haemorrhages at 26–34 weeks [1]. Since, in ordinary circumstances, an infant or adult is not completely deprived of vitamin C, it can be assumed that at least 6–9 months would elapse before clinical scurvy appears even with gross deficiency.

Pathology. The basic pathological change in scurvy is defective formation of collagen. The lining of blood vessels is defective because the cells are not cemented together. The bony matrix or framework is poorly formed for the same reasons.

Subclinical Scurvy

Before the development of clinical signs of scurvy, vague general symptoms such as lassitude, fatigue, weakness, irritability, a tendency to recurrent infections and aching of bones are noted.

Clinical Scurvy

Clinical symptoms appear when the body pool decreases to 300 mg [2]. Clinical scurvy is manifest by changes in: (1) blood vessels; (2) skin; (3) bones; (4) teeth and gums; (5) anaemia; and (6) general symptoms.

1. *Blood vessels.* The blood vessels become fragile and porous due to defective formation of collagen in the lining of the wall. This leads to spongy gums, haemorrhages into the skin, seen as petechiae and ecchymoses, and haemorrhages into the alimentary and urinary tract. Conjunctival haemorrhages occur by 74–95 days in experimental human scurvy. Muscular and subperiosteal haemorrhages may also occur.

2. *Skin.* The skin becomes rough and dry. Early hyperkeratotic changes are seen in the hair follicles, and are most marked on legs and buttocks. The occurrence of petechial haemorrhages around hair follicles and of larger haemorrhages, ecchymoses, have already been referred to.

3. *Bones.* During normal growth, cartilage cells at the growing end of bones proliferate. These are invaded by osteoblasts to form the bony matrix, also known as osteoid tissue. Ossification occurs when calcium salts are deposited in this matrix, forming bone.

In the absence of vitamin C the formation of bony matrix (osteoid tissue) is defective. Instead of osteoblasts, fibroblasts develop and bone formation is retarded. This gives rise to osteoporosis and spontaneous fractures. The periosteum is not attached firmly to the bone and subperiosteal haemorrhages occur, usually at the lower end of the femur and upper end of the humerus. These bony changes are found in infants and children with scurvy.

4. *Teeth and Gums.* Deficiency of vitamin C in children leads to defective formation of the teeth. The dentine becomes porous, the alveolar bone is absorbed and the teeth may fall out. The gums become

spongy and bleed easily if slight pressure is applied. Hypertrophy of the gums tends to bury the teeth and infection and ulceration of the unhealthy gums is common. These changes in the gums may not be seen in an edentulous subject.

5. *Anaemia.* Microcytic hypochromic anaemia is a common feature in scurvy. The anaemia is partly due to deficient absorption of iron, with a low intake of vitamin C and partly due to blood loss from haemorrhages. Deficiency of vitamin C also disturbs folic acid metabolism and a megaloblastic anaemia may develop.

6. *General manifestations* of scurvy are pyrexia, rapid pulse and susceptibility to infection. Wound healing is delayed.

Aspirin is more likely to produce gastric mucosal bleeding in a vitamin C-deficient subject.

Infantile Scurvy

Infantile scurvy occurs in babies fed on powdered milk. Mother's milk contains 3 mg of vitamin C per 100 ml so breast-fed infants do not show manifestations of scurvy unless the diet of the mother is very low in vitamin C. Boiling fresh milk destroys a considerable amount of vitamin C, while evaporation destroys it in the preparation of powdered milk.

The symptoms of infantile scurvy are loss of appetite, failure to gain weight, irritability and pallor. These symptoms may be followed by clinical manifestations in the skin as seen in adults, defective growth of bones and haemorrhages in the subperiosteum and viscera. Separation of the costochondral junction results in a prominence at the ends of the ribs (scorbutic rosary). These changes can be distinguished clinically from those of rickets as the scorbutic rosary has a sharp edge because it marks a separation of rib and cartilage whereas the rachitic rosary is rounded because of an overgrowth of the cartilage. The sternum appears to retract due to lack of support. The X-ray appearances are characteristic.

Capillary Resistance Test (Hess Test). This test gives a measure of resistance of the capillary walls. A circle 2·5 cm in diameter is marked on the skin in the antecubital region and a blood pressure armlet is applied to the upper arm. The cuff is inflated to a pressure between systolic and diastolic blood pressure and this is maintained for 5 minutes. Three minutes after releasing the armlet, the number of petechiae are counted in the circle with a magnifying glass. More than

20 denotes diminished capillary resistance, which may be due to deficiency of vitamin C.

Treatment

Infantile Scurvy. PROPHYLAXIS. The best way to prevent deficiency is to give one teaspoonful of fresh orange juice starting in the second week of life, gradually increasing the amount till the juice of one whole fruit is given.

CURATIVE. (a) *Oral.* 50 mg of vitamin C with food, or preferably in orange juice, are administered three or four times a day. (b) *Intravenous.* During an acute bleeding episode in scurvy, three or four injections of vitamin C, 50 mg each, intravenously at intervals of six hours will produce rapid recovery. This must be followed by oral therapy. As vitamin C is a reducing agent it is inadvisable to mix it with other substances during intravenous therapy.

AFTER-CARE. General instructions on dietetic requirements and methods of cooking are necessary. A diet inadequate enough to produce a deficiency disease will also lack other nutritional components.

Adult Scurvy. PROPHYLAXIS. One hundred grammes of germinated pulses may provide 10 mg vitamin C. Poor people can be taught to increase the vitamin C content of food by soaking cereals and pulses in water for about 48 hours so as to germinate them before cooking. About 10 mg vitamin C per day, which is adequate to prevent clinical manifestations of scurvy, is easily derived from a diet containing fresh fruits and vegetables.

CURATIVE. Two to four intravenous injections of vitamin C, 100 mg each, at intervals of six hours will control the haemorrhagic tendency. This is followed by vitamin C, 100 mg orally three or four times a day. The patient is also advised on the general principles of dietetics.

Other Uses of Vitamin C

1. *Wound healing.* In the absence of vitamin C, wound healing is defective and formation of scar tissue is delayed. Oral vitamin C 100 mg three times a day is administered before and after surgical operations, particularly in patients with poor nutrition and duodenal ulcer.

2. *Common cold.* Vitamin C has gained a reputation for being useful in reducing the severity of the common cold, but controlled studies have not proved this claim [3].

3. *Rheumatic fever.* In a controlled clinical study, the incidence of common cold was not greater in a group deficient in vitamin C, and yet morbidity caused by streptococcal infection was high and acute rheumatism was noted only in this group [4].

4. *Pregnancy and lactation.* The plasma vitamin C values in normal pregnancy were 0·35–0·4 mg per 100 ml as compared to a level of 1·1 mg in non-pregnant women [5]. At parturition, the concentration of vitamin C in cord blood is greater than that in the maternal plasma.

During lactation the vitamin C requirement of the mother is increased.

5. *Threatened and habitual abortion.* In cases of abortion, vitamin C deficiency has been reported, and therapeutic administration has been advocated in these cases [5].

6. *Haemorrhagic disease of newborn.* If the cord blood values are very low (below 0·3 mg), then marked deficiency in the maternal blood is presumed and such infants are likely to develop haemorrhagic disease of the newborn. As there is an associated low prothrombin concentration, administration of both vitamins C and K to the mother may diminish the incidence of haemorrhage in the newborn.

7. *Prickly heat* improves with vitamin C intake [6].

Patients with *fevers* and *diarrhoea* require increased amounts of vitamin C.

In all the above-mentioned conditions oral vitamin C, 100 mg three times a day, is adequate.

Methaemoglobinaemia is treated with ascorbic acid 100 mg three times daily.

Toxicity

High doses of vitamin C, 500–1000 mg daily, have been administered over a prolonged period without evidence of toxicity. Except in acute deficiency states, a dosage over 100 mg has no value, as it is rapidly excreted in the urine.

REFERENCES

[1] MEDICAL RESEARCH COUNCIL (1948) Vitamin C requirement of human adults —Experimental study of vitamin C deprivation in man, A preliminary report by the Vitamin C Sub-Committee of the Accessory Food Factors Committee, *Lancet,* **i,** 853.

[2] HODGES, R.F., *et al.* (1969) Experimental scurvy in man, *Amer, J. clin. Nutr.,* **22,** 535.

[3] WALKER, G.H., BYNOE, M.L., and TYRRELL, D.S.J. (1967) Trial of ascorbic acid in prevention of cold, *Brit. med. J.,* **1,** 603.

[4] GLAZEBROOK, A.J., and THOMSON, S. (1942) The administration of vitamin C in a large institution and its effect on general health and resistance to infection, *J. Hyg.* (*Lond.*), **42,** 1.

[5] JAVERT, C.T., and STANDER, H.J. (1943) Plasma vitamin C and prothrombin concentration in pregnancy and in threatened, spontaneous, and habitual abortion, *Surg. Gynec. Obstet.,* **76,** 115.

[6] HINDSON, T.C. (1968) Ascorbic acid for prickly heat, *Lancet,* **i,** 1347.

14. VITAMIN A
(RETINOL)

A growth factor present in fat was demonstrated by McCollum and Davis and by Osborne and Mendel. Later Goldblatt and Zilva found two factors in cod-liver oil: one, now known as vitamin A, was easily inactivated by heat in the presence of air, while the other, now known as vitamin D, was more stable. Thus the presence of two vitamins in animal fat was demonstrated. They also showed that the growth promoting factor in spinach, *provitamin A* or *carotene,* was not antirachitic.

Chemistry

The general term 'vitamin A' includes all compounds which have vitamin A activity. *Retinol is the generally accepted chemical name for vitamin A.*

Retinol (Vitamin A_1). This is vitamin A *alcohol* found in mammals and is abundant in the liver oils of *salt-water* fish. It has the empirical formula $C_{20}H_{29}OH$. The transport form is retinol while its ester is stored in the tissues.

Retinal (Retinene). This is vitamin A aldehyde (retinaldehyde) which combines with the protein *opsin* in the retina to form a photosensitive pigment *rhodopsin.*

Retinoic Acid (Vitamin A Acid). This is the active form of retinol. It has local therapeutic action when applied to the skin.

Dehydroretinol (Vitamin A_2). This is found mostly in *fresh-water* fish. The biological activity is only 40 per cent that of retinol.

Carotene (Provitamin A). Carotene derives its name from the plant pigment present in carrots. Carotene is a precursor of vitamin A in the body and is therefore known as 'provitamin A'. It is abundant in green and yellow vegetables as well as in yellow fruits, but it is never produced in animals. Chemically it is $C_{40}H_{56}$ and may be hydrolysed to 2 molecules of vitamin A:

$$C_{40}H_{56} + 2H_2O = 2C_{20}H_{29}OH$$

Carotene has *alpha, beta* and *gamma* isomers of which *beta* carotene is the most widely distributed in food and more effectively converted into vitamin A.

Synthesis. Vitamin A, *beta* carotene and other carotenoids have been chemically synthesized.

Stability. Destruction of vitamin A by oxidation led McCollum to separate the fat-soluble antixerophthalmic vitamin A, from the fat-soluble antirachitic vitamin D which resisted oxidation. Ordinary cooking does not destroy vitamin A but overcooking does. There is usually no appreciable loss of vitamin A in canned foods. Oxidation of fat destroys vitamin A and hence it is lacking in rancid butter and *ghee*. Vitamin E is an anti-oxidant and helps in preserving vitamin A.

Unit

Vitamin A. Vitamin A acetate is obtained in a pure crystalline form and its weight is expressed in terms of International Units. One International Unit of vitamin A is 0·3 micrograms of crystalline vitamin A alcohol (retinol), or 0·344 micrograms of crystalline vitamin A acetate.

The FAO/WHO have recommended that *crystalline retinol expressed in micrograms* should be used as the reference standard instead of the International Units (IU) hitherto used.

Carotene. One International Unit of carotene is the biological activity of 0·6 micrograms of *beta* carotene, which is better absorbed than other carotenoids. Only one third of *beta* carotene is absorbed and only one-half of what is absorbed is converted to vitamin A. Thus only one-sixth of dietary *beta* carotene is converted to vitamin A, i.e. 1 microgram *beta* carotene in the diet has the same biological activity as 0·167 microgram retinol. Since other carotenoids are less well utilized, their activity is half that of *beta* carotene.

IU of vitamin A   0·3 microgram retinol.

0·6 microgram *beta* carotene.

1·2 microgram of other mixed carotenoids with vitamin A activity.

Absorption

Vitamin A.   Vitamin A is absorbed along with fat from the proximal part of the small intestine; its absorption is more rapid in men than women [1]. It is poorly absorbed in all conditions accompanied by diarrhoea. The oral administration of unabsorbable mineral oil like liquid paraffin may produce deficiency because fat-soluble vitamin A dissolves in paraffin and is excreted unabsorbed. Commercially-obtainable water-dispersible forms of oral vitamin A are absorbed independently of fat absorption. There is no apparent relationship between the absorption following a test dose and the fasting plasma concentration of vitamin A. Ingestion of food during the test period enhances the absorption of vitamin A.

Retinol Binding Protein (RBP).   Retinol is absorbed from the intestine predominantly esterified as palmitate. It circulates in the plasma with the specific retinol binding protein [2]. The synthesis of this protein is reduced in protein deficiency (kwashiorkor), and hence vitamin A deficiency is increased.

Carotene.   Edible fats and bile salts aid, while liquid paraffin inhibits, the absorption of carotene. *Crystalline beta* carotene is completely absorbed. Carotene absorption from vegetable foods is about 50 per cent [3] but the FAO/WHO Expert Group has considered the absorption rate to be 33 per cent from *beta* carotene.

Conversion of Carotene to Vitamin A.   The conversion of carotene to vitamin A occurs primarily in the intestinal wall and not in the liver as was originally believed. The conversion is influenced by the thyroid gland. Thyroidectomy and thiourea drugs inhibit this conversion.

Plasma Vitamin A and Carotenoids.   The plasma values markedly fluctuate depending upon the season and the diet. Retinol is measured by the formation of blue colour with antimony trichloride. The normal plasma value of *retinol* is about 39 µg (130 IU) per 100 ml, although lower values are found during pregnancy and childbirth. The total *carotenoid* content of human plasma averages about 130 μg per 100 ml but varies considerably depending upon the vegetables and fruits in season.

Storage

Vitamin A is almost entirely stored in the liver in the form of an ester. A well-nourished healthy person stores 60–100 micrograms retinol per g of liver, i.e. about 120,000 micrograms retinol in the whole liver, which is sufficient to last for years.

Excretion

Unlike water-soluble vitamins, vitamin A is not excreted in the *urine* in healthy persons but it is found if there is proteinuria. *Stools* contain small amounts of carotene and vitamin A. Excretion in *milk* varies according to the ability of the animal to convert carotene into vitamin A. Human and cow's milk contain both carotene and vitamin A, while buffalo's milk contains vitamin A alone.

The mode of *destruction* of vitamin A is not known.

Source [TABLE 17]

The ultimate source of all vitamin A is carotene. Animals and fishes eat plant carotene which is converted into vitamin A and stored in the liver. Carnivorous animals or fishes derive the preformed vitamin A from the livers of their victims.

The usual sources of retinol are cod-, shark- and halibut-liver oils, and the livers of goat, sheep and cow. Eggs contain vitamin A as well as carotene.

Cow's milk contains 45 μg (150 IU) and buffalo's milk 72 μg (240 IU) retinol per 100 ml. Since vitamin A is concentrated in fat, skimmed milk contains little retinol. The retinol content of human milk is high in early lactation, 14 μg (45 IU) per g of fat, and gradually falls to 9 μg (30 IU) per g of fat [4].

Vegetables and fruits provide carotene but no preformed vitamin A. The carotene content is high in green vegetables (spinach), yellow vegetables (carrots, tomatoes), and yellow fruits (papaya, mangoes).

Vegetable oils such as olive oil, *til* oil and groundnut oil *do not* contain vitamin A. *Red palm oil* is probably the only vegetable oil rich in carotene. The red palm is grown in Africa, Brazil and Indonesia. Under Government of India regulations all vegetable oil products

TABLE 17

VITAMIN A OR CAROTENE CONTENT OF VARIOUS FOODS

FOOD	VITAMIN A IU/100 G*	RETINOL µg
Halibut-liver oil	4,000,000	1,200,000
Cod-liver oil	200,000	60,000
Liver, sheep	45,000	13,500
Liver, ox	15,000	4500
Liver, pig	5000	1500
Liver, calf	4000	1200
Butter	3500	1050
Cheese (whole fat)	1500	450
Eggs, hen	1100	330
Kidney, ox	1000	200
Salmon, canned	250	75
Milk, summer	150	45
Herrings, fresh	100	30
Milk, winter	75	22
Beef or mutton	20	6

FOOD	CAROTENE IU/100 G*	CAROTENE µg	RETINOL µg
Carrots, mature	20,000	12,000	6000
Spinach	13,000	7800	3900
Spinach beet leaves	11,000	6600	3300
Carrots, young	10,000	6000	3000
Cress	8000	4800	2400
Kale	8000	4800	2400
Sweet potato	6000	3600	1800
Watercress	5000	3000	1500
Apricot	2000	1200	600
Lettuce	2000	1200	600
Tomato	1200	720	360
Peach	800	480	240
Brussels sprouts	700	420	210
Cabbage	500	300	150
Maize, yellow	350	210	105

* Moore, T. (1959) Vitamin A, *Practitioner*, **185**, 5.
1 IU vitamin A = 0·3 µg of retinol
0·6 µg of β-carotene.

(*vanaspati*) for consumption must contain 210 μg (700 IU) of retinol per 30 g of vegetable oil product.

Commercial sources are from natural vitamin A extracted from the livers of fish like the shark in India and the cod and halibut in colder regions. Halibut-liver oil is the richest source of vitamin A, containing 200 μg (600–700 IU) per drop, while a teaspoonful of cod and shark-liver oil contains 600 μg (2000 IU) and 300 μg (1000 IU) respectively.

Injectable water-dispersible forms of vitamin A are also available commercially.

Requirements

The recommendations for vitamin A requirements differ. The only available data are based on human studies from the Medical Research Council of Great Britain [5]. As mentioned before, requirements for men are greater than those for women [1].

Vitamin A requirements can be expressed as: (1) total vitamin A requirements; (2) total carotene requirements; or (3) estimated combined requirements of vitamin A derived from animal foods and carotene derived from vegetable foods.

RECOMMENDED INTAKE OF RETINOL AT VARIOUS AGES*

AGE	RECOMMENDED INTAKE μg RETINOL PER DAY	AGE	RECOMMENDED INTAKE μg RETINOL PER DAY
0–6 months	**	10–12 years	575
6–12 months	300	13–15 years (boys/girls)	725
1 year	250	16–19 years (boys/girls)	750
2 years	250	Adults (man/woman)	750
3 years	250	Pregnancy	750
4–6 years	300	Lactation	1200
7–9 years	400		

Note: For diets containing both carotene and retinol.

  * *Wld Hlth Org. techn. Rep. Ser.*, No. 362 (1967).

  ** For infants of 0 to 6 months, it is accepted that breast feeding by a well-nourished mother is the best way to satisfy the nutritional requirements for vitamin A.

The vegetarian gets preformed vitamin A from milk and the required amount of carotene is easily supplied by 100 g of fruits (mango, papaya) or from green or yellow vegetables.

Action

On the Retina. The retina of most vertebrates contains two kinds of light receptors—rods for vision in dim light, and cones for vision in bright light and for colour vision. The rods and cones contain a photosensitive pigment which bleaches on exposure to light. This leads to nervous excitation which is transmitted to the brain and produces visual sensations [6]. The oxidation of retinol forms *retinal* (retinaldehyde) and its combination with the protein *opsin* forms *rhodopsin* or *visual purple*. It is unstable, and with light breaks down again into retinal and opsin. In the dark rhodopsin is formed again, but with vitamin A deficiency the resynthesis is delayed.

On the Body. 1. *Mucous membrane.* Vitamin A maintains the mucous membranes in the healthy state but the mode of action is not fully understood. Vitamin A is therefore credited with 'anti-infective' action, as an unhealthy mucous membrane is easily invaded by bacteria.

2. *Bone.* Vitamin A is also concerned with growth of bone and takes part in the formation of bony matrix.

3. Vitamin A has some role in the *steroid metabolism.*

DEFICIENCY

Deficiency occurs when the *intake* of vitamin A, or its precursor carotene, is poor. *Deficient fat ingestion* may also impair carotene absorption. Intestinal *malabsorption,* fatty diarrhoea, and habitual intake of *liquid paraffin* cause vitamin A deficiency. In advanced *liver diseases,* such as cirrhosis of the liver and *biliary obstruction,* there is vitamin A deficiency.

Vitamin A deficiency is very common in India, especially in children, due to inadequate intake [7] aggravated by a low-protein diet that probably reduces the synthesis of retinol binding protein.

Basic Pathology

Epithelial cells do not differentiate and undergo squamous metaplasia with vitamin A deficiency. The basal cells of the mucous membrane proliferate but the more superficial cells do not differentiate. In the absence of cilia in the superficial layers of mucous membrane, stagnation of secretion occurs where bacteria proliferate. Infection persists, as the circulating antibodies cannot reach the invading bacteria. *In the bone*, suppression of osteoclastic function decreases bony resorption. The bones become thick, compressing the brain, optic nerves and spinal cord.

Clinical Manifestations

Clinical manifesttions of vitamin A deficiency are found in the eye, mucous membranes of the respiratory, alimentary and genito-urinary tracts, and the skin.

Eye. Deficiency of vitamin A commonly produces changes in the eyes. Low intake of carotene and vitamin A in 436 children in labour camps showed marked eye changes in 27 per cent [8].

(1) *Night blindness (nyctalopia)*. In dim light visual purple (rhodopsin) in the rods is converted into chemical energy. With vitamin A deficiency rhodopsin is not formed and vision in dim light is not possible, so-called 'night blindness'. (2) *Xerophthalmia (xeros=dry)*. In this condition the conjunctiva becomes dry and lustreless. The glistening transparent appearance is lost. When the eyeball is rotated to one side, the conjunctiva appears in folds due to the loss of elasticity. (3) *Bitot's spots*. These are localized elevated areas formed on the temporal and sometimes on the nasal side of the conjunctiva. If they are scraped and examined under the microscope, corneal epithelial debris and xerosis bacilli are found. These bacilli are saprophytes and of no aetiological significance. (4) *Keratomalacia (softening of the cornea)*. The cornea may be affected in severe vitamin A deficiency. It becomes dull and vascularization takes place at the periphery. Ulcers are formed due to infection; these may perforate and vision is lost.

Mucous Membranes. (1) *Respiratory tract*. In vitamin A deficiency the mucous membranes of the nose, throat, trachea and bronchi become rough and dry, resulting in stasis and bacterial infection. (2) *Alimentary tract*. Thickening and dryness of the alimentary tract results in diminished secretion of digestive juices, impaired absorption and increased liability to intestinal infection and diarrhoea. Patients with nutritional diarrhoea due to vitamin A deficiency respond to vitamin A therapy in 48 hours.

Genito-urinary Tract. Vaginitis in females, urinary tract infection and a tendency to stone formation have been ascribed to vitamin A deficiency

Skin. Deficiency of vitamin A produces changes in the epithelium. The skin becomes dry (xeroderma) and scaly. The prominence of hair follicles on the extensor surface of the arms, legs and buttocks is known as *follicular keratosis, toad skin* or *phrynoderma*. A rough and gritty sensation is felt when the hand is passed over the skin. Some authorities maintain that phrynoderma is due to deficiency of essential fatty acids and vitamin B complex factors, and is cured with safflower oil 5 ml three times daily and oral vitamin B complex [9].

Treatment

Prophylactic. A balanced diet, containing vegetables, fruits and milk, supplies adequate vitamin A. Vitamin A deficiency, particularly in malnourished children, may produce severe eye damage including blindness, and prophylactic measures are therefore most vital. The majority of Indians have a very poor intake of carotene and vitamin A during the major part of the year. However, even among the poor in India the ingestion of the popular carotene-rich *mango* in season builds up hepatic stores of vitamin A that helps tide over the deficiency during the rest of the year.

The recommended prophylactic measures include: (1) 1 teaspoonful of cod-liver oil daily. (2) Feeding children daily 30 g *green vegetables* for 12 weeks, which maintains adequate serum levels for a subsequent 24 week carotene deprivation [10]. The carotene absorption is aided by fat in the diet. (3) *Red palm oil,* 4 ml daily providing 3000 IU carotene, is also useful for school children as it reduced the incidence of xerophthalmia in Indonesia [11]. (4) As a preventive measure at welfare clinics an oral dose of 100,000 micrograms vitamin A palmitate in 5 ml arachis oil serves to maintain a high serum vitamin A level for 6–3 months [12, 13]. Hepatic storage is better with *oral oil-soluble* vitamin A, rather than parenteral injection in oil, because the injected carrier fat is poorly absorbed. Thus, 6 monthly oral prophylaxis to children in undernourished areas could be highly effective.

Curative. 1. *Eye.* In night blindness a single dose of 300–1500 μg (1000–5000 IU) of vitamin A produces dramatic improvement.

In *xerophthalmia*, a higher dose of 7500–15,000 μg (25,000–50,000 IU) is advisable.

2. *Gastro-intestinal disorders.* If diarrhoea is present, vitamin A 3000–7500 μg (10,000–25,000 IU) daily in a water-dispersible form should be given parenterally.

3. *Skin lesions.* The skin manifestations of vitamin A deficiency may require larger dosage for prolonged periods. About 15,000 μg (50,000 IU) a day or more may be necessary for several weeks. Mistaken diagnosis of hypovitaminosis A for skin diseases frequently results in high vitamin A dosage and toxicity. A simple guide to the correct diagnosis of hypovitaminosis A is the fact that severe skin manifestations of deficiency are not likely without night blindness.

Topical application of 0·1–0·3 per cent of vitamin A acid (*retinoic acid*) has been effective in diseases associated with epidermal cell hyperplasia, e.g. psoriasis, lamellar ichthyosis and epidermolytic hyperkeratosis [14].

Sunlight sensitivity (erythropoietic porphyria) due to ultraviolet rays prevents outdoor sports activity. In such patients the tolerance to sunlight is increased with 100,000 IU *beta* carotene daily [15]. *Retarded wound healing* due to corticoid therapy can be improved with vitamin A therapy [16]

4. *Common cold, renal stones, etc.* Vitamin A is frequently prescribed for common cold and renal calculi. Unless there is a definite deficiency, the routine administration of vitamin A for these diseases is of no value.

Toxicity

Carotenaemia. Carotenaemia is manifested as a yellow discoloration of skin associated with a high carotene content of the blood. The condition should be distinguished from jaundice since in carotenaemia the sclera is not coloured yellow. Excessive ingestion of carotene-containing foodstuffs, such as carrots, papayas or mangoes may produce carotenaemia. In anorexia nervosa, hypercarotenaemia may be noted. In hypothyroidism and diabetes, carotene is not converted to vitamin A and carotenaemia may develop.

Hypervitaminosis A. Hypervitaminosis A occurs with a massive intake. It has occurred in explorers by eating the livers of fish (halibut) or polar bears. Ingestion of 4–5 ounces of halibut-liver oil (6 million IU vitamin

A) daily for 5 days produces toxicity. The symptoms of chronic toxicity include headache, blurred vision, nausea, vomiting, coarse hair, alopecia and liver enlargement. X-ray of the bones shows periosteal thickening. In children there may also be bulging of the fontanelle. *Treatment* consists in stopping the foods or preparations causing hypervitaminosis A.

Liver biopsy displays large lipid-laden Kupffer's cells.

CONGENITAL MALFORMATION. Congenital malformations have been experimentally produced in rats by massive dosage of vitamin A during pregnancy. The incidence is greatly enhanced by simultaneous administration of cortisone [17].

REFERENCES

[1] MOORE, T. (1959) Vitamin A, *Practitioner,* **185**, 5.

[2] KANAI, M., RAZ, A., and GOODMAN, DE W.S. (1968) Retinol binding protein. The transport protein for vitamin A in human plasma, *J. Clin. Invest.,* **47**, 2025.

[3] RAO, C.N., and RAO, B.S.N. (1970) Absorption of dietary carotene in human subjects, *Amer. J. clin. Nutr.,* **23**, 105.

[4] KON, S.K., and MAWSON, E.H. (1950) Human milk, *Spec. Rep. Ser. med. Res. Coun. (Lond.),* No. 269.

[5] HUME, E.A., and KREBS, H.A. (1949) Vitamin A requirements of human adults. An experimental study of vitamin A deprivation in man, *Spec. Rep. Ser. med. Res. Coun. (Lond.),* No. 264.

[6] WALD, G. (1953) Vision, *Fed. Proc.,* **12**, 606.

[7] CHANDRA, H., *et al.* (1960) Some observations on vitamin A deficiency in Indian children, *Indian, J. Child Hlth.,* **9**, 589.

[8] AYKROYD, W.R., and KRISHNAN, B.G. (1936) The carotene and vitamin A requirements of children, *Indian J. med. Res.,* **23**, 741.

[9] GOPALAN, C. (1967) Malnutrition in childhood in the tropics, *Brit. med. J.,* **4**, 603.

[10] PEREIRA, S.M., and BEGUM, A. (1968) Studies in the prevention of vitamin A deficiency, *Indian J. med. Res.,* **56**, 362.

[11] LIAN, O.K., *et al.* (1967) Red palm oil in the prevention of vitamin A deficiency. A trial in preschool children in Indonesia, *Amer. J. clin. Nutr.,* **20**, 1267.

[12] PEREIRA, S.M., and BEGUM, A. (1969) Prevention of vitamin A deficiency, *Amer. J. clin. Nutr.,* **22**, 858.

[13] SRIKANTIA, S.G., and REDDY, V. (1970) Effect of a single massive dose of vitamin A on serum and liver levels of the vitamin, *Amer. J. clin. Nutr.,* **23**, 114.

[14] FROST, P., and WEINSTEIN, G.D. (1969) Topical administration of vitamin A acid for ichthyosiform dermatosis and psoriasis, *J. Amer. med. Ass.,* **207**, 1863.

[15] MATHEW-ROTH, M.M., *et al.* (1970) Beta-carotene as a photoprotective agent in erythropoietic porphyria, *New Engl. J. Med.,* **282**, 1231.

[16] HUNT, T.K., *et al.* (1969) Effect of vitamin A on reversing inhibitory effect of
      cortisone on healing of open wounds in animals and man, *Ann. Surg.*,
      170, 633.
[17] MILLEN, J.W., and WOOLLAM, D.H.M. (1957) Influence of cortisone in terato-
      genic effects of hypervitaminosis A, *Brit. med. J.*, **2**, 196.

15. VITAMIN D

Deficiency of vitamin D was common in infants and children of
industrial towns in the temperate regions. The value of sunlight in
the prevention of rickets was demonstrated by Palm as early as 1890 [1].
He made an extensive geographical survey of rickets in many parts
of the world, including India, and concluded: 'A sunshine recorder
at an observatory on some hill-top is no guide to the amount of sunshine that reaches the street and alleys of smoky cities. It is important
that the sunshine recorder be of the form which indicates the chemical
activity of the sun's rays rather than the heat.' He recommended
the removal of rachitic children as early as possible from large towns
to a locality where sunshine abounds and the air is dry and bracing.

McCollum *et al.* in 1922 demonstrated that cod-liver oil contained
two forms of vitamins. One which easily got oxidized, cured xerophthalmia in rats, and the other, which resisted oxidation, was antirachitic. The former is known as vitamin A and the latter as vitamin D.

Chemistry

Antirachitic substances are those which prevent or cure rickets.
There are many substances having antirachitic activity, but of these,
only two, vitamins D_2 and D_3 are of importance.

Provitamins : Ergosterol and 7-Dehydrocholesterol.

Ergosterol, derived
from plants, was originally isolated from ergot, while 7-dehydrocholes-
terol is found in the skin. Structurally, ergosterol and 7-dehydrocholes-
terol have the same nucleus but different side chains, both act as pro-
vitamins and when irradiated with ultraviolet rays, become active
antirachitic substances.

Vitamin D_1.

An impure substance was named vitamin D_1, but this
term is now obsolete.

Vitamin D$_2$ (Calciferol). When *ergosterol* of vegetable origin found in ergot, fungi and yeast, is exposed to ultraviolet light, one of the several products formed is *calciferol,* or vitamin D$_2$. The name calciferol is derived from the fact that it helps to calcify bone and it is a sterol.

Dihydrotachysterol (A.T. 10). Dihydrotachysterol is another derivative of ergosterol. Like vitamin D it increases calcium absorption from the gut. It also aids in the excretion of phosphate in the urine and this action is similar to the parathyroid hormone. Since the excretion of phosphate is necessary for the maintenance of the calcium level in the blood, A.T. 10 is used for counteracting a low serum calcium level in hypoparathyroidism, but less expensive vitamin D is preferred.

Vitamin D$_3$ (Cholecalciferol). Vitamin D$_3$ is produced by the action of ultraviolet rays of sunlight on *7-dehydrocholesterol* which is present in the skin, and this forms the natural source of vitamin D$_3$ in man. Clothing and window glass interfere with exposure of skin to the ultraviolet rays of the sun.

25-Hydroxycholecalciferol (25-HCC) and 25-Hydroxyergocalciferol (25-HEC) [2]. The activity of vitamin D is due to its conversion into hydroxy forms. *Vitamin D$_3$* is converted in the liver to 25-hydroxycholecalciferol (25-HCC), which is metabolically quicker-acting and more potent than vitamin D$_3$. 25-HCC has been *isolated, identified* and *synthesized,* and has been located in the intestinal mucosa at subcellular level, where it takes part in the formation of DNA to produce alpha globulin which is a specific calcium-binding protein. *Vitamin D$_2$* is converted to metabolically active 25-hydroxyergocalciferol (25-HEC).

25-HCC and 25-HEC are useful in cases of vitamin D resistance, particularly in renal failure where there is a defect in the conversion of vitamin D into these active forms.

Biological Test of Vitamin D. In the prevention of human rickets there is no difference between vitamin D$_2$ and D$_3$. Experimentally, vitamin D$_3$ is probably more active than D$_2$ since 50,000–100,000 Units vitamin D$_3$ administered to monkeys results in toxicity that is not noted with similar doses of vitamin D$_2$ [3]. The biological test of vitamin D is the 'line test'. This consists of observing the line of calcification of bones by X-rays in rachitic rats fed on an unknown substance and comparing it with that produced by a standard, which is now taken to be calciferol.

Stability. Vitamin D is heat stable and ordinary boiling does not destroy it.

Unit. One International Unit of vitamin D is the activity of 0·025 micrograms of pure crystalline vitamin D_2 (calciferol). Thus 1 mg calciferol = 40,000 International Units of vitamin D (1 microgram = 40 Units).

Absorption

Vitamin D is absorbed together with fat from the intestine. Bile emulsifies fat and aids absorption by intestinal lymphatics. Within 2–3 hours after oral administration of radioactive vitamin D_3 plasma activity is mostly located in the chylomicrons [4]. In fat malabsorption vitamin D absorption is reduced.

Storage

Vitamin D is stored mainly in the liver hence its high concentration in cod-, halibut- and shark-liver oils. It is also found in the brain, skin and bones.

Excretion

Vitamin D is excreted in milk; the oral dose is excreted through bile in the faeces and only about 3 per cent of titrium-labelled vitamin D_3 is excreted in an inactive form in the urine after 48–72 hours.

Action

There is a complex relationship between vitamin D and *parathyroids*. Changes in serum calcium due to vitamin D alters parathyroid function; hence the exact role of vitamin D is difficult to assess.

1. *Absorption of calcium.* The action of vitamin D helps in the DNA synthesis to form a calcium-binding protein, alpha$_2$ globulin [5] that also forms the transport protein.

2. *Maintenance of calcium and phosphorus levels.* Vitamin D maintains a proper concentration of calcium and phosphorus in the blood by reabsorption of phosphorus from the urinary tubules. The calcium level is normally maintained at 10 mg and phosphorus at 3·5–5 mg per 100 ml serum.

3. *Bone formation.* Vitamin D is claimed to help deposition of crystalline rather than amorphous calcium phosphate in bones by supplying calcium and phosphorus in proper concentration to the bony matrix. The latter is formed with the aid of proteins, vitamins A and C and the sex hormones, androgen and oestrogen. The exact role of vitamin D in this process is not known.

In animals vitamin D increases hepatic cholesterol, total fat and fatty acids [6].

Source

1. FOOD. Only few food-stuffs contain vitamin D. The natural sources are egg yolk, milk and butter. A vegetarian diet does not contain vitamin D unless milk is taken. The vitamin D content of food depends upon the exposure of the fowl or milch animal to sunlight. Vitamin D is found in livers of all animals and is plentiful in oils derived from fish liver. Vitamin D is usually added to commercial baby food milk powders.

2. SUNLIGHT. The best and unlimited source of vitamin D is natural sunlight, which converts 7-dehydrocholesterol in the skin into vitamin D.

3. COMMERCIAL. (a) *Calciferol* provides a highly concentrated form of vitamin D.

(b) *Liver oils.* Cod-, shark- and halibut-liver oils form a good source of vitamin D for therapeutic administration.

Many commercial preparations of vitamin D are available with calcium salts. Vitamin D deteriorates rapidly when mixed with minerals like calcium, which may cause a loss in the vitamin content within one to two months.

Requirements

RECOMMENDED DAILY INTAKE OF VITAMIN D[*]

	μg	UNITS[**]
Birth — 6 years	10	400
7 years and over	2·5	100
Pregnancy (second and third trimesters)	10	400
Lactation	10	400
Adults	2.5	100

[*] *Wld Hlth Org. techn. Rep. Ser.,* No. 452 (1970), p. 33.
[**] 1 μg of cholecalciferol = vitamin D 40 IU.

In tropical countries a considerably lower quantity than the above recommended intake can be taken orally, provided the skin is exposed to sunlight for $\frac{1}{2}$–1 hour daily.

DEFICIENCY

Deficiency of vitamin D leads to diminished absorption of calcium and consequent low plasma calcium which may produce tetany [p. 191]. Low plasma calcium stimulates the parathyroids to mobilize bone calcium for raising the plasma calcium level. The bones are thus depleted of calcium salts. The symptoms of vitamin D deficiency are more commonly manifested as: (1) *rickets* during skeletal growth in children; or (2) *osteomalacia* in adults due to increased demand of calcium during pregnancy or deficient intake in old age.

Rickets

Rickets is common in the economically poorer countries but is noted even in Glasgow [7] and New York, among the Negroes and slum dwellers, more frequently due to *breast feeding* for over 9 months by poorer people and immigrants. Rickets is due to lack of deposition of calcium phosphate in the bones. During normal bone growth there is first proliferation of epiphyseal cartilage of the growing end of the bones and this is followed by invasion of the cartilage by blood vessels and deposition of calcium and phosphate (phosphate is abundant in the diet, and its deficiency does not occur). In rickets, bone formation is impeded but the proliferating activity of the cartilage becomes excessive giving rise to palpable swelling at the growing ends of long bones and at the costochondral junctions, producing the classical clinical deformities of rickets.

The manifestations of rickets include neuromuscular irritability, failure to thrive, and bony deformities. There are prominent frontal bosses with a large head, softened cranial bones (craniotabes) and delayed closure of cranial sutures. In the ribs there are prominent costochondral junctions (rickety rosary), depression of the ribs along the attachment of the diaphragm (Harrison's sulcus) and retraction of the chest (funnel chest). There is prominence of wrists, knees and ankles. Deformity of the weight-bearing bones give rise to kyphoscoliosis, bowing of the legs and knock knees.

Osteomalacia

In osteomalacia (*malacia* = softening) there is decrease in the mineral content due to lack of deposition of calcium phosphate. There is also bony resorption of minerals due to increased parathyroid activity following low plasma calcium. Osteomalacia occurs when there is less calcium in the body than required due to one or more of the following factors: (1) deficient intake; (2) deficient absorption as with fatty diarrhoea; (3) excessive excretion as occurs during lactation or sometimes with diseases of the kidneys; and (4) excessive demand as in pregnancy.

Osteomalacia used to be common in Eastern countries amongst women, particularly those observing *purdah*. The reasons for their low calcium level are: (1) a poor diet and a low intake of milk; (2) the calcium in the diet is not well absorbed because the *purdah* and the clothing completely protect them from exposure to sunlight and so vitamin D is also deficient; and (3) repeated pregnancies and prolonged lactation further deplete the calcium stores.

Dietary osteomalacia occurs in food faddists and in old women living alone whose dietary vitamin D intake is less than 70 IU, a not uncommon occurrence even in affluent Great Britain. The osteomalacia is entirely due to deficient intake, as small doses of vitamin D are adequate for therapy. *Epileptics* treated with phenobarbitone and phenytoin may develop osteomalacia. The liver enzyme induction probably increases vitamin D destruction [8]. *Post-gastrectomy* osteomalacia may occur in 3 per cent of women and 1 per cent of men. The remarkable response even to injection of 100 Units daily or 1000 Units weekly results in disappearance of bone pains and healing of pseudo-fracture. The response to small dosage denotes primary deficiency of vitamin D [9].

Clinically, osteomalacia manifests as skeletal pain, bony tenderness and fractures. Tetany may occur when the level of ionizable serum calcium is low. X-ray of the bones shows the normal bony matrix but the density is less, the bones may be deformed and pseudo-fractures (Looser's zones) may be seen. This is in contrast to the reabsorption of bone in hyperparathyroidism where calcium as well as the bony matrix are absorbed giving rise to a cystic appearance of the bones (osteitis fibrosa cystica).

Vitamin D Resistance in Chronic Renal Diseases

Chronic uraemic states produce metabolic defects that *prevent* vitamin

D_3 *conversion* to metabolically active 25-hydroxycholecalciferol. There is also *urinary loss* of protein-bound vitamin D_3 and 25-hydroxy-cholecalciferol [10]. If high doses of vitamin D are required, however, one should be guided by the serum level which should be kept below 10 mg.

Treatment

Prophylactic. The amount of vitamin D required to prevent rickets in infants and children will depend upon their exposure to sunlight and diet. A total daily intake of 400 Units of vitamin D from cod-liver oil protects against rickets. Vitamin D-enriched milk, sold in Western countries, containing 400 Units per litre, meets the daily requirements.

Curative. For the therapy of rickets and osteomalacia 5000 to 10,000 Units of vitamin D in the form of calciferol is given daily by mouth. Natural vitamin D_3 can also be given as cod-, halibut- or shark-liver oil.

INJECTION OF CALCIFEROL (D_2). Concentrated vitamin D injections for the routine treatment of tetany, osteomalacia or rickets are not advised as oral administration is quite effective.

Massive doses of vitamin D are useful in the treatment of the Fanconi syndrome which is a rare disease with congenital defects of the renal tubules resulting in excessive excretion in the urine of phosphates, amino acids and sugar (without hyperglycaemia). The mineral disturbance results in defective bone formation.

Hypoparathyroidism requires 1–2 mg (40,000–80,000 Units) vitamin D daily, along with liberal milk intake to supply calcium. The blood calcium level should determine the dosage of vitamin D.

Hypervitaminosis D

Massive therapy can be harmful. With increasing dosage of vitamin D almost all the dietary calcium is absorbed. Excess of vitamin D probably also causes reabsorption of calcium from the bones, exhibiting on X-ray generalized or localized osteoporosis. There is a tendency for drug manufacturers to prepare vitamins of high concentrations for parenteral injection. Many over-anxious mothers often give their children large doses of vitamin D with a view to forming strong bony structure. The serum calcium level is, therefore, raised. The parathyroid gland is concerned in the excretion of phosphorus in the urine, but with the rise in the serum calcium level, the activity of the parathyroid gland is depressed and the serum phosphorus level rises. The increased serum level of both calcium and phosphorus results in abnormal calcification in the kidneys, blood vessels and other organs.

Clinical Manifestations of Hypervitaminosis D. The commonest symptoms are anorexia (which may prompt the mother to give more vitamins), nausea, vomiting and constipation. Kidney involvement results in retention of urea and impaired renal function tests. The serum calcium and phosphorus values are high.

Vitamin D intoxication has been reported after 12 and 17 days of massive therapy with 750,000 International Units daily in two cases of fracture. In one fatal case, a doctor overdosed with vitamin D his own child suffering from pulmonary tuberculosis.

A committee of the British Paediatric Association estimated that following food fortification with vitamin D, a British infant consumed 4000 International Units daily, and strongly advocated steps to safeguard against the possible risks of an unnecessarily high intake of vitamin D. They recommended a reduction in the content of vitamin D in cod-liver oil, dried milk and cereal for infants [13, 14].

Treatment. This consists of stopping vitamin D intake, administration of plenty of fluids, low calcium diet and, if necessary, administration of cortisone to reduce the serum calcium level. Cortisone acts antagonistically to vitamin D by: (1) increasing vitamin D turnover rate; (2) diminishing production of active metabolites of vitamin D, thus diminishing intestinal calcium absorption [15]. Calcium cellulose phosphate 15 g daily in divided doses is also useful.

Hypoparathyroid patients during treatment may get vitamin D poisoning, but thereafter may become more sensitive to vitamin D, requiring a tenth of their former dose [16].

REFERENCES

[1] PALM, T.A. (1890) The geographical distribution and aetiology of rickets, *Practitioner,* **45,** 270 and 321.

[2] DE LUCA, H.F. (1969) Vitamin D, *New Engl. J. Med.,* **231,** 1103.

[3] HUNT, R.D., GARCIA, F.G., and HEGSTED, D.M. (1969) Hypervitaminosis D in New World monkeys, *Amer. J. clin. Nutr.,* **22,** 358.

[4] THOMPSON, G.R., LEWIS, B., and BOOTH, C.C. (1966) Absorption of vitamin D_3-3H in control subjects and patients with intestinal malabsorption, *J. clin. Invest.,* **45,** 94.

[5] WASSERMAN, R.H., CORRADINO, R.A., and TAYLOR, A.N. (1968) Vitamin D-dependent calcium-binding protein: Purification and properties, *J. biol. Chem.,* **243,** 3978.

[6] DALDERUP, L.M. (1968) Vitamin D, cholesterol and calcium, *Lancet,* **i,** 645.

[7] RICHARDS, I.D.G., SWEET, E.M., and ARNELL, G.C. (1968) Infantile rickets persists in Glasgow, *Lancet,* **i,** 803.

[8] DENT, C.E., RICHENS, A., ROWE, D.J.F., and STAMP, T.C.B. (1970) Osteomalacia with long-term anti-convulsant therapy in epilepsy, *Brit. med. J.,* **4,** 69.

[9] MORGAN, D.B., *et al.* (1965) Osteomalacia after gastrectomy. A response to very small doses of vitamin D, *Lancet,* **ii,** 1089.

[10] AVIOLI, L.V., BIRGE, S.J., and SLATOPOLSKY, E. (1969) The nature of the vitamin D resistance in patients with chronic renal disease, *Arch. intern. Med.,* **124,** 451.

[11] ANDERSON, D.C., COOPER, A.F., and TAYLOR, G.J. (1968) Vitamin D intoxication, with hypernatraemia, potassium and water depletion and mental depression, *Brit. med. J.,* **4,** 744.

[12] DEBRE, R. (1948) Toxic effects of overdosage of vitamin D_2 in children, *Amer. J. Dis. Child.,* **75,** 787.

[13] BRITISH MEDICAL JOURNAL (1956) Hypercalcaemia in infants and vitamin D, *Brit. med. J.,* **2,** 149.

[14] BRITISH MEDICAL JOURNAL (1957) Welfare foods, *Brit. med. J.,* **2,** 284.

[15] AVIOLI, L.V., BIRGE, S.J., and LEE, S.W. (1968) The effects of prednisone on vitamin D metabolism in man, *J. clin. Endocr.* **28,** 1341.

[16] LEESON, P.M., and FOURMAN, P. (1966) Increased sensitivity to vitamin D after vitamin D poisoning, *Lancet,* **i,** 1182.

16. VITAMIN E (Tocopherols)

Evans and Bishop in 1922 found that female rats required a factor for normal pregnancy which was known as the antisterility vitamin. However, the role of vitamin E in human nutrition remained in doubt. It is only during the last few years that the role of vitamin E in erythrocyte survival in *premature* infants has been recognized. 'Born into the vitamin family 40 years ago ... it has had a long uphill struggle to attain the present status and dignity' [1].

Chemistry

Substances which promote fertility in animals are called tocopherols (*tocos* = childbirth, *phero* = to bear) and are grouped as vitamin E. There are several (about 8) naturally occurring tocopherols with vitamin E activity. *Alpha* tocopherol is the most active and is the main tocopherol in animal tissue. The tocopherols are fat-soluble and inhibit oxidation (*anti-oxidant*). Vegetable oils are protected from rancidity by their tocopherol content.

Stability. Although they act as reducing agents and prevent oxidation, tocopherols are nevertheless easily destroyed by oxidation and ultraviolet light. The acetate is not so easily oxidized, however, and is therefore marketed as tocopherol acetate. *Loss* during ordinary cooking is less, but deep frying destroys about 75 per cent of vitamin E. In the presence of dilute *hydrogen peroxide, erythrocyte haemolysis* occurs more easily in vitamin E deficiency. *Synthesis* of vitamin E has been accomplished.

Standardization. One mg of synthetic *alpha* tocopherol acetate is used as a standard. An unknown substance is compared to it for fertility in vitamin E-deficient female rats. *One International Unit* is the potency of 1 mg *alpha* tocopherol acetate.

Absorption. *Alpha* tocopherol is readily absorbed along with fats. Normal *plasma* tocopherol values are about 1 mg per 100 ml in adults. In newborn infants the level is low, 0·25–0·4 mg per 100 ml. *Peroxidase* haemolysis test is a useful index of plasma vitamin E level. *Storage* sites are the liver and adipose tissue.

Excretion. Intravenously administered radioactive vitamin E is excreted in the course of a week, mainly by the liver and to a lesser extent in the urine.

Source [TABLE 18]

Tocopherols are found in fats, oils, cereals, poultry, meat and fish. They are not synthesized in the body. The tocopherol content of human milk is higher than that of cow's milk.

Requirements

For *males* 30 IU and for *females* 25 IU daily are recommended.

TABLE 18

ALPHA TOCOPHEROL CONTENT OF TYPICAL FOODS AS SERVED ON THE TABLE*

	SERVING g	ALPHA TOCOPHEROL mg
FRUITS AND VEGETABLES		
Apple, 1 medium (fresh)	150	0·46
Banana, 1 medium	150	0·33
Cantaloupe, ½ medium	150	0·21
Celery, 3″ × 5″ (stalk)	50	0·19
Onion rings (French fried)	50	0·36
Peas, ½ cup (fresh)	80	0·44
Potatoes, 10 pcs (French fried)	50	0·22
Strawberies, ½ cup (frozen)	100	0·21
Tomato, 1 medium	150	0·60
Tomato juice, ½ cup	100	0·22
CEREAL, PULSE AND BEANS		
Beans, ½ cup (baked)	130	0·18
Bread, 2 slices (whole wheat)	46	0·20
Cornmeal, 1 cup (cooked yellow)	28**	0·18
Rice, 1 cup (white)	168	0·30
MEAT, FISH AND POULTRY		
Bacon, 3 strips	23	0·12
Chops, 2 lamb	70	0·12
Chops, 2 pork	140	0·24
Chicken, ¼ (broiled)	85	0·31
Haddock, 1 fillet	105	0·63
Ham, 2 slices	60	0·17
Hamburger, 1 large	82	0·30
Liver, 2 slices (beef)	74	0·47
Liverwurst, 3 slices	90	0·33
Scallops, 5–6 (deep fried)	145	0·87
Shrimp, 4–6 (deep fried)	50	0·30
Steak, salmon	100	1·35
Steak, T-bone	120	0·16
DAIRY PRODUCTS		
Butter, 3 pats	30	0·30
Chocolate bar, 1	50	0·55
Egg, 1	54	0·25
Ice-cream, ⅙ chocolate	95	0·34

TABLE 18 *(Contd.)*

ALPHA TOCOPHEROL CONTENT OF TYPICAL FOODS AS SERVED ON THE TABLE*

	SERVING g	ALPHA TOCOPHEROL mg
DESSERTS		
Apple pie, 1 slice	160	4.00
Blueberry, 1 slice	160	4.99
Cookies, 3 wafer type	75	0.39
Cup cakes, 2 chocolate	120	0.16
Cookie, 1 peanut butter/oatmeal	75	1.50
NUTS		
Peanuts, 15–17 (roasted)	15	1.16
Pound cake, 1 slice	30	0.33

* *Adapted from:* Bunnell, R.H., Keating, J., Quaresimo, A., and Parman, G.K. (1965) The alpha tocopherol content of foods, *J. clin. Nutr.,* **17,** 17.
** Dry weight.

Human milk provides adequate tocopherol for *infants.* An average adult diet contains enough tocopherol, and this tocopherol content is directly related to the diet's fat and caloric content. The low fat diet sometimes recommended for heart disease may result in vitamin E deficiency.

Action

As it is anti-oxidant, vitamin E may act by preventing oxidation of cellular constituents and thereby prevent accumulation of toxic oxidation products. It is also possible that vitamin E has its action linked with enzyme systems. Adult humans maintained on a low tocopherol diet for years, exhibit increased erythrocyte susceptibility to peroxidase haemolysis and later to decreased erythrocyte survival time.

DEFICIENCY

In Animals

Experimental deficiency in female rats causes foetal death and frequently reabsorption of the foetus. A male rat develops irreversible testicular changes and sterility. Animals have also been shown to develop muscular dystrophy and paralysis.

In Man

Deficiency occurs on low fat diet, malabsorption syndrome, or after gastric surgery. Innumerable claims for the use of vitamin E in man are made in sterility and abortion. Good results in habitual abortion are obtained with general measures alone [2] without the use of vitamin E. Large doses of vitamin E have also been administered to patients with muscular dystrophies and coronary heart disease, although without definite effect.

Human vitamin E deficiency results in:

(1) *Macrocytic megaloblastic anaemia* in *protein-calorie malnutrition* in children [3]. It does not respond to any other haematinic, but responds to vitamin E. (2) *Premature infants* have tocopherol deficiency resulting in *oedema* and *haemolytic* anaemia. The deficiency may not exist at birth but may occur with formula diet. Vitamin E administration results in rise in haemoglobin, a fall in reticulocytes [4] and disappearance of oedema. (3) *Malabsorption syndrome* from any cause may be associated with poor fat and consequent tocopherol absorption. There is decreased erythrocyte survival time, increased sensitivity to hydrogen peroxide and low plasma tocopherol that responds to *alpha* tocopherol administration [5]. (4) *Acanthocytosis* is a familial disease with inability to manufacture the *beta* globulin required for the formation of *beta* lipoprotein. In this disease the spiny erythrocytes are known as acanthocytes. Autohaemolysis is corrected with the administration of tocopherol, but the cell morphology does not change. (5) *Brown muscle pigment deposition* called *ceroid* occurs with tocopherol deficiency, resulting in brown bowel syndrome and myopathy.

Low plasma vitamin E is noted after gastric surgery.

Alpha tocopherol acetate preparation can be administered as tablets, capsules or in injectable form. The daily dose is 30–100 mg.

Toxic Effects

No toxic effect has been noted from administration of large doses of vitamin E.

REFERENCES

[1]　MASON, K.E. (1968) Haematologic aspects of vitamin E, Foreword, *Amer. J. clin. Nutr.*, **21**, 1.

[2] JAVERT, C.T., FINN, W.F., and STANDER, H.J. (1949) Primary and secondary spontaneous habitual abortion, *Amer. J. Obstet. Gynec.*, **57**, 878.

[3] WHITAKER, J., FORT, E.G., VIMOKESANT, S., and DANNING, J.S. (1967) Haematologic response to vitamin E in the anaemia associated with protein-calorie malnutrition, *Amer. J. clin. Nutr.*, **20**, 783.

[4] OSKI, F.A., and BARNESS, L.A. (1968) Haemolytic anaemia in vitamin E deficiency, *Amer. J. clin. Nutr.*, **21**, 45.

[5] HORWITT, M.K., CENTURY, B., and ZEMAN, A.A. (1963) Erythrocyte survival time and erythrocyte level after tocopherol depletion in man, *Amer. J. clin. Nutr.*, **12**, 99.

17. VITAMIN K

Dam and his associates working in Copenhagen demonstrated a haemorrhagic tendency in chicks fed on a fat-free diet. This was later found to be due to a specific vitamin deficiency, originally called *Koagulations vitamin* and now known as vitamin K. Vitamin K takes part in the formation of prothrombin and factors VII, IX and X by the liver. It is the discovery of vitamin K which enables surgeons to operate on cases of jaundice without fear of bleeding.

Chemistry

Natural and *synthetic* analogues of vitamin K are effective in maintaining normal coagulation of blood. The active substances are derivatives of naphthoquinone.

1. *Naturally* occurring forms of vitamin K are: (a) *vitamin K_1*, which is derived from plants (phylloquinones), is 2-methyl-3-phytyl-1. 4-naphthoquinone and is also known as *phytomenadione* (BP) or *phytonadione* (USP); it is available for therapy; (b) *vitamin K_2* is produced by *bacterial synthesis* (putrefied fish meal). Structurally, vitamin K_2 has a difarnesyl group instead of the phytyl group of vitamin K_1.

Vitamin K_1 is oil-soluble and so it is given orally or intramuscularly. Aqueous preparations of vitamin K_1 (aquamephyton) can also be given intravenously.

2. *Synthetic vitamin K_3* has antihaemorrhagic activity. The most potent substance is 2-methyl-1, 4-naphthoquinone known as *menadione* (USP) or *menaphthone* (BP). It is only slightly water-soluble. Water-

soluble synthetic preparations are also available for intravenous use (*Synkavit*).

All forms of vitamin K are equal in potency on a molar basis but menadione is the most active on weight basis.

Standardization. Many methods are advocated for the standardization of vitamin K. The best suggestion is that the potent synthetic menadione (2-methyl-1, 4-naphthoquinone) be adopted as a standard. This can be compared with the test substance in vitamin K-deficient animals.

Absorption

Vitamin K is absorbed from the small intestine with the aid of *bile salts*. In obstructive jaundice and malabsorption syndromes, lack of absorption of vitamin K leads to lowered coagulation activity in the blood.

Storage

Vitamin K is not stored in the body.

Excretion

Vitamin K is found in the faeces. The faecal vitamin K may be the result of that produced by the bacteria and may not indicate excretion through the intestine. Vitamin K is not excreted in the urine.

Action

The action of vitamin K is obscure. It probably acts as an enzyme in the formation of prothrombin and factors VII, IX and X. Vitamin K does *not* form a part of these coagulation factors and has no direct effect on the blood. The modes of action of all vitamin K derivatives are not identical. Vitamin K_1 and K_1 oxide (intravenous) are effective in counteracting the effect of the anticoagulant drug dicoumarol, but the action of the *synthetic* vitamin K analogue, *menadione,* against dicoumarol is not uniform, although *menadione* is a more potent anti-haemorrhagic compound.

Source

1. *Food.* Green vegetables, cereals and animal foods are sources of vitamin K.

2. *Bacterial synthesis.* Vitamin K is synthesized by the intestinal bacteria. The normal synthesis is inhibited by the intake of oral

antibiotics and vitamin K deficiency may be produced. A newborn infant has a sterile intestinal tract, and hence a low blood prothrombin level for about a week.

Requirements

It is not possible to estimate the daily human requirement as the intestinal flora synthesize this vitamin. A lowered prothrombin level can be corrected by even 1 or 2 mg of vitamin K if there is no liver damage. However, with liver damage more may be needed.

DEFICIENCY

Vitamin K deficiency manifests itself clinically as a tendency to bleed from the skin and mucous membranes, or as profuse oozing during a surgical operation. Two simple laboratory procedures are used to detect vitamin K deficiency: (1) microscopic examination of the urine for the presence of red blood cells, which is a very simple procedure to arouse suspicion of prothrombin deficiency due to deficient vitamin K; and (2) a laboratory test for prothrombin.

Causes of Deficiency

Deficiency of vitamin K occurs in:

1. Deficient *production* by bacteria in the gut: (a) in newborn infants; (b) with prolonged antibiotic therapy.

2. Deficient vitamin K *absorption* due to malabsorption of fats.

3. Deficient *synthesis* of prothrombin due to liver disease or *anticoagulant therapy*.

Deficient Production by Bacteria in the Gut

(a) Newborn infants:

Normal. A newborn infant has a low plasma prothrombin and factors VII, IX and X levels due to sterile intestinal content, but by the end of the first week the bacterial flora synthesizes vitamin K. In *premature* infants the deficiency of blood coagulation factors is more marked.

Haemorrhagic diseases of the newborn. In diseases of the newborn such as icterus gravis neonatorum, anaemia neonatorum and hydrops congenitus, deficiency of vitamin K produces a lowered prothrombin level.

Treatment. (1) *Prophylactic.* Vitamin K, 2–5 mg, is administered orally to the mother every day for a week before delivery. (2) If the mother is seen just before labour, then 2–5 mg vitamin K is administered intravenously. (3) The infant is given a single dose of 1–2 mg vitamin K intramuscularly immediately after birth.

(b) Prolonged use of oral antibiotics:
Oral antibiotics given for more than a few days prevent the growth of intestinal bacteria and hence synthesis of vitamin K.
TREATMENT. Oral or parenteral synthetic vitamin K, 2–5 mg, is administered daily.

Deficient Absorption of Vitamin K

(a) *Diarrhoea* due to malabsorption of fats diminishes absorption of vitamin K and produces a tendency to haemorrhage. (b) *Biliary obstruction* by calculi, carcinoma of external biliary tract, results in deficient absorption of vitamin K.
TREATMENT. During an emergency, *fresh* blood transfusion helps for a few hours by supplying prothrombin. With prolonged diarrhoea or biliary obstruction, vitamin K, 5 mg, is administered parenterally every day.

Deficient Synthesis of Prothrombin

Synthesis of prothrombin by the liver is impaired in diseases such as viral hepatitis and cirrhosis. In prolonged obstructive jaundice, liver cell damage impairs prothrombin formation even if vitamin K is given parenterally.
TREATMENT. Administration of vitamin K, 10 mg orally with bile, or parenterally, in obstructive jaundice may help. Fresh blood transfusion may also be temporarily effective.

Anticoagulant Therapy. These drugs interfere with the synthesis of prothrombin and factors, VII, IX and X, and the levels may fall suddenly if: (1) there is coexistent liver damage; (2) oral antibiotics are administered simultaneously; (3) large doses of aspirin, salicylate, or para-aminosalicylic acid, which interfere with the formation of prothrombin, are also given. *Phenobarbitone* and *alcohol* stimulate the microsomal enzyme of the hepatic cell, thereby interfering with the action of anticoagulants.

During anticoagulant therapy it may be necessary to administer vitamin K if: (1) bleeding occurs; (2) prothrombin time is over 36 seconds (if normal, this is 12 seconds) or when the prothrombin ratio is over 3; or (3) tooth extraction or surgery is contemplated.

TREATMENT. (1) During an emergency the quickest prothrombin is provided by fresh blood transfusion and the effect lasts for 12 hours. (2) To counteract the effect of anticoagulants only vitamin K_1 is a reliable antidote and restores the prothrombin level within a few hours [1]. Other synthetic and more potent vitamin K derivatives have variable action even when given intravenously. It is not advisable to give a large dose of vitamin K to a patient on anticoagulant therapy as, with the restoration of plasma prothrombin activity to normal, the original risk of thrombosis remains and the subsequent anticoagulant therapy becomes more difficult. In these circumstances vitamin K_1, 5–10 mg, is effective and even a small oral dose of 2·5 mg has been found to correct the prothrombin level in 18 hours [2].

Unnecessary use of Vitamin K. No purpose is served by administering vitamin K in haemorrhagic diseases with a normal prothrombin time.

Toxicity

Excess of vitamin K does not raise the plasma prothrombin level above normal nor cause increased tendency to thrombosis [3], though it may produce nausea and vomiting. Paradoxically, excessive administration of vitamin K over a period has been reported to produce *hypoprothrombinaemia and alteration in liver function* [4]. Vitamin K analogue should be given with caution to infants and mothers in late pregnancy and should not exceed the usual therapeutic doses for prophylaxis or treatment [5], as otherwise hyperbilirubinaemia and kernicterus in premature infants may occur. The infant's liver capacity is limited for glucuronide formation, which is required for bilirubin conjugation as well as vitamin K excretion, and with excessive vitamin K, unconjugated bilirubin level may be markedly raised (kernicterus). The naturally occurring vitamin K_1 is less likely to result in haemolysis.

Moreover, in patients with glucose-6-phosphate dehydrogenase (G-6-PD) and deficiency of erythrocytes, a large dose of vitamin K results in haemolysis. For therapy more than 10 mg daily of vitamin K is best avoided as it is liable to depress liver function.

REFERENCES

[1] DOUGLAS, A.S., and BROWN, A. (1952) Effect of vitamin K preparations on hypoprothrombinaemia induced by dicoumarol and tromexan, *Brit. med. J.*, **1**, 412.

[2] SCHIRGER, A., Spittel, J.A., and Ragen, P.A. (1959) Small doses of vitamin K_1 for correction of reduced prothrombin activity. *Proc. Mayo Clin.*, **34**, 453.

[3] DAM, H., and GLAVIND, J. (1938) Determination of vitamin K by the curative blood-clotting method, *Biochem. J.*, **32**, 1018.

[4] SMITH, A.M., JR., and CUSTER, R.P. (1960) Toxicity of vitamin K induced hypoprothrombinaemia and altered liver function, *J. Amer. med. Ass.*, **173**, 502.

[5] LUCEY, J.F., and DOLAN, R.G. (1959) Hyperbilirubinaemia of new-born infants associated with the parenteral administration of a vitamin K analogue to the mothers, *Pediatrics*, **23**, 553.

18. BIOFLAVONOIDS (Vitamin P)

A group of substances found in nature which correct abnormal capillary permeability were collectively called permeability vitamins or vitamin P. These compounds when extracted have a yellow colour and are known as flavonoids. The flavonoids have biological activity and so are now called 'bioflavonoids'. During recent times, in the absence of dramatic claims by enthusiastic research workers, bioflavonoids are facing extinction.

Citrin. The original substance isolated by Szent-Györgyi from the rind of the citrus fruit lemon was named citrin. It was an impure substance. Later, one of the active principles, hesperidin, was isolated.

Hesperidin. It is the best known of the flavonoids derived from oranges and lemons.

Source

The best source of flavonoids are citrus fruits, particularly lemon.

Action

Bioflavonoids are claimed to aid in the absorption of vitamin C or act as anti-oxidants, thus sparing vitamin C.

Bioflavonoids may act by: (1) Maintaining or restoring the capillary permeability to normal. Capillary weakness results from the deficiency of these substances. (2) Counteracting the effect of other factors which injure the tissues [1].

Bioflavonoids in Clinical Medicine

In diseases associated with damage of the capillary wall there is exudation of plasma and red blood cells. In such diseases an adequate supply of vitamin C and bioflavonoids presumably reduce exudation in the skin, mucous membrane, central nervous system (poliomyelitis) and decidua (pregnancy).

Rheumatic Fever. The initial damage in rheumatic fever is injury and swelling of the ground substance of connective tissue particularly of the heart valves, heart muscles and joints. Vitamin C and bioflavonoids are important in maintaining the health of connective tissue and ground substance [2]. Good results were observed in cases of rheumatic fever by the administration of crude hesperidin, 0·75–1·5 g daily.

Poliomyelitis. In acute anterior poliomyelitis capillary integrity is lost, leading to oedema and damage to the nervous system. Daily administration of 600 mg each of hesperidin and vitamin C in divided doses in the acute stage enhances recovery [3].

Habitual Abortions. Some cases of habitual abortions have shown increased capillary permeability due to vitamin C and bioflavonoid deficiency. The use of hesperidin together with other measures improved the salvage rate in one series [4].

Anticoagulant Therapy. During the course of anticoagulant therapy, capillary leakage may occur. Without discontinuing the anticoagulant therapy the administration of vitamin C and bioflavonoid can clear minor purpuric areas [5]. With gross bleeding the anticoagulants must be stopped and administration of vitamin C and bioflavonoids forms a useful adjunct to vitamin K_1.

REFERENCES

[1] YOUMANS, J.B. (1955) Summary of the clinical aspects of bioflavonoids and ascorbic acid, *Ann. N.Y. Acad. Sci.*, **61**, 729.

[2] RINEHART, J.F. (1955) Rheumatic fever: observations on the histogenesis, pathogenesis and use of ascorbic acid and bioflavonoids, *Ann. N.Y. Acad. Sci.*, **61**, 684.

[3] BOINES, G.J. (1955) A rationale for the use of hesperidin and ascorbic acid in the management of poliomyelitis, *Ann. N.Y. Acad. Sci.*, **61**, 721.

[4] GREENBLATT, R.B. (1955) The management of habitual abortion, *Ann. N.Y. Acad. Sci.*, **61**, 713.

[5] BRAMBEL, C.E. (1955) The role of flavonoids in coumarin anticoagulant therapy, *Ann. N.Y. Acad. Sci.*, **61**, 678.

19. MINERALS

Minerals are inorganic substances like sodium, potassium, chloride, calcium, phosphorus, magnesium, iodine, iron, cobalt, copper, etc. Minerals resemble vitamins in not supplying any heat or energy to the human body. Minerals like sodium, potassium and chloride, play a vital role in the regulation of body fluids and acid base balance. The body can tolerate a deficiency of vitamins for a relatively long period but slight changes in the blood concentration of the important minerals may rapidly endanger life. A diminution in the plasma sodium level by 20–30 per cent may be fatal. Calcium helps to maintain neuro-muscular excitability, blood coagulation and bone formation. Phosphorus aids in tissue metabolism and bone formation. Iodine is concerned with the function of the thyroid gland. Iron is incorporated in the haemoglobin molecule. Cobalt helps in the formation of vitamin B_{12}.

In recent years the advances in antibiotics and other new drugs, and the rapid strides made in surgery, have tended to overshadow one of the most important developments in the last few decades, the clearer understanding of the fluid and electrolyte requirements of the body, an advance which owes much to the pioneering work of Gamble [1]. Many patients with haematemesis used to die of starvation and dehydration rather than of bleeding. The progress of major surgery owes more to better physiological management than to any other single factor. Many patients have died because food, water and electrolytes were withheld during prolonged fevers, particularly of the enteric group.

REFERENCE

[1] GAMBLE, J.L. (1947) *Chemical Anatomy, Physiology and Pathology of Extra-cellular Fluid*, Cambridge, Mass.

20. SODIUM

Atomic weight	= 23
Conversion factor	
mg per cent × 0·435	= mEq/1
Total body content	= 3900 mEq in 60 kg man [1]
	= (92 g expressed as sodium or 235 g expressed as NaCl)
Normal serum concentration	= 142 mEq/1
Daily requirement	= 4 g Na
	= 10 g as sodium chloride
Easy figures to remember—	
1 g NaCl	= 17 mEq
6 g NaCl	= 100 mEq
1 litre 0·85 per cent (isotonic saline)	= 140 mEq Na

Sodium forms 90 per cent base (cation) of the extracellular compartment (vascular and interstitial fluid). The osmotic pressure of extracellular fluid is almost entirely due to sodium. The total base of the extracellular fluid is 155 mEq per litre out of which sodium constitutes 142 mEq per litre (325 mg per cent).

Absorption and Administration

The body requirements of sodium are derived from food-stuffs and from the extra salt added during cooking or at the table. *Jejunal* sodium absorption is stimulated by the simultaneous presence of actively transported glucose, galactose, bicarbonate [2] or amino acids. During cholera epidemics, *oral* water, and sodium with the addition of glucose and glycine, help adequate intestinal absorption and are preferred to cumbersome intravenous therapy [3]. In the *ileum* there is an active efficient sodium absorption across the intestinal membrane. The human rectum does not absorb sodium, chloride and water while the rest of the *colon* does [4]. Sodium can be administered *subcutaneously* (as 0·45 per cent NaCl) or *intravenously* (often as 0·85 per cent NaCl, isotonic saline, but more concentrated solutions even up to 10 per cent can be given).

Excretion

Sodium is filtered by the glomeruli of the *kidneys* but is reabsorbed by the tubules. The suprarenal cortex maintains the plasma sodium level by reabsorption of sodium from the kidney tubules. A healthy kidney can conserve sodium and during extreme deficiency no urinary sodium is excreted. In *postural hypotension* diuresis occurs with recumbency [5].

Sweat contains 0·1 to 0·3 per cent sodium chloride. A healthy person in cold weather sweats little and 95 per cent of the total sodium excretion is through the kidneys. In hot weather with excessive sweating as much as 5 g of sodium (12·5 g sodium chloride) may be lost daily in the sweat. With acclimatization to heat much less sodium chloride is excreted in the sweat even in the hot weather because the sodium concentration of sweat decreases. In hypertensive patients sweat sodium excretion is reduced.

Function

Sodium is concerned in the maintenance of:
1. Fluid balance.
2. Muscle irritability.
3. Acid-base balance.
4. Osmotic pressure.

Requirement

The average requirement of sodium is 4 g (10 g as sodium chloride) a day which is easily supplied in a normal diet. Persons who sweat profusely require an additional 10 g sodium (25 g sodium chloride) per day which can be supplied as extra salt at the table.

The maintenance sodium requirement in infants, children and adults has been given in TABLE 19.

Sources

Salt added during cooking is the commonest source of sodium. Processed cheese, ham, bacon, sausages, dried fish, butter and nuts are rich in sodium as salt is *added* to them.

TABLE 19

NORMAL DAILY MAINTENANCE REQUIREMENT*

AGE	SODIUM mEq/KG	AS G OF SODIUM CHLORIDE PER KG BODY WEIGHT
3 days	0·88	0·052
1 to 3 years	0·80	0·047
4 to 6 years	0·72	0·042
10 to 12 years	0·56	0·033
15 years +	0·40	0·027
Adult	0·32	0·019

* Modified from Frank, H.A., Hastings, T.N., and Brophy, T.W. (1952) Fluid and electrolyte management in pediatric surgery, *West. J. Surg.*, **60**, 25.

DEFICIENCY

Sodium deficiency occurs when the intake is poor or when an excessive amount is lost. Sodium loss through profuse sweating causes sodium deficiency if the salt intake is not correspondingly increased. With the rapid industrialization in the tropics salt deficiency poses a problem in heavy manual workers and stokers. They suffer ill health, lassitude and tiredness, leading to lack of enthusiasm. This situation could be easily corrected by giving extra salt in food, drinks or as salt tablets.

The concentration of sodium in the various fluids in the body is given in TABLES 20 and 21. During an illness or surgical operation the total loss of sodium can be assessed by measuring all the fluids lost from the body.

Deficiency of sodium occurs due to:

Inadequate intake: (1) starvation; (2) therapeutic low salt diets as in cardiac failure, hypertension, cirrhosis of the liver and generalized oedema.

TABLE 20

THE APPROXIMATE CONCENTRATION OF SODIUM, POTASSIUM AND
CHLORIDE IN VARIOUS FLUIDS*

	SODIUM mEq/L	POTASSIUM mEq/L	CHLORIDE mEq/L
Urine, normal	40–90	20–90	40–120
Urine, pathological	0·5–312	5–166	5–210
Formed stool	10	10	15
Gastric	60	9	84
Small bowel (Miller-Abbott suction)	111	5	104
Ileostomy (recent)	130	11	116
Ileostomy (adapted)	46	3	21
Caecostomy	53	8	43
Bile fistula	149	5	101
Pancreatic fistula	141	5	77
Transudate	130–145	2·5–5	90–110

If an intake and output chart is accurately kept the above information helps in assessing the sodium loss and approximate amount of sodium chloride therefore required to replace the loss.

N.B. Figures are rounded up for convenience.

* Lockwood, J.S., and Randal, H.T. (1949) The place of electrolyte studies in surgical patients, *Bull. N.Y. Acad. Med.,* **25,** 228.

TABLE 21

TOTAL BODY SODIUM, SODIUM LOSS AND REPLACEMENT FLUID
EXPRESSED IN mEq, AND AS SODIUM CHLORIDE

	TOTAL mEq	APPROXIMATE WEIGHT AS SODIUM CHLORIDE
Body sodium (60 kg man)	3900	235 g
Sodium in blood vessels and interstitial space	3510	210 g
Excretion in stool	10	0·6 g
Excretion in urine	68	4 g
Mild sweat	10	0·6 g
Profuse sweating for a stoker	400	25 g
1 litre (1000 ml) 'normal saline'	140	9 g
1 pint normal saline	70	4·5 g

Excessive loss: (1) sweat; (2) gastro-intestinal secretions, e.g. vomiting, diarrhoea, intubation and suction, fistulae; (3) renal, e.g. diuretics, salt-losing renal disease; (4) endocrine, e.g. Addison's disease.

Estimation of Sodium Deficiency

The sodium deficit during an *acute* episode like surgical operation or gastro-enteritis may be about 400 mEq which depletes the body sodium by 10 per cent. Acute depletion of sodium by 30 per cent will lead to circulatory collapse and death. *Chronic* sodium loss as from continuous drainage from the gastro-intestinal tract may well be over 100 mEq per day.

In assessing sodium deficiency, a knowledge of the patient's recent food intake and of the quantity of all excreta and discharge is indispensable. *Pure sodium deficiency* causes giddiness, anorexia, cramps in muscles which are exercised the most, particularly calf muscles, collapsed veins, cold extremities and low blood pressure. *Associated water deficiency* is common. This produces in addition to the above symptoms oliguria, dry mouth, inelastic skin and disorientation. Electrolyte studies may be done to corroborate the existence of sodium deficiency. 'None of these, perhaps least of all, the chemical analysis, gives by itself all the information which we require for considered treatment.' The best guide for the diagnosis and therapy for fluids and electrolytes in an acute state is twelve-hourly evaluation of the patient with a complete intake and output chart.

Management of Salt Deficiency in an Emergency with Poor Facilities

When a physician is faced with the problem of seeing a patient with sodium deficiency where hospital facilities are not available the best guide is to *estimate the number of days* the patient has gone without food. The approximate minimum sodium chloride needs should be estimated as 500 ml of isotonic saline for each day of fasting, to this should be added about 100 ml of isotonic saline for each small stool the patient has passed. If the patient perspires moderately additional 500 ml isotonic saline should be given.

Example: A patient has been off food for two days, passing 5–6 small liquid stools daily and has not been visibly perspiring. He, therefore, requires at least 4 pints (2 litres) of isotonic saline (0·85 per cent).

Mode of Supplying Sodium Chloride

1. *Oral feeds.* Two to four ounces of vegetable soup with added salt to be given every two to three hours. If other foods are also taken liberally, no fluid or electrolyte disturbance need be feared if the total daily urinary output is over 1000 ml.

2. *Nasogastric intubation.* If the patient cannot be fed orally, a nasogastric tube should be passed and liquid feeds given.

3. *Rectal drip.* Oral or nasogastric feeds should always be aimed at. If they are not feasible when the patient is vomiting, a rectal drip can be resorted to. Some clinics use rectal saline at room temperature routinely after abdominal surgery. A teaspoonful of salt added to four glasses of boiled drinking water and put in as an enema can be given at room temperature. This approximates to 1000 ml of water with 5 g of sodium chloride. Before starting the rectal drip a low enema to evacuate the faecal matter from the lower bowel is advised. The flow of the drip is regulated at 15–20 drops a minute before inserting the tube high in the rectum. The amount of saline given is according to the amount of estimated loss.

Management in Hospital

When hospital facilities are available, the history, physical examination, a well-kept chart of fluid intake and output, and estimation of the serum electrolytes by flame photometer are of help in assessing the sodium loss and guide the therapeutic programme.

Intravenous. ISOTONIC SALINE. It is best to give sodium as sodium chloride either orally or through a nasogastric tube as advised above. If necessary, during an acute sodium deficiency such as with severe diarrhoea and vomiting, intravenous isotonic saline (0·85 per cent sodium chloride) infusion is given. One litre of isotonic saline contains 140 mEq sodium, hence approximately 3 litres (6 pints) may replace sodium loss of moderate degree such as 400 mEq, i.e. about 10 per cent loss of total body sodium.

HYPERTONIC SALINE. When sodium deficiency is marked it is not feasible to give adequate amounts of sodium as isotonic saline. In order to correct sodium deficiency the total fluid supplied as isotonic saline may be excessive for patients with pulmonary congestion, cardiac failure or when the volume of fluid required exceeds three litres. Hypertonic solution of 5 or even 10 per cent sodium chloride is then indicated. A patient with protracted vomiting was given 1700 mEq of sodium (100 g sodium chloride) in a single infusion with benefit.

Hyponatraemia (Water Introxication)

Hyponatraemia is usually defined as serum sodium below 130 mEq per litre and may be without symptoms. The *symptoms* occur due to overhydration of cells of the central nervous system, producing fatigue, weakness, confusion, twitchings, muscle cramps and convulsions.

Dilutional hyponatraemia occurs with excessive water *intake* or *absorbed* water through enema or bowel washes, or *impaired water excretion* in oedematous states of congestive cardiac failure, cirrhosis, nephrotic syndrome, hypo-albuminaemia, acute renal failure and chronic renal failure. In such patients, a low serum sodium in the absence of known deficient intake or excessive sodium loss is not an indication for saline therapy. The *treatment* is water restriction only.

SODIUM RETENTION

A healthy kidney regulates the excretion of sodium according to the intake, but oedema results when there is excessive retention of sodium. Sodium retention occurs with *kidney diseases* and with the use of *drugs* such as *liquorice,* cortisone and *sodium-containing drugs* as massive sodium penicillin therapy or antacids used for the therapy of peptic ulcer. Antacids, when analysed, contained between 12 and 270 mg sodium per 30 g (1 ounce) [6]. There is also a potential danger of sodium retention and pulmonary oedema in cases of rheumatic fever who are given *sodium salicylate* as well as cortisone. *Oestrogens* given in large doses for carcinoma of the prostate, and *reserpine* are also known to produce retention of sodium.

Hypernatraemia [7]

Hypernatraemia is the presence of serum sodium 150 mEq per litre and above. It is commoner in *infants* than in adults, as about 50 per cent of water loss in infants is from the skin and respiration. *Deficient water intake* is more often the cause of hypernatraemia, rather than increased intake of sodium.

Hypernatraemia may occur due to: (1) *decreased water intake:* in the postoperative state in elderly debilitated people, due to nausea, vomiting, difficulty in swallowing with sore throat, oesophageal diseases and cerebral impairment; (2) *increased water loss* through respiration, diarrhoea, vomiting or excessive urination in diabetes mellitus or chronic renal diseases; (3) *increased sodium intake;* (4) *deficient sodium excretion,* due to corticosteroid therapy, Cushing's syndrome or aldosteronism.

There is usually raised blood urea, raised extracellular osmolarity, and rapid transfer of water from cells which result in cellular dehydration. Shrinkage of brain in infants is believed to cause rupture of the cerebral veins and consequent intracranial haemorrhage of various types, cerebral venous and sinus thrombosis. The neurological symptoms, including convulsions, are more likely to occur 24 hours after commencing therapy with glucose or hypotonic saline during the stage of rapid *overhydration* and *oedema of the brain.* Therefore, to avoid overhydration, hypovalaemia is corrected immediately but total fluid replacement should be much more gradual [7].

Treatment. This is with oral salt-free fluids, or oral or intravenous 5 per cent glucose to combat hypovolaemia.

LOW SODIUM DIET

Retention of sodium in the body causes fluid retention producing oedema or ascites. A low sodium diet is indicated in oedema due to congestive cardiac failure, renal diseases, hepatic cirrhosis with ascites, toxaemia of pregnancy, and during prolonged administration of corticosteroids. In marked hypertension a very low sodium diet is of value.

It is not the concentration of sodium in the food-stuffs alone but also the total amount of the food-stuff consumed which determines the total sodium intake. Compared to milk, spinach has twice the concentration of sodium but an occasional helping of 60–100 g of spinach supplies far less sodium than the daily consumption of 500 ml of milk.

The diets can be divided into:

1. SODIUM-POOR DIET. Sodium-poor diet consists of foods which contain only a trace of sodium. As protein-rich foods contain an appreciable amount of sodium, a sodium-poor diet (0·2 g sodium) must necessarily be vegetarian. Milk is allowed for the preparation of beverages like tea or coffee. Cream and unsalted butter are permitted. An appreciable amount of protein can be given by allowing cereals and preparations made from cereal flour, pulses

(*dal*) and nuts (unsalted). Depending upon the clinical improvement, the sodium-poor diet may be changed to a 'low sodium diet' in order to prevent symptoms of sodium deprivation.

FOODS LOW IN SODIUM	FOODS HIGH IN SODIUM
Cereals, as wheat, rice, *bajra, jowar,* maize chappatis*, bread* *Fruits,* fresh *Fats,* oils, butter* cream *Nuts** *Sugar,* honey, jam *Vegetables,* brinjals, cabbage, cauliflower, cucumber, french beans, lettuce, tomato, peas, onion, potato, pumpkin Vinegar, pepper, sourlime.	Biscuits†, pastries†. Egg white *Fruits,* dried, raisin, sultana *Meat,* meat, extracts, fish, poultry Milk, cheese, butter* Nuts, salted *Vegetable,* beetroot, carrot, radish, spinach or Any food that is salted.

* Unsalted. † Salted.

2 LOW SODIUM DIET. Low sodium diets restrict food-stuffs rich in sodium. It is more liberal and easily observed [see Hypertension]. This diet may have to be modified in cardiac or renal failure, ascites due to hepatic cirrhosis and obesity, according to the requirements for calories and protein, described in the respective sections.

Prolonged Deprivation of Sodium

In a resistant case of oedema, drastic reduction of sodium intake may be necessary. Prolonged use of sodium-poor diet when combined with mercurial diuretics leads to the salt depletion syndrome and impaired renal function, which aggravates oedema formation. It may then be difficult to decide whether the persistent oedema is due to sodium retention in the body or due to kidney failure with sodium depletion. Raised blood urea helps the detection of deteriorating kidney function.

Salt Substitutes

Salt-free diets are not so palatable, and potassium chloride is unpleasant as a salt substitute because of its taste. As a compromise,

1 : 1 ratio of sodium chloride to potassium chloride improves the taste.
Such mixtures contain about 20 per cent sodium and 26 per cent potassium and provide potassium during thiazide therapy in oedematous patients.

REFERENCES

[1] FORBES, G.B., and LEWIS, A.M. (1956) Total sodium, potassium and chloride in adult man, *J. clin. Invest.*, **35**, 596.
[2] FORDTRAN, J.S., RECTOR, F.C., JR., and CARTER, N.W. (1968) The mechanism of sodium absorption in the human small intestine, *J. clin. Invest.*, **47**, 884.
[3] NALIN D.R., CASH, R.A., RAHMAN, M., and YUNUS, M.D. (1970) Effect of glycine and glucose on sodium and water absorption in patients with cholera, *Gut*, **11**, 768.
[4] DEVROEDE, C.J., and PHILLIPS, S.F. (1970) Failure of human rectum to absorb electrolytes and water, *Gut*, **11**, 438.
[5] SHEAR, L. (1963) Renal function and sodium metabolism in idiopathic postural hypotension, *New Engl. J. Med.*, **268**, 347.
[6] RIMER, D.G., and FRANKLAND, M. (1960) Sodium content of antacids, *J. Amer. med. Ass.*, **173**, 995.
[7] MORRIS-JONES, P.H., HOUSTON, I.B., and EVANS, R.C. (1967) Prognosis of the neurological complications of acute hypernatraemia, *Lancet*, **ii**, 1385.

21. POTASSIUM

Atomic weight	= 39
Conversion factor	
mg per cent × 0·256	= mEq/1
Total body potassium [1]	= 3000 mEq in 60 kg man
	= 120 g as potassium
	= 245 g potassium chloride
Normal serum concentration	= 20 mg/100 ml
	= 5 mEq/1
Daily requirement	= 70 mEq
	= 3 g as potassium (approx.)
	= 5·5 g as potassium chloride
Easy figures to remember	
100 mEq potassium	= 4 g potassium or
	= 7·5 g as potassium chloride.

Potassium is an important constituent of the animal and vegetable cells. It is the main base of the cellular compartment just as sodium is of the extracellular compartment [TABLE 22] [1].

TABLE 22

APPROXIMATE POTASSIUM CONTENT IN THE BODY

SOURCE	mEq/L	MG PER CENT
Blood plasma	5	20
Red blood cells	100	390
Body tissue cells	150	586
Gastric juice	10	40
Bile	5	20
Intestinal juices	5	20

The body cells form the main potassium pool, so that out of a total body potassium of 120 g, 117 g is found in the cells and 3 g in the extracellular compartment. *A 1-month-old infant* has about 7·5 g (190 mEq) potassium or 1·8 g (46 mEq) per kg body weight [2]. In clinical practice, cellular potassium is not usually estimated but the serum level of the potassium can be used as an indirect guide to the intracellular body potassium. During venepuncture for serum potassium estimation exercise of the forearm should be avoided and blood flow should not be restricted, otherwise false high values are obtained [3].

Absorption
The absorption of potassium is mainly from the small intestine.

Excretion [TABLE 23]
About 90 per cent of potassium is excreted by the *kidneys*. Adreno-cortical hormones, chiefly aldosterone, increase the urinary excretion of potassium. During prolonged administration of cortisone there is retention of plasma sodium and increased urinary excretion of potassium. In Addison's disease on the other hand the function of the

TABLE 23

TOTAL BODY POTASSIUM, INTAKE AND OUTPUT

	mEq	APPROXIMATE WEIGHT IN TERMS OF KCl FOR REPLACEMENT
Total body potassium in 60 kg man	3000	245·0 g
Daily intake	70	5·5 g
Faecal excretion	8	0·6 g
Urinary excretion	70	5·5 g
Sweat	Negligible	

suprarenal gland is depressed and there is increased excretion of sodium and retention of potassium. Administration of mercurial or chlorothiazide diuretics increase the urinary excretion of potassium.

Potassium is actually excreted by the colon (unlike sodium which is absorbed) under adrenal control and this mechanism is similar to that of the kidney.

About 8 mEq of potassium is excreted daily through the faeces. Sweat contains little potassium.

Functions

Potassium is concerned with cellular excitability. The irritability of the nerves, skeletal and cardiac muscles is determined by the relative amounts of potassium, calcium and magnesium. Muscular irritability is increased by increase in potassium or diminution of calcium and magnesium. Potassium is necessary for the proper functioning of the involuntary muscle hence the electrocardiogram shows changes when there are alterations in the potassium level of the myocardium. Potassium is also necessary for the maintenance of acid-base balance.

Sources

Almost all food-stuffs contain potassium; cereals, dried fruits, fruit juices and vegetables are good sources. Fruit juices or vegetable soups should, therefore, be given during acute illness or surgical convalescence.

Requirements

A normal adult requires daily 60–80 mEq of potassium which is equivalent to 2·5–3·3 g of potassium or 4–6 g expressed as potassium chloride. Infants and children require daily about 1 mEq/kg body weight, i.e. 75 mg potassium chloride per kg body weight.

Potassium in Tissue Breakdown

During tissue breakdown either due to trauma as in surgery or to a deficient supply of calories, as in starvation of diabetic coma, potassium is released from the cells. With the tissue breakdown the concentration of nitrogen and potassium in the blood rises and the renal excretion is increased. During the formation of cellular protoplasm as with recovery from diabetic coma, potassium is withdrawn from the blood into the cells and symptoms of potassium deficiency may occur.

DEFICIENCY (HYPOKALAEMIA)

Deficiency of potassium occurs in the following conditions:

1. *Deficient intake.* Potassium excretion in the urine continues even during starvation. Deficiency, therefore, occurs when food cannot be eaten, as after surgery when a patient is maintained for long periods on parenteral therapy without the administration of potassium.

2. *Excessive loss from gastro-intestinal tract.* Loss of digestive juices leads to loss of potassium. This may occur with persistent vomiting, continuous aspiration of gastro-intestinal fluids, fistulae or diarrhoea.

Non-insulin-secreting islet cell tumours of pancreas produce low serum potassium with: (1) Zollinger-Ellison syndrome associated with *gastrin*-secreting tumour resulting in marked increase in hydrochloric acid that makes intestinal contents acid. Pancreatic and intestinal digestive enzymes do not act in acid medium, resulting in diarrhoea and potassium loss. (2) *Pancreatic cholera* with profuse diarrhoea, hypokalaemia and achlorhydria may occur due to excessive secretion of peptide-secreting tumour that may also secrete *secretin* [4].

3. *Potassium deficiency in surgical practice.*

Before operation. Not infrequently the patient is on a poor diet or is starved before an operation. An enema or a bowel wash if given may cause a further loss of 100 mEq of potassium.

During operation. The trauma to the tissues during surgery releases potassium from the cells.

After operation. The stress of operation liberates increased amounts of corticosterioids which enhance the excretion of potassium from the tubules resulting in increased excretion.

Surgical drainage. The loss of potassium through surgical drainage of the biliary tract, pancreas or ileostomy may amount to about 100 mEq a day which is 3 per cent of the total body potassium. If no potassium is given, as during parenteral administration of fluids containing only glucose and sodium chloride, then the total body depletion becomes considerable and even dangerous within a few days. It is, therefore, necessary to prevent or recognize early potassium deficiency in surgical practice.

4. *Diabetic acidosis.* In diabetic acidosis potassium is lost from the cells due to dehydration, acidosis and tissue breakdown and it is excreted by the kidneys. When insulin is given for the treatment of diabetes, sugar is converted into glycogen and is deposited in the cells. During the formation of glycogen, potassium is withdrawn from the extracellular fluid, thus the serum potassium level falls. In the management of diabetic ketosis a close watch has to be kept on the serum potassium level as in the early stage of tissue breakdown it may rise and with insulin therapy it may fall.

5. *Diuretics.* There is a considerable loss of potassium through the urine when oral or parenteral diuretics are administered. The kidneys can lose potassium even during gross body deficiency. The loss of potassium during polyuria is due to the inability of the kidneys to retain potassium during deficiency (unlike sodium which is conserved by the kidneys as required). Potassium salts should therefore be supplemented during diuretic therapy.

With the prolonged administration of diuretics the excretion of potassium is regulated by the amount of sodium in the diet. When a high sodium diet is given there is diminished production of endogenous aldosterone, consequently there is increased urinary excretion of sodium and chloride but potassium excretion or serum potassium levels are unchanged. When a low sodium diet (1 g sodium chloride daily) is given, there is increased secretion of aldosterone which increases the urinary excretion of potassium chloride and reduces the serum potassium level without an appreciable rise in sodium excretion.

6. *Potassium deficiency with purgatives and bowel washes.* Potassium in the lumen of the alimentary tract is part of the body pool of cation and is included in the determinations of exchangeable potassium [5]. Potassium can also be lost through the intestinal mucous membrane. When liquid stools are passed with purgation an appreciable amount of potassium, representing the requirement of 3–4 days, may be lost. During bowel washes and enemas the longer the enema fluid remains in contact with the colon, the more potassium is excreted [6].

7. *Conn's syndrome.* Conn has described a syndrome due to an aldosterone-secreting adrenal cortical neoplasm. This hormone causes excessive loss of potassium from the kidneys, leading to intracellular acidosis and extracellular alkalosis, with retention of sodium without oedema formation. Clinically there are episodes of tetany, paraesthesiae, periodic severe muscle weakness and paralysis, polyuria, polydipsia and hypertension. Histologically there is tubular vacuolation in the kidneys. The kidney loses the power of concentration and acidification of urine [7]. *Intestinal potassium loss* is also increased [8]. Recovery occurs if the adenoma is removed surgically. Conn recommends that in cases of hypertension, serum potassium and bicarbonate estimations be done routinely so as to recognize these cases earlier, but forearm exercise, for collecting blood for potassium estimation, may fail to show low values. Low salt diet may show increased plasma renin concentration. A high plasma aldosterone is therefore of greater help in the diagnosis [9]. Measuring *erythrocyte potassium level* is a useful pointer to potassium depletion and aldosteronism [10].

8. *Potassium-secreting tumours of large intestine.* Villous tumours of the large intestine may result in excessive loss of potassium by secretion of mucous containing a high concentration of potassium.

9. *Potassium-losing nephritis.* This is a condition in which large amounts of potassium are lost in the urine. It is difficult to distinguish it from Conn's syndrome because hyperaldosteronism also causes renal damage.

10. *Familial periodic paralysis.* This disease runs in families and periodic attacks of paralysis occur. During the attack lower potassium values are found and the patient improves on administration of potassium.

11. *Potassium loss during treatment with steroids and similar drugs.* Prolonged administration of corticosteroids produces retention of sodium and excretion of potassium which may produce clinical manifestations. Even administration of liquorice (Liquorice Liquid Extract,

BP) which has a steroid-like action can produce considerable diminution in the serum potassium level.

Potassium deficiency also occurs with heat stroke, violent exercise, kwashiorkor, and during recovery from megaloblastic anaemia.

Potassium and Digitalis

In congestive cardiac failure, potassium depletion may occur spontaneously due to concurrent malnutrition, gastro-intestinal disorder and mercurial or chlorothiazide diuretics which produce excessive urinary loss. With potassium deficiency the cardiac muscle becomes more irritable and predisposes to arrhythmias during digitalis therapy. Premature beats due to digitalis therapy can be abolished by the oral administration of 5–10 G of potassium salts which raises the serum potassium level. It is possible that even if the serum potassium level is normal there may be deficiency of intracellular potassium in the myocardium which makes the heart muscle more irritable.

Patients with *valvular heart failure* are frequently depleted of exchangeable cellular potassium though the plasma level may not exhibit this deficiency. Supplements of potassium of 48 mEq daily for a month prior to heart surgery have shown a rise in exchangeable potassium [11].

Clinical Manifestations of Potassium Deficiency

Symptoms of deficiency become manifest when about 300 mEq, which is about 10 per cent of the total body potassium, is lost. Unfortunately the clinical manifestations of potassium deficiency are not clear cut and they may remain unrecognized due to the gravity of the primary disease process. The clinician must be alert for the symptoms of anorexia, nausea and muscular weakness, particularly in a patient whose food intake is disturbed. Loss of intestinal tone due to potassium deficiency causes abdominal distension and finally ileus. Paralytic ileus after surgery is often due to potassium deficiency.

Alkalosis is common with potassium deficiency. Decreased serum potassium causes the cellular potassium to enter extracellular space while hydrogen replaces potassium in the cells. In the *urinary tubules*, sodium is normally reabsorbed by exchange with potassium and hydrogen ions. With potassium deficiency more hydrogen is exchanged for tubular sodium reabsorption, resulting in increased urinary hydrogen excretion. Extracellular alkalosis therefore results from hydrogen entering the cells and also being excreted in urine. Thus, paradoxically, despite extracellular alkalosis the urine is acid. Potassium administration corrects alkalosis.

Glucose tolerance deteriorates with fasting due to potassium depletion, and potassium therapy increases the ability of the pancreas to secrete insulin [12].

Typical Electrocardiographic Changes. The electrocardiogram may show changes when the serum potassium levels fall well below 3 mEq per litre:

T waves	lowered or inverted
ST segment	depressed
QT	prolonged as a result of a wide and depressed T wave. (In calcium deficit the QT is also prolonged but the ST segment is wide.)
U waves	prominent

The electrocardiogram is not as reliable a measure of the serum potassium level as the flame photometer but the former is very useful when electrolyte studies cannot be done. The characteristic changes may not always be seen on the electrocardiogram even with a low serum potassium level. The explanation may be that electrocardiographic changes are seen only when the potassium content of the cardiac muscle cells is appreciably decreased, which may not correspond to the serum potassium level.

Treatment

Prevention. Potassium deficiency should be prevented in all operated or unconscious patients by giving feeds orally or with the gastric tube. Three or four helpings daily of fruit juice or vegetable soup can avoid a lot of highly complicated and even dangerous procedures later.

Potassium Therapy. *Oral administration.* Potassium, if possible, is best given orally. If potassium is given by mouth to a patient who passes over 1000 ml of urine a day then no gross disturbance need be feared. To correct minor depletion the patient should be given 4–6 helpings of fruit juice and vegetable soup. If more vigorous replacement is needed, any one of the following potassium salts provide about 100 mEq in 24 hours:

(a) Potassium chloride 3 G (45 grains) dissolved in fruit juice given every 8 hours.

(b) Potassium citrate (or acetate) 4 G (60 grains)
    Syrup of lemon   5 ml (one teaspoon)
    Water   30 ml (one ounce)
            (2 tablespoons every 8 hours)

(c) Potassium bicarbonate   1 G (15 grains)
    Potassium citrate   1 G (15 grains)
    Potassium acetate   1 G (15 grains)
    Water   30 ml (one ounce)

Two tablespoons are given three times a day. It is less nauseating than potassium chloride and makes a good drink with fruit juice.

(d) Effervescent potassium-containing granules can be prepared from the following formula:

   Potassium bicarbonate   50 G
   Potassium acid tartrate 30 G
   Citric acid   10 G
   Sodium saccharin   0·5 G
   Sucrose powder   20 G

Slow-K provides 600 mg potassium chloride (8 mEq potassium) per tablet.

The prepared granules are kept in an airtight container. One teaspoon (4 G) supplying 26 mEq of potassium could be rapidly dissolved in a glass of water making it a comparatively pleasant drink which could be flavoured with fruit juice.

Tube feeding. If the patient is unconscious and cannot be fed orally it is best to pass a nasogastric tube and administer food or administer potassium salts as mentioned above through a gastric tube.

Intravenous. If the patient cannot be fed orally or when potassium salts cannot be given by intragastric tube due to the need for continuous gastric suction or due to vomiting, then intravenous administration of potassium is resorted to, provided there is adequate kidney function and the volume of urine exceeds 1000 ml daily.

Potassium chloride is given by slow intravenous infusion at a rate not exceeding 10 mEq/hour. The usual strength given is 30–40 mEq per litre in 5 per cent glucose or isotonic saline. Ampoules of 1·5 G (20 mEq) potassium chloride are kept in stock. One ampoule in a pint or 2 ampoules in a litre of solution provides 40 mEq potassium per litre. Alternatively an ampoule of 2·2 G potassium chloride can be added to a litre of 5 per cent glucose or isotonic saline providing

30 mEq. It is advisable not to give more than 6 G (80 mEq) potassium chloride by the intravenous route in 24 hours. If the solution containing potassium chloride is given too rapidly cardiac arrest can occur.

Caution. Potassium is never given undiluted as a sudden concentrated solution will stop the heart. If a patient excretes less than about 1000 ml of urine daily then intravenous administration of potassium should not be undertaken without frequent estimations of serum potassium level.

When required, intensive potassium therapy up to 860 mEq in 24 hours, of which 600 mEq is administered intravenously, has been given successfully [13].

Not infrequently the inadequately acquired knowledge in this field of electrolytes does more harm. Mystically, the patient may survive only until the laboratory electrolyte values are normal. This demonstrates that electrolyte problems are only manifestations of the overall complexity of the clinical situation and may not be the primary factor [14] *One does not treat the laboratory electrolytes report, but the patient.* A careful and experienced clinical assessment is vital. A neglected patient at home may die of deficiency of fluid and electrolytes. In modern hospitals, enthusiastic but *inexperienced clinicians contribute to fatality due to abundance of fluid and electrolytes.*

POTASSIUM EXCESS (HYPERKALAEMIA)

1. The potassium level in the serum can be high due to: (a) forearm exercise; and (b) obstructing venous flow for collection of blood for potassium estimation; (c) *diminished urine volume;* (d) *intake* of potassium salts of penicillin, iodide; (e) endogenous *tissue breakdown* with trauma; and (f) *acidosis.*

2. *Addison's disease.*

3. *Kidney failure* due to causes like lower nephron nephrosis or in chronic renal failure.

4. *Rapid intravenous potassium administration.*

5. *Mismatched transfusion* where the breakdown of red blood cells may release excess of potassium.

6. *Stored blood transfusions.* Cardiac arrest due to a very high serum potassium level during blood transfusions has been observed [15, 16]. Storage of blood for 15 days increases the serum potassium level from 5 mEq to 25 mEq per litre because potassium leaves the red blood cells

which are very rich in it. Thus during rapid blood transfusions with large volumes of stored blood an excessive amount of potassium may reach the heart but the estimation of potassium in the peripheral venous blood may not reflect the high concentration reaching the heart. In 50 patients in whom massive transfusion was the cause of cardiac arrest an average of 77·7 mEq of potassium was administered. Administration of fresh blood avoids this danger. In stored blood the serum concentration of potassium reaches dangerous levels within 10 days.

Clinical Manifestations of Hyperkalaemia

It is unfortunate that the clinical manifestations of potassium deficiency and of potassium excess are similar, both manifesting as anorexia, weakness of the muscles, diminished deep tendon jerks and general apathy. In the management of a patient on prolonged parenteral therapy, therefore, estimation of the serum potassium level with a flame photometer is helpful.

Electrocardiogram in Potassium Excess. When the serum level reaches a level of 7 mEq per litre (28 mg per 100 ml) the electrocardiographic changes seen are as follows:

T waves	high peaked
ST segment	depressed
QRS	wide
PR	interval prolonged.

There may be AV dissociation and finally cardiac arrest when the serum level rises above 10 mEq per litre.

Treatment

The high potassium level which usually accompanies kidney failure is treated by the administration of protein-free diet by nasogastric or intravenous administration of 10–20 per cent glucose. Simultaneous administration of insulin for the deposition of glycogen helps potassium from the blood being stored in the cells. A bowel wash can get rid of over 100 mEq of potassium. Cation exchange resin (*Resonium-A* or *Kayexalate*) 10 G 4-hourly by mouth is useful in mild cases as a temporary measure to tide over the crisis, but haemodialysis is the best measure in severe cases or those with crush injury involving muscle tissue.

POTASSIUM ULCERS IN THE SMALL INTESTINE

Potassium chloride enteric coated tablets are administered with thiazide diuretic therapy to prevent potassium deficiency. Potassium chloride released over the small segment of the bowel acts upon the mucosal or submucosal veins to produce venous spasm, and blood stagnation results in haemorrhagic circumferential ulceration and stenosis [17]. The patient may have gastro-intestinal bleeding, obstructive symptoms or perforation.

REFERENCES

[1] FORBES, G.B., and LEWIS, A.M. (1956) Total sodium, potassium and chloride in adult man, *J. clin. Invest.*, **35**, 596.

[2] NOVAK, L.P., HAMAMOTO, K., ORVIS, A.L., and DURKE, E.C. (1970) Total body potassium in infants: Determination by whole body counting of radioactive potassium (40 K), *Amer. J. Dis. Child.*, **119**, 419.

[3] SKINNER, S.L. (1961) A cause of erroneous potassium levels, *Lancet,* **i**, 478.

[4] CLEATOR, I.G.M., *et al.* (1970) Bio-assay evidence of abnormal secretin-like and gastrin-like activity in tumour and blood in cases of 'choleraic diarrhoea', *Gut.*, **11**, 206.

[5] SPENCER, R.P. (1959) Potassium metabolism and gastrointestinal function. A review, *Amer. J. dig. Dis.*, **4**, 145.

[6] DUNNING, M.F., and PLUM, F. (1956) Potassium depletion by enemas, *Amer. J. Med.*, **20**, 789.

[7] CONN, J.W. (1955) Primary aldosteronism, a new clinical syndrome, *J. Lab. clin. Med.*, **45**, 3.

[8] SHIELDS, R., MULHOLLAND, A.T., and ELMSLIE, R.G. (1966) Action of aldosterone upon intestinal transport of potassium, sodium and water, *Gut.*, **7**, 686.

[9] BROWN, J.J., *et al.* (1968) Plasma electrolytes, renin and aldosterone in the diagnosis of primary hyperaldosteronism, *Lancet,* **ii**, 56.

[10] BOYD, D.W. (1970) Red-blood-cell potassium and aldosteronism, *Lancet,* **i**, 594.

[11] WHITE, R.J. (1970) Effect of potassium supplements on the exchangeable potassium in chronic heart disease, *Brit. med. J.*, **3**, 141.

[12] ANDERSON, J.W., HERMAN, R.H., and NEWCOMER, K.L. (1969) Improvement in glucose tolerance of fasting obese patients given oral potassium, *Amer. J. clin. Nutr.*, **22**, 1589.

[13] PULLEN, H., DOIG, A., and LAMBIE, A.T. (1967) Intensive intravenous potassium replacement therapy, *Lancet,* **i**, 809.

[14] TAKACS, F.J. (1969) Nephrologic emergencies—fluids and electrolytes, *Med. Clin. N. Amer.*, **53**, 407.

[15] LE VEEN, H.H., SCHATMAN, B., and FALK, G. (1959) Cardiac arrest produced by massive transfusions, *Surg. Gynec. Obstet.*, **109**, 502.

[16] LE VEEN, H.H., *et al.* (1960) Haemorrhage and transfusion as the major cause of cardiac arrest, *J. Amer. med. Ass.*, **173**, 770.

[17] ALLEN, A.C., BOLEY, S.J., SCHULTZ, L. and SCHWARTZ, S. (1965) Potassium-induced lesions of the small bowel. II. Pathology and pathogenesis, *J. Amer. med. Ass.*, **193**, 1001.

22. IRON

Atomic weight   = 56
Total body iron   = 4 g
Daily requirement   = 10 mg (15–20 mg in women during child-bearing period)
1 g haemoglobin   = 3·4 mg iron
1 per cent rise in total blood
    haemoglobin   = 25 mg iron

Iron is a vital component of haemoglobin which transports oxygen to the various tissues of the body.

Absorption

Iron in food exists as organic porphyrin or as inorganic salts. *Haemoglobin iron* is absorbed intact as haem, even at neutral pH, and is not affected by the dietary phosphate or phytate. Iron of meat and liver is better absorbed than eggs and leafy vegetables. Absorption is least from cereals. *Inorganic* ferrous or ferric salts, as they are soluble, are absorbed, but ferrous iron is better absorbed. Gastric acidity maintains the solubility of inorganic iron and allows it to combine to form small molecules with ascorbic acid, citrate, fructose or amino acids, which allow iron absorption in the duodenum and jejunum. In animals the only site of active transport is the duodenum and iron is absorbed by a process of diffusion through the small intestine.

The observation that iron-deficient patients absorbed more iron than normals led to the hypothesis of a receptor protein in the intestinal mucosa which could be saturated when sufficient iron had entered the body. This receptor was identified as *apoferritin* which then combined with iron to form *ferritin*. Doubt has been cast on this idea by the observation [1] that experimentally no saturation of the carrier could be demontsrated. However, it is of interest that the duodenum, with its active transport of iron, contains the most ferritin.

Phosphates and phytates in large amounts in the diet inhibit iron absorption by precipitating ionized iron. *Vitamin C* reduces ferric iron to the ferrous state, which remains soluble even at neutral pH and increases absorption. Dietary iron is better absorbed with vitamin C supplements [2]. It is possible that the habit of ingesting lime or orange juice with food results in better absorption of iron. When radio-active iron salts were added to flour to provide 6–8 mg of iron per pound of bread the absorption was satisfactory. Thus, fortification of flour with iron is helpful [3]. However, iron from *brown* bread is absorbed better than *iron from enriched white bread* 'fortified' to provide 1·65 mg iron per 100 g flour as is required by the British regulation [4].

About 10 per cent food iron is normally absorbed. However, iron absorption is increased with iron deficiency anaemia, low plasma iron or increased erythropoietic activity in the bone marrow, and pancreatic deficiency.

Oral administration of iron impairs *tetracycline* absorption [5].

Plasma Iron. The absorbed iron in plasma occurs in the ferric state and combines with a specific iron-binding *beta* globulin fraction of protein called *siderophyllin* or *transferrin*. The *plasma iron level* is about 60–100 micrograms per 100 ml. The *total iron-binding capacity* (TIBC) of plasma is about 300 micrograms per 100 ml. The *normal plasma iron saturation* is about 30 per cent.

Body Iron. The total iron in the body is 3–5 g, of which more than half is in haemoglobin. The storage iron in the liver, spleen and bone marrow exists as *ferritin* and *haemosiderin* (made up of several ferritin molecules). Muscle haemoglobin (*myohaemoglobin*) and the tissue enzyme cytochrome also contain iron.

Excretion

Absorbed iron is tenaciously bound to protein and the little excretion that occurs is in an organic form. The total daily excretion of iron cannot be correctly assessed as it is also lost through the desquamation of epithelium of the mucous membrane. (1) *Faecal* iron is mostly *unabsorbed* dietary iron. Some *absorbed* iron is lost through bile and in the 50–80 g of intestinal epithelium which desquamates every day. (2) *Desquamation of the skin* increases with sweating in the hot humid climate of the tropics. Cell-rich sweat contains 1·61 mg while cell-free sweat contains 0·44 mg iron per litre [7]. Depending upon the percentage absorption of iron, about 10–15 mg additional iron may have to be taken in food to replace the loss through 1 litre of cell-rich sweat. (3) The *urinary* loss of iron is negligible.

Desferrioxamine is a chelating agent that binds iron, and excretes it in the urine. The urinary excretion of iron is thus easily measured and this method is utilized to estimate the iron stores. Parenteral injection of desferrioxamine in patients with decreased iron store shows diminished urinary iron excretion [8].

Iron Loss in Women.   A woman loses additional iron during her *reproductive life*. (1) During each *menstrual cycle* 30–60 ml of blood is lost which involves a monthly loss of 15–30 mg of iron. (2) During *pregnancy,* the foetus, placenta and loss during parturition drains the mother of over 500 mg of iron, which would require an increase in the daily absorption by 2 mg. (3) During *lactation* there is an additional daily loss of 1·5 mg of iron. Due to such losses women even of Western countries have low iron stores [9].

Conservation of Iron

The normal life span of red blood cells is 120 days. About 20 mg of iron is released daily from the breakdown of haemoglobin. It is oxidized to the ferric form and incorporated into ferritin or haemosiderin until it is re-utilized.

Requirements

The daily requirement of iron is determined by the type of food taken. Animal food iron is better absorbed than iron from vegetable foods, and a predominantly meat diet therefore decreases, while a predominantly cereal diet increases, the iron requirement.

About 1 mg of iron is lost daily by the adult *male* and about 2 mg is lost daily by the adult *female during her reproductive life*. Assuming that about 10 per cent of ingested iron is absorbed, then a diet supplying 10 mg of iron daily is adequate for a man. About 15 mg of iron daily is required by a woman between puberty and the menopause, as with increased requirement the absorption rate may rise by 20 per cent. The diet usually does not provide enough iron for women and iron supplements are desirable.

An infant at full term is born with about 242 mg of iron which is adequate to last for 6 months, after which a daily intake of 8 mg of iron is required. A full term infant born with iron deficiency, say with 190 mg, requires 8 mg a day at the third month [10]. A premature infant is born with even less iron, for example 132 mg, and requires 8 mg daily at the second month. As this amount can be supplied only with an optimal food intake, it is best to give iron supplements to an iron-deficient infant from the third month and to a full term infant from the sixth month. About 30 mg of ferrous sulphate provides 8 mg of elemental iron.

Source

The average diet in Western countries provides 12–15 mg iron which is adequate even with 10 per cent absorption. In the tropics, the ordinary staple diet of cereals is rich in iron. Iron intake was adequate in South Indian plantation workers [11]. Iron deficiency anaemia in Indians, despite adequate intake, may partly be due to poor absorption, due to the high phosphate content of cereals, and the low intake of vitamin C.

Vegetables. Cereals, beans, lentils, vegetable leaves, spinach, water-cress, cauliflower, radish, dried peach, dried apricots and pomegranate, all contain iron. Though the iron content of spinach is high (12 mg per cent) it is not easily absorbed.

Non-vegetarian Foods. Liver, kidney, brain, egg yolk, meat, oysters, shrimps and fish contain iron.

When food is cooked in iron utensils, some iron is added from the utensils. When aluminium and stainless steel utensils are used, this source is lost.

DEFICIENCY

The commonest cause of ill health in women, particularly in India, is iron deficiency anaemia. Women seeking admission to charitable hospitals usually have subnormal haemoglobin values. Occasionally the haemoglobin level is about 20 per cent, rarely even less than 10 per cent. This anaemia is probably the result of many factors, such as poor intake and absorption, together with loss of iron during menstruation, repeated pregnancies, prolonged lactation, parasitic infestation and through sweat in hot kitchens.

The manifestations of iron deficiency are weakness, lack of energy, particularly during the evenings, and absence of enthusiasm for work or play. There may be brittle nails, koilonychia, sore tongue, pharyngeal web and gastritis. In the more severe cases there may be palpitations, dyspnoea and even congestive cardiac failure.

The *sequence of changes in iron deficiency is:* (1) depletion of bone marrow iron; (2) elevation of serum iron-binding capacity over 350 micrograms per 100 ml; (3) decrease in serum iron concentrated below 50 micrograms per 100 ml; and (4) low haemoglobin. A haemoglobin level below 12 g, therefore, shows depleted iron stores.

Treatment

Prophylaxis. It would help organizations with female employees, for instance hospitals, to provide daily one tablet of 100 mg of ferrous sulphate which would improve efficiency.

Curative. 1. ORAL. An inexpensive ferrous preparation should be prescribed with benefit to all pregnant and lactating women, who are always on the borderline of iron deficiency. It is best to administer iron between two meals, as during that period insoluble phytates and phosphates derived from other foods are not formed. Simultaneous administration of vitamin C, 100 mg, enhances iron absorption. The initial dose of ferrous sulphate should be 300 mg and in divided doses gradually increased to about 1000 mg a day. Despite all claims, the cheapest ferrous sulphate is as effective as any other preparation. Ferrous compounds are 4–6 times as easily absorbed and utilized as ferric compounds [12]. The *initial high dose* of over 1 G a day results in vomiting, intestinal colic, diarrhoea or constipation. In severely anaemic patients the response to iron therapy appears in 1 week; thereafter, the haemoglobin rises at the rate of 0·15–0·2 g a day.

2. PARENTERAL. *Iron is best administered orally* as the rate of haemoglobin formation does not significantly differ from that administered parenterally [13]. Parenteral therapy is indicated in patients with diarrhoea, malabsorption syndrome, ulcerative colitis, or in pregnancy with severe anaemia or persistent vomiting. Iron injections are not helpful in conditions where utilization of iron is defective unless the bone marrow iron stores are absent [14].

Advantages of parenteral therapy are: (1) Once iron is introduced directly into the body it is stored and utilized when necessary. (2) The amount introduced is known. (3) An adequate amount of iron can be given to a markedly anaemic patient within a few days. (4) When the necessary amount is given the excretion is not increased, as occurs with other minerals. (5) Parenteral injection of iron may avoid the necessity of blood transfusions. Blood transfusion of 500 ml provides over 200 mg of iron. This amount can be given by parenteral iron injection and the dangers of transfusion reactions, the possibility of initiating antibody responses and the transmission of homologous serum jaundice, are all avoided.

DOSAGE. About 25 mg of elemental iron is required to raise the haemoglobin level of blood by 1 per cent, and an additional 1000 mg should be given to compensate for the deficiency of storage iron in the liver, spleen and bone marrow. A patient with 40 per cent haemoglobin therefore requires a maximum of 2500 mg of parenteral iron. A larger amount is contra-indicated.

1. *Intramuscular iron.* Low molecular *iron-dextran complex* is available for intramuscular use, supplying 50 mg of elemental iron per ml. Initially, 100 mg may be injected in the gluteal region and if necessary may be increased to 200 mg a day (2 ml in *each* gluteal region). Sometimes toxic reactions such as high fever, tachycardia, painful enlargement of inguinal lymph nodes and severe pain in the lumbosacral region may occur.

An *iron-sorbitol complex* (*Jectofer*) is rapidly removed from the injection site. It is, therefore, quickly utilized and leaves less skin staining. Urinary excretion of iron-sorbitol complex may exacerbate undiagnosed renal infection. Fatality due to iron-sorbitol injection may occur [17]. Anaemic females administered intramuscular iron in the gluteal region prior to pelvic surgery may exhibit large siderotic lymph nodes, which the surgeon is liable to mistake for secondary metastasis [18].

Carcinogenicity of iron-dextran complex. Iron-dextran given intramuscularly in large dosage to experimental animals has produced local sarcomata. This has produced a scare in the medical profession about the use of intramuscular iron [19]. The dosage which produced these tumours was out of proportion to that used in clinical practice. Some authorities, therefore, have stated that, 'after carefully considering the available data in connection with the carcinogenicity of iron-dextran complex we have concluded that its use in the clinical dosage recommended carries a negligible risk and is probably less hazardous in other respects than intravenous iron preparations and blood transfusions' [20].

2. *Intravenous iron.* Iron dextran (*Imferon*) is given intravenously. An initial dose of 50 mg of elemental iron is given, which is subsequently increased to 100 mg a day. Local inflammation is produced when the preparation leaks outside the vein. With rapid injection there may be

flushing of the face, nausea, headache and abdominal pain. Fatal reactions have even been reported.

A single total dose of intravenous iron-dextran (Imferon) iron therapy is occasionally advocated for grossly anaemic patients in the tropics who attend the hospital irregularly. It is rather a dangerous practice and anaphylactic reactions are likely; hence it is not recommended, except in the hands of an experienced person who personally supervises the injection. The incidence of local venous thrombosis is high but is minimized by mixing hydrocortisone hemisuccinate. The *intra-peritoneal route* for administering iron-dextran has been occasionally used [21]. Usually 2 G is injected in 500 ml (5 per cent dextrose or isotonic saline).

Blood transfusions for iron deficiency anaemia are seldom required unless the patient is actively bleeding.

EXCESSIVE IRON STORAGE
(Iron over-load, siderosis)

Unlike most inorganic substances, iron, once absorbed, is not readily excreted. When iron is introduced into the body by injection or blood transfusion, then the normal absorption mechanism is by-passed and the unutilized excess iron is stored. Various terms are employed to denote this excessive iron storage.

Siderosis (sideros = iron) is a comprehensive term denoting excess of iron in the body. Abnormal iron deposits can occur with increased iron *absorption* or after iron *injections*, without definite indications or without calculating the required dosage. The absorption of iron also depends on the dietary ratio of iron to phosphorus. Raising the iron phosphorus ratio increases iron absorption. Africans who eat maize cooked in iron pots and drink local beer may ingest 100 mg of iron per day. This staple food of Africans of low economic status contains little phosphorus and an excessive amount of iron is absorbed, leading to considerable iron deposition in the liver and subsequent cirrhosis.

Haemosiderosis denotes iron which has been converted into haemoglobin and subsequently broken down and deposited in excess in the body. This occurs during intravascular haemolysis as in aplastic and haemolytic anaemias, especially with repeated transfusion. With each transfusion of 500 ml of blood over 200 mg of iron is supplied and stored. Transfusions supplying 4·3 to 30·0 g of iron may cause haemosiderosis and occasionally cirrhosis [22].

Haemochromatosis (bronze diabetes) is a rare error of metabolism with deposition of the pigments, haemosiderin and haemofuchsin, in the *skin, liver, pancreas* and other viscera. Deposition of iron in the liver leads to cirrhosis. The pancreatic involvement leads to fibrosis, diminished production of insulin and resultant diabetes. Deposition in the skin gives an abnormal pigmentation, which in the later stages produces a bronze colour (bronze diabetes). The serum iron level is raised, with an average of 224 micrograms per 100 ml (normal 100 micrograms, and the maximum capacity of 100 ml of serum is to bind 300 micrograms of iron). A low residual serum iron-binding capacity is a good diagnostic test.

Normally, iron is not absorbed unless it is needed by the body, but in haemochromatosis abnormal amounts are absorbed. Since increased iron absorption is noted in some relatives of patients, it is suggested that haemochromatosis is a genetic defect of iron absorption. Haemochromatosis occurs in a significant number of *alcoholics* after the age of 40 and is rarely seen in females. Pancreatic deficiency increases iron absorption. Pancreatic damage in an alcoholic may be an associated factor in producing haemochromatosis.

The treatment of haemochromatosis is repeated phlebotomies.

REFERENCES

[1] Smith, M.D., and Pannacciulli, I.M. (1958) Absorption of inorganic iron from graded doses: its significance in relation to iron absorption tests and the 'mucosal block' theory, *Brit. J. Haemat.*, **4**, 428.

[2] Apte, S.V., and Venkatachalam, P.S. (1965) The effect of ascorbic acid on the absorption of iron, *Indian J. med. Res.*, **53**, 1084.

[3] Steinkamp, R., Dubach, R., and Moore, C.V. (1955) Studies in iron transportation and metabolism. VIII. Absorption of radioiron from iron-enriched bread, *Arch. intern. Med.*, **95**, 181.

[4] Callender, S.T., and Warner, G.T. (1970) Iron absorption from bread, *Lancet*, **i**, 546.

[5] Neuvonen, P.J., Gothoni, G., Hackman, R., and Bjorksten, K. (1970) Interference of iron with absorption of tetracyclines in man, *Brit. med. J.*, **4**, 532.

[6] Rath, C.E., and Finch, C.A. (1949) Chemical, clinical, and immunological studies on the products of human plasma fractionation, XXXVIII. Serum iron transport, measurement of iron-binding capacity of serum in man, *J. clin. Invest.*, **28**, 79.

[7] Hussain, R., and Patwardhan, V.N. (1959) Iron content of thermal sweat in iron-deficiency anaemia, *Lancet*, **i**, 1073.

[8] Losowsky, M.S. (1966) Effects of desferrioxamine in patients with iron-loading with a simple method for estimating urinary iron, *J. clin. Path.*, **19**, 165.

[9] COUNCIL OF FOOD AND NUTRITION (1968) Iron deficiency in the United States, *J. Amer. med. Ass.*, **203**, 407.

[10] SCHULMAN, I. (1961) Iron requirements in infancy, *J. Amer. med. Ass.*, **175**, 118.

[11] RAMALINGASWAMI, V., and PATWARDHAN, V.N. (1949) Diet and health of the South Indian plantation labourer, *Indian J. med. Res.*, **37**, 51.

[12] MOORE, C.V., DUBACH, R., MINNICH, V., and ROBERTS, H.K. (1944) Absorption of ferrous and ferric radioactive iron by human subjects and by dogs, *J. clin. Invest.*, **23**, 755.

[13] McCURDY, P.R. (1965) Oral and parenteral therapy: a comparison, *J. Amer. med. Ass.*, **191**, 859.

[14] DAVIS, A.G., BEAMISH, M.R., and JACOBS, A. (1971) Utilization of iron dextran, *Brit. med. J.*, **1**, 146.

[15] HAGEDORN, A.B. (1957) The parenteral use of iron in the treatment of anaemia, *Proc. Mayo Clin.*, **32**, 705.

[16] BEN-ISHAY, D. (1961) Toxic reactions to intramuscular administration of iron dextran, *Lancet*, **i**, 476.

[17] KARHUNEN, P., HARTEL, G., KIVIKANGAS, V., and REINIKAINEN, M. (1970) Reaction to iron sorbitol injection in three cases of malabsorption, *Brit. med. J.*, **2**, 521.

[18] DeSOUZA, A.E.J. (1968) Iatrogenic siderosis, *Indian J. Cancer*, **5**, 246.

[19] BRITISH MEDICAL JOURNAL (1960) Carcinogenic risks of iron-dextran, Editorial, *Brit. med. J.*, **1**, 788.

[20] DUTHIE, J.J.R., *et al.* (1960) Carcinogenicity of iron-dextran complex, Letter to the Editor, *Lancet*, **ii**, 155.

[21] MEHTA, B.C., and PATEL, J.C. (1969) Total dose iron therapy using iron dextran by intra-peritoneal route, *Indian J. med. Sci.*, **23**, 587.

[22] SINNIAH, R. (1969) Transfusional siderosis and liver cirrhosis, *J. clin. Path.*, **22**, 567.

23. CALCIUM

Contributed by R. H. Dastur

Atomic weight   = 40
Conversion factor for converting
  mg/100 ml to mEq/1   = × 0·5
Total body calcium 60 kg man   = 1200 g approx.
Daily requirement   = See p. 189

Calcium is a very important mineral for the maintenance of neuro-muscular function. Calcium constitutes 2 per cent of the total body weight and 26 per cent of the dry weight of bones and teeth in the form of phosphates and carbonates.

Absorption
The absorption of calcium depends upon the following factors:

Body Needs. The absorption of calcium is according to the needs of the body. On a normal diet only 30 per cent calcium is absorbed but on a low calcium diet the proportion of calcium absorbed is higher.

Concentration. Other factors being equal the higher the concentration of calcium in the intestine the greater the absorption of calcium.

Time of Administration. Commercial calcium preparations are best absorbed if given an hour before meals because insoluble salts with other food-stuffs are not formed.

Intestinal Motility. Intestinal hurry diminishes the absorption of calcium. With chronic diarrhoea and prolonged use of purgatives, calcium absorption is considerably diminished.

Fat. When there is deficient fat absorption as in steatorrhoea, calcium combines with fatty acids to form insoluble calcium soaps. Decreased fat absorption also diminishes absorption of vitamin D.

Ingested Food. Cereals contain phytic acid (inositol hexaphosphate) which combines with calcium to form insoluble calcium *phytate* which is not absorbed. Similarly foods containing *oxalate* such as spinach, combine with calcium to form insoluble calcium oxalate. An excess of magnesium apparently diminishes absorption of calcium.

Vitamin D. The most important factor in promoting calcium absorption is vitamin D. When vitamin D is not taken, as with a strict vegetarian diet, e.g. 'vegans' (who exclude even milk as it is considered to be of animal origin) and also if there is no exposure of the skin to sunlight then severe hypovitaminosis D occurs. This in turn leads to poor absorption of calcium. With high doses of vitamin D the absorption of the calcium from the food can be almost complete and it is possible to maintain a positive calcium balance even on a low intake. Absorption from the proximal intestine in the first two to four hours is not influenced by vitamin D. After four hours the absorption of calcium is from the distal part of the intestine and is dependent on vitamin D. However, the ability to concentrate calcium against a gradient in an everted sac preparation of the jejunum depends upon the presence of vitamin D. *Parathyroids* also play a part in calcium absorption.

Calcium-Phosphorus Ratio. The ratio of calcium to phosphorus in the food has an important influence on the metabolism of the elements Most foods containing calcium have also a proper proportion of phosphorus. Milk, eggs, some leafy vegetables like spinach, lettuce, etc. provide these elements in the required proportions

SERUM CALCIUM

Calcium is present in the plasma but not in the red blood cells. The serum level is about 10 mg per 100 ml and is partly composed of ionized and partly of protein bound calcium. *Ionized calcium* is diffusible, its normal serum level of 4–5 mg per 100 ml is controlled by the parathyroid glands. Alkalosis reduces the level of ionizable serum calcium. Diminution of ionic calcium leads to increased muscle irritability and tetany. The rest of the plasma calcium is bound to proteins, mainly albumin, so that when the plasma albumin level falls very low the total level of serum calcium drops. Since this decrease is only in the non-diffusible form tetany does not develop.

Serum Calcium Estimation. In clinical practice the ionizable calcium level alone is of importance. However, routine methods measure the total serum calcium. Simultaneous estimation of serum proteins, particularly the albumin level, will indirectly reflect the amount of non-ionizable protein bound calcium. There is also a reciprocal relationship between the level of serum calcium and phosphorus; a rise in the serum phosphorus leads to a fall in the serum calcium.

Factors Regulating Serum Calcium

Parathyroid Hormone. The serum calcium level is the resultant of dietary calcium, bone resorption and urinary calcium excretion. The action of *parathyroids* on *renal tubular reabsorption* of calcium is mainly responsible for plasma calcium homeostasis in man [1]. There is a 'theoretical urinary calcium threshold' at 9 mg per 100 ml of serum. The threshold is reduced in hypoparathyroidism and increased in hyperparathyroidism. Low calcium diet increases the threshold, which is reduced with high calcium diet [2].

Mobilization of calcium and phosphorus from the bones. Parathyroid hormone mobilizes calcium and phosphorus from the bones to maintain the blood level. Hyperparathyroidism causes reabsorption of minerals together with the bony matrix, giving an X-ray appearance of cysts in the bones, known as osteitis fibrosa cystica. Hyperparathyroidism may also manifest as renal stones without detectable bone changes.

Parathyroid hormone also aids in the absorption of calcium from the gut.

Vitamin D also increases the serum calcium level by: (1) increased absorption; (2) mobilization of calcium from the bones even in physiological doses.

Calcitonin. Calcitonin is secreted by the C cells of the thyroid gland (thyrocalcitonin) and also of the parathyroids and thymus. Having a very short half life it is continuously secreted. The secretion increases with rising serum calcium and helps to maintain the blood level by *preventing calcium release* from the bone and also by *increasing urinary calcium excretion*. These actions are antagonistic to parathyroids. *Therapeutically, calcitonin* used in hypercalcaemia due to Paget's disease reduces the blood calcium level by decreasing bone reabsorption, while in hyperparathyroid and breast carcinoma the calcium lowering effect is essentially due to increase in urinary calcium excretion [3]. Excessive calcitonin is secreted by the C cells in medullary carcinoma of the thyroid.

Hypercalcaemia

An increased serum calcium level is seen in:

1. *Hyperplasia or neoplasm of the parathyroid gland.* Mobilization of the calcium from the bones occurs with increased parathyroid activity and the serum calcium may rise to 12 mg and in advanced disease over 15 mg per cent. There is increased urinary excretion of calcium. The resulting decalcification allows bending of the long bones and compression of the vertebrae whereby the height is diminished. There is weakness, nausea and vomiting. Deposition of calcium in the kidneys may give rise to calculus formation and even renal failure. X-rays of the bone shows cystic cavities (osteitis fibrosa cystica), most apparent in the skull.

2. *Hypervitaminosis D.* Over-dosage of vitamin D results in excessive absorption of calcium from the gut. In large doses vitamin D is also known to produce mobilization of calcium from the bones.

3. *Dihydrotachysterol (A.T.* 10) *overdosage* due to vitamin D-like action produces hypercalcaemia.

4. *Milk-alkali syndrome.* When soluble alkalies (e.g. sodium bicarbonate) are given with large amounts of milk for the treatment of peptic ulcer, systemic alkalosis and hypercalcaemia may occur which may eventually lead to renal failure. It is possible that some of these cases were hyperparathyroidism with peptic ulcer. Increased vitamin D intake in milk may also have been the cause.

5. *Sarcoidosis.* In this condition a vitamin D-like factor operates to raise the serum calcium.

6. *Bone destruction* due to carcinomatous deposits and more particularly from carcinoma of the breast or myelomatosis increases the serum calcium level which may even prove fatal.

7. *Idiopathic infantile hypercalcaemia. Clinical symptoms* of hypercalcaemia are constipation, lethargy, lassitude, easy fatigability and sometimes polyuria. *Hypercalcaemic crisis* occurs with intractable nausea, vomiting, dehydration, stupor, coma and azotaemia.

The treatment is administration of corticosteroid. Furosemide (*Lasix*), used as a diuretic, increases urinary calcium excretion. Furosemide administered intravenously in doses of 80–100 mg every 1–2 hours, along with adequate replacement of fluids and electrolyte losses, is an effective therapy for lowering the serum calcium level [4]. Calcitonin by intravenous infusion has also been suggested as a treatment for hypercalcaemia. Maintenance of a low calcium diet by excluding milk and dairy products is helpful. Intestinal calcium absorption is decreased with the oral administration of sodium cellulose phosphate 15 G (5 G three times) with meals. Inorganic phosphate taken orally as disodium or potassium phosphate is also effective. Sodium phosphate can also be administered intravenously, but extraskeletal precipitation of calcium phosphate is a possibility.

Hypocalcaemia

Low serum calcium levels are seen in:

1. *Hypoparathyroidism* and pseudohypoparathyroidism.

2. *Vitamin D deficiency* due to a poor diet or in regions where women do not expose themselves to the sunlight or due to a possible diminished absorption in steatorrhoea.

3. *Hypoproteinaemia,* in which the non-diffusible fraction bound to albumin is reduced. Some cases of hypocalcaemia after gastric surgery may be due to hypoproteinaemia.

4. *Renal disease* in which there is retention of phosphate or failure to acidify the urine leading to systemic acidosis and loss of calcium.

5. *Acute pancreatitis* where the pancreatic enzyme lipase is released into the peritoneum and blood, splitting fat into glycerol and fatty acid and the latter combines with calcium to form soaps lowering serum calcium level.

6. *Transient hypoparathyroidism* in the neonatal period.

7. *Drugs and toxins* like sodium fluoride and viomycin.

8. Following *hypothermia* for cardiac surgery.

9. Following *gastric surgery,* probably due to deficient vitamin D absorption. These patients respond to small daily oral doses of 100 units or weekly injection of 1000 units of vitamin D.

Storage

Most of the body calcium is stored in the bones and teeth. The skeleton is the dynamic reservoir where calcium is continuously deposited and reabsorbed. This turnover activity is high in the young and declines with age. About 1 per cent of total body calcium occurs in the circulation and soft tissue.

Excretion

About half the daily calcium is excreted in the *faeces,* representing unabsorbed calcium and calcium from endogenous sources. If a high dose of vitamin D is taken the calcium content of the stools decreases. When absorption from the intestine is diminished, faecal excretion of calcium rises.

About half of the total daily calcium is excreted in the *urine.* The urinary excretion is under the control of the parathyroid glands and represents mostly the 'endogenous' calcium. The normal range of urinary calcium in adults on a normal diet is 100–300 mg per day for men and 100–250 mg per day for women. The kidneys conserve calcium during deficiency and very little is excreted.

Increased urinary calcium excretion (hypercalcinuria) may result in kidney stones (see Renal Calculi).

Function

1. Calcium and phosphorus are necessary for bone formation.

Ninety-nine per cent of the body calcium is stored in the bones. If necessary for the body needs, calcium can be mobilized from the bones to maintain a normal serum level by the action of parathyroid hormone. The extent of this mobilization is seen by the fact that even when large amounts of calcium are removed by haemodialysis, normal serum calcium is soon restored.

Bones consist of the protein *matrix* or framework in which calcium phosphate is deposited. Protein, vitamins A and C and sex hormones are necessary for the formation of matrix. Calcium in the bones, once deposited does not remain fixed but is always being turned over with calcium in the blood and other tissues. In a normal person new bone salt is formed at the rate of 0·5 g of calcium per day and a corresponding amount is reabsorbed. This exchange corresponds to 0·04 per cent of the total body calcium.

2. Calcium is necessary for the *growth* of children.

3. *Ionic calcium* affects *neuromuscular excitability* of both voluntary and involuntary muscles. When the ionic serum calcium concentration is diminished, the neuromuscular excitability is considerably increased, as seen in tetany.

4. Calcium probably aids in the absorption of vitamin B_{12}. In the malabsorption syndrome deficiency of free calcium ion is one of the causes of poor vitamin B_{12} absorption. With the oral administration of calcium lactate the absorption of vitamin B_{12} significantly improves but this observation requires confirmation.

Physiologically calcium is necessary in proper functioning of the heart muscle, clotting of blood and maintenance of capillary permeability.

Source

Milk and milk products are the best sources of calcium and there is evidence that calcium in milk is better absorbed than in other foods, because lysine and lactose enhance calcium absorption. Fatty preparations like butter, cream and *ghee* are poor in calcium but contain an adequate amount of vitamin D which aids in better calcium absorption. The daily calcium requirements of an adult male are easily supplied by a cup of buffalo milk. *Molasses and vegetables* like peas, beans, pulses, potatoes, cauliflowers and dried figs supply calcium. Pumpkin leaves are edible with a calcium content of 240–300 mg per 100 g [5]. Chewing betel leaves with *lime* (calcium hydroxide), a common practice in India, augments the dietary calcium. Hard water contains calcium which can be better absorbed in tropical countries with vitamin D derived from exposure to sunlight. Those who chew fish bones are also assured of adequate calcium intake.

Tropical diet which is rice, wheat or millet is deficient in calcium but exposure to sunlight produces vitamin D which improves absorption and tends to compensate for the low intake. In Western countries, the compulsory addition of calcium (fortification) to wheat flour ensures an adequate calcium intake.

Requirements

The daily requirements of calcium vary according to factors favourable or otherwise for its absorption. In the tropics, with exposure to sunlight a positive calcium balance is maintained even on a calcium intake lower than is generally recommended. Calcium absorption is also regulated by the intake of certain foods. The retention of calcium was more when *ragi* was substituted for rice supplying the same amount of calories [6].

Man has a remarkable capacity to adapt to low calcium intake, when there is not only diminished urinary excretion but also increased intestinal absorption.

With an average Indian vegetarian diet containing little milk the calcium intake is about 0·3 g [7]. When calcium supplies are limited, the available calcium should be reserved for infants and women of child-bearing age as far as possible. For an adult male, therefore, 0·3 to 0·5 g calcium per day is adequate.

Adolescents require more calcium during their bony growth and a supply of 0·6 to 0·7 g per day is adequate.

Pregnancy increases the demand for calcium. An infant at birth has more than 20 g calcium, the major portion of which is accumulated in the last three months when the bones of the foetus are ossifying. Even if extra calcium is not taken by the mother during pregnancy, the foetus still derives calcium from the bones of the mother. When there is marked deficiency of calcium the mother may suffer from osteomalacia. About 1·0–1·2 g calcium per day is adequate for the mother during the last trimester.

Lactation involves loss of calcium in milk. Human milk contains 20–30 mg calcium per 100 ml. If 1000 ml of milk is secreted, 300 mg extra calcium has to be absorbed by the mother. Even if the mother's intake of calcium is not adequate the concentration of calcium in her milk is maintained at the necessary level by mobilization from her bones. To allow for losses and daily needs, a lactating mother requires 1·2 g of calcium daily.

Infants who are breast fed require daily 50 mg calcium per kg of body weight. Artificially fed infants require two to three times the quantity of calcium as the calcium from the mother's milk is more absorbed.

Conclusions. The recommended daily calcium allowance:

Adults	0·3–0·5 g
10–15 years	0·6–0·7 g
16–19 years	0·5–0·6 g
Pregnancy	1·2 g
Lactation	1·2 g
Infants (breast fed)	50 mg per kg
Infants (artificially fed)	100–150 mg per kg

With exposure to sunlight and formation of vitamin D the recommended oral intake may be reduced as the absorption of calcium increases.

Calcium Supplements for Children.   Calcium supplements for children did not contribute to better growth [8]. This should not be taken as conclusive, however, as we do not know the value of calcium supplement at an earlier period of life or when combined with other food supplements.

DEFICIENCY

Since the absorption and metabolism of calcium is closely related to that of vitamin D and also because disease processes like steatorrhoea may prevent the absorption of both these factors, there is a lack of clarity in the manifestations of pure calcium deficiency in contrast to the effect of both calcium and vitamin D deficiency. Furthermore, pure vitamin D deficiency will also cause calcium deficiency. However, in the present state of knowledge the only condition which appears to be due to pure calcium deficiency is *osteoporosis*. This may be due to inadequate intake, renal acidosis, Cushing's syndrome or disuse atrophy. In all these conditions the serum calcium and phosphorus are normal but the body calcium stores are markedly reduced and the skeleton decalcified. In contrast, calcium and vitamin D deficiency are operative in the production of osteomalacia and rickets and in both these conditions the serum calcium and/or phosphorus levels are abnormal.

Tetany

The syndrome of tetany is characterized by hyperexcitability of the nervous system. It is due to lowering of the ionizable serum calcium. The ionizable serum calcium may be lowered in:

1. Lack of *absorption* of calcium from the gut. This may be due to lack of intake of vitamin D or non-exposure to sunlight, or to small intestinal diseases characterized by malabsorption of fat as in sprue and coeliac disease.

2. *Late pregnancy and lactation* where there is increased demand for calcium.

3. *Alkalosis* which lowers ionizable calcium. Alkalosis occurs due to hyperventilation, prolonged gastric lavage or intake of excessive soluble alkalies particularly when the kidneys are damaged. The alkalosis of pyloric stenosis is now thought to be due mainly to potassium deficiency which produces an intracellular acidosis and an extracellular alkalosis.

4. *Hypoparathyroidism*, either due to diminished function of parathyroids or more commonly due to accidental removal of the parathyroids during surgery of the thyroid gland in hyperthyroidism.

5. *In acute pancreatitis*, the pancreatic enzymes released in the peritoneal cavity and blood, split fat all over the body into fatty acids which combine with circulating calcium and this may appreciably lower the level of ionizable calcium.

The manifestations of tetany depend not so much upon the absolute level of calcium in the blood as upon the ionizable calcium and decrease in the normal ratio of calcium to phosphorus. Marked symptoms may be produced by only slight lowering of serum calcium with a rise in serum phosphorus over 5 mg per 100 ml of serum (normal 3·5 mg per 100 ml). High serum phosphorus values are found in hypoparathyroidism and nephritis. Tetany does not usually occur in renal failure because of the associated acidosis.

Clinically tetany may be seen as: (1) latent tetany; (2) manifest tetany.

Latent Tetany

In the latent form of tetany there may be *hyperexcitability only* on stimulation. Tapping the facial nerve anterior to the external auditory meatus causes contraction of the facial muscles on that side (Chvostek's sign). Inflating a sphygmomanometer cuff around the arm to a pressure just above the systolic level and obstructing the circulation produces spasm of the fingers and hand in the accoucheur position (Trousseau's sign) within 5 minutes.

Manifest Tetany
Manifest tetany may be: (1) acute; or (2) chronic.
1. *Acute.* The acute form of tetany may occur after thyroidectomy if the parathyroids are accidentally removed. There is irritation, confusion, paraesthesia, pain and carpopedal spasm. Involuntary *muscle spasm* may result in dyspnoea due to bronchial spasm; spasm of the laryngeal muscles produces cyanosis, convulsions and collapse; spasm of the gastro-intestinal tract produces dysphagia, vomiting and pain simulating intestinal or biliary colic.
2. *Chronic tetany* is usually seen in hypoparathyroidism. There may be irritability, depression, impairment of memory, changes in the hair and nails, roughness of the skin, pitting of teeth, cataract and epileptic fits.

Treatment of Calcium Deficiency
The dietetic treatment consists of providing regular milk and milk products so as to supply adequate calcium.

Oral Calcium. Calcium salts such as calcium lactate are administered orally. Three grammes of calcium lactate is best given one hour before meals, three times a day.
The amount of available calcium in therapeutically administered calcium preparations is:

	Percentage of available calcium
Calcium chloride	36
Calcium lactate	18
Calcium gluconate	9

Management of Acute Tetany. During an attack of tetany it is best to give calcium gluconate, 10 per cent, 10 ml intravenously. Injection of vitamin D is of no value in relieving the acute manifestations. *Calcium chloride* by the intravenous route is best avoided as a leak into the surrounding tissues causes necrosis.

Vitamin D. Vitamin D is indispensable for better absorption of oral calcium. Vitamin D can be given orally as calciferol, 5000 Units a day. Intramuscular injections of vitamin D are rarely required except when the malabsorption syndrome or renal disease is present.

Osteoporosis

Osteoporosis has gained in importance due to increasing expectancy of life, which increases debilitating deformities. It is not necessary to segregate *post-menopausal* and *senile* osteoporosis. Bone loss occurs in both sexes, beginning with the fifth decade, but progresses twice as fast in females who also have a small bone mass; in such cases the *demand* for calcium increases during repeated pregnancies which diminish calcium stores.

Aetiology. Osteoporosis is due to a combination of nutritional, hormonal, physical and circulatory factors: (1) *Nutritional. Calcium intake* is low and *calcium absorption* is diminished (sometimes due to vitamin D deficiency) in both sexes after the age of 60 and most markedly after 80 [9]. *Lactose* increases absorption of intestinal calcium and phosphorus [10]. Lactase-deficient patients avoid milk that decreases calcium intake. (2) *Hormonal* disturbances in menopausal women, or removal of ovaries in earlier life, cause osteoporosis. The *oestrogens* are claimed to inhibit the bone-resorptive function of parathyroid. Female sex hormones also aid intestinal calcium absorption [11]. Osteoporosis is also noted in *Cushing's syndrome* and *corticosteroid* therapy. (3) *Bed rest* and immobilization increases resorption from the weight-bearing bones and increases urinary and faecal calcium excretion [12].

Clinically, there is low back pain, loss of weight, fracture of the vertebrae, neck of the femur, distal radius and ulna, and loss of teeth due to lack of bone support. The serum calcium and phosphorus values are normal. Radiologically, the second metacarpal bone is usually observed to indicate the progress of the disease.

Prophylactic measures both in the young and old include adequate intake of calcium and proteins with daily 1 or 2 cups of milk or milk products, outdoor exercise, and at least 100 Units of vitamin D in the aged.

Therapy is aimed at supplying calcium and retarding the rate of bone reabsorption. Calcium 2·5 G daily is advised [13]. Since intestinal calcium absorption is decreased in the aged, intravenous calcium therapy is also advocated. Oestrogen in females and testosterone in males inhibit bone resorption [14]. The female sex hormones also increase intestinal calcium absorption [11].

Generalized Osteosclerosis (Osteopetrosis). This is a rare hereditary disease where there is increased intestinal calcium absorption, normal bone formation, but defective bone resorption with few osteoclasts in the bone. The treatment is severe restriction of dietary calcium.

Calcium in General Practice

Placebo Effect. A sense of warmth is produced during the intravenous administration of calcium. It is given to a patient by a physician with a 'pep talk' that an injection is required 'to warm up the blood'.

Acute Haemorrhage. During an acute bout of bleeding from oesophageal varix or duodenal ulcer intravenous calcium is enthusiastically administered.

Blood coagulation is not improved by administering calcium to a bleeding patient, as even during severe reduction in serum calcium level seen in tetany, haemorrhage is not a feature because the amount of calcium required for the clot formation is very small and this amount is always present in the blood.

Multiple transfusions, particularly with damaged liver, result in *citrate intoxication*. Raised serum citrate decreases serum *ionic* calcium and aggravates bleeding tendency. This is corrected by administering 10 per cent calcium gluconate, 10 ml for each litre of blood transfused.

Calcium in Allergy. Calcium may be helpful in allergic states as it diminishes the capillary permeability.

Calcium and Digitalis. Therapeutic administration of calcium is avoided during digitalis therapy. Digitalis makes the heart muscle irritable and if calcium is administered it further irritates the cardiac muscle producing premature beats and fibrillation.

REFERENCES

[1] NORDIN, B.E.C., and PEACOKC, M. (1969) Role of kidney in regulation of plasma-calcium, *Lancet*, **ii**, 1280.

[2] PEACOCK, M., ROBERTSON, W.G., and NORDIN, B.E.C. (1969) Relation between serum and urinary calcium with particular reference to parathyroid activity, *Lancet,* **i,** 384.

[3] COCHRAN, M., PEACOCK, M., SACHS, G., and NORDIN, B.E.C. (1970) Renal effect of calcitonin, *Brit. med. J.,* **1,** 135.

[4] SUKI, W.N., *et al.* (1970) Acute treatment of hypercalcaemia with furosemide, *New Engl. J. Med.,* **283,** 836.

[5] INDIAN COUNCIL OF MEDICAL RESEARCH (1951) *Wheat and Wheat Products as Human Food,* Special Series No. 24, New Delhi, p. 41.

[6] JOSEPH, K., KURIEN, P.P., SWAMINATHAN, M., and SUBRAMAHNYAN, V. (1959) The metabolism of nitrogen, calcium and phosphorus in undernourished children, *Brit. J. Nutr.,* **13,** 213.

[7] GOPALAN, C. (1970) Some recent studies in the Nutrition Research Laboratory, Hyderabad, *Amer, J. clin. Nutr.,* **23,** 35.

[8] BHALSAL, P., RAU, P., VENKATACHALAM, P.S., and GOPALAN, C. (1964) Effect of calcium supplementation on children in a rural community, *Indian J. med. Res.,* **52,** 219.

[9] BULLAMORE, J.R., *et al.* (1970) Effects of age on calcium absorption, *Lancet,* **ii,** 535.

[10] CONDON, J.R., *et al.* (1970) Calcium and phosphorus metabolism in relation to lactose tolerance, *Lancet,* **i,** 1027.

[11] CANIGGIA, A., *et al.* (1969) Intestinal absorption of calcium-47 after treatment with oral oestrogen-gestogens in senile osteoporosis, *Brit. med. J.,* **4,** 30.

[12] DONALDSON, C.L., *et al.* (1970) Effect of prolonged rest on bone mineral, *Metabolism,* **19,** 1071.

[13] COHN, S.H., DOMBROWSKI, C.S., HAUSER, W., and ATKINS, H.L. (1968) High calcium diet and the parameters of calcium metabolism in osteoporosis, *Amer. J. clin. Nutr.,* **21,** 1246.

[14] RIGGS, B.L., *et al.* (1969) Effect of sex hormones on bone in primary osteoporosis, *J. clin. Invest.,* **48,** 1065.

24. PHOSPHATE

Phosphate is widely distributed in all the cells and body fluids, and plays a vital role in enzyme reactions and tissue metabolism. The metabolism of phosphate and calcium is closely linked and both the minerals usually occur together in food. Their absorption, excretion, blood levels and functions in bone formation are interrelated.

Absorption

Most of the phosphate in food is in organic form. It is present, for example, in milk casein, vitellin of egg yolk and neuroproteins.

The organic phosphates are digested in the intestines to form inorganic phosphates of sodium, calcium and potassium and absorbed from the upper small intestine. The factors which favour absorption are similar to those influencing calcium absorption. Excess calcium and aluminium form insoluble phosphate, diminishing phosphate absorption.

Distribution

Phosphorus is widely distributed in the body tissues and fluids. The serum level is 3·5–5 mg per 100 ml in adults and 5–6 mg per 100 ml in infants. It is reduced in rickets, osteomalacia, sprue and hyperparathyroidism. It is increased in renal failure and hypoparathyroidsm.

Excretion

Phosphate is excreted in the urine and faeces. When the calcium intake is low, the urinary phosphate excretion rises. On an average diet the kidney excretes about 750 mg of phosphate daily. Parathyroid hormone decreases tubular reabsorption of phosphate in kidney leading to increased excretion of phosphates in the urine. However, the amount of dietary phosphate is the major factor in the tubular handling of the phosphate and, therefore, the measurement of phosphaturia is an unreliable guide to parathyroid function. [1]

Function

(1) Phosphate and calcium are necessary for bone formation. (2) Carbohydrates and fats require phosphate for their intermediate metabolism. (3) Many enzyme systems require phosphate for their action. (4) Phosphate is the principal anion in the cell. (5) High energy phosphate bonds provide a source of metabolic energy.

Requirement

The daily requirement is about 1 g which is easily supplied in an average diet. Dietary deficiency, therefore, never occurs under normal circumstances.

Source

As calcium and phosphate exist together their sources are similar.

Vegetarian. Milk and milk products (except its fatty parts like cream, butter and *ghee*), beans, carrot, cauliflower, corn, peas, potato and banana are good sources.

Non-vegetarian. Liver, egg, fish and meat products.

Phosphate Diabetes

Fanconi [2] has described a syndrome with renal tubular insufficiency and dwarfism. This condition is due to excessive excretion of phosphate by the proximal tubules and the excess loss has been labelled as 'phosphate diabetes'. It has no relation to diabetes mellitus but renal glycosuria without hyperglycaemia may coexist. There is also excessive excretion of amino acids in the urine. It is a rare cause of oestomalacia in adults.

Hypophosphataemia

Low plasma phosphate may be a *familial* or *non-familial* isolated disorder. There may be *defective intestinal absorption* of phosphate [3] or excessive renal loss due to defective urinary phosphate reabsorption. Hypophosphataemia also occurs when non-absorbable antacids, aluminium and magnesium hydroxide are administered in large doses for hyperphosphataemia [4] or peptic ulcer. Low serum phosphate is more likely in Gram-negative than in Gram-positive septicaemia [5].

Clinically, with hypophosphataemia there is anorexia, nausea, weakness and malaise, vitamin D-resistant rickets in children, and osteomalacia in adults. There is increased intestinal calcium absorption and urinary calcium excretion, while urinary phosphate excretion is diminished.

The therapy for persistent hypophosphataemia is oral phosphate and vitamin D to aid phosphate absorption [3]. Inorganic phosphate is administered either orally as disodium or potassium phosphate, or even intravenously [6]. Phosphate supplements reduce the high dosage of vitamin D and the dangers of its toxic effects [7].

Bony fractures heal more quickly in patients receiving phosphate supplement [8].

REFERENCES

[1] FAIRHURST, B.J. (1963) Urinary phosphate excretion in hypoparathyroidism, *Lancet*, **i**, 302.
[2] FANCONI, G. (1954) Tubular insufficiency and renal dwarfism, *Arch. Dis. Childh.*, **29**, 1.
[3] CONDON, J.R., NASSIM, J.R., and RUTTER, A. (1970) Defective intestinal phosphate absorption in familial and non-familial hypophosphataemia, *Brit, med. J.*, **3**, 138.

[4] LICHMAN, M.A., MILLER, D.R., and FREEMAN, R.B. (1969) Erythrocyte adenosine triphosphate depletion during hypophosphatemia in uremic subjects, *New Engl. J. Med.,* **280,** 240.

[5] RIEDLER, G.F., and SCHEITLIN, W.A. (1969) Hypophosphataemia in septicaemia: Higher incidence in gram-negative than in gram-positive infection, *Brit. med. J.,* **1,** 753.

[6] GOLDSMITH, R.S., and INGBAR, S.H. (1966) Inorganic phosphate treatment in hypercalcemia of diverse etiologies, *New Engl. J. Med.,* **274,** 1.

[7] WILSON, D.R., YORK, S.E., JAWORSKI, Z.F., and YENDT, E.R. (1965) Studies in hypophosphataemic vitamin D-refractory osteomalacia in adults, *Medicine,* **37,** 99.

[8] GOLDSMITH, R.S., WOODHOUSE, C.F., INGBAR, S.H., and SEGAL, D. (1967) Effect of phosphate supplements in patients with fracture, *Lancet,* **i,** 687.

25. MAGNESIUM

Atomic weight	=	24·3
Conversion factor	=	mEq/1
mg per cent × 0·823	=	mEq/1
Total body content	=	2000 mEq
Daily requirement	=	0·3 g
	=	25 mEq
	=	1·5 g magnesium sulphate

The role of magnesium in the body is imperfectly understood, as chemical estimation is difficult and requires an atomic spectrophotometer. Better understanding and correction of sodium, potassium and chloride imbalance has revealed disturbances due to magnesium deficiency or excess.

The total body magnesium is about 2000 mEq (24 g) of which 66 per cent is in the bones. The gastro-intestinal secretions contain about 3 mEq per litre.

Absorption
Magnesium is easily absorbed from the small intestine.

Plasma Level
In normal persons the level varies from 1·5 to 1·8 mEq per litre [1]

but this plasma value does not necessarily reflect the cellular concentration.

Excretion

Magnesium is excreted in the *faeces,* probably derived from intestinal secretions and bile. *Urinary* excretion is variable, being 35–224 mg for males and 55–213 mg in females in 24 hours [2]. The kidneys can conserve magnesium even more efficiently than sodium, so deficiency is slow to develop. Urinary excretion for 24 hours could be a reliable index of magnesium deficiency, and primary hyperparathyroidism due to bone reabsorption is sometimes associated with a negative magnesium balance and increased urinary loss.

Functions

Magnesium plays an important role in normal calcium and potassium metabolism in man. Despite adequate calcium and vitamin D, magnesium depletion produces hypocalcaemia and hypocalcinuria, a positive Trousseau sign and low body potassium [3]. Magnesium is essential for neuromuscular irritability, intracellular enzymes, the metabolism of carbohydrates, and the structure of DNA and RNA.

Requirements

About 0·3 g (25 mEq) magnesium is required daily.

Sources

Whole grain cereals and chlorophyll-containing vegetables, like cabbage and cauliflower, are good sources of magnesium.

DEFICIENCY

Magnesium deficiency occurs due to: (1) *Deficient intake,* usually with prolonged starvation and when parenteral therapy is given which omits magnesium. (2) *Alimentary loss* of magnesium may occur in vomiting, ileostomy dysfunction, or intestinal fistulae. (3) *Urinary loss* of magnesium may occur in prolonged diuresis with the administration of ammonium salts, chlorothiazides or mercurials. In primary hyperparathyroidism there may be reabsorption of magnesium from the bone with increased urinary excretion, which may result in a negative magnesium balance. This could be restored to normal after parathyroidectomy [4]. However, with the deposition of magnesium in the bone during the postoperative period clinical manifestations due to low serum magnesium may occur. (4) *Malabsorption* of magnesium may occur after massive bowel resection, and in the malabsorption syndrome [5] and regional enteritis. Diabetic acidosis is associated with raised serum levels but with insulin therapy the serum level is markedly decreased (changes similar to potassium). A low serum magnesium may also be noted in toxaemia of pregnancy [6] and with excessive lactation. In proteincalorie malnutrition magnesium deficiency is common [7].

The *clinical features* of magnesium deficiency are related to neuromuscular irritability and mental changes. *Neuromuscular irritability* may manifest as: (1) An aimless plucking at the bed clothes. (2) Tremors, best seen in the hand with outstretched palm. The tremors may disappear for several hours and then reappear; they may sometimes be accentuated by asking the patient to maintain a steady grasp of the examiner's hands. (3) Cramps, twitchings and choreo-athetoid movements. (4) Convulsions may be an early manifestation. (5) The reflexes are hyperactive and bilateral plantar extensor response may be noted. (6) There may be a positive Chvostek's sign. The clinical picture of magnesium deficiency may be indistinguishable from tetany produced by a low serum calcium, and in fact there is low serum calcium level as well [8]. (7) Low voltage on electrocardiogram. The *mental changes* may be confusion, disorientation, and hallucinations which are visual rather than auditory.

Treatment

Prophylaxis. Magnesium deficiency can be prevented by giving feeds of cereals and vegetables or by the oral administration of magnesium as Magnesium Hydroxide, B.P., 5 ml three times a day (each ml contains 3 mEq) or magnesium citrate or magnesium sulphate, 2 G (16 mEq) three times a day. Oral supplements are necessary after parathyroidectomy.

Curative. With clinical deficiency, 2 ml of 50 per cent magnesium sulphate is injected intramuscularly twice a day. Magnesium chloride, 100 mEq (1·67 G) in 1 litre of 5 per cent dextrose can be administered intravenously over a period of 4 hours. Associated calcium and potassium deficiencies also require correction.

INTOXICATION

Retention of magnesium occurs when there is scanty flow of urine due to kidney disease. During oliguria, magnesium salts, such as magnesium sulphate for purgation, should be avoided. The clinical manifestations of magnesium intoxication are drowsiness when the serum level is 8 mEq per litre, stupor and coma when the serum level is about 14 mEq per litre. The electrocardiogram shows increased PR and QRS duration and increased height of T waves.

REFERENCES

[1] Hanna, S. (1961) Plasma magnesium in health and disease, *J. clin. Path.*, **14**, 410.

[2] Evans, R.A., and Watson, L. (1966) Urinary excretion of magnesium in man, *Lancet,* **i**, 522.

[3] Shils, M.E. (1968) Experimental magnesium deficiency in man and associated calcium and potassium abnormalities, *Amer. J. clin. Nutr.,* **21**, 536.

[4] Hanna, S., North, K.A.K., MacIntyre, I., and Fraser, R. (1961) Magnesium metabolism in parathyroid disease, *Brit. med. J.,* **2**, 1253.

[5] Booth, C.C., Babouris, N., Hanna, S., and MacIntyre, I. (1963) Incidence of hypomagnesaemia in intestinal malabsorption, *Brit. med. J.,* **2**, 141.

[6] Achari, G., *et al.* (1961) Serum magnesium in women in the normal state and in certain conditions, *J. Indian med. Ass.,* **36**, 93.

[7] Caldwell, J.L., and Goddand, D.R. (1967) Studies in protein-calorie malnutrition. I. Chemical evidence of magnesium deficiency, *New Engl. J. Med.,* **276**, 533.

[8] Hanna, S., Harrison, M., MacIntyre, I., and Fraser, R. (1960) The syndrome of magnesium deficiency in man, *Lancet,* **ii**, 172.

26. MANGANESE

Atomic weight	=	55
Total body content	=	35 mg
Daily requirement	=	5 mg

Manganese exists as a trace metal in the body. Estimation of manganese in the body is difficult and a neutron activation technique may have to be used for its estimation.

Absorption

Manganese given orally is absorbed from the gut. Chemical workers and miners exposed to manganese dust absorb it from the lungs.

Distribution

The manganese content of the body is about 35 mg of which 20 mg in bone acts as a body reserve [1]. The serum level in Indians is 0·5–2·6 micrograms per 5 ml serum [2]. Manganese is found mainly in the pancreas, pituitary, liver, kidney and in the bones which contain the greatest concentration (3–5 mg/kg wet tissue). Most of the cellular manganese is in the mitochondria [3] and is rapidly exchangeable [4].

Excretion

Manganese is mainly excreted in the bile and thus in the faeces. It is also excreted in the urine.

Source

About 5 mg or more of manganese is ingested daily. Cereal, bran, nuts, coffee and particularly tea are good sources of manganese. Sea foods, milk products, meat and vegetables, are low in manganese.

Requirement

The daily requirement of manganese is roughly estimated to be 5 mg.

Action

The role of manganese in the human body is little understood. It is a cofactor in several enzyme systems [5]. The concentration of manganese in the pancreas and pituitary points to some role in carbohydrate metabolism [1]. In one unusual type of insulin-resistant diabetes 10 mg of manganese chloride by mouth was shown to have a definite hypoglycaemic action. After pancreatectomy the patient responded to insulin but not to manganese [6].

DEFICIENCY

Experimental manganese deficiency has been produced in birds and mammals but it has not been described in man. There is slowing of growth, with the development of bony abnormalities, and dysfunction of the reproductive organs. Neurologically there is weak-

ness of the limbs, ataxia and lack of balance. A classical and spontaneously occurring defect in birds known as *perosis* is due to deficiency
of manganese, and consists of bony deformities and dislocation of the
tendo Achillis.

EXCESS

In man excessive inhalation may occur in those miners and chemical
workers who are exposed to manganese compounds. The lung probably
acts as a depot and the blood manganese level is raised.

Pathological studies are few but changes occur in the basal ganglia,
posterior part of the hypothalamus and upper midbrain.

The disease affects mainly the central nervous system and the
respiratory system. The *initial symptoms* [2] are anorexia, asthenia,
apathy, depression, irritability, impotence, body aches, sleep disturbances, either as insomnia or somnolence, and occasionally bouts of
temporary insanity and violence. Pathological laughter called, 'sham
mirth' and causeless weeping may be noted.

On examination [2, 7] a form of *Parkinsonism* with a mask-like face,
low indistinct monotonous speech, abnormal gait in which the patient
walks on the ball of his feet with the heels raised (cock-walk), retro-
pulsion, micrographia and fine tremors (not the coarse tremor of classical Parkinsonism) form the essential picture. There is no paralysis
but mild pyramidal signs have been recorded. Sensory changes are
uncommon. The intellect is not usually impaired.

The *respiratory* manifestations are repeated bronchitis, dry pleurisy
and even acute pneumonia. Chronic emphysema and bronchitis,
pulmonary tuberculosis, and pneumoconiosis also occur.

The red blood cell count and haemoglobin estimation are higher
in those affected than in people of the same social background not
exposed to manganese.

The disease can be *prevented* by dust extraction and by vigilance for
early symptoms with removal of the affected person from any manganese dust. There is no specific *treatment*. British anti-lewisite (BAL)
is of no value. Dicalcium disodium ethelenediamine tetra-acetate (ED
TA) has been tried without definite success.

REFERENCES

[1] FORE, H. (1963) Manganese-induced hypoglycaemia, Letter to the Editor.
Lancet, i, 274.

[2] MINISTRY OF LABOUR AND EMPLOYMENT (1960) *Report of the Manganese Poisoning Enquiry Committee,* Government of India Press, Faridabad.

[3] MAYNARD, L.S., and COTZIAS, G.C. (1955) The partition of manganese among organs and intracellular organelles of the rat, *J. biol. Chem.,* **214,** 489.

[4] BORG, D.C., and COTZIAS, G.C. (1958) Manganese metabolism in man: Rapid exchange of Mn[56] with tissue as demonstrated by blood clearance and liver uptake, *J. clin. Invest.,* **37,** 1269.

[5] COTZIAS, G.C. (1961) Manganese versus magnesium: Why are they so similar in vitro and so different in vivo?, *Fed. Proc.,* **20,** Part 2, 98.

[6] RUBENSTEIN, A.H., LEVIN, N.W., and ELLIOTT, G.A. (1962) Manganese-induced hypoglycaemia, *Lancet,* **ii,** 1348.

[7] CHARLES, J.R. (1927) Manganese toxaemia; with special reference to the effects of liver feeding, *Brain,* **50,** 30.

27. IODINE

Atomic weight	=	127
Total body iodine	=	10 mg
Serum protein bound iodine	=	4–8 micrograms/100 ml
Daily requirement	=	150 micrograms
	=	197 micrograms potassium iodide
1 mg potassium iodide	=	765 micrograms iodine
1 drop Lugol's iodine	=	8433 micrograms iodine

Iodine is the essential constituent of the hormone thyroxine produced by the thyroid gland. For centuries seaweeds were used for the treatment of goitre but it was only at the turn of the nineteenth century that iodine was recognized as its active principle. With the advent of radio-iodine there is better understanding of physiology of iodine and its action on the thyroid gland.

Absorption and Incorporation into Hormone

Organic iodine in the diet is reduced to inorganic iodide before absorption from the small intestine. The circulating iodide is then selectively 'trapped' by the thyroid. Thyroxine, tri-iodothyronine and di-iodotyrosine may be absorbed intact.

Thyroxine. The exact mechanism by which the trapped iodide is incorporated into thyroxine is not yet certain. However, the following is the generally accepted pathway for hormone formation. Trapped iodide first combines with tyrosine to form mono-iodotyrosine. Two mono-iodotyrosine molecules combine to form di-iodotyrosine and two di-iodotyrosine molecules combine to form *tetra-iodothyronine* also called *thyroxine*. *Tri-iodothyronine* and *thyroxine* are the active principles circulating in the blood. The combination of one mono-iodotyrosine with one di-iodotyrosine produces *tri-iodothyronine*. It is chemically more potent than thyroxine and may be the ultimate active hormone utilized by the tissues.

Unless iodine is *trapped and incorporated* into hormone it has no action. (1) The thyroid gland can be *prevented from trapping* iodine by perchlorate. It is therefore sometimes used in the treatment of hyperthyroidism during pregnancy, as during this period the administration of either thiourea compounds or radio-iodine is not advisable. (2) The trapped iodine can be *prevented from being incorporated into hormone* by the thiourea group of drugs which are used in the treatment of hyperthyroidism.

Serum Protein Bound Iodine (PBI)

Thyroxine in the plasma is mainly bound to a specific thyroxine-binding globulin and a small amount to albumin. Serum protein bound iodine (PBI) estimation is a good indicator of the amount of circulating hormone and consequently the thyroid function. The normal range of serum PBI is 4–8 micrograms per 100 ml. It is increased in hyperthyroidism and diminished in hypothyroidism. It is only well-organized laboratories that can undertake reliable PBI estimation.

Storage

Almost the entire body store of 10 mg iodine is in the thyroid gland.

Excretion

Excretion is best studied by the administration of radioactive iodine. The amount of ingested iodine trapped by the thyroid gland does not depend upon the body requirement but only upon the activity of the gland. A hyperfunctioning gland traps more while a hypofunctioning gland traps less. Thus after administering a known amount of radio-iodine and measuring the quantity retained by the thyroid gland its activity is estimated. Iodine that is not trapped by the thyroid gland is mostly excreted in the *urine*. Measuring urinary excretion after orally administering a known amount of radio-iodine also gives an indication of the activity of the thyroid gland.

A small amount of iodine is lost through the *faeces, sweat* and *milk*. In a hyperthyroid lactating mother, therapy with radio-iodine is not advisable as its excretion in milk damages the thyroid gland of the breast-fed baby.

Action

Iodine acts in the body only when it is incorporated into hormone thyroxine which: (1) increases metabolism and oxygen consumption of tissues; (2) converts glycogen to glucose thereby raising the blood sugar level; since that depletes liver glycogen the organ becomes more vulnerable to injury; (3) increases the heart rate; and (4) depletes the bones of calcium and phosphorus and increases urinary calcium excretion.

Source

The richest food source of iodine is sea foods like fish, shell-fish and fish oil. The iodine content of vegetables, fruits and cereals depends upon the iodine content of the soil. Spinach is a source of iodine but it also has an anti-thyroid effect. The inorganic salts of iodine have a high iodine content. One drop of Lugol's iodine contains enough iodine to supply the body needs for 8 weeks.

Other sources of iodine in the tropics, where diarrhoea is common, are iodine-containing *drugs* (iodoxy-quinoline compounds) which are used as a household remedy by most people. These drugs provide appreciable amounts of iodine that usually vitiate the result of radio-iodine uptake. Radiological contrast media, digestives and tonics also contain large amounts of iodine.

Requirement

The mean daily human consumption of iodine in non-endemic goitre areas of the world lies above 75 micrograms [1]. The total amount of iodine required during the life time of a 70 year old man is less than 4 g, that is a mere teaspoon of potassium iodide.

Pregnancy increases the basal metabolic rate and need for iodine. The requirements also increase at puberty, during menstruation and in the cold weather.

IODINE DEFICIENCY AND GOITRE

A goitre is an enlargement of the thyroid gland associated with either normal, hypo- or hyper-function. Iodine deficiency may produce goitre with a normal or hypofunctioning gland.

Aetiology

One of the causes of thyroid enlargement is deficient output of the thyroid hormone which produces hypersecretion of thyroid stimulating hormone of the pituitary with consequent enlargement of the thyroid. Deficient thyroid hormone secretion occurs due to: (1) *Deficiency of iodine* which produces endemic goitre as seen in the Himalayan regions [2]. (2) Deficient *trapping of iodine* by the thyroid gland by goitrogens like thiocyanates (they were used for the treatment of hypertension), or perchlorate. (3) *Insufficient hormone formation* because of foods or thiouracil compounds even after iodine is adequately trapped. With radioactive iodine studies the following foods are found to be goitrogenic: beans, beet, cabbage, carrot, lettuce, peach, spinach, strawberry, turnip. These foods contain a substance known as thio-oxazolidone present only in the raw vegetables but cooking destroys it. Cabbage was the first vegetable proved to be responsible for goitre formation and the goitrogenous vegetables are labelled 'cabbage family'. (4) *Hereditary deficiencies of specific enzymes* needed in the thyroid synthesis pathway also produce goitre.

Prophylaxis. It is generally believed that those living near the sea are assured of an adequate iodine supply. However, a survey of school children in Bombay showed a high incidence of goitre with low urinary iodide excretion due to iodine deficiency. Those living in the mountains may not get an adequate amount. One gramme potassium iodide added to 10,000 parts of common salt supplies 1 mg potassium iodide with the daily intake of 10 g of salt. In the mountainous regions of the advanced countries this simple precaution solves the problem of iodine deficiency. Incorporation of 2 parts per million potassium iodate in bread is an effective prophylactic against endemic goitre [3].

Hypothyroidism

Hypothyroidism results from diminution in the circulating thyroid hormone. The term *myxoedema* is not synonymous with all hypothyroid states but is used where there is an associated thickening of the skin and submucosal tissues. Hypothyroidism encountered clinically is usually not due to a primary deficiency of iodine. It may be due to atrophy of the thyroid gland due to auto-immune antibodies or deficient secretion of thyroid stimulating hormone with pituitary diseases. The commonest cause of hypothyroidism is treatment of thyrotoxicosis either with radio-iodine or with surgery.

The usual *complaints* are: tiredness, lethargy, constipation and increase in weight. There may be a history of feeling cold, requiring warmer clothing even in the hot weather, dryness of the skin and hair, lack of perspiration and difficulty in hearing. In women a characteristic hoarseness of voice may be the first sign to draw the attention of the physician. *Examination* may reveal puffiness of the face, a slow pulse rate, slow cerebration and dry skin. The area of cardiac dullness may be increased and the electrocardiogram shows low voltage.

It is of utmost importance to suspect hypothyroidism from the history, otherwise the patient may be labelled as a neurotic. The clinical manifestations of hypothyroidism are far more helpful in the diagnosis than the basal metabolic rate or radioactive iodine studies which may sometimes be misleading.

Treatment. Administration of desiccated thyroid is useful. Chemically pure L-thyroxine is also used. Tri-iodothyronine is rapid acting and is used under certain circumstances.

Hyperthyroidism with Iodine

According to some reports administration of iodine to goitre patients produces thyrotoxicosis, known as 'iodine-Basedow' because with iodine deficiency the gland becomes overactive in an attempt to produce the hormone. When iodine is supplied, excess of hormone is produced resulting in thyrotoxicosis. Not all clinicians agree that thyrotoxicosis could be produced with the administration of iodine to a goitre patient.

REFERENCES

[1] STANBURY, J.B. (1960) *Endemic Goitre, Wld Hlth Org., Geneva,* p. 261.
[2] RAMALINGASWAMI, V., SUBRAMANIAN, T.A.V., and DEO, M.G. (1961) The aetiology of Himalayan endemic goitre, *Lancet,* **i**, 791.
[3] CLEMENTS, F.W., GIBSON, H.B., and HOWLER-COY, J.F. (1970) Goitre prophylaxis by addition of potassium iodate in bread, *Lancet,* **i**, 489.

28. COPPER

Atomic weight	=	63
Total body content	=	100–150 mg
Serum concentration	=	122 micrograms per 100 ml
Daily requirement	=	2 mg

Copper in the body is stored mainly in the liver, muscles and bones.

Absorption

Copper is absorbed from the stomach and proximal intestine.

Serum

The mean concentration of copper in the serum of healthy persons is about 122 micrograms per 100 ml but spontaneous variations of up to 30 micrograms may occur.

When radioactive copper is administered, it appears initially in the circulation loosely bound to albumin, but later transfers to the protein *ceruloplasmin* which is a blue *alpha$_2$*-globulin. The normal serum level of ceruloplasmin is about 34 micrograms per 100 ml.

Low serum copper occurs in nephrosis, protein-calorie malnutrition, exclusive milk diet, and Wilson's disease. High serum copper occurs with excessive intake from food cooked in copper vessels, in leukaemia, Hodgkin's disease, haemochromatosis, myocardial infarct and hyperthyroidism.

Store

About 90 per cent is stored in the liver.

Excretion

Absorbed copper is mainly excreted through bile in the faeces. The normal urinary excretion is about 48 micrograms in 24 hours. Some copper is excreted through sweat.

Source [TABLE 24]

Nuts, dried fruits, cereals, pulses, meat products, fruits and vegetables are the usual sources of copper.

TABLE 24

COPPER CONTENT OF FOODS (IN MG)

FOOD-STUFF	EDIBLE PORTION/ 100 g	FOOD-STUFF	EDIBLE PORTION/ 100 g	FOOD-STUFF	EDIBLE PORTION/ 100 g
CEREALS AND PULSES					
Bajra	0·55	Vermicelli	0·29	Cow gram	0·75
Barley	0·34	Wheat (whole)	0·49	Green gram (whole)	0·97
Cholam	1·78	Wheat flour (whole)	0·49	Green gram (dal)	1·13
Italian millet	0·55	Wheat flour (refined)	0·19	Khesari (dal)	0·77
Maize (dry)	0·19	Bengal gram		Lentil	0·66
Ragi	0·59	(whole)	0·76	Mothbeans	0·85
Rice (raw) milled	0·72	Bengal gram (roasted)	0·74	Peas (dried)	0·85
Rice, parboiled (milled)	0·33	Bengal gram (dal)	0·98	Peas (roasted)	1·32
Rice flakes	0·37	Black gram		Red gram (dal)	1·25
Rice (puffed)	0·32	(dal)	0·72	Soya bean	0·88
		'Bhetmas'	0·88		
		Chavli (small)	1·42		
VEGETABLES					
Amaranth (tender)	0·33	Drumstick (leaves)	0·62	Raddish (pink)	0·19
Celery leaves	0·30	Neem (tender)	0·60	Drumstick	0·60
Colocasia — (green leaves and stem)	2·38	Tamarind (leaves tender)	2·09	Peas, (English)	0·23
		Beetroot	0·20	Tomato (green)	0·19
Coriander (leaves)	0·53	Potato	0·20	Vegetable marrow	0·22
FRUITS					
Banana (ordinary)	0·40	Orange	0·58	Sapota (Hyderabad chiku)	0·36
Guava (country)	0·34	Pears (country)	0·40		
		Pineapple	0·36	Sithaphal (Hyderabad)	0·85
Malta sweet (lime)	0·51	Pomegranate, (Punjab			
Mango	0·23	Anar lal)	0·21		

* AYKROYD, W.R. (1966) *Nutritive Value of Indian Foods and the Planning of Satis-factory Diets,* 6th rev. ed., eds. GOPALAN, C., and BALASUBRAMANIAN, S.C., Indian Council of Medical Research, New Delhi.

Requirement

The daily requirement of copper is about 2 mg but more is ingested in normal diet.

DEFICIENCY

In *swine*, copper deficiency causes anaemia and the administration of copper increases the intestinal absorption of iron [1]. However, parenteral administration of iron does not cure the anaemia when copper is deficient, which suggests that copper is *not* primarily concerned with the absorption of iron. Copper probably helps to release the iron store for haemoglobin synthesis [2]. Ceruloplasmin is also claimed to mobilize iron from stores such as the liver to the bone marrow for erythropoiesis [3]. Copper also aids in vital enzymatic body functions. In *man*, low serum copper values are noted in malnutrition, but a specific copper deficiency disease is not known. Copper is concerned in the formation of myelin sheath [4] by allowing phospholipid formation.

HEPATOLENTICULAR DEGENERATION
(Wilson's disease)

This is a hereditary disease due to abnormal deposition of copper in the body. The disease is probably due to an inherited defect in the synthesis of the copper-binding protein ceruloplasmin. The serum ceruloplasmin level may be only 9 micrograms compared to the normal 34 micrograms per 100 ml serum, so circulating copper remains loosely bound to albumin from which it is readily dissociated and excreted in the urine or deposited in the tissues. The *urinary excretion* of copper may increase to 100 micrograms per day. There is over a sixfold increase in the copper content of the brain and liver. The liver copper content is over 250 micrograms per g of dry weight (normal 15–55 micrograms) [5]. Increased intestinal absorption of copper has also been observed in this disease, and isolated tissue removed at surgery shows an increased avidity for copper [6]; hence avidity of tissue protein for copper is also suggested as a probable mechanism of Wilson's disease.

The *renal dysfunction* is probably due to deposition of copper in the proximal tubule and resembles that found in poisoning with other heavy metals. Renal tubular defect results in amino-aciduria, glycosuria, phosphaturia and uricosuria, such abnormalities being associated with a correspondingly low level of blood glucose, phosphate and uric acid respectively.

The *pathological* changes are demyelination, and degeneration and cavitation of the *basal ganglia in the brain,* and *cirrhosis of the liver.* *Clinically,* the disease is seen in young adults, and presents as neurological or hepatic disease, with a ring of brown or olive-green pigmentation due to copper deposits at the margin of the cornea (*Kayser-Fleischer ring*). There may be personality changes and mental defect; 'flapping' tremors of the upper extremities, at first only seen on outstretched hands, and later also at rest; choreo-athetoid movements, dysarthria, rigidity and muscular wasting may also occur. The pyramidal tracts and the sensory system are not affected. The liver abnormality may present first as hepatic enlargement and later as cirrhosis with associated splenomegaly, ascites and jaundice.

Treatment

The brain damage appears to be due to excessive deposition of copper and treatment depends upon preventing copper absorption, mobilizing these deposits and promoting their excretion. *Potassium sulphide,* 20 mg three times a day with meals, prevents copper absorption. Penicillamine (*Cuprimine*), a degradation product of penicillin, has a sulfadryl (SH) group capable of binding copper [7] and increases the urinary excretion. It is started as 250 mg capsules, 1 hour before meals four times daily, and increased to a total of 2 G daily.

REFERENCES

[1] WINTROBE, M.M., CARTWRIGHT, G.E., and GUBLER, C.J. (1953) Studies on the function and metabolism of copper, *J. Nutr.,* **50,** 395.

[2] MARSTON, H.R., and Allen, S.H. (1967) Function of copper in the metabolism of iron, *Nature (Lond.),* **215,** 645.

[3] FRIEDEN, E. (1970) Ceruloplasmin, a link between copper and iron metabolism, *Nutr. Rev.,* **28,** 87.

[4] EVERSON, G.J., SHRADER, R.E., and WANG, T. (1968) The chemical and morphological changes in the brain of copper deficiency in guinea pigs, *J. Nutr.,* **96,** 115.

[5] SMALLWOOD, R.A., WILLIAMS, H.A., ROSENOER, V.M., and SHERLOCK. S. (1968) Liver copper levels in liver disease. Studies using neutron activation analysis, *Lancet,* **ii,** 1310.

[6] UZMAN, L.L., IBER, F.L., CHALMERS, T.C., and KNOWLTON, M. (1956) The mechanism of copper deposition in the liver in hepatolenticular degeneration (Wilson's disease), *Amer. J. med. Sci.,* **231,** 511.

[7] WALSHE, J.M. (1956) Penicillamine, a new oral therapy for Wilson's disease, *Amer. J. Med.*, **21**, 487.

29. COBALT

The biological function of cobalt came to light with the discovery of vitamin B_{12} (cyanocobalamin). When radioactive cobalt is given it is absorbed and quickly excreted by the kidneys. How the human body utilizes cobalt is obscure. In herbivorous animals, the intestinal bacteria take up cobalt and synthesize vitamin B_{12} which becomes available for the animal. In man and carnivora this does not occur and they depend on preformed vitamin B_{12} in the food.

The cobalt content of our food is high [1]. Cereal grains usually have 0·006–0·008 mg (6–8 micrograms) per 100 g. Beans have 0·018–0·0475 mg (18–47 micrograms) per 100 g; peas 0·014–0·042 mg (14–42 micrograms) per 100 g. It is unlikely that cobalt deficiency occurs in man and pernicious anaemia, which responds to vitamin B_{12}, is not due to deficiency of cobalt. Cobalt given in high doses to premature infants produces a moderately large goitre [2].

REFERENCES

[1] AHMED, B., and McCOLLUM, E.V. (1939) Cobalt content of some food materials from different parts of the United States , *Amer. J. Hyg.*, Sect. A, **29**, 24.
[2] GAIRDNER, D., MARKS, J., and ROSCOE, J.D. (1954) Goitrogenic hazard of cobalt, *Lancet*, **ii**, 1285.

30. CHLORIDE

Chloride is the main anion of the extracellular compartment. The total anion of the extracellular fluid amounts to 155 mEq per litre, of which chloride constitutes 103 mEq per litre (365 mg per 100 ml of plasma or 600 mg expressed as sodium chloride in 100 ml of plasma). The total body chloride content, based on the analysis of Forbes and Lewis [1], is about 2150 mEq in a 60 kg man.

The absorption and excretion of chloride is similar to that of sodium. Since chloride is absorbed from the colon, the water content of stool is only 15 mEq/1 chloride.

Functions

Sodium chloride is concerned in the maintenance of extracellular acid-base equilibrium and osmotic pressure. The mechanism of chloride shift from the plasma to the red blood cells enables carbon dioxide to be carried from the tissues and excreted by the lungs. Plasma chloride is required for the secretion of hydrochloric acid by the stomach.

Chloride and sodium deficiency usually occur under similar conditions, and so the treatment is similar. However, in vomiting due to pyloric obstruction, chloride is lost as hydrochloric acid without the corresponding loss of sodium. In loss of alkaline secretions, as from a pancreatic fistula, the converse occurs, sodium being lost as bicarbonate without chloride.

Congenital Chloridiarrhoea. This condition, due to malabsorption of chloride in the ileum and colon, results in watery diarrhoea from birth, metabolic alkalosis and excessive chloride excretion in stools [2].

REFERENCES

[1] FORBES, G.B., and LEWIS, A.M. (1956) Total sodium, potassium and chloride in adult man, *J. clin. Invest.*, **35**, 596.
[2] EVANSON, J.M., and STANBURY, S.W. (1965) Congenital chloridiarrhoea or so-called congenital alkalosis with diarrhoea, *Gut,* **6**, 29.

31. FLUORIDE

In the human body fluoride is detected in the teeth, bones, thyroid gland, skin and blood. The bones contain 110 mg fluorine per 100 g ash. Less than 0·15 mg per 100 ml is excreted in the urine. Normal blood contains only traces of fluoride.

Sources

The fluoride content of water depends upon the soil. Soft water contains little fluoride, while significant amounts may be present in

hard water. The most desirable amount of fluoride in drinking water
is 1 part per million (ppm), i.e. 0·1 mg per 100 ml, in Great Britain.
However, the desirable amount varies in different countries, partly
dependent upon the volume of water consumed. Vegetables, sea-fish
and tea also supply fluoride. The daily intake of fluoride may be 2–3 mg
[TABLES 25 and 26].

Absorption
Fluoride is easily absorbed from the intestine. The *plasma level* is
0·4–0·19 ppm. Fluoride is easily excreted by the kidneys.

Function
Fluoride is necessary in early life for the formation of caries-resistant

TABLE 25

FLUORIDE ION LEVELS (PPM) IN MAJOR FLUORIDE ION-CONTAINING FOODS*

FOOD	FLUORIDE ION (PPM)
VEGETABLE ORIGIN	
Tea	3·2 — 4·0
Grain	About 1·0
Vegetables	0·10— 0·30
Potatoes	0·4 — 5·20
Spinach	0·1 —20·3
Citrus fruit	0·07— 0·36
Non-citrus fruit	0·35— 2·1
Nuts	0·3 — 1·45 (maximum 7·8)
Wine	0·05— 0·3 (maximum 18·1)
Beer	0·2 — 1·2
ANIMAL ORIGIN	
Bone meal	146—770
Meat	0·2 — 2·0
Dried meat	3·3 — 7·7
Fish	1·0 — 8·0 (maximum 84·5)
Milk	0·09— 0·32
Cheese	0·16— 1·31
Egg	0·2 — 0·4

*Waldbott, G.L. (1963) Fluoride in food, *Amer. J. clin. Nutr.*, **12**, 455.

TABLE 26

FLUORIDE ION IN WATER*

SOURCE	LOCATION	FLUORIDE (PPM)
Sea water		1·0—1·4
Sea water	Persian Gulf	8·72
Rain water	Germany	Up to 3·4
Well water	U.S.A.	Less than 0·5
River water		0·0—25 and more
Maximum allowable limit	In warm climate In cool climate	1·4 2·4

* Waldbott, G.L. (1963) Fluoride in food, *Amer. J. clin. Nutr.*, **12**, 455.

teeth. The principal action of fluoride on bone is to slow the resorption, with additional function of promoting calcification [1].

DEFICIENCY

Fluoride is deposited in the enamel of the developing teeth. Its deficiency in children leads to *dental caries*. Fluoride acts probably by preventing the growth of acid-forming bacteria or calcium phosphate fluoride compound in teeth which is resistant to acids.

Treatment

In the fluoride-deficient areas in the United States and Great Britain dental caries in children has been prevented by the addition of fluoride to drinking water. Such water cannot be beneficial to adults as fluoride cannot be incorporated in their teeth. Fluoride added to toothpaste is now a recognized method for preventing caries of teeth.

TOXICITY
(Fluorosis)

Fluorosis is excessive deposition of fluorine particularly in the bones and teeth. It occurs in many parts of the world. In India it is reported from Madras, Hyderabad-Deccan, and Punjab. The fluorine content of water in an endemic area may be as high as 14 parts per million (ppm). People over the age of 30 years are usually affected. Some immigrants to endemic areas are known to develop symptoms within a few years depending upon the fluoride content of the soil, climate, occupation and nutrition. Heavy manual workers in hot, humid climates who drink much water with high fluoride content develop symptoms earlier. In experimental animals fluorosis is less readily produced on a diet high in vitamin C and calcium. In humans oral administration of sodium fluoride results in increased calcium retention.

Teeth. The deciduous teeth are more easily affected. The upper incisors are first involved. In an endemic area up to 67 per cent of children may show mottling of teeth enamel. In the adults the teeth are lustreless and may have opaque white areas which appear as transverse ridges, localized or diffuse spots. In the advanced stage the teeth appear chalky white.

Bones. The bones most effected are of the vertebral column, particularly the cervical spine, pelvis and bones of the lower extremities. The bones are heavier and show exostosis particularly at the site of tendon attachment. The vertebrae are compressed anteroposteriorly, reducing the size of the vertebral canal and compressing the spinal cord. The nerves also are compressed due to fusion of the vertebrae, diminution of intervertebral foramina with osteophytes and calcification of intervertebral ligaments. Clubbing of fingers may occur.

Clinical Manifestations. Initially there is stiffness and pain in the spine. The *motor* system involvement produces weakness, spasticity of lower limbs, wasting of the distal muscles of hands, exaggerated deep jerks in the lower extremities with plantar extensor response. The *sensory* symptoms are paraesthesia, numbness or girdle pain. Examination may reveal involvement of the spinothalamic tract and posterior column. A transverse level of sensory loss up to the umbilicus, and *sphincter* disturbances may occur. *Deformities* such as kyphosis or flexion of the hips and kness produce difficulty in standing, sitting or lying prone. Fluorotic myelopathy therefore clinically resembles cervical spondylitis, spinal cord tumour, syringomyelia or subacute combined degeneration of the cord. *Radiologically* the bones show increased density, osteophytes and calcification of ligaments. The blood, urine and bones show high fluorine content. In one series the maximum fluorine content was, blood 0·61 mg/100 ml (6·1 ppm), urine 2·5 mg/100 ml (25 ppm) and 680 mg/100 g bone ash [2]. Due to decreased urinary excretion ingested calcium is retained [3].

Treatment. There is no specific treatment. Water supply with low fluoride content from canals and tube wells is the only effective prophylactic measure. In advanced crippling fluorosis, a low calcium diet of 200 mg a day increases urinary fluoride excretion, the bone pain is lessened, the spine straightened, and mobility is sufficiently improved to permit resumption of the daily routine [4].

FLUORIDE THERAPY FOR BONE DISEASES

Osteoporosis. Though it is conceded that fluoride up to 4 ppm is probably beneficial in the *prevention* of osteoporosis, the value of fluoride *therapy* in osteoporosis remains controversial. The intestinal absorption of calcium and calcium balance was not improved with daily intake of 20·6 mg sodium fluoride [5], and fluoride therapy for several months did not help [6]. On the other hand decreased bone absorption and increase in bone mass is reported with prolonged therapy with fluoride, a high calcium diet and vitamin D [7].

Therapeutically, sodium fluoride produces subjective improvement in patients with *Paget's disease*. In *multiple myeloma* fluoride and calcium therapy is claimed to be of benefit [8]. *Optic neuritis* is reported with the oral administration of sodium fluoride, 20 mg three times a day for 6 weeks [9].

Organic compounds with high fluoride content can retain much oxygen and have been experimentally used as erythrocyte substitutes [10].

REFERENCES

[1] SHAMBAUGL, G.E., and PETROVIC, A. (1968) Effects of sodium fluoride on the bone, *J. Amer., med. Ass.,* **204,** 969.
[2] SINGH, H.A., and JOLLY, S.S. (1961) Endemic fluorosis, *Quart. J. Med.,* **30,** 357.
[3] SRIKANTIA, S.G., and SIDDIQUI, A.H. (1965) Metabolic studies in skeletal fluorosis, *Clin. Sci.,* **28,** 477.
[4] TEOTIA, S.P.S. (1969) Report on meeting on biological action of fluoride, *Amer.*

J. clin. Nutr., **22**, 1409.

[5] SPENCER, H., LEWIN, I., FOWLER, J., and SAMACHSON, J. (1969) Effect of sodium fluoride on calcium absorption and balance in man, *Amer. J. clin. Nutr.*, **22**, 381.

[6] ROSE, G.A. (1965) A study of the treatment of osteoporosis with fluoride therapy and high calcium intake, *Proc. roy. Soc. Med.*, **58**, 436.

[7] JOWSEY, J., and KELLY, P.J. (1968) Effect of fluoride treatment in a patient with osteoporosis, *Proc. Mayo Clin.*, **43**, 435.

[8] COHEN, P. (1966) Fluoride and calcium therapy for myeloma bone lesions, *J. Amer. med. Ass.*, **198**, 583.

[9] GEALL, M.G., and BEILLIN, L.J. (1964) Sodium fluoride and optic neuritis, *Brit. med. J.*, **2**, 355.

[10] SLOVITER, H.A., PETKOVIC, M., OGOSHI, S., and YAMADA, H. (1969) Dispersed fluorochemicals as substitutes for erythrocytes in intact animals, *J. appl. Physiol.*, **27**, 666.

32. WATER

Water is the largest constituent of the body; the proportion of total body water varies with the proportion of fat. Whole body analysis as carried out by Widdowson, McCance and Spray [1] and Forbes and Lewis [2] suggests that water comprises 55–60 per cent of body weight in an average person. Thus a 60 kg man has approximately 34 litres of water in his tissues.

In tropical countries the supply of wholesome drinking water in villages is still a problem. Villagers depend upon rivers, rivulets, streams or wells as the sole source of water for agriculture, animal husbandry and their personal needs for cooking, drinking, bathing and for washing clothes and utensils. Not uncommonly the same contaminated water which is used for washing clothes and utensils or animals, is drawn for the purpose of drinking and cooking. This is likely to spread water-borne epidemics like typhoid, cholera, dysentery and virus jaundice. These epidemics are likely to occur during the summer months when the rivulets and streams are dry and water is stagnant.

Composition

Water is a simple compound containing two parts of hydrogen with one of oxygen (H_2O). Good drinking water has no odour and is pleasant to taste. Water contains traces of sodium, calcium, magnesium and iron depending upon the soil from which it is obtained. Soft water contains small amounts of minerals and lathers easily. Hard water contains a higher proportion of calcium salts and does not lather easily. Drinking hard water does not lead to formation of stones in the urinary tract unless excessive intake of vitamin D or prolonged exposure to sunlight cause increased absorption of calcium. One of the possible causes of urinary calculi in hill-people of Maharashtra is that they drink hard water and are excessively exposed to the sun. On the other hand, people drinking soft water are more likely to have coronary heart disease than those drinking hard water.

Absorption

Water is absorbed only slightly from the stomach but it is rapidly absorbed from the small intestine and to a lesser extent from the large intestine. Water given as an enema can be absorbed. The maximum capacity for water absorption from the entire human bowel is 20 litres a day [3].

Balance

There is a balance between the intake and the output of water. The kidneys of a healthy person excrete within a few hours any excess water ingested.

Daily intake	ml	Daily excretion	ml
As fluids like water, tea, coffee, aerated waters, sherbet, milk and soup	1500–1750	Urine	1200–1500
		Perspiration	700– 900
Water contained in solid food	600– 900	Respiration	400– 400
Water of oxidation of carbohydrate, protein and fat	300– 350	Faeces	100– 200
Total	2400–3000	Total	2400–3000

The above figures are approximate and vary considerably with different environments. In the tropics more fluids, especially water, is ingested during the hot season because of increased loss through perspiration.

Almost all food-stuffs except pure fat contain varying amounts of water. Thus cooked rice contains about 70 per cent and cucumber about 97 per cent water. When food is metabolized the ultimate breakdown products are carbon dioxide and water. Approximately 55, 40 and 100 ml of water are released when 100 g of carbohydrate, protein and fat respectively are metabolized. The total water available from oxidation of food is about 300 ml per day.

Excretion

Kidneys. About 170 litres of fluid pass through the glomeruli of the kidneys each day, of which only 1·5 litres are excreted as urine while 168·5 litres are reabsorbed by the tubules. If the body is deprived of water or water loss for any reason is high, the amount of urine formed is reduced. The average output of urine on a cool day is about 1500 ml which is more than adequate to excrete the waste products of metabolism. The capacity of the kidneys to concentrate the urine is limited. The limit of concentration for urea, which forms the bulk of the waste products, is 4 per cent. In order to excrete 30 g of urea which is the daily average, 750 ml of urine must be passed. If less urine is formed then waste products are retained in the body.

Sweat. With excessive sweat much water is lost from the body and so less urine is formed. Excessive sweating occurs with increased external temperature and humidity, fever and exercise. During violent exercise the body weight can fall by as much as 2–4 kg in an hour due to sweating. An obese person may lose 1–2 kg in weight when he sweats profusely in a steam bath but immediately afterwards he regains this weight by drinking to quench the thirst produced by dehydration. Dehydration is always corrected by retention of water to replace losses before any excess is excreted by the kidneys. Attempts to reduce weight by sweating are useful only to prize-fighters and jockeys who have to remain within a certain weight for the weighing in. In the summer months in the hot Persian gulf patients had a daily loss of 2–4 litres of fluid [4].

Insensible Loss. Apart from visible sweating, water constantly evaporates from the surface of the skin, a process referred to as 'insensible perspiration' and independent of the sweat glands. During respiration moisture is also being constantly lost from the respiratory epithelium. When humidity is low, evaporation from the alveolar surfaces is high; if moist air is inhaled evaporation is less. The total water loss through respiration amounts to about 400 ml a day.

Function

Water is concerned in all metabolic processes and correction of dehydration is therefore a most important aspect of treatment. In many conditions secondary dehydration is a cause of death even when the primary condition has been treated. All the vital functions of the body depend on the presence of a proper amount of water. The high water content of various tissues serves to illustrate its importance in the body. For example, blood plasma contains 92 per cent and the red blood cells 70 per cent of water; digestion depends upon the secretion of juices which are mainly water; urine contains about 97 per cent water.

Water also helps in the regulation of body temperature. Evaporation of water by respiration and sweat is an efficient mechanism regulating body heat. Sweating is the chief mode of heat loss when the atmospheric temperature is higher than the body temperature. Evaporation of sweat is rapid when the air is dry but with increasing humidity, sweat does not evaporate so rapidly. The hot dry plains, even with high atmospheric temperature, are therefore much more tolerable than the humid atmosphere near the sea.

Source

All liquids taken by man are water, with or without other constituents; solid foods, particularly fruits and vegetables, also contain a high proportion of water.

Requirement

A person's water requirements vary considerably according to the climate, dietetic habits, activities and body build and so it is impossible to specify the daily requirement. The basic minimum under most circumstances has been discussed. Healthy kidneys regulate body water efficiently. With an excess there is increased formation of urine, and during deprivation the secretion of urine is diminished. As a working rule, a person should take enough fluid to excrete 1200–1500 ml of urine per day. In the tropics, where much water is lost through perspiration, about 7–10 glasses (2400–3000 ml) of fluids as water, aerated water, tea, coffee, etc. are needed to maintain this urine volume. The colour of the urine is a practical guide to the adequacy of fluid intake; in a healthy person a pale yellow urine indicates an adequate intake while a high coloured urine indicates an insufficient fluid intake. In acute vomiting and diarrhoea excessive loss of water and electrolytes may have to be replaced by parenteral administration. Water intake also affects the bowels, the commonest cause of constipation in the tropics is an inadequate intake of water.

In oliguric kidney diseases and hyponatraemia due to retention of water the intake may have to be restricted.

Water with Meals. It is a popular notion that if water is taken with meals it tends to dilute the digestive juices and impair digestion. Moderate amounts of water, about one glass, taken with meals, has no harmful effect. Soups, milk, beverages like tea and coffee, and most of our so-called solid foods like cucumber, tomatoes and fruits contain a large proportion of water but no one has ever claimed that these should not be taken with meals.

Pure Dehydration

Pure dehydration without salt loss, occurs in deserts, after ship-wreck and in acutely ill or unconscious patients. In these circum-stances the daily loss of water as insensible perspiration continues even though no water is taken, only a little being replaced by the water of oxidation. Water deprivation leads to thirst, weakness, loss of weight, dryness of the skin and mucous membranes, tachycardia, disorienta-tion, delirium and coma. The urine is scanty, high coloured and of high specific gravity. The serum levels of end products of metabolism like urea are elevated. The excretion of salt is also diminished and the serum sodium and chloride levels are elevated. In an attempt to com-pensate, water is drawn from the cellular compartment of the body leading to cellular dehydration and loss of function by vital organs.

Pure water deficiency should be corrected by the administration of water by mouth. In an unconscious patient a gastric tube can be passed and fluids given. If the patient vomits, a rectal drip of boiled tap water is useful. The rectum is first cleaned by a low enema. A rectal tube lubricated with vaseline is then gently inserted to about

15 cm and a slow drip started so as to infuse 15–20 drops of water per minute. Where better facilities are available 5 per cent glucose solutions can be given intravenously. Pure water deficiency should not be corrected with normal saline.

The best and simplest guide to determine the adequacy of water replacement is to measure the urine output. It should exceed 1000 ml in 24 hours.

Combined Salt and Water Depletion

This is more common than pure water depletion in clinical practice especially in acutely ill patients with fever, diarrhoea, diabetic coma or after surgical operation.

Water Intoxication

When excess of water is taken, especially when water excretion is deficient as in oliguric renal failure or adrenal failure, water intoxication occurs. During an over-enthusiastic bowel wash an excessive amount of water may be absorbed from the gut. The commonest cause of water intoxication is intravenous therapy, particularly in children in whom the margin of error is small. Water intoxication may also occur during tests for adrenal cortical deficiency or after administration of an antidiuretic to psychotic patients who drink an excessive amount of water. A patient who has almost pure salt depletion develops water intoxication if given parenteral isotonic saline or glucose (only hypertonic saline is indicated). Excessive fluid intake during oliguric renal failure can be a dangerous cause of water intoxication.

The *symptoms* of water intoxication are weakness, lethargy, confusion, vomiting, coma and convulsion. An epileptic is likely to get a fit even with moderate water retention. The serum sodium level is low.

The condition is treated by withholding water and giving a dry diet. In severe cases hypertonic saline may have to be administered intravenously.

REFERENCES

[1] WIDDOWSON, E.M., McCANCE, R.A., and SPRAY, C.M. (1951) The chemical composition of human body, *Clin. Sci.*, **10**, 113.
[2] FORBES, G.B., and LEWIS, A.M. (1956) Total sodium, potassium and chloride in adult man, *J. clin. Invest.*, **35**, 596.

[3] LOVE, A.H.G., MITCHELL, T.T., and PHILLIPS, R.A. (1968) Sodium and water absorption in the human intestine, *J. Physiol. (Lond.)*, **195**, 133.

[4] TINCKLER, L.F. (1966) Fluid and electrolyte observations in tropical surgical practice, *Brit. med. J.*, **1**, 1263.

PART II

FOODS

33. WHEAT

Wheat is the most widely used cereal in the world. It is the main cereal of the Punjab, Uttar Pradesh and West Pakistan, providing over 70 per cent of the total calorie intake.

Structure

It is necessary to understand the structure of wheat because during processing the parts that may be removed are of importance for nutrition.

1. *Bran.* This is the outer protective brown coat of the grain. It consists of cellulose and minerals and constitutes about 12 per cent of the weight of the whole grain. The term bran is generally used a little loosely for the residue left after the removal of milled flour. This residue includes both the outer coat and the underlying layer of cells called the aleurone layer.

2. *Aleurone layer.* This single layer of cells, on the inner side of bran, is the outer layer of the endosperm and is rich in proteins. During milling this layer is removed—because it is firmly attached to the bran.

3. *Endosperm (kernel).* This is the main constituent of wheat, forming about 85 per cent of the whole grain. It is rich in starch and proteins and when milled yields flour.

4. *The germ (embryo).* The embryo, which is situated at the base of the grain, is rich in proteins, fats, the fat-soluble vitamin E (wheat germ oil), and thiamine. The germ is usually removed in milling as otherwise the fat in it rapidly turns the flour rancid.

5. *Scutellum.* This is a thin layer between germ, at the base of the grain, and the main body, the endosperm. It contributes 1·5 per cent of the total weight of the grain, but contains 59 per cent of all the thiamine (vitamin B) in the whole wheat [1]. To derive vitamin B_1 from a wheat diet, it is thus very important to preserve the scutellum in the flour.

Milling

Most wheat is processed to make flour for bread. After grinding, the coarser part of the grain, which contains cellulose, is removed and the white flour remains. The amount of flour remaining from the original wheat is called the percentage extraction. Thus 95 per cent extraction means that 95 per cent of the grain has been extracted as flour while the remaining 5 per cent has been removed as bran. The lower the extraction rate of flour the smaller the amount of bran and the whiter the flour—thus 70 per cent extraction flour is whiter than 85 per cent extraction. Bakers prefer the more refined flour (lower extraction flour) which is whiter and can be made into better looking bread or cake, than the high extraction flour which is more nutritious.

The percentage extraction and its effect on nutrition and growth particularly in the children was a problem in Great Britain during and after the Second World War when the import of wheat was restricted. An experimental study on the effects of feeding flour of different extraction rates was undertaken on German children by McCance and Widdowson [2, 3]. Wheat supplied 75 per cent of the calories for these children and 20 per cent of the calories were derived from potatoes and vegetables. All flours were fortified with calcium carbonate to supply adequate calcium. Fortifying 70 per cent flour with thiamine, riboflavine, nicotinic acid and iron did not increase the rate of growth nor did an additional pint of milk make any difference. There was no significant difference in growth rates between groups of undernourished German children who were fed either on 100 per cent or 70 per cent extraction wheat flour.

This excellent study appears to have settled once and for all the dispute as to whether the wheat extraction rate makes difference to man as long as adequate calories are provided. How far we should accept this for the Indian conditions is impossible to answer without a parallel experiment. The German children were well provided with calories and variety of foods. Whether the same results hold good among the semi-starved millions of India has yet to be proved. As McCance and Widdowson themselves have said 'how important it is not to generalise too widely from any experiment carried out within limiting condition' [2]. It is well known that when a deficiency of any nutrient exists in the body the absorption rate rises. In the present state of knowledge it is logical to assume that to starving millions the higher extraction rate, which contains a higher proportion of calcium, iron and vitamin B, would be a distinct advantage.

In many Eastern countries there are no regulations about the percentage extraction of wheat. According to the local demand the miller may process wheat to various degrees of extraction and coarseness.

Flour is the general name used for milled wheat containing little bran. *Atta* is wheat flour containing variable amounts of bran. *Maida* is finely ground flour for making bread, cakes, or biscuits. *Semolina* (*suji*) is granular, and is used in the preparation of sweets.

Fortification of wheat flour with inexpensive calcium carbonate is advocated, particularly in areas where milk intake is low and little calcium is available from other food sources. Indian children showed nearly the same rate of growth on a daily supplement of 1 g calcium lactate as on a supplement of 30 g skimmed milk powder (1 cup liquid milk) [4].

Chappatis (*unleavened bread*). In India, Pakistan, Bangladesh and Ceylon most people prefer *chappatis* which are made by adding water (some fat as *ghee* or oil may also be added) to wheat flour, forming dough. Small pieces of dough are then rolled evenly flat with a rolling pin by the housewife with amazing dexterity and speed. The thin flat rolled dough is then toasted on a heated pan to make brown *chappatis*. To what extent the proteins and vitamins are destroyed by direct toasting of *chappatis* on a heated pan is not known. Bread as made in the Western countries tastes better if made from more refined flour but *chappatis* are relished only if prepared with an appreciable quantity of bran (90–95 per cent extraction). *Chappatis* made from refined flour (*maida*) are not palatable.

Wheat bran. Bran is highly prized by some. They add it to wheat flour because the chemical analysis of bran shows that it contains a large proportion of proteins and vitamins. As mentioned previously the term bran is used rather loosely to include both the outer seed coat and the aleurone layer rich in proteins, both of which are removed during milling.

The proteins of wheat bran are albumin, globulin and an alcohol-soluble protein [5]. Taken collectively, the proteins of bran are richer in amino acid than those of wheat flour. Immature rats thrive better for the first few weeks on bran than on wheat flour [6]. These results of experiments on young rats cannot be applied directly to man. Adult rats did not show the same difference between high extraction flour and bran.

Bran contains cellulose which is digested by cattle but not by humans. The high phosphorus and phytate content of bran interferes with the absorption of calcium and iron.

Bran in constipation. The unabsorbed cellulose of bran forms bulk in the intestine which stimulates peristalsis and helps evacuation of the bowel. For constipation, bran is helpful though it interferes with absorption of other foods. In some people bran irritates the bowel and produces diarrhoea.

COMPOSITION

Calories

Wheat flour provides 350 Calories per 100 g (100 Calories per oz).

Proteins

Wheat flour is derived mainly from the endosperm (kernel) which contains polypeptides, *gliadin* and *glutenin,* which are collectively known as *gluten* and constitute about 12 per cent of the flour. Gluten, and particularly the gliadin fraction, has been found to be the substance responsible for *coeliac disease* in children in whom complete exclusion of wheat and wheat preparations results in remarkable improvement. Wheat is perhaps the only cereal eaten in the East which contains gluten but in the Western countries bread is also made from 'rye' which contains gluten. Gluten is relatively poor in the amino acid lysine which is necessary for proper growth. Animals thrived when bread was fortified with lysine [7]. If lysine is supplied to a wheat diet by other vegetable proteins then nutrition improves. Pulses, soya bean, groundnut and cotton-seed flours provide a good supplement to wheat and partially replace an absence of animal protein of high biological value [8, 9]. Milk is probably the best supplement of all for providing the amino acids missing in a purely wheat diet [10].

Properties of Gluten. Gluten is a protein which becomes viscous when water is added to it. Thus a good dough can be made from wheat flour. This property of wheat is not shown by rice, *bajra* or *jowar* flour which form an amorphous mass with water and do not form a good dough. Carbon dioxide can be bubbled into wheat dough to make a spongy mass suitable for making bread or cake. Bakers use brewers' yeast or baking powder as a source of carbon dioxide. Many Indians make delicious spongy preparations by fermenting wheat flour with *toddy*.

The hard Indian wheat contains more gluten than the Western variety. The gluten content of wheat flour can be greatly reduced, even to 3–4 per cent by infestation with weevils [11].

Fats
Wheat flour contains 1·7 per cent fat derived from the germ.

Carbohydrates
Whole wheat flour provides 72 per cent carbohydrates.

Vitamins
Thiamine, riboflavine and nicotinic acid values diminish considerably as the extraction rate is increased.

Minerals

Calcium. Wheat is poor in calcium. The calcium requirement of Indians is assumed to be 0·3–0·5 g a day for an adult male [see CHAPTER 23]. The calcium content of Indian whole wheat flour is 40 mg per 100 g so that 750–1250 g (1½–2½ lbs) of wheat must be eaten to meet the calcium requirements. This figure is based on the assumption that all the calcium in wheat is absorbed, in fact only about 30 per cent is absorbed because wheat flour contains an excess of phosphorus and phytate which prevent calcium absorption. Taking this factor into account, 2500–3750 g (5–8 lbs) of whole wheat flour has to be eaten to satisfy the calcium requirement. Refined flour contains only 20 mg calcium per 100 g but this lower content is offset by better absorption. The best and most inexpensive way of solving the problem of calcium deficiency in wheat is to add calcium carbonate, 14 ozs to 280 lbs flour, as is done in the United Kingdom.

Iron. The iron content of whole wheat flour is high, while refined flour has considerably less iron. In Great Britain flour regulations require not less than 1·65 mg iron per 100 g flour. Thus, 70 per cent extraction white flour requires the addition of iron. However, iron from brown bread is absorbed better than iron-enriched white bread [12]. The addition of iron to flour in Great Britain appears in effect to fulfil the policy of restoration, as intended, and not one of fortification [13].

Phosphorus. Whole wheat flour is rich in phosphorus, as compared to refined flour. The high content of phosphorus prevents the absorption of other minerals like iron and calcium.

Gluten Sensitivity
[See Malabsorption Syndrome]

REFERENCES

[1] HINTON, J.J.C. (1944) The chemistry of wheat germ with particular reference to scutellum, *Biochem. J.*, **38**, 214.

[2] McCANCE, R.A., and WIDDOWSON, E.M. (1955) Old thoughts and new work on breads white and brown, *Lancet*, **ii**, 205.

[3] WIDDOWSON, E.M., and McCANCE, R.A. (1954) Studies on the nutritive value of bread and on the effect of variations in the extraction rate of flour on the growth of undernourished children, *Spec. Rep. Ser. med. Res. Coun. (Lond.)*, No. 287, London, H.M.S.O.

[4] AYKROYD, W.R., and KRISHNAN, B.G. (1939) A further experiment on the value of calcium lactate for Indian children, *Indian J. med. Res.*, **27**, 409.

[5] JONES, D.B., and GERSDORFF, C.E.F. (1923) Proteins of wheat bran. I. Isolation and elementary analysis of globulin, albumin and prolamine, *J. biol. Chem.*, **58**, 117.

[6] MURPHY, J.C., and JONES, D.B. (1926) Proteins of wheat bran. III. The nutritive properties of the proteins of wheat-bran, *J. biol. Chem.*, **69**, 85.

[7] ROSENBERG, H.R., RHODENBURG, E.L., and BALDINI, J.T. (1954) The fortification of bread with lysine. III. Supplementation with essential amino acids, *Arch. Biochem.*, **49**, 263.

[8] JONES, D.B., and DIVINE, J.P. (1944) The protein nutritional value of soyabean, peanut and cottonseed flours and their value as supplements to wheat flour, *J. Nutr.*, **28**, 41.

[9] PHANSALKAR, S.V., and PATWARDHAN, V.N. (1956) Utilization of animal and vegetable proteins: Nitrogen balances at marginal protein intakes and the determination of minimum protein requirements for maintenance in young Indian men, *Indian J. med. Res.*, **44**, 1.

[10] HENRY, K.M., and KON, S.K. (1942) The effect of the method of feeding on the supplementary relationships between the proteins of dairy products and those of bread or potato, *Chem. and Ind.*, **61**, 97.

[11] INDIAN COUNCIL OF MEDICAL RESEARCH (1952) *Wheat and Wheat Products as Human Food*, Special Report Series No. 23, New Delhi, p.34.

[12] CALLENDER, S.T., and WARNER, G.T. (1970) Iron absorption from brown bread, *Lancet*, **i**, 546.

[13] ELWOOD, P.C., NEWTON, D., EAKINS, J.D., and BROWN, D.A. (1968) Absorption of iron from bread, *Amer. J. clin. Nutr.*, **21**, 1162.

34. RICE

Rice is the staple food in South India, Assam and Kashmir. It is also the staple food of Bangladesh, Ceylon, Burma, China and Japan. When rice forms the major source of calories, the nutritive value of the diet depends upon the processing undertaken before it is marketed. Depending upon the mode of processing, different parts of the rice grain may be removed. The effect of each process can be clearly understood by a study of the structure of the rice grain.

Structure

1. *Husk.* The husk is the loose covering of rice. It has no nutritive value and is always removed before cooking. The process of removing the husk is called *milling*.

2. *Bran.* It is the outermost coat of the grain. It contains nutrients and cellulose. The latter interferes with the absorption of other foods, hence this layer is best removed.

3. *Aleurone layer.* It is a thin layer underneath the bran. It cantains vitamins, minerals, proteins and fats.

4. *Embryo or the germ.* It is at the base of the grain and is rich in nutrients and vitamin E.

5. *Endosperm.* It forms 75 per cent of the grain. It consists mainly of starch which is the principal source of calories.

COMPOSITION

Rice is rich in starch, moderate in proteins and poor in fat, iron and calcium. During cooking rice absorbs a considerable amount of water.

Calories

Rice provides about 350 Calories per 100 g dry weight (100 Calories per oz).

Proteins

Rice contains about 7 per cent proteins; these are deficient in the amino acid lysine. When rice is supplemented with lysine the growth rate of animals is rapid. Soya bean and pulses form an excellent supplement to the rice diet [1]. The Chinese custom of eating rice with soya bean provides proteins of high biological value. Eating rice with *dal* (pulses) or a preparation of rice and *dal* (*khichdi*) or eating rice with milk or milk products like curd and buttermilk are also helpful in balancing the diet.

PROCESSING

For the removal of the husk and bran the following processes are employed: (1) hand pounding; (2) machine milling; (3) parboiling followed by hand pounding or machine milling [2].

Hand Pounding

This is mainly done by farmers who cultivate rice for their own consumption. Rice is placed in a big mortar and pounded with wooden or iron pestles. The hand pounding does not remove the bran as completely as milling, so vitamins are better preserved.

Machine Milling

Most of the rice sold in the market is machine milled, a process which removes bran, aleurone layer and embryo. These components are collectively called the *polishings;* they are nutritious and constitute 10 per cent of the weight of the grain.

Advantages of Milling. (1) Milled rice keeps better as it is less likely to be contaminated by insect pests which destroy the stored grain; (2) it looks clean and attractive for marketing; (3) it is easily digested and absorbed; (4) it contains little phytate and hence minerals from other foods are better absorbed.

Disadvantages of Milling. According to the mode of milling variable proportions of vitamin B complex, calcium, iron, proteins and fats are removed. It is possible to remove over 75 per cent of thiamine during milling. When rice constitutes the main source of food this loss leads to beriberi. In Western countries vitamin B is supplied from other sources consequently an occasional helping of highly polished rice has no deleterious effect.

Parboiling followed by Hand Pounding or Machine Milling

In the States of Madras, Bengal and Goa parboiled rice is consumed. The methods of parboiling vary but essentially consist of: (1) soaking paddy (rice with husk) in water; (2) the water is then brought to the boil; (3) the water is drained off and the paddy is dried; (4) the dried paddy is later either machine milled or hand pounded, as described above, to separate the husk.

Advantages of Parboiling. (1) The grain after parboiling is harder. (2) Parboiled rice can be preserved better both in the uncooked as well as in the cooked state than the rice which has not been parboiled. (3) When parboiled rice is processed the outer bran is more easily removed without the aleurone layer so polishing is easier and the nutrients are better preserved. It is, therefore, better to machine mill parboiled rice than raw rice. (4) When parboiled rice is washed prior to cooking the loss of nutrients is far less than from raw rice.

Disadvantages of Parboiling. (1) It involves an additional process before polishing. (2) Parboiled rice may give off an unpleasant smell during cooking.

Washing

Washing rice before cooking is another step in which up to 33 per cent of vitamins are lost. Repeated rigorous washing before cooking is best avoided if vitamins are to be preserved.

Cooking

The method of cooking also determines the loss of nutrients. Cooking with extra water which is later drained off is uneconomical and up to 33 per cent of thiamine is lost. Only just sufficient water should be used so that no excess need be thrown away.

Stored Rice

Stored rice cooks better than the fresh crop. When kept over six to twelve months it is well dehydrated and on cooking absorbs about double the quantity of water and the grains remain separate, making an attractive dish when served.

Digestion

Rice is well digested. When chewed well the digestion begins with ptyalin in the mouth and is completed by the pancreatic and intestinal juices. It is assumed by some that rice is difficult to digest and should be avoided during an acute illness. The reason for this notion is that amongst the rice eaters it forms the main course and an average helping is at least a plateful. If eaten with *dal* (pulses) it produces too big a bulk. Smaller feeds of a couple of tablespoons of rice with milk or milk products are easily digested even during an acute illness.

Absorption

Almost all the rice is completely absorbed from the intestine as the polished grain has no covering of cellulose. Since rice leaves no residue it is advised for a low residue diet. The low phosphorus content of rice allows better absorption of minerals, calcium and iron, and thus partly compensates for the low content of these elements.

Fermented Rice

Fermented rice gives better nutrition. Rats fed on 2 parts rice and one part black gram (*urd dal*) with a high fat, low protein diet, showed fatty changes in the liver but when rice was previously fermented (*idli*) the fatty changes in the liver were prevented. The fermented rice has a higher content of choline and folic acid [3]. The fact that Tamils in Southern India often eat fermented rice as *idli* may be a factor in the prevention of liver damage despite a low intake of proteins.

BERIBERI

The vitamin B content, mainly thiamine, is high in rice. Despite this the discovery that deficiency diseases could occur due to lack of vitamins was made in rice-eating populations suffering from clinical beriberi [see CHAPTER 5]. When rice is the principal food then it also becomes the main source of the vitamin B group. During the process of milling, washing and cooking of rice over 75 per cent thiamine may be lost. Added to this, when the main source of calories is carbohydrate the demand for vitamins of the B group is increased. Subclinical or clinical vitamin B deficiency can occur when a diet consists mainly of highly polished rice.

KEMPNER'S RICE DIET

In hypertension a diet with rice and fruit has been described by Kempner. There is no hypotensive factor in rice and the benefits are due to the low intake of proteins and sodium.

REFERENCES

[1] DESIKACHAR, H.S.R., SANKARAN, A.N., and SUBRAHMANYAN, V. (1956) The comparative value of soyabean and Bengal gram as supplements to the poor South Indian rice diet, *Indian J. med. Res.*, **44**, 741.

[2] NARAYANSWAMI, C.K. (1956) *The Rice We Eat,* All India Khadi and Village
     Industries Board, Bombay.
[3] KHANDWALA, K.P. (1960) *Studies in Fermented Foodstuffs,* M.Sc. Thesis,
     University of Bombay.

35. PULSES AND BEANS

Pulses is a general name given for plants which provide dried edible
seeds. Pulses when split are known as *dal.* Dried peas and beans have
about the same composition as *dal.* Groundnut should also be included
here but the taste as well as the composition are akin to nuts and
so for convenience they are considered as nuts. In the tropics, pulses
are second only to cereals as important sources of calories and proteins
for the masses.

COMPOSITION

Calories

Pulses supply the same amount of calories as cereals, i.e. 350 Calories
per 100 g dry weight (i.e. 100 Calories per oz).

Proteins

The protein content of pulses is 20–25 per cent, about twice as
much as cereals, and the most economical source of proteins. There is
less of amino acid methionine in pulses than in animal proteins, but
the higher lysine content makes them a good supplement to rice. The
combination of cereals with pulses can provide enough protein of high
biological value [1]. The usual habit of eating rice with *dal* (*khichdi*), or
wheat *chappati* with pulses, is nutritionally sound. The addition of a
cup of milk greatly enhances the biological value of a meal of pulses
with cereals.

Fats

The fat content of pulses is negligible, being 1–2 g per 100 g. Bengal
gram (*chana*) contains 5 per cent fat.

Carbohydrates

Pulses provide about 60 g of carbohydrate per 100 g.

Vitamins

Pulses are a fair source of *thiamine, riboflavine* and *nicotinic* acid. The *vitamin C* content of pulses can be greatly increased by soaking them in water and allowing them to germinate. The *carotene* content appreciably increases on the third day after germination when the shoots change from yellow to green, probably with an increase in the chlorophyll content [2].

Minerals

The *iron* content of pulses is high, being 8–10 mg per cent (less in lentils and split peas). The *calcium* content is between 100 and 200 mg per cent.

Germination

The simple measure of soaking the pulses for a couple of days improves their nutritive value and vitamins A and C content. Black gram (*urd dal*) and lentils (*masur dal*) when germinated contain a definite growth promoting factor. Its nature is not known [3].

COOKING AND DIGESTIBILITY

Pulses are most completely digested and absorbed if made into flour. The usual practice is to eat pulses in the form of *dals* (split pulses). Unless cooked well, split pulses are not easily digested and are incompletely absorbed. Pulses contain an antidigestive factor (trypsin inhibitor) which is destroyed by cooking. Green gram (*mung dal*) is better digested than other pulses because its smaller size facilitates cooking. In persons suffering from diarrhoea, undigested pulses in the large intestine are acted upon by gas-producing bacteria. Even in a healthy person, the consumption of more than 100 g (dry weight) of pulses gives rise to marked flatulence. Beans are acted upon by the intestinal anaerobic bacteria, which results in hydrogen and carbon dioxide production. This gas production can be inhibited by decreasing the bacterial flora with antibiotics and bacteriostatic agents [4].

Bengal gram consumed over a period of several weeks may reduce serum cholesterol levels by increasing faecal excretion of total bile acids [5].

Palatability

Most people in the tropics like pulses and they are relished even by the rich. Some pulses, notably field beans (*val dal*) have a bitter taste but a taste can be acquired for them just as for a bitter drink of beer.

LATHYRISM [6]

Lathyrism is a disease, seen in India and in Spain, peculiar to regions where there is a high consumption of the pulse known as *Lathyrus sativus* (*khesari dal*). In India, lathyrism is seen in Madhya Pradesh and the border districts of Uttar Pradesh, Bihar and Orissa. In the district of Rewa and Satna in Madhya Pradesh 2·6 per cent of the population are affected. It is 10 times more common in males and in females the disease does not set in during the reproductive period of life.

Aetiology

Lathyrus sativus requires little water and is sown with wheat as a para-crop in the winter so as to guard against drought. It is cheap and is consumed by the labourers of the lowest economic group. Among these people, *Lathyrus sativus* usually contributes about 40 per cent of the diet, but, during drought and famine the consumption increases to 95–100 per cent. At these times there is a marked increase in the prevalence of the disease. The incidence of the disease is increased if the husk is eaten. A diet of *Lathyrus sativus* provides over 3000 Calories and 140 g of protein daily, which is a high intake. There is no specific nutritional deficiency and, even in 1926, McCarrison reported that lathyrism affected the better fed men.

Clinical Manifestations

Clinically the disease affects the pyramidal tracts only. The onset is sudden, usually after exertion or exposure to cold, with contraction of the calf muscles, usually during sleep, and pain in the lower back. A spastic paralysis of the lower limbs develops with rigidity, weakness, exaggerated knee and ankle jerks, and ankle clonus. Progress of the disease results in paraplegia in flexion. The sensory system and sphincters are spared.

The serum albumin values are normal, the serum globulin may show a slight increase. There is an increase in the urinary excretion of glutamic acid.

A *latent form* of the disease also occurs manifested only by exaggerated knee and ankle jerks. In this type the progress can be prevented if lathyrus seed is removed from the diet.

The patients survive for many years but the severe cases do not improve.

The toxic factor of *L. sativus* is water-soluble *beta* (N)-oxalylamino alanine (BOAA) that produces neurotoxicity. *Prevention* of lathyrism is now possible. The contaminated *dal* is made safe for consumption by the following: (1) Steeping the pulse in four times its volume of hot water for an hour removes not only 90 per cent of the BOAA but also the water-soluble vitamin B complex. The water is removed and the pulse is sun-dried and ground to make flour for *chappatis* (unleavened bread). (2) Parboiling the pulses (a process similar to that for rice) [see p. 236], preserves the B complex vitamins [8].

REFERENCES

[1] PHANSALKAR, S.V., and PATWARDHAN, V.N. (1956) Utilization of animal and vegetable proteins, *Indian J. med. Res.*, **44**, 1.

[2] CHATTOPADHYAY, H., and BANERJEE, S. (1951) Effect of germination on the carotene content of pulses and cereals, *Science*, **113**, 600.

[3] CHATTOPADHYAY, H., and BANERJEE, S. (1953) Effect of germination on the biological value of proteins and the trypsin-inhibitor activity of some common Indian pulses, *Indian J. med. Res.*, **41**, 185.

[4] RICHARDS, E.A., STEGGERDA, F.R., and MURATA, A. (1968) Relationship of bean substrates and certain intestinal bacteria to gas production in the dog, *Gastroenterology*, **55**, 502.

[5] MATHUR, K.S., KHAN, M.A., and SHARMA, R.D. (1968) Hypochlolesterolaemic effect of Bengal gram: A long-term study in man, *Brit. med. J.*, **1**, 30.

[6] NAGARAJAN, V. (1970) *A Decade of Progress* 1960–1970, *National Institute of Nutrition, Hyderabad, India*, Indian Council of Medical Research, New Delhi, p. 20.

[7] McCARRISON, R. (1926) A note on lathyrism in the Gilgit Agency, *Indian J. med. Res.*, **14**, 379.

[8] NAGARAJAN, V., and GOPALAN, C. (1967) *Annual Report*, Nutr. Res. Lab., Hyderabad, p. 14.

36. SOYA BEAN
(*Glycine hispida, Glycine max*)

Soya bean is extensively consumed in Japan and China and has been increasingly grown in the United States. It has drawn considerable attention from nutritionists in Asia, because it is cheap to grow yet is rich in calories, proteins and fats.

COMPOSITION

Soya bean contains 19·5 per cent fat, 21 per cent carbohydrate and provides 432 Calories per 100 g.

Proteins

Soya bean contains 43 per cent protein which is a higher proportion than other protein-rich foods, including meat and fish which contain about 20–25 per cent. The proteins of soya bean yield all the essential amino acids in adequate amounts except for methionine and cystine which are deficient. Soya bean is rich in lysine and can be used to supplement a staple rice diet. A mixture of fifteen parts soya bean with 85 parts wheat flour promotes growth experimentally [1].

Digestion and Absorption

Cooking. Soya bean contains a factor which inhibits the action of the digestive enzyme trypsin and this factor can be destroyed by heat. Soya bean should thus be well cooked to aid digestion and absorption. The biological value of soya bean protein can be increased by autoclaving it in steam at 125°C for 2 hours.

The trypsin-inhibiting factor of raw soya bean fed to animals enlarges the pancreas and enhances pancreatic enzyme secretion. This excessive enzyme is excreted through faeces, producing loss of protein and amino acid with resultant stunted growth [2].

Soya Bean Milk

Milk can be prepared from soya bean [3], and has the following composition:

Total solids	10·15 per cent
Protein	4·2 ,,
Fat	3·4 ,,
Carbohydrate	1·8 ,,
Salts	0·75 ,,

The vitamin content of soya milk is similar to that of cow's milk.

	Soya milk per litre	Cow's milk per litre
Vitamin A	750 IU	1,050 IU
Thiamine	0·82 mg	0·43 mg
Riboflavine	1·10 mg	1·32 mg
Nicotinic acid	2·49 mg	1·16 mg
Ascorbic acid	21·6 mg	17.8 mg

For the normal growth of babies soya bean milk requires to be supplemented by animal milk, minerals and vitamins.

Soya Bean in the Indian Diet

The possibility of using soya bean in large quantities for the Indian population has been studied [4]. The report concludes that although soya bean contains more fat, minerals, vitamins and available proteins than other pulses, it has for some unknown reason not proved itself superior to other pulses. To an Indian palate, a diet of pulses, with 20–25 per cent proteins, and cereals is more acceptable than soya bean.

SOYA BEAN GOITRE

McCarrison noted goitre in rats fed on soya bean flour [5]. Infants given preparations containing soya bean develop goitre [6, 7]. The mechanism of soya bean goitre is not understood. The metabolism of iodine is probably interfered with because the goitre can be largely prevented by supplementing a soya bean diet with iodine.

REFERENCES

[1] JONES, D.B., and DIVINE, J.P. (1944) The protein nutritional value of soyabean, peanut, and cottonseed flours and their value as supplements to wheat flour, *J. Nutr.*, **28**, 41.

[2] MELMED, R.N., and BOUCHIER, I.A.D. (1969) A further physiological role for

naturally occurring trypsin inhibitors: the evidence for a trophic stimulant of the pancreatic acinar cell, *Gut*, **10**, 973.

[3] SUBRAHMANYAN, V. (1946) Quoted in *Report on Soya Bean by the Soya Bean Sub-Committee of the Nutrition Advisory Committee*, Indian Research Fund Association, Spec. Rep. No. 13, Kanpur.

[4] INDIAN RESEARCH FUND ASSOCIATION (1946) *Report on Soya Bean by the Soya Bean Sub-Committee of the Nutrition Advisory Committee*, Spec. Rep. No. 13, Kanpur.

[5] McCARRISON, R. (1933) The goitrogenic action of soyabean and groundnut, *Indian. J. med. Res.*, **21**, 179.

[6] VAN WYK, J.J., ARNOLD, M.B., WYNN, J., and PEPPER, F. (1959) The effects of a soybean product on thyroid function in humans, *Pediatrics*, **24**, 752.

[7] SHEPARD, T.H., PYNE, G.E., KIRSCHVINK, J.F., and McLEAN, M. (1960) Soybean goitre, *New Engl. J. Med.*, **262**, 1099.

37. MAIZE (*Zea mays*)

Maize or *makai* is also known as 'corn' or Indian corn in the United States. It can be cultivated under varied climatic conditions without much care and labour and in this respect it is similar to millet. Maize provides more calories per acre of cultivated land than rice and about 33 per cent more calories than wheat [1]. Although the United States cultivates nearly half the total world output of maize, most of it is used for feeding livestock and proportionately very little is used for human consumption. Other maize-growing regions are South America, South East Europe, Africa, China and Java.

Structure

Like other cereals, maize has the following structure: (1) *Bran,* the outer cover of cellulose comprising about 5 or 6 per cent of the grain. (2) The *aleurone layer,* a single layer of cells beneath the bran contains 20 per cent protein. The aleurone layer is rich in vitamins of the B group. (3) The *endosperm* or kernel is mainly starch and constitutes 80 per cent of the whole grain. The separated starchy portion removed after steaming is known as 'hominy' in the United States. (4) The *germ* or embryo, is at the lower end and constitutes about 10 per cent of the grain. It is rich in fats, minerals and proteins, mainly glutelin.

COMPOSITION

The composition of maize depends on its variety. The approximate composition is:

Calories

Like other cereals maize provides about 350 Calories per 100 g (100 Calories per oz).

Proteins

Maize contains about 11 per cent protein. There are two principal types of protein in maize: (1) *Zein* forms 50 per cent of the maize proteins and is mostly present in the endosperm. Zein is a poor protein, being deficient in tryptophan and the growth promoting amino acid, lysine. (2) *Glutelin* is found mainly in the germ and is rich in essential amino acids. If the endosperm with its predominant protein zein is eaten alone then deficiency of tryptophan and lysine may occur but grinding the whole grain reduces such deficiencies by including glutelin from the germ. Maize also contains a small quantity of globulin and albumin.

Since maize protein contains a large amount of the sulphur-containing amino acids, cystine and methionine [1] a diet of maize and pulses gives a reasonable intake of essential amino acids at a low cost.

A variety of maize, *opaque*-2, has a higher content of lysine and tryptophan and less leucine. It promotes better growth in children subsisting mainly on a maize diet. In adults, nitrogen equilibrium and positive nitrogen balance can be maintained on 250–300 g of *opaque*-2 [2].

Fats

Maize contains 3·6 per cent fats, mostly as unsaturated fat in the germ. Maize oil has been extracted commercially (*mazola* oil).

Carbohydrates

Carbohydrate comprises two-thirds of the grain and it is found mainly as starch in the endosperm.

Vitamins

Compared to the endosperm, the aleurone layer and the germ are rich in vitamins. Maize contains 0·4 mg per 100 g of thiamine and 0·1 mg per 100 g of riboflavine. It is a poor source of nicotinic acid, containing only 1·4 mg per 100 g, and cannot fulfil the daily requirement. About 63 per cent of the nicotinic acid in maize is in the aleurone layer. The vitamin C content is negligible. Maize contains vitamin A precursor carotene, more of which is found in the yellow variety.

Minerals

Iron in maize (2 mg per cent) is probably well absorbed due to the low phosphate content. Since *calcium* content is only 10 mg per cent a predominantly maize diet would be deficient in calcium. In Mexico this deficiency is overcome by adding lime water in the preparation of *tortillas* (maize bread).

MILLING

As with rice and wheat, the method of milling has a great effect on the nutrients, particularly vitamins, and they are best preserved by grinding the whole corn. Much of the maize used for human consumption in the world is eaten without the removal of some of the more nutritious parts of the grain.

MODE OF SERVING

Tender maize is boiled or toasted and eaten as 'corn on the cob'. The whole grain may be cooked as such or its flour may be used to make *chappatis* (unleavened bread) or *tortilla*. The popular breakfast cereal known as corn flakes is made from maize.

Digestion and Absorption

Maize is easily digested and well absorbed.

DISEASES ASSOCIATED WITH A MAIZE DIET

Pellagra

Maize is deficient in nicotinic acid and a predominantly maize diet, specially one using flour obtained from the endosperm alone, will produce pellagra unless it is supplemented by groundnuts, animal protein or nicotinic acid. The daily requirement of niacin is increased on a maize diet [3] because there is a concurrent deficiency of tryptophan, an amino acid used by the body to synthesize nicotinic acid. If an adequate source of tryptophan is supplied in a predominantly maize diet, then nicotinic acid deficiency does not occur [4].

Kwashiorkor

African children fed on maize develop a nutritional deficiency known as 'infantile pellagra' [5], malignant malnutrition or kwashiorkor [6]. This condition is due to dietary protein deficiency.

Siderosis

Siderosis (deposition of iron) in the liver is seen in poor Africans subsisting on maize [7]. This has been ascribed to an excessive intake of iron because: (1) the maize is cooked in iron vessels; and (2) the low content of phosphorus in maize facilitates iron absorption [8].

REFERENCES

[1] FOOD AND AGRICULTURE ORGANIZATION (1953) *Maize and Maize Diets*, Nutritional Studies No. 9. FAO, Rome.

[2] CLARK, H.E., *et al.* (1967) Nitrogen balance of adults consuming *opaque-2* maize protein, *Amer. J. clin. Nutr.*, **20**, 825.

[3] KREHL, W.A., TEPLY, L.J., and ELVEHJEM, C.A. (1945) Corn as an etiological factor in the production of a nicotinic acid deficiency in the rat, *Science*, **101**, 283.

[4] KREHL, W.A., TEPLY, L.J., SARMA, P.S., and ELVEHJEM, C.A. (1945) Growth-retarding effect of corn in nicotinic acid-low rations and its counteraction by tryptophan, *Science*, **101**, 489.

[5] TROWELL, H.C. (1940) Infantile pellagra, *Trans. roy. Soc. trop. Med. Hyg.*, **33**, 389.

[6] TROWELL, H.C. (1949) Malignant malnutrition (kwashiorkor), *Trans. roy. Soc. trop. Med. Hyg.*, **42**, 417.

[7] GILLMAN, J., and GILLMAN, T. (1945) Structure of the liver in pellagra, *Arch. Path. (Chic.)*, **40**, 239.

[8] MOORE, C.V., and DUBACH, R. (1956) Metabolism and requirements of iron in the human, *J. Amer. med. Ass.*, **162**, 197.

38. MILLETS

Millets are the cheapest cereals consumed by the poorer masses of the Peninsular region of India. They are known as 'coarse grains' because, as compared to wheat the outer coat is thicker and contains more cellulose. Little care or water are needed for cultivation and so they can be grown in hilly regions where water is scarce. Unlike wheat and rice, different types of millet are grown in different areas. The following are the main varieties of millet grown in India.

1. *Bajra* or *bajri* (*Pennisetum typhoideum*), also known as *cambu* in the Southern states cf India. Compared to other Indian cereals it has a high fat content of 5 per cent and is also rich in iron (14·3 mg per cent) and nicotinic acid (3·2 mg per cent).

An epidemic in Poona of increased thirst and urine excretion was ascribed to contamination of *bajra* with the fungus *Phizopus nigricans* [1] but this has not been confirmed.

2. *Jowar* or *juar* (*Sorghum vulgare*) known as *cholam* in the Southern Indian states.

3. *Ragi* or *nachni* (*Eleusine coracana*). It is poor in protein (7·3 per cent) but the calcium content 344 mg per 100 g is the highest amongst cereals.

Composition

Millets provide approximately 350 Calories per 100 g (100 Calories per oz), which is about the same as wheat or rice. The protein content is about 10 per cent. The gluten content is negligible which is obvious from the amorphous dough produced by the addition of water. Millets can be allowed in a gluten free diet from which wheat is excluded.

Millets are ground into flour and moulded with water into flat 'chappatis'. These are toasted on an iron pan and then over an open fire. An average farmer takes one or two such big *chappatis,* each weighing about 150 g and eats them with cooked vegetables and *chutney* at the two main meals.

Digestion and Absorption

These cereals are rather coarse. Those unaccustomed to them may get abdominal discomfort after eating a large quantity. The high proportion of cellulose interferes with the absorption of minerals.

REFERENCE

[1] Deodhar, N.S., *et al.* (1970) An epidemic of 'polyuria and polydipsia syndrome'. Epidemiology of the Poona disease, *Indian J. med. Sci.,* **24,** 626.

39. MILK

Milk is rich in proteins, fats, carbohydrates, vitamins and minerals and is therefore an important source of nutriment. One pint (20 ounces)[1] of milk supplies $\frac{7}{8}$ of the calcium, slightly less than $\frac{1}{3}$ of the riboflavine, over $\frac{1}{4}$ of the proteins and just under $\frac{1}{5}$ of the vitamin A requirements of a moderately active man for one day [1]. If we also consider that one pint of cow's milk supplies about $\frac{1}{5}$, and buffalo's milk about $\frac{1}{3}$, of the daily calorie requirement, then the importance of milk in our nutrition becomes apparent. In countries like India daily milk consumption is very low.

COMPOSITION OF MILK

The proportion of proteins, fats and carbohydrates in human, cow or buffalo milk forms an ideal diet for growth. The composition of milk varies appreciably according to the breed of the animal, the season and the time of the year, fodder supplied and the stage of lactation. Analysis shows wide fluctuations in composition even when samples are collected from well organized dairies. Animal milk forms an excellent adjunct to other foods.

Calories

The analysis of Coonoor Research Laboratory reports 65 Calories per 100 g of cow's milk, while the Dairy Science College, Karnal (Punjab) reports 80 Calories, a difference of 22 per cent.[2] A greater variation is expected from random samples collected from the village farms.

Proteins

The protein content of cow's milk is 3·5 per cent and of buffalo's milk is 4 per cent. The proteins of milk are *casein, lactalbumin* and a trace of *lactoglobulin*. Cow's milk contains about 3 and buffalo's milk about 3·5 per cent casein. Casein, combined with calcium exists in milk in collodial form and is known as caseinogen. It can be precepitated at its isoelectric point of pH 4·6 by the addition of acids and

[1]In the United States one pint represents 16 fluid ounces.

[2]Data supplied by Dr. N. N. Dastur, Principal, Dairy Science College, Karnal, Punjab.

further acidification redissolves it. Fermentation of milk or the addition of rennet leads to precipitation of insoluble calcium caseinate curds. There is a higher proportion of calcium and casein in animal milk than in human milk, the curds are therefore harder and more difficult to digest.

Lactalbumin is akin to plasma albumin and is easy to digest. It is present in solution and is precipitated by heating to 60°C. When milk is heated the white coat noted on the bottom and sides of the vessel is precipitated lactalbumin.

Biological Value of Milk Proteins. The proteins of milk are of a high biological value. Indeed, when one considers the rapid growth, with a doubling in weight in 6 months, of an infant fed only on milk, its growth promoting and tissue building properties are easily appreciated. The nutritive value of milk proteins exerts a supplementary effect when fed with vegetable proteins like bread or potato, but when these proteins are fed separately on alternate days no such effect is noted [2]. Serving milk with cereals or preparing milk pudding of sago or rice is more nutritive than serving the same amount of each product at different times.

Fats

The caloric value of milk is proportionate to the fat content. Cow's milk has 3·6–4·5 and buffalo's milk 7–8·8 per cent fat. Fat in milk exists as a fine emulsion which can be separated by allowing milk to stand. By removing cream or 'malai' (clotted cream) the fat content of milk can be varied to suit individual requirements. In dairies the fat is separated by centrifugation. Milk fat is two thirds saturated and one-third unsaturated. The linoleic acid content of human milk is about four times that of cow's milk.

Carbohydrates

The concentration of *lactose* (milk sugar), the carbohydrate in milk, is about 4·5 per cent in cow and also buffalo's milk. The group of bacilli called *lactic acid bacilli* ferment lactose and advantage is taken of this to produce fermented milk. This keeps longer than fresh milk and imparts various flavours to milk products. As intestinal *lactase* deficiency is widely prevalent, milk is frequently not well tolerated.

Vitamins

The vitamin content of milk varies with the breed of the animal, the season, the available sunlight and the food supplied. Animals fed on green pasture and exposed to sunlight yield the greatest concentration of fat-soluble vitamins.

Vitamin A. The yellow colour of the cow's milk is due to *carotene* derived from the fodder. Animals vary in their ability to convert carotene into vitamin A. Buffalo's milk contains only *vitamin A*. Cow's milk contains 45 μg (150 IU) and buffalo's milk 72 μg (240 IU) of vitamin A per 100 ml. As this vitamin is fat-soluble, skimmed milk is poor in vitamin A.

Thiamine (Vitamin B$_1$). The thiamine content of cow and buffalo's milk is 0·04 mg per 100 ml.

Riboflavine. The riboflavine content of milk is high —0·17 mg and 0·14 mg per 100 ml in cow's and buffalo's milk respectively.

Nicotinic Acid. The nicotinic acid content of 0·1 mg per 100 ml in animal milk is low but the high content of the essential amino acid tryptophan compensates for the deficiency.

Vitamin C. The vitamin C content of cow's and buffalo's milk is 1 mg per 100 ml. Up to 50 per cent of this vitamin is destroyed within 30 minutes if the milk is exposed to sunlight on a doorstep in transparent bottles [1]. It is also easily destroyed by boiling. However, it is not worthwhile trying to preserve this vitamin at the risk of infection with pathogenic organisms through consuming unboiled milk.

Vitamin D. Cow's milk has 4 IU, and buffalo's milk 7 IU of vitamin D per 100 ml. Vitamin D is absent in skimmed milk as it is concentrated in the fatty milk products like cream and butter. The vitamin D content of milk is greatly enhanced if the animals graze in the open; sunlight acting on 7-dehydrocholesterol in their skin converts it into vitamin D. The vitamin D content of milk is thus higher in summer than in winter.

In the United States, three methods are employed to increase the vitamin D content of cow's milk [1]: (1) direct irradiation of milk; (2) addition of vitamin D concentrate to milk; and (3) feeding irradiated yeast to the cows.

Vitamin E content is about 1 mg per litre.

Minerals

The important minerals of milk are calcium, phosphorus, iron, sodium and potassium.

Calcium. The calcium content of cow's milk is 122 mg, and of buffalo's milk 150 mg per 100 ml. The calcium is combined with casein.

Phosphorus. The phosphorus content of cow's milk is 92 mg, and of buffalo's milk 100 mg per 100 ml. The phosphorus is in the form of calcium and potassium phosphate.

Iron. The iron content of cow and buffalo milk is 0·1 mg per 100 ml. It has always been argued that milk is not a 'perfect food' because its iron content is low. If milk is consumed with cereals the iron intake is adequate.

Sodium and Potassium. Milk contains 50 mg of sodium and 160 mg of potassium per 100 ml. The sodium in milk becomes significant if a patient with oedema requires a low sodium diet. Sodium can be removed from milk by dialysis.

Water. Milk contains about 85 per cent water. It thus supplies both food and fluid.

COLOSTRUM

Colostrum is secreted by the mammary glands before and for about 5 days after parturition. The lactose and fat content is lower than in milk but the protein content is higher, being 12 per cent in cow's and 21 per cent in buffalo's colostrum. Half of the protein in colostrum is lactoglobulin. Colostrum is easily coagulated by heat due to its high lactalbumin content.

BACTERIOLOGY OF MILK

Milk is an excellent culture medium for many organisms and unboiled milk is never sterile. The bacterial count gives information about the method of milking and handling, the cleanliness of utensils and the temperature at which the milk has been preserved. The longer milk is allowed to stand the more it is influenced by temperature [3]. The usual standard plate count for certified milk is 10,000 bacteria per ml.

The average bacterial count for milk drawn aseptically from the udder is less than 1500 per ml. Some bacteria therefore enter milk from the normal udder. They are chiefly *micrococci* and small rod forms, both types being harmless to humans [4].

FERMENTATION OF MILK

Milk Fermenting Organisms

During fermentation 40 per cent of the lactose is changed into lactic acid. Bacteria which ferment lactose are known as *lactic acid bacteria*. They are not present in milk when it leaves the udder but are present by the time milking has been completed [3]. Besides bacilli, other organisms like moulds and yeast also ferment milk, and they are collectively known as *lactic acid organisms*. Lactic acid bacilli are of various types, the commonest being *Streptococcus lactis, Lactobacillus acidophilus,* and *Lactobacillus bulgaricus. Streptococcus lactis* is easily grown and is usually found in household fermented milk.

Fermentation of lactose produces lactic acid which combines with calcium to form calcium lactate. The calcium is thus removed from caseinogen, and the casein, thus set free, coagulates when its isoelectric point of pH 4·6 is reached. Depending upon the type of bacteria causing fermentation distinctive tastes and flavours are imparted to fermented milk products like butter, *ghee* and cheese. For domestic fermentation of milk in India pure cultures of bacteria are not used. The cultures consist of mixed lactic acid organisms and so the fermented products are of different standards and tastes [5].

Advantages of Fermentation

Fermented milk has the following advantages: (1) It is the starting point for products like curd and *ghee*. (2) Its products are tolerated better by some people than unfermented milk which produces flatulence. (3) It is said to be more nutritious than fresh milk. The riboflavine and thiamine are both increased [6]. (4) Fermented milk is reported to partially inhibit the growth of *B. typhosus, B. dysenteriae* and *Vibrio cholerae* [7]. Typhoid infection can still be a source of potential danger as the organisms can grow in curd [8].

MILK-BORNE DISEASES

As milk is an excellent culture medium for the growth of potentially lethal pathogens, it can be a source of epidemics, especially in the hot humid climate of the tropics. The commonest milk-borne diseases are (1) typhoid; (2) paratyphoid; (3) amoebic dysentery; (4) bacillary dysentery; (5) tuberculosis; (6) diphtheria; (7) brucellosis; (8) poliomyelitis; and (9) cholera; (10) anthrax; (11) Q-fever; (12) vaccinia; and (13) staphylococcal enterotoxin.

PASTEURIZATION AND BOILING

To make milk safe for drinking it should be heated to kill pathogenic organisms. The common methods adopted are: (1) pasteurization and (2) boiling.

Pasteurization

Pasteurization is extensively used in the dairy industry of Western countries. Three methods are employed: (1) Milk is heated to between 63° and 66°C (145°–150°F) and kept at this temperature for 30 minutes. (2) The high-temperature short time process (HTST) in which the milk is heated to 72°C (160°F) for 15 seconds and chilled rapidly. (3) Flash pasteurization in which the milk is heated momentarily to between 74° and 77°C (165°–170°F) and cooled immediately. Whichever method of heat processing is used, the milk is cooled rapidly and stored at a low temperature until it is distributed.

Boiling

In tropical countries milk supplied direct from the farm is not always safe. The best safeguard against drinking contaminated milk is to boil it.

The advantages of boiling milk are much greater than the trifling objection that vitamins are destroyed, since they can so easily be replaced. (1) Pathogenic organisms are killed. (2) Lactic acid organisms are killed and the milk can thus be kept longer without fermentation. (3) The digestibility of casein is enhanced, raw casein being less digestible than cooked casein. Observations on the stomach contents of dogs with a Mann-Bolman fistula showed that after unboiled milk the stomach contained hard curds and emptied slowly; whereas after boiled milk the curds were smaller and the stomach emptied faster [9].

Pasteurization alone, even with the 'Flash' process does not alter the nature of curds. Patients with dysentery who cannot tolerate unboiled milk may be able to tolerate boiled milk from which fat has been removed. (4) When boiled milk is cooled, clotted cream floats to the top and over 70 per cent of the milk fat can be easily separated. This allows the high fat content of buffalo milk to be reduced to suit individual requirements.

Alteration in Food Value by Pasteurization and Boiling

Pasteurization does not appreciably alter the food value of milk. The vitamin C is diminished by 20 per cent and the vitamin B_1 content by 10 per cent. *Boiling* milk destroys $\frac{1}{3}$ of the vitamin B_1 and about $\frac{1}{2}$ of the vitamin C. The caloric value is not reduced provided the top scum and residue at the bottom are not discarded.

PRESERVATION OF MILK

Milk is a perishable commodity. In a hot humid climate bacteria grow rapidly and ferment or putrefy it. Milk can be preserved for variable periods by: (1) pasteurization or boiling soon after milking, followed by storage in a cool place, like a refrigerator or near an earthen pot (*matka*) used in the tropics for storing drinking water. (2) Evaporation and preparation of *khoa*. In Western countries evaporated milk (condensed milk) is produced by partially evaporating the water from milk in a closed chamber in the absence of oxygen. Addition of cane sugar (sweetened condensed milk) aids in preventing bacterial growth. (3) Fermentation and conversion of milk into products like curd, buttermilk, butter, *ghee* (clarified butter). (4) Production of dried milk powder by a drum or roller process.

MILK PRODUCTS

Milk products preserved for variable lengths of time can be served in a liquid, semi-solid or solid form and vary in their composition and nutritive value. Fermentation by various types of bacteria imparts specific tastes. The common milk products are:

Unfermented Products. (1) Skimmed milk and skimmed milk powder (2) toned milk; (3) cream; (4) *malai* (clotted cream; Devonshire cream); (5) *khoa* (*mava*: evaporated milk); (6) *chana* (cottage cheese);

(7) whey; and (8) junket.

Fermented Products. (1) *Dahi* (curd) and yoghurt; (2) *lassi* (buttermilk); (3) butter[1] (*desi butter*); (4) *ghee*[1] (clarified butter, butter fat); and (5) cheese.

UNFERMENTED PRODUCTS

Skimmed Milk and Skimmed Milk Powder

Countries like New Zealand, Australia and the Netherlands with a highly organized dairy industry make cream and butter. The remaining skimmed milk, low in fat and fat-soluble vitamins but retaining the other nutrients, can be preserved as skimmed milk powder.

Skimmed Milk Powder. To preserve milk for a long period it can be dried and packed in tins. The dry powder is made by: (1) the drum or roller process in which a thin layer of milk is run over a heated cylinder and the dried powder is removed by scraping; or (2) the spray process in which minute droplets of milk are sprayed into a heated chamber and powder falls to the bottom. In order to *reconstitute* this powder into milk one part of powder is added to eight parts of water.

Skimmed milk is deficient in fat and fat-soluble vitamins but the proteins, sugar, minerals and vitamin B factors (except pyridoxine) are well preserved. If skimmed milk powder is supplemented with vitamins A, D and pyridoxine then it is a comparatively cheap food of high nutritive value, rich in proteins, and suitable for children. It is useful for the treatment of malnutrition, the nephrotic syndrome and cirrhosis of the liver. The addition of about six tablespoons of skimmed milk powder during the preparation of *chappatis,* custard, curd, etc. will supply additional 35 g of protein.

Toned Milk

Milk is in short supply in India. The Government of Bombay has introduced a system by which 'toned' milk is supplied to the public at a cheaper rate. It is prepared by mixing equal part of fresh buffalo's milk (which is rich in fat) with reconstituted skimmed milk powder. The fat, protein, carbohydrate, vitamin and mineral content, and

---

[1]Butter and *ghee* need not be fermented products but farmers usually ferment milk for the purpose.

thus the *nutritive value is the same as that of fresh cow's milk*, yet it costs only half as much. It is a useful source of protein for malnourished children, pregnant mothers, schools, hospitals and other public institutions. 'Double toned' milk contains only 1·5 per cent fat. The prejudice which some people have against 'toned' milk is due to its slightly altered taste and to the fact that they do not understand its composition.

Cream

Milk fat floats to the surface if milk is allowed to stand for several hours and it can be separated as cream. Commercially, cream is produced by centrifugation. Light, medium, heavy and extra heavy cream contain 16, 25, 34 and 38 per cent fat respectively.

Malai (Clotted Cream—Devonshire Cream)

After boiling the milk and allowing it to cool, a thick layer of fat and coagulated proteins collect at the surface and can be skimmed off, and by repeating the process twice, most of the fat is removed. Buffalo's milk being richer in fat produces better *malai*. Good *malai* supplies protein 3·5 per cent; fat 30 per cent; carbohydrate 3·8 per cent and 300 Calories per 100 g or 43 Calories per tablespoon.

Khoa (Mava)

Khoa is milk in which the water content is reduced to between 20 and 25 per cent. *Khoa* is prepared by vigorously boiling milk, stirring it continuously so as to avoid burning at the bottom of the pot or overflowing at the top. When cooled, *khoa* forms a uniform mass, containing fats, heat coagulated proteins and lactose. It can be stored for about 3–5 days and with the addition of sugar can be kept longer. It can be eaten as such but is more often used for preparing sweets. *Khoa* supplies protein 24 per cent; fat 41 per cent; carbohydrate 28 per cent; 580 Calories per 100 g or 82 Calories per tablespoon.

Chhana (Cottage Cheese)

Chhana is prepared by adding lemon juice to boiling milk (when commercially produced, a previous residual preparation of *chhana* is used) which precipitates casein, lactalbumin and fat. The liquid part (whey) is strained through a cloth and *chhana* is collected. *Chhana* is not a fermented product of milk so it cannot be ripened like cheese as all the organisms are destroyed by boiling. *Chhana* supplies protein

15 per cent; fat 22 per cent; carbohydrate 5 per cent; 280 Calories per 100 g or 40 Calories per tablespoon.

Whey

When the proteins and fats in milk are precipitated by acids, rennet or bacterial fermentation, liquid whey, which contains lactose and minerals, separates. Whey, which is a by-product of butter and cheese production, is frequently discarded. However, when dried it can be preserved and forms a good source of nutrition for poorer countries. *Liquid whey* provides protein 1 per cent; fat 0·3 per cent; carbohydrate 5 per cent; 50 Calories per cup. *Dried whey* provides protein 11 per cent; fat 1 per cent; carbohydrate 73 per cent; 350 Calories per 100 g.

Sodium and Potassium Content of Whey. The administration of whey has for many years helped in maintaining the electrolyte balance of patients suffering from prolonged pyrexia. Whey contains 21 mEq per litre of sodium and 35 mEq per litre of potassium [10]. Four cups of whey daily during acute fever thus not only provide about a quarter of the daily requirement of sodium and half of the potassium but also one-third of the daily requirement of fluid, as well as some water-soluble vitamins.

Junket

Milk clotted with rennet is called 'junket'. Junket is made by warming milk to 37°C (98°F), stirring in a small amount of rennet, and leaving the mixture to cool and set. Boiled milk is not used owing to a change in the calcium caseinate. Rennet is derived from the enzyme rennin which is present in normal human gastric juice. Commercially, rennet is derived from animal or vegetable sources and is sold in Western countries as liquid rennet or as junket powder.

The *composition of junket* is the same as milk.

FERMENTED PRODUCTS

Dahi

Solid *dahi* may be termed curd. For the preparation of curd, the milk is boiled because: (1) the bacteria already present in the milk are killed, providing a sterile culture medium for the 'starter' organisms which are added. (2) Softer curd is formed after boiling and the water content is reduced by about 5 per cent. When the boiled milk cools to about 37°C (body temperature), 'starter', which is usually residual *dahi* from a previous preparation, and which is rich in lactic acid organisms, is added. These organisms ferment lactose to lactic acid. When the acidity reaches about 1·1 per cent, fermentation ceases. The mode of preparation of *dahi* varies considerably, as does its flavour because the flavour depends upon the type of lactic acid organisms predominating in the starter.

Dahi is eaten as such with salt or sugar added to taste. It is also eaten with rice or converted into a drink called *lassi*. *Dahi* is also the intermediate product of milk in the preparation of butter and *ghee*. Sweetened *dahi* is made by adding cane sugar. *Dahi* has the same caloric value as the milk from which it is prepared even though 40 per cent of the lactose may have been converted to lactic acid.

Yoghurt

Yoghurt is the name given to milk curdled by a specific type of lactic acid bacillus called *Lactobacillus bulgaricus*. At the beginning of this century, yoghurt was thought to be panacea for all intestinal diseases. No extraordinary benefits have been shown to accrue from taking yoghurt, though it is likely that the *Lactobacillus* aids digestion of the milk and is responsible for the formation of vitamins in the gut.

Feeding rats with commercial yoghurt that contains a high galactose and low fat content produces *cataract*. The high incidence of cataract amongst Indians may have a bearing on the consumption of defatted yoghurt [11].

Lassi (Buttermilk)

When *dahi* is churned with water and fat removed the residual acid buttermilk is called *lassi*. *Dahi* and *lassi* can be prepared from whole or skimmed milk.

Ghee (Clarified Butter: Butter-fat)

Ghee is the Indian name for clarified butter. It is extensively used and accounts for over 50 per cent of the total milk produced. *Ghee* is not necessarily a fermented product and is prepared in many ways in different parts of India. A kind of butter is produced from *dahi,* which is boiled to evaporate the moisture. This helps to preserve *ghee* for several months.

The *composition* of cow and buffalo *ghee* is similar. It contains 99 per cent fat, mostly saturated. The vitamin A content of *ghee* is about

1,114 µg (3800 IU) per 100 g, varying with the cattle food, the mode of preparation and the freshness. The vitamin D content of *ghee* is about 30 µg (99 IU) per 100 g and it varies with the exposure of the cattle to sunshine. *Ghee* contains practically no calcium, phosphorus, iron, vitamin B or vitamin C.

Ghee derived from milk or *vanaspati* (hydrogenated vegetable fat) has the same calorie value. *Vanaspati* fortified with vitamins A and D has the same nutritive value as *ghee*.

Cheese

In India, cottage cheese (*chhana*) is an unfermented milk product, but in Western countries cheese produced commercially is a fermented product. Cheese making is a specialized art. There are 400 varieties of cheese. The flavour of cheese varies according to the quality of the milk, whether skimmed or whole; the mode of heating; the type of bacterial culture used for fermentation; the method of storage, and the temperature and humidity used for 'ripening'. Cheese contains casein, some or all of the fat from milk (depending upon the type of cheese produced), vitamin A, calcium and phosphorus, thiamine and riboflavine.

Caution : Monoamine oxidase (MAO) inhibitors, (*Parnate, Niamid, Nardil, Marplan*) therapy inhibits the liver from deaminating the tyramine in cheese. Circulating tyramine releases norepinephrine producing a sudden rise in blood pressure that may occasionally even prove fatal. Other foods reported to have similar effect with MAO inhibitors include beer, wine, pickled herring, chicken liver, yeast, marmite, bovril, coffee, broad-bean pods, and canned figs [12].

DIGESTION AND ABSORPTION OF MILK

In the stomach, milk curdles due to the action of the enzyme rennin and hydrochloric acid. The toughness of the clot increases with the amount of casein and calcium in the milk and with concentration of gastric acid. Clot formation delays digestion and tough clot formation can be prevented by: (1) boiling the milk for 3–5 minutes; (2) mixing the milk with cereals like porridge, which also increases the biological value of milk proteins; (3) adding sodium citrate to the milk, so forming calcium citrate; and (4) producing fermented milk products like curds and buttermilk which do not clot during digestion.

Milk is usually well *absorbed* from the intestine.

Milk Intolerance

Though milk is one of the most nutritious foods, some people cannot tolerate it. *Constipation* with milk may partly be due to its complete absorption leaving little residue. *Flatulence* and *borborygmi* occur if indigestible hard curds are formed from casein and also if there is deficiency of any of the enzymes, lipase, amylase and lactase. Deficiency of *lactase* is one of the commonest digestive troubles that results in abdominal discomfort and *diarrhoea* (see Lactase Deficiency, p. 373).

Diverticulitis of the colon may be associated with the passage of blood and mucus in the stools and this may be relieved by omitting or reducing milk and cream in the diet.

Those who get dyspepsia with milk or milk products should be treated for any intestinal infestation which may be present. The patient is then started on a small quantity, say half a cup of milk which has been boiled for 3–5 minutes, cooled and the fat removed. Milk products made from skimmed milk, including curd, buttermilk or custard may also be tolerated. The quantity taken is gradually increased until whole milk can be tolerated.

Milk Allergy

Milk allergy may produce acute abdominal colic [13], persistent rectal bleeding lasting for several years [14], and recurrent rhinorrhoea and bronchitis [15]. Milk may contain *penicillin,* if cattle have been treated with this antibiotic, leading to penicilin sensitivity, bacterial resistance, or alteration of intestinal bacterial flora. In a highly sensitive individual even penicillin in milk results in allergy [16].

Milk Protein Allergy. In some individuals malabsorption of lactose and fat also occurs with milk *protein* allergy and its withdrawal results in cure [17]. *Protein-losing gastro-enteropathy* with oedema, anaemia, hypo-albuminaemia, hypo-gammaglobulinaemia, eosinophilia, stunted growth, allergic asthma, rhinitis or eczema may occur in some due to milk allergy [18], with remarkable clinical improvement on withholding milk and deterioration on its reintroduction. Milk *precipitins in stools* are not necessarily due to sensitivity to milk as they are also found in normal infants [19].

Milk and Ulcerative Colitis. Milk may cause ulcerative colitis [20]. Some patients improve when milk is eliminated from their diet. High titre reactions to milk protein, found in the serum of patients with ulcerative colitis [21] may only be due to protein absorption from the inflamed bowel and not due to true allergy. *Lactase* deficiency in ulcerative colitis may aggravate diarrhoea on taking milk.

MILK IN THE TREATMENT OF DISEASE

Milk is used in the treatment of many diseases:

Peptic Ulcer. Milk buffers the acid in gastric juice. During the intestinal digestion of milk fat, enterogastrone is secreted which inhibits gastric secretion.

Protein Deficiency. When a high protein diet is indicated, as in malnourishment, nephrosis or cirrhosis of the liver, milk and milk products form the usual source of concentrated protein. Milk is indispensable when treating vegetarians suffering from protein deficiency as other foods like pulses and cereals may not be sufficiently well tolerated to supply enough protein.

Acute Illness and Convalescence. It is easy to cater for any taste or whim during an acute illness and convalescence, with the many varieties of milk and milk products available. Milk and milk products can be served hot or cold; solid, semi-solid or liquid; sweet or sour; mixed with cereals or other proprietary foods, like chocolate; served with beverages like tea or coffee. The relative amounts of fat, protein and carbohydrate can be easily changed by preparing various milk products to suit individual requirements.

Increasing Weight. If it is well tolerated, milk, and fatty preparations of milk like cream, butter and *ghee,* help to provide the extra calories needed for a thin person to gain weight.

MILK SUBSTITUTES

Milk is in short supply in tropical countries. An attempt has therefore been made to prepare milk substitutes of vegetable origin. Milk prepared from soya bean has been used in some parts of the world. In India, vegetable milk and its products are prepared from cheaper foods like groundnut and coconut. These vegetable products have almost the same composition as animal milk and are very nutritious but they are not popular, partly due to scepticism and partly to the unpalatable flavour which they impart to tea and coffee.

Filled milk is a product made by combining *fats* or *oils* (other than milk fats), with milk solids. Variable amounts of vitamins are added. *Imitation milk* contains no milk at all. It contains water, corn syrup, sugar, a vegetable fat, and a protein such as sodium caseinate or soyabean protein with added vitamins, specially A and D. Such milk substitutes cost less but their value is not yet clear. They are not claimed to be as nutritious as whole milk [22].

Vegetable cream substitutes are available in North America as liquids, semisolids and dry powders, sweetened or soured, the fat content varying from 10–55 per cent. They can be preserved longer and taken by those who have an allergy to milk, or on the *assumption* that their intake of saturated fats will be restricted, although the lipids on analysis are almost exclusively saturated fatty acids [23]. Thus, cream substitutes provide only saturated fatty acids while milk fats are over 33 per cent unsaturated.

REFERENCES

[1] KON, S.K. (1943) The chemical composition and nutritive value of milk and milk products, *Chem. and Ind.*, **62**, 478.

[2] HENRY, K.M., and KON, S.K. (1942) The effect of the method of feeding on the supplementary relationships between the proteins of dietary products and those of bread or potato, *Chem. and Ind.*, **61**, 97.

[3] HAMMER, B.W. (1948) *Dairy Bacteriology*, 3rd ed., New york.

[4] ELLIKER, P.R. (1949) *Practical Dairy Bacteriology*, 3rd ed., New York, p. 132.

[5] RANGAPPA, K.S., and ACHAYA, K.T. (1948) *The Chemistry and Manufacture of Indian Dairy Products*, Bangalore, p. 66.

[6] CHITRE, R.G., and PATWARDHAN, V.N. (1945) The nutritive value of milk and curds, *Curr. Sci.*, **14**, 320.

[7] NICHOLLS, L., NIMALASURIYA, A., and DE SILVA, R. (1939) The preparation of fermented milk (curds), *Ceylon, J. Sci.*, **5**, 17.

[8] BHAT, J.V., and REPORTER, R.N. (1949) Fate of some intestinal pathogenic bacteria in Dahi, *Indian J. Dairy Sci.*, **2**, 99.

[9] ANTIA, F.P. (1949) *The Effect of Vagotomy on the Gastric Function in the Dog*, Thesis, Master of Science in Physiology, Graduate College of the University of Illinois, Chicago.

[10] RINDANI, T.H., BILLIMORIA, F.R., and ANTIA, F.P. Unpublished data.

[11] RICHTER, C.P., and DUKE, J.R. (1970) Yoghurt-induced cataracts: comments on their significance to man, *J. Amer. med. Ass.*, **214**, 1878.

[12] JARVIK, M.E. (1970) Drugs used in the treatment of psychiatric disorders, in *Pharmacological Basis of Therapeutics* 4th ed., ed., Goodman, L.S., and Gilman, A., London, p. 185.

[13] ANTIA, F.P. (1953) Gastrointestinal allergy to milk, *Indian J. med. Sci.*, **7**, 247.

[14] ANTIA, F.P., and COOPER, S.H. (1955) Chronic rectal bleeding due to milk, *Brit. med. J.*, **1**, 1416.

[15] GERRARD, J.W. (1966) Familial recurrent rhinorrhoea and bronchitis due to cow's milk, *J. Amer. med. Ass.*, **198**, 605.

[16] WICHER, K., REISMAN, R.E., and ARBESMAN, C.E. (1969) Allergic reaction to penicillin present in milk, *J. Amer. med. Ass.*, **208**, 143.

[17] LIU, H.Y., TSAO, M.U., MOORE, B., and GIDAY, Z. (1968) Bovine milk protein-induced intestinal malabsorption of lactose and fat in infants, *Gastroenterology*, **54**, 27.

[18] WALDMANN, T.A., WOCHNER, R.D., LASTER, L., and GORDON, R.S. (1967) Allergic gastro-enteropathy: a case of excessive gastrointestinal protein loss, *New Engl. J. Med.*, **276**, 761.

[19] DAVIS, S.D., *et al.* (1970) Clinical nonspecificity of milk coproantibodies in diarrhoeal stools, *New Engl. J. Med.*, **282**, 612.

[20] GRYBOSKI, J.D. (1967) Gastrointestinal milk allergy in infants, *Pediatrics*, **40**, 354.

[21] TAYLOR, K.B., and TRUELOVE, S.C. (1961) Circulating antibodies to milk proteins in ulcerative colitis, *Brit. med. J.*, **2**, 924.

[22] BRINK, M.F., BALSLEY, M., and SPECKMAN, E.W. (1969) Nutritional value of milk compared with filled and imitation milks, *Amer. J. clin. Nutr.*, **22**, 168.

[23] MONSEN, E.R., and ADRIANENSSENS, L. (1969) Fatty acid composition of total lipid of cream and cream substitutes, *Amer. J. clin. Nutr.*, **22**, 458.

40. EGG

An appreciable number of vegetarians do not object to eating eggs. Non-vegetarians usually eat them at breakfast, and use them in the preparation of many dishes. It is estimated that 200,000,000,000 eggs are consumed in the world every year, the United States alone consuming about 30 per cent. The eggs consumed are mostly hen's, duck eggs are eaten to a lesser extent. An average hen can lay 150–200 eggs a year. In the tropics the average *per capita* consumption is negligible because production is low. In hot climates preservation and transport are difficult.

Structure of the Shell

The outer shell of calcium carbonate constitutes about 10 per cent of the total weight. The pigment of the shell is white or brown and bears no relation to the nutritive value; and the same hen may lay eggs of different shades. The porous shell allows passage of air and hence the egg may imbibe the flavour and taste of the material in which it is stored. Eggs preserved in salt, for instance, may have a salty taste.

Composition

The composition of eggs is influenced by the food of the fowl. In the tropics an average hen's egg is small, about 30–37 g compared to 50 g in temperate countries. The white of an egg constitutes about 60 per cent and the yolk 30 per cent of the total weight.

The white of an egg consists of protein, mainly egg albumin (albus= white). When fresh it is transparent and turns milky white on cooking because the albumin is coagulated. It contains vitamins of the B group.

The yolk of egg is rich in finely emulsified, easily digestible fats. Carotenoid pigments make the yolk yellow, with less pigment the colour is paler. Artificial colours can be imparted to the yolk by feeding the foul with oil or alcohol-soluble dyes. An average egg contains 100 mg of cholesterol. It also contains proteins and is rich in fat-soluble vitamins as well as minerals like calcium, phosphorus and iron. The yolk being a perfect food is an excellent nutrient for the growth of organisms and hence is used for the culture of tubercle bacilli and viruses.

A duck's egg is larger but has a similar composition to a hen's egg.

Digestion

Soft boiled and poached eggs are better digested than eggs cooked in other ways. They are most easily digested when albumin is coagulated at 70°C. Raw albumin contains anti-digestive factors which are destroyed when heated. The yolk is easily digested compared to other fats, even by infants. Frying an egg or making an omelette from it delays its digestion; *boiling* delays digestion a little. Blackness around the yolk of a boiled egg is due to iron sulphide, hydrogen sulphide in the white having combined with iron in the yolk.

Absorption

A cooked egg, even a hard boiled egg, is completely absorbed.

Clinical Uses

Easy digestibility and complete absorption make eggs the ideal nutritive food for acutely ill and convalescent patients. In diseases of the gastro-intestinal tract, particularly in diseases of the colon, eggs are the best food because of their nutritive value and lack of residue.

Testing a Fresh Egg

Fresh eggs have the best nutritive value. Eggs stored in a cool place away from any odour, will keep for a long time but changes do occur with age. Evaporation of water during storage reduces the weight and specific gravity. The ancient method of testing fresh eggs is to dip them into water before purchase. A rotten egg, due to evaporation and liberation of gases like carbon dioxide and ammonia, floats while a fresh egg sinks to the bottom.

Raw Egg

Raw egg is believed by some to be more nutritious than cooked egg, but this is not so. Egg albumin contains an anti-digestive factor which is destroyed by heat. Unless it is cooked, the undigested albumin is excreted in the faeces.

Avidin. Egg white contains a protein called avidin (avidin=avid albumin) which exists in combination with biotin, a vitamin of the B group. This avidin-biotin complex is not absorbed from the intestine. When an egg is cooked, this combination is broken down and biotin is released for absorption. Animals fed on raw eggs develop dermatitis, roughening of the fur, loss of weight and a spastic gait. This syndrome is known as 'egg white injury' and is due to deficiency of biotin [1]. With cooking, avidin is destroyed and absorption of biotin cures the deficiency. The biotin deficiency syndrome has also been produced in humans by giving desiccated egg white [2].

EGG IN DISEASES

Allergy

Egg is a common allergen in infants, children and adults, producing urticaria or asthma. In all allergic patients a careful search should be made not only to exclude egg, but also egg preparations such as biscuits or cakes.

Atherosclerosis

Eggs contain about 100 mg cholesterol. Hypercholesterolaemia is found in a higher proportion of patients suffering from atherosclerosis and coronary heart disease than in normal subjects. The present state of knowledge does not prove that mere restriction of the cholesterol intake is the answer to the problem.

Fats in egg yolk contain saturated fatty acids. Fowls fed with unsaturated fatty acids (sunflower seed oil) produce eggs containing unsaturated fatty acids. On feeding these eggs to humans, their serum cholesterol level does not rise [3] as it does after eating eggs containing saturated fatty acids.

Gall-bladder Disease

Fats in eggs cause contraction of the gall-bladder and this may produce pain and discomfort if the gall-bladder is diseased. Such patients should avoid taking eggs. Patients with a diseased gall-bladder who do not experience pain should be advised to take one or two eggs a day in order to prevent stasis of bile in the gall-bladder.

Egg-borne Infections

Because the shell is porous, eggs are not always sterile. When eggs are laid on dirty marshy land, micro-organisms permeate the shell. Ducks usually lay their eggs near moist areas where they are likely to be infected. The commonest infection is by the salmonella group of organisms giving rise to typhoid fever and gastro-enteritis. If eggs are well cooked this danger is prevented.

Egg and Rheumatic Susceptibility

A low consumption of eggs is related to a high incidence of rheumatic disease. Egg consumption, particularly egg yolk, diminishes susceptibility to rheumatic fever [4]. Whether an alcohol-soluble fraction or some other factor provides this beneficial effect is not clear.

Hypoglycaemic Effect of Egg Yolk

Oral or parenteral administration of hen's egg yolk may cause hypoglycaemia and reduce the glycogen content of the liver. The active substance producing these effects is not insulin because it is equally effective whether administered orally or parenterally and is not destroyed by ordinary cooking. A similar extract with hypoglycaemic properties has been isolated from the eggs of fish (fish roe) [5].

REFERENCES

[1] EAKIN, R.E., MCKINLEY, W.A., and WILLIAMS, R.J. (1940) Egg-white injury in
     chicks and its relationship to a deficiency of vitamin H, *Science*, **92**, 224.
[2] SYDENSTRICKER, V.P., SINGAL, S.A., BRIGGS, A.P., DEVAUGHN, N.M., and ISBELL,
     H. (1942) Observations on the 'egg white injury' in man, *J. Amer. med.
     Ass.*, **118**, 1199.
[3] HORLICK, L., and O'NEIL, J.B. (1958) The modification of egg-yolk fats by
     sunflower-seed oil and the effect of such yolk fats on blood-cholesterol
     levels, *Lancet*, ii, 243.
[4] COBURN, A.F. (1960) The concept of egg-yolk as a dietary inhibitor to rheumatic
     susceptibility, *Lancet*, i, 867.
[5] SHIKINAMI, Y. (1928) On hypoglycemia produced by material from various
     animal substances especially from the egg yolk of hens' eggs, *Johoku
     J. Expr. Med.*, **10**. 1.

41. MEAT AND SOUPS

Animal flesh and organs like liver, kidney, spleen, pancreas, and brain
contain protein of high biological value and provide a palatable source
of food for many. In India the majority of people are vegetarian and
even amongst the meat-eaters, the consumption of meat is only 50–
100 g a week or fortnight because of the high cost. The majority of
non-vegetarians consume so little meat for this reason, that from the
nutritive point of view they should be considered vegetarians.

It is often assumed that for stamina it is essential to eat meat.
There is no scientific basis for this belief. As long as a person takes
enough protein to supply the essential amino acids the nutrition of a
vegetarian can be favourably compared with a meat-eater.

Varieties

Mutton derived from sheep is most commonly eaten in India. *Beef*
is extensively consumed in Western countries and by the Mohamedans
and Christians in India. Beef is less expensive in the tropics than
mutton because cattle yield twelve times as much flesh as sheep. Pork,
ham, and bacon are derived from the pig. *Pork* is pig meat which has
not been processed; *ham* is processed meat derived from the sides,
belly and back of the animal. There are various ways of processing
ham and bacon. The consumption of pork, ham and bacon is low in

the tropics. Beef is forbidden amongst meat eating Hindus. Pork is forbidden amongst the Mohamedans but is freely consumed by the Christians and Sikhs.

Structure

Meat consists of muscle fibres bound together by a connective tissue matrix. The meat fibre is a tubular structure containing protein, mineral salts, extractives and water. The connective tissue is composed mainly of collagen which yields gelatin on boiling. The amount of fat in the connective tissues depends upon the part of the animal from which the flesh has come and on the nutrition of the animal prior to slaughter.

Composition

Meat contains about 15–25 per cent protein, variable amounts of fat, thiamine, riboflavine, nicotinic acid, phosphorus, sulphur and iron. Animals in the tropics are usually not so well fed as those on farms in Western countries and so the quality of the meat is inferior.

Liver, kidney and sweetbread are greatly relished by some in the form of a mixed grill. These highly cellular organs are rich in protein and nucleoprotein, the latter are broken down in the body to uric acid. As vitamin A is stored in the liver over 22,000 Units of vitamin A are found in 100 g of sheep liver. Liver contains over 6 mg of iron per 100 g.

Preservation

In the tropics meat is not usually stored due to lack of facilities for refrigeration. The animal is slaughtered the same day or the day prior to marketing. If meat is kept longer without refrigeration, autolysis followed by bacterial putrefaction rapidly begins in the hot weather. For storage at home, meat should always be kept in the freezing compartment of the refrigerator.

Cooking

Cooking improves the flavour of meat and affects its structure. During cooking, the protein of meat fibres is coagulated and the collagen of connective tissue swells up and is converted into gelatin. The fat is melted to a varying extent depending upon the heat applied and frying removes a considerable proportion of it. The water content is reduced by 40 per cent during roasting and by 60 per cent during frying. Thus cooked meat weighing one ounce has more nutritive value than raw meat of the same weight.

The flavour of meat depends partly on the acids it contains. These acids increase during muscular exertion so meat from an animal killed after a chase is particularly delicious.

Digestion and Absorption

The digestibility of meat depends upon the rate of gastric emptying, the toughness of its muscle fibres and the amount of fat. The coarser fibres of beef are more difficult to digest than mutton. The fat delays emptying of the stomach. Meat is almost entirely absorbed from the intestinal tract leaving very little faecal residue. If undigested meat passes into the colon, as in patients with malabsorption, it is acted upon by bacteria giving rise to putrefaction and the formation of foul smelling flatus.

Clinical Uses

High meat diet is indicated in anaemia, nephrosis, hepatic cirrhosis without portosystemic encephalopathy, and protein malnutrition.

Contra-indications. Meat is contra-indicated in acute liver failure and in oliguric renal failure. Organs like the liver, kidney, and pancreas (sweetbread) are rich in nucleoprotein and are best avoided by patients with gout.

Meat-borne Diseases

Meat-borne diseases may occur due to chemicals like boric acid and benzoic acid used for its preservation. Bacterial diseases transmitted by meat are bovine tuberculosis, brucellosis, salmonella and shigella infections. Pork transmits *Trichinella spiralis* and the tape worm *Taenia solium;* beef transmits the tape worm *Taenia saginata*. Putrefied meat produces staphyloccocal gastro-enteritis and botulism.

Poultry

The word poultry is derived from the French word 'poulet' (fowl). Poultry includes domestic birds like chicken, duck, goose, and turkey which are reared for the sake of their eggs and flesh. It is a relatively expensive type of food as there is much waste from a small bird in the form of inedible parts like feather, head, bones and feet. The flesh of poultry is similar to meat but more tender and appetizing; the breast particularly is fleshy and yields tender white meat. The meat of duck and goose contains more fat and is less digestible than that of chicken.

White and Red Meat

White meat is generally more tender than red meat and is readily digested. Red meat is made up of coarser fibres and has a higher fat content making it less digestible. After digestion and absorption there is no difference in their metabolism, their end products being similar. Because of its easy digestibility white meat is generally prescribed for ill and convalescent patients.

SOUPS

In the tropics meat soup is a luxury. It is also an item of diet very enthusiastically prepared for the sick and is always recommended for convalescence after an acute illness. It is believed that as soups are extracts of food-stuffs they are concentrated food.

Nutritive Value

Thick soups made from potatoes, almonds, peas, etc. are nourishing but thin clear soups have little caloric value. Soups contain factors of the vitamin B group and minerals like potassium and sodium.

When meat soup comes in contact with the pyloric gland mucosa of the stomach a powerful hormone, gastrin, is secreted which stimulates gastric secretion. If soup is taken in a small quantity at the beginning of a meal it induces appetite but a bigger quantity reduces appetite by giving a sense of repletion. Meat becomes tasteless after the extractives have been removed in the making of soup. Frequently expensive commercial extracts of meat and chicken are advised but it is better for patients to eat chicken and derive the full nutritive value than to take an extract.

Clinical Uses

Soup is prescribed to provide extra fluid and minerals in a pleasant form for patients with fever. Thin soup taken in a large quantity at the beginning of a meal can fill the stomach and helps patients to keep to a reducing diet.

42. FISH

The importance of fish as a source of food varies with the geographical factors and with the availability of other foods. People living near the sea or on banks of rivers are likely to be fish-eaters. In many parts of India and Japan, fish is a staple food, but in North America, where meat and milk are freely consumed, relatively less fish is eaten.

Fish is relatively expensive for the low income people in the tropics who may afford it only once a week. Fish need not be cultivated like vegetables or reared like cattle. The oceans abound in fish and can provide an almost unlimited supply at all times. Fish also could be cultured to yield more nutrition per acre than any other foodstuff. This method of providing nutrition gives tremendous scope for private or public enterprise.

The taste of fish depends upon its origin whether from salt or fresh water, its fat content, and whether it is eaten fresh or preserved.

Preservation

Unless well preserved, fish deteriorates rapidly. Without facilities for preservation and storage, supplies and the market price vary considerably with the season, fish being cheap with a big haul and expensive at other times. The various methods employed for preservation are: (1) drying ; (2) salting; (3) freezing; (4) canning; and (5) pickling.

1. *Drying.* Drying fish in the sun is extensively practised in India. Sun drying is a gradual process. Fish is sometimes salted prior to drying. Drying by mechanical dehydration is expensive but useful for an organized fishing industry.

2. *Salting.* Salt can be used for preserving fish for short periods of time.

3. *Freezing.* Fish is kept among blocks of ice and this is the usual way in which it is sent in small quantities from coastal areas to the interior. Freezing below zero is practised extensively in places where the fishing industry is well organized.

4. *Canning.* Canning after cooking is a good method of preservation but not very practicable for economically poor countries.

5. *Pickling.* Fish can be preserved by pickling in vinegar and spices.

Composition

Many parts of a fish, including the head, scales, fins, bones, and usually the skin, are not edible and there is a wastage which may be as much as 50 per cent of the total weight purchased.

Calories. The caloric value of the edible portion depends upon its fat content, and thus on the season. During the spawning season the fat content may rise and the caloric value increases. The variable results of analysis are partly due to analysis at different times of the year.

Proteins. Fish contains 16–20 per cent protein of high biological value.

Fats. Some fish are rich in fat which raises the caloric value. Hilsa (*Colupea ilisa*), a common fish in Bengal, contains 19.4 per cent fat, most of which is unsaturated.

Vitamins. Fish which contains much fat is rich in vitamins A and D. Oil from shark, cod and halibut liver is very rich in these vitamins. Vitamins of the B group, mainly nicotinic acid, and vitamin C are present in raw fish, but the latter is largely destroyed by cooking. The habit of eating raw fish, as in Japan, provides a useful supplement to the total vitamin C intake, particularly if fish liver or roe is eaten.

Minerals. *Iodine.* Salt water fish is particularly rich in iodine. Those who regularly eat salt water fish rarely suffer from iodine deficiency. *Phosphorus and calcium.* The phosphorus content of fish is high, and those who chew fish bones can absorb a fair amount of phosphorus and calcium. Fish also contains *copper*.

Fish has been described as a 'food for the brain' but there is no reason to believe that a fish-eating population is in any way mentally superior to those who do not eat fish or those who are vegetarians.

Cooking [1]

Steaming is generally assumed to be the best form of cooking for the retention of calories, vitamins and minerals. This is a fallacy, as a considerable loss in nutritive value occurs during steaming. The maximum loss occurs when fish is boiled and the water thrown away.

Cooking in vinegar increases the available calcium as the bones become soft and can be eaten. Fried fish has a high caloric value due to the retention of fat and by frying the nutritive value as well as the flavour of fish can be preserved.

SHELLFISH

Lobsters, crabs, shrimps and prawns are common salt water shellfish. They are highly valued by gourmets for their characteristic flavour, but as a daily article of food they are expensive and a considerable portion of the shell and head are discarbed as offal. Shellfish is rich in proteins and minerals, particularly iodine.

DISEASES PRODUCED BY FISH

Fish, and especially shellfish, is one of the commonest causes of food *allergy* which is usually manifest as urticaria. Consuming fish which has not been properly stored or carefully cured is a common cause of gastro-intestinal upset resulting in abdominal *colic* and *diarrhoea*. Fish, particularly the roe, is rich in purines and likely to precipitate an attack of *gout* in those who are predisposed to it. *Diphyllobothrium latum* is conveyed to humans by eating fish infested with this tape worm. Human infestation of this parasite occurs in 20 per cent of the population in Finland but only about 1 in 3000 of such carriers of the worm has anaemia morphologically indistinguishable from pernicious anaemia. Expulsion of this worm is usually followed by a cure [2].

REFERENCES

[1] CALLOW, A.B. (1951) *Cooking and Nutritive Value,* Oxford, p. 54.
[2] CASTLE, W.B. (1959) Factors involved in the absorption of vitamin B_{12}, *Gastroenterology,* **37,** 377

43. VEGETABLES

A vegetable is defined here as a non-woody plant cultivated for the table; the roots, tubers, stems, leaves or fruits being consumed. Unlike cereals and pulses, vegetables in India are relatively expensive and their consumption amongst the poorer class is very low. The high cost is due to the amount of labour needed to grow them, for they require constant attention and frequent watering and the fact that vegetables tend to perish on the way to the cities if transport facilities are poor. Vegetables are very rich in carotene, vitamin C, and potassium.

CLASSIFICATION

No useful purpose is served by following a botanical classification and when discussing nutrition, vegetables can be conveniently divided into the following groups:

1. *Green and leafy.* Cabbage, cauliflower, coriander, lettuce, spinach.

2. *Other vegetables.* Brinjal, cucumber, drumstick, bitter gourd (*karela*), *parwar,* white pumpkin, red pumpkin, *tindola,* tomato.

3. *Roots and Tubers.* Potato, sweet potato, onion, beetroot, carrot, radish, yam.

4. *Legumes.* Double beans, french beans, green peas, cluster beans (*guar phalli*).

Green and Leafy Vegetables and other Vegetables

Vegetables contain a high proportion of cellulose and the intestinal juices of man, unlike those of herbivorous animals, cannot digest it. Vegetable cellulose thus remains unabsorbed and increases the bulk of the intestinal contents.

Vegetables are helpful in weight-reducing diets as they provide bulk and give a feeling of satiety but provide few calories. The bulk and water content of green vegetables also help in the treatment of constipation.

Vegetables supply very few calories but they are a rich source of carotene, vitamin C and potassium.

Vegetables	Vitamin C per 100 g
Bitter gourd	96
Cabbage	124
Cauliflower	66
Coriander	135
Drumstick	120
Drumstick leaves	220
Tomato	31

Spinach

Methaemoglobinaemia may rarely be seen after consuming spinach. Fresh spinach contains a high proportion of nitrate that is converted to nitrites 24–48 hours after gathering leaves and also by the intestinal bacteria. In susceptible individuals nitrites cause methaemoglobinaemia [1].

Roots and Tubers

The root of a plant serves two functions, it acts as an anchor and it absorbs water and minerals. A tuber is a storage organ and is a short thickened portion of an underground stem, a common example being the potato. More calories can be derived from an acre of potatoes than from growing most other crops.

Potatoes and Sweet Potatoes

Potatoes and sweet potatoes are rich in starch.

Cooking. The potato cell has a cellulose envelope which is broken down on cooking, allowing digestion of the starch by intestinal juices. Cooking potatoes unpeeled, conserves most of the vitamins B, C and salts in the skin. Peeling the potato and cutting it into pieces before it is boiled reduces its vitamin content considerably. If cooked potatoes are reheated there is a further loss of vitamins.

Digestion. Proper mastication helps the ptyalin of saliva to begin the conversion of starch into maltose and dextrose. Mashed potato is most easily digested.

Beet

Beeturia may occur after consuming beet, due to excretion of the pigment betanin. The pigment appears red in an acid and yellow in an alkaline medium. Beeturia is claimed to be more commonly seen in iron deficiency anaemia in children [2].

Carrots

Carrots are rich in carotene and the red variety contains 10–15 times more carotene than the yellow variety [3]. Food faddists who eat a large quantity of carrots to improve their eyesight may develop carotinaemia which can be confused with jaundice unless it is noted that the sclera of the eye is not yellow.

Onion

Onion is widely used in tropical countries. The white variety contains more water than the brown or the red variety, and cannot be stored as well. Onions have a pungent taste and as water evaporates during storage the pungency is increased.

The principal chemical constituent in onion which gives it its taste, the pungent odour and brings tears to the eyes, is the sulphur-containing volatile oil, allyl propyl disulphide. If uncooked onion is eaten the volatile oil is excreted through the lungs and saliva, giving a characteristic odour to the breath. This does not happen if cooked onion is eaten as the volatile oil evaporates with heat.

The vitamin C content is higher in green onions especially in their central parts than in stored ones.

Clinical Uses.   Raw fresh onion can be a good and cheap source of vitamin C particularly for poor villagers. As its volatile oil is excreted by the lungs a stored red onion can be used as an expectorant.

A fat-rich meal decreases blood fibrinolytic activity. The ingestion of fried onion not only prevents this decrease but may actually increase fibrinolytic activity [4]. It is therefore hoped that eating onions may inhibit the tendency to blood coagulation and help to prevent coronary and cerebral thrombosis.

Legumes

Dried legumes like gram, peas and beans are considered as pulses. The green legumes like green peas, french beans and cluster beans are used as vegetables and are considered here. Green peas contain about 7 per cent protein and supply about 100 Calories per 100 g.

DAILY REQUIREMENTS

The green, leafy and root vegetables form an important item in a balanced diet. The former supply vitamins A and C and iron, and the latter supply calories and vitamin C.

For a well balanced diet a daily consumption of 30 g of green leafy vegetables, 100 g of roots or tubers and 100 g of other vegetables is recommended.

REFERENCES

[1] BRITISH MEDICAL JOURNAL (1966) Spinach: a risk to babies, *Brit. med. J.*, **1**, 250.

[2] TUNNESSEN, W.W., SMITH, C., and OSKI, F.A. (1969) Beeturia: a sign of iron deficiency, *Amer. J. Dis. Child.*, **117**, 424.

[3] SADANA, J.C., and AHMAD, B. (1947) The carotenoid pigments and the vitamin A activity of Indian carrots, *Indian J. med. Res.*, **35**, 81.

[4] GUPTA, N.N., MEHROTRA, R.M.L., and SIRCAR, A.R. (1966) Effect of onion on serum cholesterol, blood coagulation factors and fibrinolytic activity in alimentary lipemia, *Indian J. med. Res.*, **54**, 48.

44. FRUITS

The term fruit (*fructus* = to enjoy) is taken here to mean the edible envelope containing the seeds of a plant or tree. The common fruits are banana, mango, orange, sweet lime, guava, grapes, papaya, *chikoo,* apple, pineapple, pomegranate and various types of berries. In the tropics fruits are a delicacy and are relatively expensive.

Raw fruit contains varying proportions of starch, which, in the process of ripening, is converted into fructose and glucose. These impart a sweet taste and are readily absorbed. Fresh fruits also contain vitamin C. The flavour of fruits is due to the presence of various organic acids like citric, malic and tartaric. Fruits can also be eaten to quench thirst as they may contain up to 90 per cent water.

Fructose intolerance is a rare condition in which there may be severe hypoglycaemia on eating fruits [1].

Fruits should be avoided by people predisposed to types III, IV and V lipoproteinaemia, because fructose stimulates more lipid synthesis as opposed to glucose.

BANANA

Banana is perhaps the cheapest and the most extensively-eaten fruit in the tropics. An average green banana weighs about 150 g of which two-thirds is edible, the rest being inedible skin. It supplies more calories than other fresh fruits, an average size banana providing 100 Calories. There are many varieties of banana each having a distinctive flavour. The word *plaintain* is generally used for the coarser types of banana.

Raw banana can be cooked but they are not usually eaten unless ripe. Ripe bananas contain carbohydrates in the form of sucrose, fructose and glucose which are readily digested. Bananas contain much 5-hydroxytryptamine (serotonin) and with a high banana diet there is a rise in its urinary excretory product 5-hydroxyindolacetic acid (5-HIAA).

Clinical Uses

In some constipated people bananas act as a mild laxative. They can be given as a source of calories in a non-residue diet, for example in diarrhoea and ulcerative colitis. A high banana diet probably increases the butyric acid concentration in the colon and this may control diarrhoea by inhibiting the growth of *B. coli*.

MANGO

Mango is a tropical fruit, available during the hot season. The flavour of mango varies with the quality, the *Alphonso* variety being the best available. Raw mango is widely used for preparing pickles and in cooking, as the *gallic acid* in it imparts a sour taste to the food.

Ripe mango is commonly eaten in large amounts and it provides a good source of calories during the season. Depending upon its size, a mango supplies 50–100 Calories, mainly derived from fructose. An average mango supplies 25 mg of vitamin C and over 10,000 Units of carotene. Eating too many mangoes may impart a yellow tinge to the skin due to carotenaemia, distinguishable from jaundice by the fact that the sclera does not turn yellow.

Clinical Uses

Mango is an excellent source of vitamin A and C and of calories. The diet of an average Indian is low in vitamin A and eating mangoes in the season may provide a store of vitamin A in the liver sufficient to last for the rest of the year.

CITRUS FRUITS

Citrus fruits contain citric acid. This is metabolized into carbonate and, if sufficient quantities are taken the urine becomes alkaline. The common citrus fruits are orange, tangerine, sweet lime, grape, sour lime and grape fruit. Tangerine (extensively grown in tropical countries) is a variety of orange with a loose skin which can be easily peeled.

Citrus fruits may precipitate an attack of allergic rhinitis in those susceptible to it. An anaphylactoid reaction to orange is described [2]. Intestinal obstruction due to the ingestion of orange pith, after partial gastrectomy, has also been described [3].

Clinical Uses

The juice of citrus fruits is a very refreshing drink during fevers and in patients with severe liver damage. It also supplies vitamin C. The high potassium content makes it unsuitable for patients with oliguric renal failure.

PAPAYA

Papaya is a common tropical fruit. The unripe fruit is a rich source of papain, which is 'vegetable pepsin' and is capable of digesting proteins in acid, alkaline or neutral medium. Because of this property raw papaya is used during cooking to soften tough meat or *dal*. Patients with *coeliac disease* who cannot digest the wheat protein gliadin, can tolerate it if it is treated with crude papain (not crystalline) [4].

Ripe papaya is rich in carotene and excessive consumption produces carotenaemia.

Clinical Uses

Papaya can be prescribed for dyspeptic patients as the pepsin may help in the digestion of proteins. Papaya seeds have an antihelminthic action [5].

APPLE AND POMEGRANATE

Apple is rich in pectin which is a hemicellulose with the capacity of absorbing water. Depending upon the quality, fresh apple may contain 2–5 per cent of pectin. Apple also contains an appreciable amount of tannin.

Pomegranate is rich in tannin which acts as an astringent in the intestine and precipitates food proteins.

Clinical Uses

Apples and pomegranates are usually advised in diarrhoea but there is no evidence to prove their efficacy in this condition.

PINEAPPLE

Bromelain is a mixture of proteolytic enzymes found in the stem of the pineapple (*Anans comosus*). In chronic pancreatitis oral bromelains aid in intestinal fat absorption [6].

GUAVA

(*Psidium guajava*)

This is a relatively cheap fruit, relished particularly by children, and a rich source of vitamin C (300 mg per 100 g). As it is grown extensively it provides the cheapest source of vitamin C. If unripe guava are eaten, intestinal colic may occur because of the acids they contain. The ripe fruit, on the other hand, may be helpful in constipation.

AMLA

Amla is the subject of much interest for tropical nutritionists because of its high content of 600 mg of vitamin C per 100 g. However, it has an extremely sour and rather unpleasant taste.

BAEL FRUIT

Bael fruit is eaten for its medicinal value. It contains pectin, mucilagenous principle and tannin, all of which are useful for the treatment of diarrhoea and dysentery.

GRAPES

Grapes are a seasonal fruit. The carbohydrate, and therefore, the calorie content varies according to the variety. The carbohydrate present is grape sugar (glucose) which is readily absorbed from the stomach and intestine without further digestion. Grapes contain 3 mg of vitamin C per 100 g and so they are a poorer source of this vitamin than citrus fruits.

Clinical Uses

Because they contain glucose, grapes are a delicious and nutritious food and drink for patients with fever and for invalids. Intestinal distension may occur if grapes are consumed in large quantities.

REFERENCES

[1] BLACK, J.A., and SIMPSON, K. (1967) Fructose intolerance, *Brit. med J.,* **4,** 138.
[2] BENDERSKY, G., and LUPAS, J.A. (1960) Anaphylactoid reaction to ingestion of orange, *J. Amer. med. Ass.,* **173,** 255.
[3] BUTLER, M.F. (1959) Orange-pith ileus after partial gastrectomy, *Brit. med. J.,* **2,** 549.
[4] MESSER, M., ANDERSON, C.M., HUBBARD, L. (1964) Studies on the mechanism of destruction of the toxic action of wheat gluten in coeliac disease by crude papain, *Gut,* **5,** 295.
[5] POHOWALLA, J.N., and SINGH, S.D., (1959) Worm infestation in infants and children of preschool age in Indore, *Indian J. Pediat.,* **26,** 459.
[6] KNILL-JONES, R.P., PEARCE, H., BATTEN, J., and WILLIAMS, R., (1970) Comparative trial of nutrizym in chronic pancreatic insufficiency, *Brit. med. J.,* **4,** 21.

45. NUTS AND DRIED FRUITS

A nut is a fruit and the edible seed or kernel is enclosed in a hard shell. The common nuts consumed in the tropics are coconut, groundnut, cashew nut, walnut, almonds and pistachios (*Pistaria vera*). They are rich in proteins, fats, carbohydrates, minerals and factors of the vitamin B complex. Nuts approach an ideal food by supplying high calories in a palatable form. The large proportion of fat which they contain is surrounded by a compact cellulose matrix and requires thorough mastication for better digestion.

COCONUT

Coconut consists of an outer husk, a middle hard shell, and inside a sweet *kernel* and coconut *water*. The kernel is the white and firm edible portion, is consumed as such, is desiccated as *copra,* or extracted as oil. A mature coconut may yield up to 225 g of kernel supplying about 1000 Calories. Coconuts provide more calories per acre of land than any other food.

Coconut Water

A tender coconut yields 500–900 ml of water and contains only a negligible quantity of soft creamy kernel. In the tropics coconut water drawn straight from the nut is a safe and sterile drink to quench thirst as it is not likely to be contaminated with pathogenic organisms.

Coconut Water for Intravenous Therapy [1].

The Japanese used coconut water in Sumatra during the Second World War as did the British in Ceylon. Coconuts are cut at seven months of age when the sugar content of the water is at its highest. The coconut water is removed under strict sterile conditions. If the shell is cracked the coconut is not used. A cut is made through the hard shell and 1–1½ inches into the soft meaty substance. Alcohol is then applied to the cut surface and when it is dry, a sterile trocar is introduced into the nut cavity. The escaping fluid is filtered through sterilized gauze and funnel, into a sterilized bottle. About 500–900 ml of fluid is usually obtained. The solution must be used immediately for intravenous therapy. The pH is 5·6 and the nutrients in the coconut water are [2]: glucose 2·1 per cent, fructose 3·8 per cent, inulin 152 mg per cent, proteins 180 mg per cent, potassium 49 mEq per litre, sodium 5 mEq per litre, calcium 12 mEq per litre, magnesium 17 mEq per litre, chloride 62 mEq per litre, phosphate 8 mEq per litre, and sulphate 5 mEq per litre.

Fresh Kernel

Less coconut water and more kernel is obtained as the nut matures. Fresh coconut is not only eaten raw but also used specially in South India for the preparation of *curries,* vegetables and sweets.

Desiccated Coconut (Copra)

Dried kernel is less liable to be contaminated with fungus and is less bulky for transport than the fresh kernel. Dried kernel is used for cooking and as a source of oil. Typhoid fever and other salmonella infections have been traced occasionally to desiccated coconut [3].

Coconut Oil

Dried coconut contains about 70 per cent of oil [4], most of which can be extracted. An acre of land can yield 250–500 kg of oil per year. Coconut oil is easily digestible and is used as fat for cooking and frying. It is extensively used in the preparation of vegetable *ghee* (*vanaspati*) and margarine.

Coconut cake is a by-product of the coconut oil industry. It provides a nutritious mash for feeding milch cows and increases the quantity and nutritive value of milk.

GROUNDNUT
(Peanut)

Groundnut is relatively inexpensive and is therefore consumed extensively in the tropics. It has a high content of proteins, fats, carbohydrates and calories. *Arachin,* the preponderant protein of groundnut is deficient in methionine.

Clinical Uses
Groundnut is palatable and cheap. Served with half to one cup of milk or a tablespoon of milk powder it can be an excellent source of food for protein-deficient children specially in schools and orphanages. When mixed with jaggery it makes a delicious sweet known as *Chikki.* Groundnut is rich in *nicotinic acid* (2·3 mg per 100 g) and is a good supplement to a maize diet for the prevention of pellagra. The quantity of groundnut consumed should be increased gradually otherwise flatulence and intestinal colic may be produced.

Groundnut Oil. This is extensively used for the preparation of vegetable *ghee* (*vanaspati*).

Aflatoxins [5]. Stored groundnut may be contaminated with the fungus *Aspergillus flavus* that produces toxins known collectively as *aflatoxins. Mung dhal,* soya bean, dried fish, etc., are also known to contain aflatoxin. The contamination is increased with atmospheric moisture and the duration of storage. Aflatoxin is also excreted in the *milk* of animals fed on contaminated groundnut cake.

Aflatoxins isolated are B (most toxic) B_2, G_1 and G_2. Feeding aflatoxins produces liver cancer in ducklings, rats and the rainbow trout. In rhesus monkeys, this produces fatty liver and periportal fibrosis. Aflatoxin is more likely to produce liver damage in protein-deficient animals. There is now an increasing awareness that aflatoxin-contaminated foods may be responsible for human *cirrhosis* and *primary liver cancer* [6], but proof which directly links aflatoxin with these diseases is lacking.

CASHEW NUT, WALNUT, ALMOND and PISTACHIO

These nuts have a high calorific value but they are expensive and are consumed only by the rich.

DRIED FRUITS

The commonly consumed dried fruits are dates, figs, currants, raisins and apricots are expensive. Dried fruits are a good source of calcium and iron but, unlike fresh fruits, the vitamin C content is poor.

Dates

Dates are the fruit of the date palm and the staple diet of the Arabs. In the tropics dates are comparatively cheap amongst the dried fruits. Dates kept exposed to flies and dust may become a source of infections like typhoid, dysentery and cholera.

Clinical Uses

Dried fruits like dates, figs and raisins are advised for lean constipated patients because of their laxative effect. As they are rich in calories they should be avoided by the obese.

REFERENCES

[1] GOLDSMITH, H.S. (1962) Coconut water for intravenous therapy, *Brit. J. Surg.*, **49**, 421.

[2] EISEMAN, B., (1954) Intravenous infusion of coconut water, *Arch. Surg. (Chic.)*, **68**, 167.

[3] BRITISH MEDICAL JOURNAL (1960) Infected coconut, *Brit. med. J.*, **2**, 589.

[4] DESHIKACER, N., (1952) Coconut products, *Indian Coconut, J.*, **5**, 101.

[5] NAGARAJAN, V. 1970) Toxins in food, in *A Decade of Progress* 1960–1970, *National Institute of Nutrition, Hyderabad, India,* Indian Council of Medical Research, New Delhi.

[6] LIN, T.Y. (1970) Primary cancer of the liver, *Scand. J. Gastroent.*, **6**, Suppl. 223.

46. SWEET FOODS AND SWEETENING AGENTS

SUGAR (Sucrose)

The word sugar is used here to denote household sugar. Sugar is made from sugar-cane in the tropics and from sugar-beet in the Western countries. In the United Kingdom and North America the average consumption of sugar is well over 100 g a day per person.

Sweets made from sugar produce a sense of satiety hence they should be taken only after a meal. If eaten at the beginning of a meal they reduce appetite and so reduce the intake of essential protein-rich foods. Sugar and sour lime added to a glass of cold water makes a very pleasant drink on a hot day. Syrup made of sugar is an excellent preservative for fruits, jam and preserves.

Composition

Sugar is almost pure sucrose, a disaccharide made up of glucose (dextrose) and fructose (laevulose). One gramme of sugar supplies 4 Calories and a teaspoonful (5 g) supplies 20 Calories. Food faddists advocate brown sugar as being more natural but it is no more nutritious than white sugar.

Digestion and Absorption

The small intestinal enzyme sucrase (invertase) breaks down sucrose into glucose and fructose both of which are rapidly absorbed. The digestion and absorption of sucrose is very rapid but perhaps not as rapid as the absorption of glucose which can be absorbed without digestion.

Sugar and Ill Health

Sugar is a cheap source of carbohydrate and supplies only energy without vitamins or minerals. An individual who is addicted to sweet tea may take 10 cups of tea a day with three teaspoonfuls of sugar to a cup providing 600 Calories, about one-third of his daily calorie requirement, without any vitamins.

Sugar and Teeth. In children, bad teeth are ascribed to excessive consumption of sweets. The sweets may take the place of foods containing calcium and vitamin D which are necessary for the development of healthy teeth. The habit of going to bed at night without brushing the teeth promotes bacterial growth on stagnant sweet food particles around the teeth and leads to tooth decay.

Sugar-cane Juice

The juice obtained by crushing sugar-cane is a popular and refreshing drink in the tropics. The addition of ginger and lemon juice improves its taste and flavour. Sugar-cane juice is often advised for patients during an attack of viral hepatitis because of its high carbohydrate content.

This pleasant drink can be a potential source of disease. The juice itself, when sold in the bazaars, is frequently contaminated by road dust and flies. The glasses may be a source of infectious diseases like typhoid, dysentery and cholera, if they are washed in filthy water.

Jaggery

Jaggery is produced by heating sugar-cane juice. It has been reputed to be a cardiac tonic because villagers who consume it in large amounts do not suffer from heart diseases. The infrequency of coronary artery disease in villagers in the tropics is more likely to be due to their short span of life.

Molasses

Molasses or treacle is a by-product in the manufacture of sugar. Fermentation of molasses produces alcohol, the most popular drink produced in this way being rum.

Honey

Honey is a golden coloured syrupy substance made by bees from the nectar of flowers. It contains a mixture of glucose and fructose which gives it a particular sweetness. The quality of honey depends on the prevailing flower blossom. Many villagers have now been taught to keep an apiary to produce honey and thus supplement their income.

Clinical Uses. Honey in warm water or milk can be a soothing drink for patients with pharyngitis and tracheitis which frequently accompanies 'common cold'.

Composition of Honey. Water 17·7 per cent, dextrose 36·5 per cent, laevulose 40·5 per cent, sucrose 1·9 per cent, 288 Calories per 100 g (82 Calories per oz).

Saccharin and Cyclamates

In our modern society physical work and exercise have been considerably reduced but calorie consciousness has arisen in an attempt to preserve a slim figure. Sweetening agents do not supply calories and are therefore popular with food manufacturers to boost their sales of low-calorie foods and drinks, while retaining their palatability.

Saccharin was discovered in 1879. It is 350 times sweeter than sugar (sucrose) but has a bitter taste in concentrated form. Excretion of saccharin is 90 per cent in the urine.

Cyclamate was discovered in 1937. It is 30 times sweeter than sucrose, is excreted in urine and faeces, and over 5 g daily causes softening of stools. Cyclamates can cross the placental barrier and are also excreted in milk. Cyclamate consumption increased in the United States, from 2·3 million kg in 1963 to 6·8 million kg in 1967, a notable increase occurring in the preparations of soft drinks.

Rats fed cyclamates in doses of 2·5 g per kg body weight developed malignant bladder tumours. This is an excessive dose that has prompted withdrawal of cyclamate in the United Kingdom and the United States, but the wisdom of such a step has been questioned [1] for cyclamate has hitherto been an important adjunct to foods for those wanting to restrict their dietary carbohydrates in obesity and heart disease, which are potentially dangerous.

Dermatitis and renal tubular acidosis are reported with excessive consumption of soft drinks containing 4 g or more of cyclamates [2].

Liquid Glucose (see p. 47).

REFERENCES

[1] BRITISH MEDICAL JOURNAL (1969) Cyclone over cyclamate, *Brit. med. J.*, **4**, 251.
[2] YONG, J.M., and SANDERSON, K.V. (1969) Photosensitive dermatitis and renal tubular acidosis after ingestion of calcium cyclamate, *Lancet*, **ii**, 1273.

47. SPICES

Since ancient times spices have been highly prized, and exported from the East to Middle Eastern and European countries. Attempts by European sailors to find new routes to the Orient to get spices resulted in many expeditions and the discovery of new lands. It is curious that spices are consumed more in hot sultry tropical climates than in colder regions. This may be partly explained by the fact that the food is frequently seasonal and monotonous in the East due to poverty and poor transport facilities.

Spices are aromatic pungent substances. *Condiments* are processed spices made into a sauce or relish. Spices do not make a significant contribution to nutrition as they are consumed in small quantities.

The saying 'one man's meat is another man's poison' applies particularly to spices. The highly spiced food taken by South Indians may upset Europeans unaccustomed to it. Spices should be used to bring out the best flavour of food and make it more appetizing, rather than to give the food a pungency which irritates the mouth and masks the original flavour.

Clinical Uses

Spices stimulate the appetite of convalescent patients and make the food more palatable for them. In constipated persons spices help evacuation of the bowel by irritating the intestines.

Contra-indications. 1. *Alimentary tract.* Condiments and spices irritate mucous membranes and should be avoided in all the inflammatory diseases of the digestive tract. In stomatitis, spices produce a sense of intense burning, and they are also best avoided in gastritis, peptic ulcer and diarrhoea. Some apparently healthy individuals get loose stools after eating spiced food because the irritation may activate a latent colonic infection. The habit of 'purging with pleasure', the consumption of highly spiced food to relieve constipation, is to be condemned.

2. *Liver and gall-bladder disease.* Spices when digested and absorbed reach the liver. It is possible that these products of absorption are an aetiological factor in hepatic cirrhosis so frequently seen in the tropics. Spices produce flatulence in sufferers from gall-bladder disease.

3. *Urinary tract.* Infections of the urinary tract like pyelitis, cystitis

and urethritis tend to relapse with spiced foods. The probable explana-
tions are: (1) irritation of the intestinal mucous membrane by spices
produces hyperaemia and favours absorption of intestinal bacteria
which are excreted by the kidneys; (2) small amounts of spices may be
absorbed into the blood stream and irritate the urinary tract, as they
are excreted in the urine.

4. *Gout.* Persons suffering from metabolic disorders like gout may
get an attack after eating spiced food.

The commonly used spices are: (1) asafoetida; (2) cardamom;
(3) chillies; (4) cinnamon; (5) cloves; (6) coriander; (7) cumin;
(8) garlic; (9) ginger; (10) mustard; (11) nutmeg; (12) pepper;
(13) tamarind; and (14) turmeric.

Asafoetida (*hing*)

Asafoetida contains an essential oil, gum and a resin. It oozes out
when the head of the plant *Farula nathrex* or *Farula foetida* is cut.
Asafoetida has a peculiar strong odour which is liked by a few people
in India who use it in cooking. It has a carminative effect and facilitates
the passage of flatus.

Cardamom (*elchi, elachi*)

Cardamom is derived from the seed of the plant *Electtaria carda-
momum*. It has an agreeable flavour and is used in cooking. Many
people put cardamom in their mouth after a meal or eat it with betel
leaf (*pan*). Cardamom has a carminative action and its tincture forms
an important ingredient of a carminative mixture.

Chillies (*mirch, mirchi, marchu*)

Chillies are the most pungent spices used in Indian cooking. The
important varieties are *Capsicum annum, Capsicum fastigiatum* and *Capsicum minimum. Green chillies,* the fresh fruit of the chilli plant, are sold
in the bazaar and used for cooking. If whole green chillies are used in
cooking and taken out before serving, then they impart flavour without
making the food unduly pungent. *Red chillies* are the dried fruit of the
chilli and are usually sold by grocers as the whole fruit or as powder.
Chillies usually form an ingredient of curry powder and *chutney.*

Capsaicin. The active principle of chillies which makes them pungent
is capsaicin. Its maximum concentration is in the inner wall of the
fruit and not in the seeds. If capsaicin is heated the vapour irritates the

eyes and the mucous membranes of the respiratory tract.

Chillies in large amounts produce gastritis and even predispose to a bout of haematemesis. Chillies are not tolerated by those who have suffered from dysentery or who have an irritable colon and pungent food usually provides a burning reminder during defaecation the next day. Chillies also produce recurrence of bleeding in persons suffering from piles.

Cinnamon (*taj: dalchini*)

Cinnamon is the dried brown inner bark of the tree *Cinnamomum zeylanicum*. It contains over 1 per cent oil, mainly cinamic aldehyde. Cinnamon is used to impart flavour to food. It also acts as a carminative.

Cloves (*lavang*)

Cloves are dried flower buds of the plant *Eugenia caryophyllata*. They are dark brown, about 1 cm long, with a bulbous end, and are used for imparting flavour to food and for their carminative action. Oil of cloves is sometimes applied to relieve toothache.

Coriander (*dhania*)

Coriander is the spherical dried fruit of the delicate plant, *Coriandrum sativum*. It is used with other ingredients during cooking.

Cumin (*jira*)

The dry fruits of *Cuminum cyminum* contain thymol. Cumin is used for cooking. Cumin water is commonly used as a carminative. It is also given to children in doses of one or two teaspoons after each feed in order to prevent intestinal colic.

Garlic (*lashan, lashun*)

Garlic is obtained from the bulb of the plant *Allium sativum*. It is used as a flavouring agent for cooking but it also has medicinal properties. An antibacterial agent with a high sulphur content called *allicin* has been isolated from garlic. Allicin inhibits the growth of Gram-negative and Gram-positive bacteria. Garlic in the natural form used in cooking, or extracted as allicin, has been given by mouth to suppress intestinal bacterial activity in diarrhoea and flatulence. The active principle of garlic is absorbed from the intestines and excreted by the lungs. It was used before the antibiotic era in the treatment of bronchitis, bronchiectasis and lung abscess. Garlic juice diluted with water has sometimes been used as lotion for cleaning septic wounds. In leprosy, oral administration of garlic has been reported to show encouraging results [1].

Ginger (*adu, adrak*)

Ginger is the root of *Zingiber officinale*. The pungency of ginger is due to the oleoresin, *gingerol*. Ginger is commonly used along with garlic, for the preparation of many dishes. Ginger preserved in syrup is eaten to aid digestion after a heavy meal. Ginger is also utilized to produce aerated beverages such as ginger ale or ginger beer.

Mustard (*rai*)

Mustard is obtained from the powdered seeds of the plant *Brassica nigra* (black mustard) or *Brassica alba* (white mustard). Mustard powder when mixed with water has a pungent taste. Mustard is extensively used on the dinner table all over the world. Good sandwiches cannot be prepared without the judicious use of mustard.

Nutmeg (*jaiphal*)

Nutmeg is a dried kernel derived from seeds of the tree *Myristica fragrans*. It is used as flavouring agent and also acts as a carminative.

Nutmeg Poisoning. Nutmeg has sometimes been self administered to induce menses or an abortion. The active toxic factor in nutmeg is *myristicin*. Even a teaspoon of nutmeg (5 g) can produce toxic symptoms. From 1–7 hours after ingestion there is abdominal burning and pain, vomiting, restlessness, giddiness and excitement. There may be fear of impending death and a feeling of a heavy weight on the chest. Later drowsiness and stupor supervene. Recovery is usual within 24 hours, but with larger doses periodic outbursts of excitement and delirium may persist for several days [2].

Pepper (*miri*)

Black pepper is the dried fruit of a plant *Piper nigrum*. White pepper is prepared by soaking black pepper and rubbing it to remove the outer coat. The pungency of pepper is due to the resin, *chavicine*.

To obtain the best flavour, pepper should be freshly ground. Pepper is added either during cooking or at the table, along with salt. Pepper added to hot tea has been endorsed by many Indian grandmothers as the best remedy for the common cold.

Tamarind (*imli*)

Tamarind is the fruit of the plant *Tamarindus indica*. Every schoolboy in India knows the location of the tree in his village and relishes the sour taste of the fruit. When ripe it also imparts a sweetish taste. Tamarind is extensively used in cooking to impart a sour taste.

Turmeric (*haldi, haladi*)

Turmeric is the root of a plant *Curcuma longa*. It has a deep yellow colour and is commonly used during cooking. It acts as a carminative and inhibits gastric secretion [3]. Even in high dilutions it has anti-bacterial properties and has therefore been used topically for cleaning wounds.

REFERENCES

[1] CHAUDHURY, D.S., SREENIVASAMURTHY, V., JAYARAJ, P., SREEKANTIAH, K.R., and JOHAR, D.S. (1962) Therapeutic usefulness of garlic in leprosy, *J. Indian med. Ass.,* **39,** 517.
[2] GREEN, R.C. (1959) Nutmeg poisoning, *J. Amer. med. Ass.,* **171,** 1342.
[3] CHOPRA, R.N., GUPTA, J.C., and CHOPRA, G.S. (1941) Pharmacological action of the essential oil of curcuma longa, *Indian J. med. Res.,* **29,** 769.

48. BEVERAGES

Beverages are drinks which subjectively refresh a person and help to supplement his fluid requirements. Beverages help to foster social contact as it is convenient to gossip, or discuss business, over a cup of tea or coffee. The commonly used beverages are tea, coffee, fruit juices, cordials and aerated waters. Individual preferences depend upon taste, habit and local culture.

TEA

Tea contains thein which has a pharmacological action similar to caffeine, tannin and an essential oil which imparts a characteristic aroma.

Caffeine. The leaves contain about 3 per cent caffeine which has a stimulating effect on the heart, nervous system and kidneys.

The amount of caffeine extracted depends upon the quality of the tea and the mode of preparation. The extraction rate increases if the leaves are infused for a long period. Boiling water makes a better infusion than hot water. When one teaspoon of tea leaves is infused in a cup of boiling water for about 5 minutes, approximately 60–120 mg (1–2 grains) of caffeine are extracted.

Tannin. Tea leaves contain 7–14 per cent tannin. After infusion for five minutes, a cup of tea contains 60–240 mg (1–4 grains) of tannin. If it is allowed to stand for a longer period the extraction of tannin is increased. The action of tannin is neutralized by adding milk.

Preparation

The preparation of tea varies with the custom and taste. Tea should be infused in a china or earthenware pot in preference to metal pots, as tannin acts on metals. Usually, the tea pot is first rinsed with boiling water and one teaspoon or less of tea leaves per cup of tea is put into it, the required quantity of *boiling* water is now poured on to the leaves. If the tea leaves are removed after 5 minutes the infusion can be kept for a long period without any change in its composition. It is better to make a stronger infusion by adding more tea leaves than by infusing for a longer period, otherwise an excess of tannin is extracted which is undesirable. In most hotels and restaurants, strong tea is prepared by boiling tea leaves with water, a process which increases the extraction of tannin.

COFFEE

Coffee is extensively consumed in Europe, America and South India. It contains caffeine, tannin and an essential oil which gives it a characteristic aroma.

Processing

In India two methods are used for processing coffee. The 'cherry' or mature red fruit is depulped, fermented, washed and dried, resulting in 'parchment' or 'plantation' coffee. Alternatively, the fruit may be dried before dehusking to produce 'cherry' coffee [1]. The two varieties of coffee grown in India are *Arabica* and *Robusta* which can be blended according to taste.

When coffee is ground it rapidly loses its aroma unless it is kept in an airtight container. It is therefore better to purchase small quantities of freshly-ground coffee than to store a big quantity. Many people grind fresh coffee at home.

Generally a cup of coffee is prepared from 2 teaspoons of ground coffee and each cup then contains approximately 60–120 mg (1–2 grains) of caffeine and 200–240 mg (3–4 grains) of tannin.

Adulteration

Because of its high price, coffee is frequently adulterated with roasted peas, cereals, tamarind seed, date seed or tapioca skin. Chicory, a plant root, imparts flavour to coffee. It can be blended with coffee in all proportions up to 50 per cent. Such coffee is known as '*French Coffee*' and the presence of chicory is declared on the container.

Test for Detecting Adulteration. About $\frac{1}{4}$ teaspoon of coffee powder is boiled with a cup of water and allowed to settle. The supernatant water is removed, the powder dried and spread on a white porous paper, and a solution of 2 per cent caustic soda is slowly dropped over it. If pinkish or coloured spots appear on the paper within 5–10 minutes, the coffee is adulterated with tamarind or date seeds.

Clinical use of Tea and Coffee

Tea and coffee are often taken first thing in the morning for their stimulant effect. These beverages, taken hot, induce intestinal peristaltic activity (the so-called gastrocolic reflex) useful for stimulating a normal bowel evacuation. For many who scarcely drink water, tea or coffee provide a large proportion of the daily fluid intake. In diarrhoea they are useful drinks to combat dehydration. They also act as diuretics.

Contra-indications to Tea and Coffee. Tea and coffee should not be given to *children* as their nervous system may be over-stimulated with caffeine. These beverages are also a poor substitute for milk in childhood. Caffeine stimulates gastric secretion, and so *strong* tea and coffee are contra-indicated in *gastritis* and *peptic ulcer*. The undesirable side-effects of strong tea or coffee are premature heart beats, tremors and nervousness. These effects are most pronounced if the beverage is taken on an empty stomach or without milk. Some people cannot sleep for several hours after a cup of coffee and should avoid taking it in the evening.

Ingestion of a moderate amount of coffee stimulates adrenocortical activity as seen by the rise in plasma free fatty acids and increased urinary excretion of corticoids [2].

Caffeine in coffee elevates fasting blood glucose and impairs glucose tolerance [3], and has a possible adverse effect in diabetics. Excess consumption of coffee is also reported to cause chronic ill health and fever [4].

Some correlation has been found between coffee drinking and bladder cancer, particularly among females [5].

Nutritional Value

Though tea and coffee *per se* do not supply any nutrition, yet the calorie content of the added sugar and milk may be surprisingly high. A person used to having about eight cups of tea daily, each containing three teaspoons of sugar and two tablespoons of milk, derives 480 Calories from sugar and 176 Calories from milk, a total of 656 Calories, approximately one-third of his daily needs.

The available *niacin* content of coffee is high. One cup of dark roasted coffee provides between 2 and 3 mg, while light roasted coffee provides 1 mg per cup [6]. The low incidence of pellagra in the State of Madras, despite poor nutrition, may be partly due to the intake of coffee.

COCOA

Cocoa is made from the seeds of a tropical tree. The chief constituents of cocoa are fat, protein, starch and 1–2 per cent theobromine which has a stimulating action similar to caffeine. Cocoa also contains caffeine, but its tannin content is considerably less than that of tea or coffee.

Cocoa is not generally used as a beverage in the tropics. Two teaspoons of cocoa provide 30–40 Calories but the calories derived from a cup of cocoa are mainly from the added milk and sugar. Cocoa is less stimulating than tea or coffee and so is suitable for children.

AERATED WATERS

For the preparation of aerated drinks carbon dioxide is dissolved in water under pressure and stored in a sealed bottle. Unflavoured aerated water is known as 'soda water', though it does not contain any sodium bicarbonate When the bottle is opened, bubbles of carbon dioxide are released. Different essences and colours like lemon, raspberry, or ginger are added in the manufacture of these drinks. Dyspeptics often like aerated drinks because belching the ingested carbon dioxide gives them a sense of relief.

REFERENCES

[1] DIVISION OF INFORMATION AND STATISTICS (1955) *Coffee: What the Consumer Should Know,* Central Food Technological Research Institute, Mysore.

[2] BELLET, S., *et al.* (1969) Effect of coffee ingestion and adrenocortical secretion in young men and dogs, *Metabolism,* **18,** 1007.

[3] WACHMAN, A., HATTNER, R.S., GEORGE, B., and BERNSTEIN, D.S. (1970) Effects of decaffeinated and nondecaffeinated coffee ingestion on blood glucose, and plasma radioimmunoreactive insulin response to rapid intravenous infusion of glucose in normal man, *Metabolism,* **19,** 539.

[4] REIMANN, R.A. (1967) Caffeinism. A cause of long-continued, low grade fever, *J. Amer. med. Ass.,* **202,** 1105.

[5] COLE, P. (1971) Coffee-drinking and cancer of the lower urinary tract, *Lancet,* **i,** 1335.

[6] GOLDSMITH, G.A., MILLER, O.N., UNGLAUB, W.G., and KERCHEVAL, K. (1959) Human studies on biologic availability of niacin in coffee, *Proc. Soc. exp. Biol. (N.Y.),* **102,** 579.

49. ALCOHOL

The word alcohol is derived from the Arabic *al-kohl,* meaning 'subtle'. Alcohol is a colourless, volatile liquid with a characteristic odour and taste. It is usually prepared by fermentation of carbohydrates like malt, hops or molasses. In India, illicit liquor is usually made from *mohwa,* rice or jaggery.

Alcohol has a specific gravity of less than 0·8, hence, for the same volume, its weight is only four-fifths that of water. 'Proof spirit' is a mixture of equal amounts of alcohol and water by weight. The strength of alcohol is usually expressed in terms of percentage of volume or weight. Ten per cent volume of alcohol denotes 10 ml of alcohol, which is 8 g by weight, in 100 ml of fluid.

Varieties

Whisky, made in Scotland from barley, is highly prized, as the Scots have a long tradition for distilling it. Beer is made from grains such as barley and hops, while rum is made from molasses. Brandy, sherry and port are made from grapes; French brandy is very popular.

In alcoholic beverages the average concentration of alcohol by volume is: brandy 43 per cent, sherry 20 per cent, and beer 7 per cent.

Absorption

The comparatively small molecular size of alcohol readily permits simple diffusion [1] through the mucous membrane of the mouth or stomach, or even when administered as an enema, douche or inhalation. *Stomach* absorption varies with the *concentration* and *emptying time,* being rapid on an empty stomach while the presence of food, particularly of fatty foods, delays stomach emptying and allows greater gastric absorption. Six per cent alcohol is absorbed at the rate of 4·7 ml per minute [2]. Up to a 6 per cent alcohol concentration, the acid output is not increased, and acid secretion is the same, as it is stimulated by the corresponding volume of water. *Small intestinal* absorption is rapid. After partial gastrectomy, a patient feels tipsy with a small quantity of alcohol that would not have affected him before the operation. This is because of the rapid entry into the small intestine, where alcohol is absorbed quickly leading to a rapid rise in the blood level.

Blood and Tissue Concentration

After a single drink the arterial blood alcohol level at an early stage is higher than the venous, while capillary blood shows intermediate values. After about 2 hours, however, the venous blood shows higher values as alcohol from the tissues is released.

The *urine* alcohol level reflects the venous blood level, provided a 30 minute sample of urine is collected after emptying the bladder, for this avoids errors due to retained urine.

The *breath alcohol* level reasonably reflects blood concentration and is a very convenient method of analysis [3]. The breath analysis may show a 'mouth effect' if the test is carried out soon after a drink or vomit.

Distribution. The distribution of alcohol in the body is proportional to the water content of the tissues. Plasma has more water than any other tissue in the body, hence the plasma concentration is the greatest. Fatty tissues contain little water and hence the concentration is low. Fat people therefore have a higher blood alcohol concentration than thin people when both consume the same amount per kilogram body weight [4].

METABOLISM

Alcohol is *not stored* in the body as whatever is ingested is oxidized. The *rate of elimination varies.* A 68 kg man can eliminate 6–8 g (7·5–10 ml) per hour [1], while a person habituated to alcohol can eliminate it faster.

About 90 per cent of ingested alcohol is oxidized into carbon dioxide and water by: (1) the enzyme alcohol *dehydrogenase,* produced mostly by the liver cells and also by the kidneys; (2) alcohol (and phenobarbitone) stimulates proliferation of the smooth endoplasmic reticulum of liver cells, enhancing the activity of the *microsomal enzyme oxidizing system* (MEOS), which destroys drugs and alcohol. Enhanced alcohol intake increases the activity of MEOS, which is why an alcoholic can tolerate increasing amounts [5]. The stimulation of MEOS also destroys sedatives more rapidly, for which reason an alcoholic who is not under the influence of liquor requires a bigger therapeutic dose of a sedative or an anaesthetic. On the other hand, when alcoholics consume liquor the MEOS is required to metabolize alcohol, and consequently other drugs if administered are not metabolized, which enhances their effect [6]. In normal persons, blood alcohol clearance is about 25 mg per 100 ml per hour while in alcoholics (without liver disease) it is about 50 mg per 100 ml [7]. Oral fructose increases the rate of alcohol metabolism in healthy humans.

The *anticoagulant* dosage for coronary infarct etc. may have been adjusted to stabilize prothrombin at a desired level. In such patients intake of alcohol alters the metabolism of the anticoagulant by stimulating MEOS resulting in marked fluctuations in the prothrombin level.

Nutritional Value

Alcohol is a pure carbohydrate and yields 7 Calories per g on oxidation. Seventy-five Calories are provided by 30 ml (1 oz) of brandy or whisky. A bottle of whisky supplies 2250 Calories [4]. Alcohol can spare protein breakdown when taken in small quantities. It can also be the *quickest source of energy,* as it does not require digestion like other foods and is absorbed from the stomach. It has poor nutritive value, contains no essential food factors, and excessive consumption leads to nutritional deficiency.

Carbohydrate Metabolism

Ingestion of alcohol is followed by a reduction in the amount of liver glycogen. A high blood sugar level, however, protects animals from a lethal dose of alcohol [4]. Alcohol is most likely to damage the liver in people who take large quantities without taking adequate food.

Hypoglycaemic Coma

Alcohol inhibits glucose formation from lactate [8] and decreases enzyme activity for glycogenesis. In those fasting for 2 or 3 days hypoglycaemia and coma may occur 6–8 hours after excessive alcohol consumption. This hypoglycaemic coma may be mistaken for drunkenness. In those admitted to hospital, hypoglycaemia may not be noted due to continuous glucose drip. Even in children, alcoholic hypoglycaemia may occur [9] following ingestion of drugs containing alcohol.

Diabetes

Diabetics taking hypoglycaemic drugs must be warned about the blood glucose lowering effect of alcohol. Alcohol stimulates the microsomal enzyme system which metabolizes drugs faster. *Tolbutamide* taken by alcoholics is metabolized twice as fast as normal [10]. *Insulin* effect is prolonged when alcohol is in the blood, and may result in hypoglycaemia [11]. Diabetics treated with *oral sulphonylureas* within 3–10 minutes of taking alcohol have facial flushing and a sense of warmth even increasing to headache, nausea, giddiness, tachycardia, breathlessness and conjunctival injection that may persist for an hour. These effects are similar to those after taking disulfiram (*Antabuse*) which is used for the treatment of chronic alcoholism.

Stomach

Alcohol stimulates the secretion of gastric juice and a 7 per cent 'alcohol meal' is used for gastric analysis. Up to 6 per cent, alcohol does not increase acid output. If taken in a concentrated form, alcohol produces *gastritis*.

Skin

Alcohol produces a sense of warmth and visible flushing. The body temperature may rise by 1–2 degrees after the ingestion of 30–60 ml

(1–2 oz) on an empty stomach. This is due to dilatation of the peripheral blood vessels. Contrary to the popular belief, ingestion of alcohol before exposure to extreme cold may be harmful, as the dilated blood vessels dissipate heat quickly.

Bone Marrow

Alcohol, even without nutritional deficiency, produces toxic effects on the bone marrow resulting in thrombocytopenia, anaemia and haemosiderosis due to iron accumulation [12]. Iron over-load in alcoholics may occur because the beverage is rich in iron and alcohol increases iron absorption [13]. Alcoholic pancreatitis reduces pancreatic secretion, which also enhances iron absorption.

Vitamin B Complex Deficiency

Vitamin B complex is required for the oxidation of alcohol by the tissues. An alcoholic develops vitamin B complex deficiency because: (1) the increased calories supplied by alcohol increase the *requirement;* (2) the *intake* of food and vitamins is decreased because alcoholic gastritis and resulting anorexia decrease food intake during drinking bouts; (3) alcoholics have diminished thiamine absorption [14] and significantly low levels of other B-complex vitamins. Deficiency of vitamin B complex is manifest as polyneuropathy and the Wernicke-Korsakoff syndrome.

Nervous System

Brain. The sense of well-being produced by alcohol is due not to stimulation of the cerebral centres but to their depression. Anxieties and worries are lessened; confidence and extrovert tendencies are increased.

Alcoholic Polyneuropathy. This is not the result of the toxic effect of alcohol on the nerves, but of vitamin B deficiency as it responds to the administration of vitamin B-complex, provided irreversible changes have not taken place.

Wernicke-Korsakoff Syndrome [15] (Amnestic Confabulatory Psychosis). This is characterized by: (1) ocular signs; (2) mental disturbance; and (3) ataxia.

 1. *Ocular signs.* There is horizontal and vertical nystagmus, with

paralysis of external recti or paralysis of conjugate gaze. Nystagmus disappears with total paralysis of external recti. Pupils are usually spared but later may be small and poorly reactive. Total ophthalmoplegia is rare.

2. *Mental disturbances.* Delirium tremens, hallucinations, disorders of perception, agitation or automatic activity may occur. Severe global confusion and mental apathy are common. Usually there is disinterest in the surroundings, disorientation and misidentification of people. Spontaneous speech is minimal.

Amnestic syndrome is characterized by difficulty in registering, retaining and recalling simple meaningful material, e.g. a simple story or even the headlines of a newspaper, or the doctor seen as little as 5 minutes before may not be recognized. Old experiences and events are stated as recent happenings and unless the examiner is aware of those events he might interpret them as 'confabulation'.

3. *Ataxia* is of stance and gait. There is difficulty in walking and the gait has a wide base, but when an individual limb is examined in bed in the reclining position, there is minimal or no ataxia in that limb.

Ocular signs respond dramatically to a parenteral dose of a potent thiamine preparation but the mental disturbance and ataxic difficulty may take weeks or months to improve.

Myopathy. *Acute alcoholic myopathy* after a binge may occur, involving muscles of the proximal extremities and thorax [16]. There may be oedema and muscle necrosis. *Chronic alcoholic myopathy* manifests as muscle wasting and weakness of the proximal group [17]. Though alcohol may affect the myocardium directly, epidemics of *cardiomyopathies* have been related to cobalt in beer.

Liver

Alcohol produces: (1) *enlarged liver* without alteration in any of the liver function tests; (2) *fatty* liver; (3) *acute alcoholic hepatitis*; (4) *cirrhosis*; and (5) *haemochromatosis*.

Fatty liver is common, as alcohol increases the rate of synthesis of fatty acids and their conversion to triglycerides. Alcohol also reduces the oxidation of fatty acids and the release of triglycerides from the liver. Fat therefore accumulates in the liver cells after alcohol intake, even in casual drinkers [18]; these changes are more marked with deficient protein intake.

Acute alcoholic hepatitis is the direct effect of alcohol on the liver and also occurs when excessive alcohol is consumed with a low intake of food. It is characterized by moderate to severe jaundice, anorexia, nausea, vomiting, fever, upper abdominal pain and splenomegaly. Such patients are easily misdiagnosed as viral hepatitis, obstructive jaundice, or as jaundice associated with alcoholic cirrhosis. The biochemical tests may suggest hepatocellular damage or cholestasis. Histologically, the liver shows focal or massive cellular degeneration and necrosis, marked fatty changes, biliary stasis and an acute inflammatory reaction. These acute changes disappear with treatment, but cirrhotic changes will persist [15], if they have already occurred. Treatment is bed rest, vitamin supplements and withdrawal of alcohol. In the acute stage of hepatic failure, proteins should be restricted and a diet as recommended for hepatic coma advised. Supplements of vitamin B complex and intravenous glucose may be necessary if anorexia is marked. Subsequently a high-calorie, high-protein diet, as recommended for cirrhosis of the liver, is prescribed.

Alcoholic cirrhosis was formerly supposed to follow fatty liver, but now an increasing number of hepatologists agree that the *initial* process is alcoholic hepatitis with necrosis of liver cells. Necrosis results in cellular regeneration, collapse, intra-hepatic shunts, fibrosis and ultimately cirrhosis.

Pancreatitis is a common accompaniment of chronic alcoholics. A mild degree of steatorrhoea and decreased pancreatic function are related to low protein intake as they are reversed with adequate protein [20].

Clinical Uses

Alcohol taken well diluted and in small quantities can be a good appetizer. It is recommended in debilitating diseases and during convalescence from an acute illness. During an acute attack of cardiac pain, alcohol can help in dilating the coronary blood vessels. A well diluted long drink serves as a diuretic.

Intravenous Alcohol. Ethanol is administered intravenously during anaesthesia. It is also administered intravenously to augment calorie intake in patients unable to take oral feeds. More than 3 per cent alcohol solution produces venous thrombosis.

Bilirubin Metabolism in Newborn. The enzyme *glucuronyl transferase* helps conjugation of bilirubin. Gross deficiency of the enzyme in the first few days in the newborn results in unconjugated hyperbilirubinaemia and even kernicterus. Glucuronyl transferase activity is increased by phenobarbitone and alcohol. In mothers given more than 100 g alcohol intravenously, 3 to 96 hours prior to delivery, the serum bilirubin level of the infant diminishes during the first 5 days of life [21].

ACCIDENTS

Road Accidents. A blood level of over 150 mg/100 ml is considered dangerous and an absolute contra-indication to driving in most countries. Three single whiskies or 1½ pints of beer give ablood level of 50 mg/100 ml, while 4 large whiskies or 4 pints of beer produce a blood level of 150 mg/100 ml. The Road Safety Act, 1967 of Great Britain considers a blood level of alcohol (ethanol) over 80 mg/100 ml as drunkenness. In road accidents, it may not always be a car driver who is drunk but may even be the pedestrian.

Alcohol contributes to home and transport accidents and higher incidence of suicide.

MALIGNANT DISEASES

Alcohol may cause pain at the site of malignant disease and that may be the earliest symptom. It is noted in lymphomas, notably Hodgkin's disease. If women, on taking alcohol, develop pain in an organ or bleeding from the cervix they must have a cancer check-up [22]. In carcinoid tumour alcohol may produce flushing, and in osteomyelitis local pain. Oesophageal carcinoma is ascribed to alcoholics in Central Africa, but such a correlation cannot be obtained from Indian Gujarati women who have a very high incidence of oesophageal carcinoma without even sniffing alcohol.

CONTRA-INDICATIONS

Peptic Ulcer and Gastritis. In these diseases it is best to prohibit alcohol to chronic drinkers as they are liable to continue heavy drinking. However, for those not habituated to liquor, half a peg well diluted does no harm.

Viral Hepatitis. Alcohol is prohibited during acute viral hepatitis and for 6 months after the serum bilirubin and hepatic function tests return to normal.

Gout. Alcohol diminishes renal uric acid excretion. In gout, red wines, beer, stout and champagne should be avoided. Brandy, whisky and white wines may be allowed in moderation, but each patient should be studied individually as one gouty patient may tolerate wines of a type which may precipitate an attack in another.

Paromomycin (intestinal antibiotic) administered to an alcoholic may induce abdominal pain.

Addiction to Alcohol

Alcoholic addiction seldom, if ever, occurs in a man who is satisfied with himself and his surroundings. Addiction is often the outcome of conflicts, worries, anxieties and frustrations in a man who drinks to 'drown his sorrows'. Alcohol has a lower specific gravity than water, but the specific gravity of sorrows is still lower, and persistent attempts at drowning them with alcohol results and in addiction.

REFERENCES

[1] MUEHLBERGER, C.W. (1958) The physiological action of alcohol, *J. Amer. med. Ass.*, **167**, 1842.

[2] COOKE, A.R. (1970) The simultaneous emptying and absorption of ethanol from the human stomach, *Amer. J. dig. Dis.*, **15**, 449.

[3] BEGG, T.B., HILL, I.D., and NICKOLIS, L.C. (1964) Breath analyser and Kitagawa-Wright methods of measuring breath alcohol, *Brit. med. J.*, **1**, 9.

[4] WESTERFELD, W.W., and SCHULMAN, M.P. (1959) Metabolism and caloric value of alcohol, *J. Amer. med. Ass.*, **170**, 197.

[5] LIEBER, C.S. and DE CARLO, L.M. (1969) Hepatic microsomes: a new site for ethanol oxidation, *J. clin. Invest.*, **47**, Abstr. No. 185.

[6] LIEBER, C.S. (1970) New pathway of ethanol metabolism in the liver, *Gastroenterology*, **59**, 930.

[7] KATER, R.M.H., CARULLI, N., and IBER, F.L. (1969) Differences in the rate of ethanol metabolism in recently alcoholic and non-drinking subjects, *Amer. J. clin. Nutr.*, **22**, 1608.

[8] KREISBERG, R.A., SIEGAL, A.M., and OWEN, W.C. (1971) Glucose-lactate interrelationship: effect of ethanol, *J. clin. Invest.*, **50**, 175.

[9] HEGGARTY, H.J. (1970) Acute alcoholic hypoglycaemia in two 4-year olds. *Brit. med. J.*, **1**, 280.

[10] KATER, R.M.H., TOBON, F., and IBER, F. (1969) Increased rate of tolbutamide metabolism in alcoholic patients, *J. Amer. med. Ass.*, **207**, 363.

[11] ARKY, R.A., VEVERBRANTS, E., and ABRAMSON, E.A. (1968) Irreversible hypoglycaemia, a complication of alcohol and insulin, *J. Amer. med.*

Ass., **206,** 575.

[12] HOURIHANE, D.O.B., and WEIR, D.G. (1970) Suppression of erythropoiesis by alcohol, *Brit. med. J.,* **1,** 1.

[13] CHARLTON, R.W., JACOBS, P., SEFTEL, H., and BOTHWELL, T.H. (1964) Effect of alcohol on iron absorption, *Brit. med. J.,* **2,** 1427.

[14] TOMASULO, P.A., KATER, R.M.H., and IBER, F.L. (1968) Impairment of thiamine absorption in alcoholism, *Amer. J. clin. Nutr.,* **21,** 1341.

[15] VICTOR, M., and DREYFUS, P.M. (1961) Nutritional diseases of the nervous system, *Wld Neurol.,* **2,** 862.

[16] LAFAIR, J.S., and MYERSON, R.M. (1968) Alcoholic myopathy: with special reference to the significance of creatine phosphatase, *Arch. intern. Med.,* **122,** 417.

[17] EKBOM, K., HED, R., KRISTEIN, L., and ASTROM, K.E. (1964) Muscular affections in chronic alcoholism, *Arch. Neurol. Chic.* **10,** 449.

[18] RUBIN, E., and LIEBER, C.S. (1968) Alcohol induced hepatic injury in non-alcoholic volunteers, *New Engl. J. Med.,* **278,** 869.

[19] BECKETT, A.G., LIVINGSTONE, A.V., and HILL, K.R. (1961) Acute alcoholic hepatitis, *Brit. med. J.,* **2,** 1113.

[20] MEZEY, E.J., JOW, E., SLAVIN, R.E., and TOBON, F. (1970) Pancreatic function and intestinal absorption in chronic alcoholism, *Gastroenterology,* **59,** 657.

[21] WALTMAN, K., NIGRIN, G., BONURA, F., and PIPAT, C. (1969) Ethanol in prevention of hyperbilirubinaemia in the newborn, *Lancet,* **ii,** 1265.

[22] BREWIN, T.B. (1967) The incidence of alcohol intolerance in women with tumours of the uterus, ovary or breast, *Proc. roy. Soc. Med.,* **60,** 1308.

PART III

CLINICAL DIETETICS

50. DIET PRESCRIPTION

Medical teachers usually refrain from imparting knowledge of dietetics to medical students. As a result, doctors seldom prescribe full dietetic instructions. For example, instructions are commonly given to a patient like 'avoid sour and spiced foods' and unless a special diet sheet is prepared the patient is not likely to follow the instructions. Where facilities are available, dietetic prescriptions are prepared by a dietitian. This facility is not available everywhere and all physicians should be able to prescribe a diet for their patients. The following may, therefore, serve as a baseline.

Dietetic History

Economic Status. The economic status is an important practical consideration in formulating a diet prescription. During an acute illness or convalescence a few expensive items may be permissible but for more prolonged or chronic illness like diabetes or peptic ulcer the recommended foods must be, as far as possible, within the means of the patient.

Vegetarian or Non-vegetarian. Whether the patient is a vegetarian or not must be known. If vegetarian then the 'degree' of vegetarianism should be assessed, e.g. 'egg vegetarians' eat egg but no flesh; 'egg and fish vegetarians' eat egg and fish but not animal flesh; 'home vegetarians' prefer to remain vegetarian at home, to keep at peace with the wife or mother-in-law, but relish meat or chicken at a restaurant or a party.

Intolerance to Food. The dietetic history should also elicit whether a patient can tolerate all foods. For example, milk may produce diarrhoea in some and constipation in others. Those with colonic disorders are likely to get flatulence with pulses. The dietetic history should, therefore, elicit reactions to milk, pulses, spices, egg, meat, fish and prawn, and such foods should be restricted or excluded as necessary.

Allergy. Allergy to food is manifest as urticaria, abdominal cramps or bleeding. Many are allergic to shellfish or egg and these foods may have to be excluded.

Occuption and Time of Meals. The occupation of the patient and the time he takes his meals have to be noted. A mill worker who works on different shifts requires more detailed instructions for a peptic ulcer diet than a clerk whose hours of work are fixed.

When planning a diet the requirement of calories, proteins, fats, carbohydrates, vitamins, minerals and fluids are assessed according to the state of health of the patient.

Calories

Bed Rest. A person confined to bed tends to consume less calories than a person doing physical exertion. Bed rest decreases appetite. For an average adult confined to bed, about 1400–1600 Calories may be adequate. Fever increases the calorie needs.

High Calories. A diet high in calories is indicated for undernourished or convalescent patients. They are advised to take more cereals, butter and oils at the principal meals and snacks of milk, sandwiches, or biscuits at mid-morning, mid-evening and before retiring.

Low calories. A low calorie diet is indicated for all obese patients. A diet consisting of raw and cooked vegetables, fruits, egg, meat, fish, chicken and skimmed milk, with a low intake of cereals, provides bulk, satiety, adequate proteins and relatively few calories.

Proteins

In a usual well planned non-vegetarian diet the total intake of proteins is adequate. For vegetarians the important sources of proteins are: (1) milk; (2) cereals and pulses. In diseases of the colon whole milk usually produces diarrhoea while pulses produce flatulence. The protein requirements of vegetarians with colonic diseases can only be met by providing commercial protein foods or by supplying skimmed milk powder which is usually more easily digested than fresh milk.

High Protein Diet in Cirrhosis, Nephrotic Syndrome, Pregnancy and Lactation. A high protein diet is prescribed when the serum albumin is low as in hepatic cirrhosis without liver failure and in the nephrotic syndrome. It is also advisable to increase the protein intake during pregnancy and lactation. For a non-vegetarian, the protein content of the diet is increased by increasing the quantity of meat, chicken, fish or egg. For the vegetarian, extra protein in the form of skimmed milk, cottage cheese and pulses is advised. All pulses, including gram (Bengal gram) and groundnut, are relatively inexpensive and palatable protein rich foods.

Protein Withheld During Hepatic and Kidney Failure. During hepatic coma or uraemia, protein has to be withheld temporarily and carbo-hydrate-rich foods like fruit juice, banana, sugar-cane juice, and lemonade with sugar, honey or jaggery are advised.

Fats
Fats are a convenient source of calories. Fats are not as indispensable as proteins though prolonged deficiency of essential fatty acids leads to skin changes. A high calorie diet should contain fatty foods like cream, butter, *ghee* and oil, and fats should be freely used in cooking. A low calorie diet contains little fat.

Carbohydrates
Carbohydrates provide bulk and, together with fats, form the chief source of calories. If a high calorie diet is to be prescribed, carbohydrates in the form of *chappatis* (of wheat or other cereals), bread and biscuits provide comparatively inexpensive yet nourishing foods. For a low calorie diet they are advised sparingly.

Vitamins
The best sources of vitamins are liver, yeast, whole grain cereals and fruits. Vitamin A is derived from egg, milk and butter, while carrots and green vegetables provide the pro-vitamin A, carotene. Vitamin B complex is derived from unrefined cereals and flesh foods. The best sources of vitamin C are fresh fruits, vegetables and germinating cereals. Vitamin D can be easily acquired by exposure to the sun for about half an hour.

Minerals
Calcium is available from milk. The usual diet is seldom deficient in *phosphorus*. *Iron* is available from cereals, liver, kidney and egg. Sodium is easily provided by common salt added to the food. A low sodium diet may have to be prescribed during fluid retention as in ascites, cardiac failure or the nephrotic syndrome. The *potassium* intake is increased when vegetables and fruits are prescribed for patients

with an acute illness. A low potassium intake is advisable for patients with oliguric renal failure.

Fluids

Many people in the tropics do not drink enough fluid and this commonly leads to constipation. The water intake should always be liberal enough to ensure the passage of light coloured urine.

Fluids need to be restricted when excretion is impaired as in acute nephritis and kidney failure. The water requirement per day is then calculated as: 1000 ml a day to replace the insensible loss in respiration and perspiration plus the volume of urine passed during the previous 24 hours.

Depending upon the disease, or intolerance to food, certain foods may have to be excluded. For peptic ulcer and gastritis *spices* and *chillies* are not permitted. For a patient confined to bed, *fried foods* and *pulses* are best avoided as they produce flatulence.

Accuracy in Diet Prescription

Reluctance to prescribe a diet usually arises from lack of confidence because it is assumed that the diet should be mathematically precise and that the balance of total calories, proteins, fats and carbohydrates should be exact. A high degree of accuracy in diet prescription is not necessary. A vegetarian diet consists of cereals, pulses, green vegetables, root vegetables, milk and milk products. Those who take a mixed diet are advised additional meat, fish, chicken and eggs. A prescription with the usual intake of these foods in the customary quantity is seldom unbalanced.

A diet prescription can never be mathematically precise because of the following factors:

Variable Standards. No two authorities agree as to the exact requirements of calories, proteins, fats, carbohydrates, vitamins and minerals. The British Medical Association (1950) recommended 30 mg of vitamin C per day for an adult, while the Food and Nutrition Board of the United States recommended 75 mg.

Variable Quality. When certain foods are prescribed, we assume that they have always the same chemical composition. This is not true as can be seen from the varying results of analysis. Thus, the Dairy Science College, National Dairy Research Institute, Karnal, Punjab and Nutrition Research Laboratory from Coonoor reported 22 and 18 Calories respectively for an ounce of cow's milk, a variation of 22 per cent. If we also consider that milk delivered at our doors may not be of the same quality as that supplied by well organized Government dairies, a greater variation in the chemical analysis may be expected. The vitamin C content of cow's milk depends upon the season, when the animals graze on green pastures the vitamin C content rises. The vitamin D content of cow's milk in Western countries rises in the summer when the animals are exposed to the sun and diminishes in the winter. Many results of chemical analysis are based on the study of one or two samples. The composition of foods varies according to the season, soil and fertilizer used.

Chemical Analysis and Intake. Food as served may not have the same chemical composition as that analysed in the raw state. Considerable alterations occur in the processing, preserving, washing, cooking and serving of food. A 10–15 per cent variation in the food served is assumed even from a well organized institution like the Mayo Clinic [1]. This variation can occur on the positive or the negative side so that 30 per cent differences may be found. Chemical analysis of a given food-stuff may give different results depending upon the method used for the estimation For example, the fat content of Horlicks malted milk was found to be 1·2 g per cent by Soxhlet's method and 8·6 g per cent by von Lieberman's method [2], a variation of 700 per cent.

Metabolism. Digestion of food may be variable not only in two persons but also in the same person at different times. The absorption of a particular vitamin or mineral is usually better during a deficiency state. That digestion, absorption and utilization and energy output are variable can be seen by keeping two women of the same age, height and weight on an identical diet. One of them may put on weight while the other may maintain a constant weight. The human body, therefore, is not to be considered in the same way as a machine, giving a precise performance.

Combination of Foods. The combinations of foods that we take may improve or impair the quality of our diet. A combination of cereals with milk provides amino acids which supplement each other. At the same time, the phytic acid in the cereals decreases the amount of calcium or iron that is absorbed.

It will be clear from this discussion that mathematical exactitude is not necessary and that general guidance suffices in formulating a diet. Just as our diet should be a combination of various foods, the diet prescription should be a blend of nutritional knowledge with common sense.

DIET PRESCRIPTION

Household measures.   Only a faddist wants to keep a scale at his dining table to weigh out his food. The dietetic prescription should express the cooked foods in terms of table measures. The food values given below for household measures are in round figures for simplicity. Variations will, therefore, be found from the exact figures mentioned in tables.

Diet sheet.   The usual meals are breakfast, lunch, afternoon tea with snacks and dinner. The following information is meant to help plan out a diet sheet.

Breakfast

Some of the following are usually taken at breakfast:

1. Cereals
2. Eggs
3. Ham or bacon
4. Toast or *chappatis*
5. Butter and jam
6. Fruit
7. Tea, coffee or milk.

Cereals.   Cereals may be taken cooked in the form of oatmeal porridge, corn flakes, puffed rice, semolina, etc. They are served with milk and sweetening agents, such as sugar, jaggery or honey, which increase the calorie intake.

Household measure.   The usual helping of breakfast cereals is about 100 Calories with 3·5 g of protein. Added milk and sugar provide additional calories.

Eggs.   They can be served half-boiled, or poached if a low calorie intake and easy digestibility is the aim. If the patient has better digestion and requires more calories then fried eggs or eggs scrambled in fat are prescribed.

Household measure. An average Indian hen's egg provides 50 Calories and about 4 g of protein while a European egg provides 80 Calories and 6 g protein.

Ham or Bacon. They are eaten at breakfast particularly in Great Britain.

Household measure. One average slice of ham weighs 50 g and provides 120 Calories. Two strips of fried bacon weigh 15 g and supply 50 Calories.

Bread or Chappatis. The amount of bread or *chappati* prescribed varies according to the calories required and the economic status of the patient. For poorer people bread or *chappatis* form the chief source of food and provide the bulk of the calories. Toasting makes no difference to the calories supplied by bread. *Chappatis* prepared from any cereal or millet supply 100 Calories for every 30 g flour used.

Household measure. One medium slice of bread, or two thin wheat *chappatis,* or one small *chappati* of millet like *bajra* or *jowar,* supply about 80 Calories and 3 g protein.

Butter and Jam. The quantity advised is variable according to the calories required.

Household measure. One teaspoon of butter provides 30 Calories. A level teaspoon of jam provides 30 Calories.

Fruit. Fruit like orange, sweet lime, apple or banana may be available according to the season.

Household measure. One average helping of fruit provides 50–100 Calories.

Tea or Coffee. One cup of tea or coffee with two tablespoons of milk and two teaspoons of sugar provides 65 Calories.

Lunch and Dinner

The prescription for lunch or dinner is selected from some of the following items according to the dietary habit:

     1. Soup

     2. Vegetable salad

     3. Cooked vegetables

4. Potatoes
5. Milk, butter-milk or curd
6. Rice
7. Curry
8. Pulses (*dal*)
9. Meat, fish or chicken
10. Bread or *chappatis*
11. Custard, pudding or ice-cream
12. Fruit.

Soup. A small quantity of thin soup may increase the appetite. A large helping of thin soup just before meals decreases the appetite for other foods and may be desirable in a low calorie diet. Thin soup is low in calories but is rich in minerals and vitamins. Thick soup prepared by the addition of cream, potatoes, peas or nuts has a high caloric value depending upon the amount of such foods added.

Household measure. One cup of thin meat or vegetable soup provides 35 Calories.

Vegetable Salad. Raw vegetable salad is prescribed in large quantities if the aim is a low calorie intake. In a high calorie diet the quantity of salad is reduced. The usual salad vegetables—cucumber, radish, lettuce, tomato, carrots, shredded cabbage—are prescribed as available in the season. Raw vegetables in large quantities are not well digested and produce flatulence.

Salad dressing. For a low calorie diet a dressing of lemon, pepper and vinegar is advised. If a high calorie intake is needed a dressing containing oil such as mayonnaise, is prescribed.

Cooked Vegetables. One or two cooked vegetables are prescribed with each meal. The usual helping of a vegetable is 100 g . There are a variety of vegetables like bitter gourd (karela), brinjals (egg plant), cabbage, cauliflower, carrots, french beans, ridge gourd (turiya), lady's fingers (okra), pumpkin, *papri,* spinach, *tindola* and yellow pumpkin. The vegetables in season are advised.

Household measure. A single good helping of vegetable salad and cooked vegetables provides 100 Calories, mainly as carbohydrate.

Potatoes. Potatoes are served in many ways: mashed, baked, boiled or fried as chips or wafers. Their availability all the year round makes them a useful item of food. The quantity may be increased or decreased depending on the calories required.

Household measure. One medium potato weighing 100 g provides 100 Calories with 20 g of carbohydrate.

Milk, Butter-milk, Curd, Yoghurt. Milk or milk products, like butter-milk or yoghurt, are indispensable for a vegetarian menu because of their protein content of high biological value. Curd or yoghurt is served as *vati,* about 100 g or a cup, 200 g. The calorie content of milk products is calculated from the original quantity of milk used for their preparation. If a low calorie diet is necessary then skimmed milk is advised.

Household measure. Two-thirds of a cup of whole cow's milk or half a cup of whole buffalo's milk provides 100 Calories. A cup of skimmed cow's milk provides 70 Calories with 7 g protein. A cup of skimmed buffalo's milk provides 90 Calories with 9 g protein.

Rice. The quantity of rice prescribed is varied according to the dietary habit. As a main dish some eat it by the plateful. Usually about four tablespoons are prescribed to increase the bulk of the diet for those who do not take it as a staple food.

Household measure. Four tablespoons of cooked rice provide 100 Calories.

Curry. Curry is made in diverse ways. It is usually made with spices and coconut with the addition of meat, fish, egg, chicken, vegetable, etc. Curry is forbidden in digestive disorders because it is usually spiced.

Household measure. Four tablespoons of curry provides 50–100 Calories.

Pulses, Lentils (Dal). Pulses are more difficult to digest than other foods. They form a rich source of protein and should be a part of the menu for vegetarians, served as liquid (thin *dal*) or semi-solid (thick *dal*). *Dal* water (ossaman), the supernatant water obtained after cooking *dal,* is taken by many as soup.

Household measure. One cup of thin *dal* or half a cup of thick *dal* provides 100 Calories and 7 g protein.

Meat, Fish or Chicken. These are prescribed for non-vegetarians.

The usual Indian custom is to cook them together with vegetables or curry. The edible portion of an average helping weighs about 100 g. Meat or chicken may be boiled, grilled, roasted, or minced and fried into cutlets.

Household measure. One average helping of 100 g provides 100 Calories with 20 g protein.

Bread or Chappatis. These are discussed above under breakfast.

Custard, Pudding, Ice-cream. Custard and pudding are usually made from milk and sugar with eggs. They are made in various ways and flavours depending on the ability of the cook.

Household measure. Half a cup of custard, pudding, blancmange or ice-cream provides 150–200 Calories.

Fruits. Fruits are prescribed according to the season.

Household measure. An average helping of one fruit provides 50–100 Calories.

Fat Allowed in Cooking. The daily amount of fat recommended for cooking depends upon the caloric requirement.

Household measure. One tablespoon of fat like butter, *ghee* or oil provides 100 Calories.

Snacks and Dry Fruits

Snacks include sandwiches, biscuits, cakes, bananas, boiled eggs or milk drinks such as chocolate. They are prescribed: (1) with tea; or (2) as substitute for a main meal where a regular cooked meal is not feasible at the place of work; or (3) between the principal meals to increase the consumption of calories.

Sugar, Honey or Jaggery. These are advised according to the taste of the patient.

Household measure. One teaspoon of sugar, honey or jaggery provides 20 Calories.

Vitamins and Minerals. As long as the menu is based on the customary food habit in the usual quantity a special calculation for vitamins and minerals is not necessary.

Fluids. A liberal intake of water, about 6–10 glasses daily, is advised unless otherwise indicated.

Adjustments

After the menu has been written down in household measures its calorie equivalent and content of proteins, fats and carbohydrates are compared with the recommended intake. The calories are increased or decreased by varying the quantity of bread or *chappatis* or fat for cooking. If the *protein* intake is not adequate the quantity of milk, skimmed milk powder, pulses (*dal*), wheat or fish is increased. The *carbohydrate* intake can be varied by adjusting the intake of cereals as bread or *chappatis*. As long as enough calories and proteins are provided, fats and carbohydrates are interchangeable.

The skill in diet prescription lies in preparing a menu within a limited budget. The doctor should always have a fair idea of what foods are available in the market and their current price. A mother advised to give apples to her child suffering from diarrhoea may consider them to be a specific cure and buy them even though they cost more than the child's weekly food budget. An inexpensive diet can only be prescribed when the doctor knows the prevailing food prices.

REFERENCES

[1] MAYO CLINIC (1961) *Mayo Clinic Diet Manual,* 3rd ed., Philadelphia.
[2] McCANCE, R.A., and WIDDOWSON, E.M. (1960) The composition of foods, *Spec. Rep. Ser. med. Res. Coun.* (*Lond.*), No. 297, London, H.M.S.O., p. 6.

51. ABDOMINAL SURGERY

The advances in the knowledge of nutrition and better understanding of fluid and electrolyte balance have contributed to a great extent towards the successful outcome of a major surgical operation. A carefully planned operation diminishes mortality, avoids complications and reduces the period of convalescence.

MANAGEMENT

Patients without Digestive Complications

If a major operation is to be performed on a patient without any digestive complication, the minimum investigations required to assess the nutritional status of the patient are estimations of blood haemoglobin and serum proteins, particularly serum albumin values. As soon as an operation is contemplated, adequate stores of proteins are ensured by instructing the patient to take a nourishing diet with plenty of milk, skimmed milk, meat and eggs. If necessary the patient is advised to take fruit and lemon juice for vitamin C, supplements of vitamin B complex and iron. Clear instructions are also given to take adequate fluids by mouth so as to see that a light coloured urine is being passed.

The normal daily gastro-intestinal secretions of 6000 ml are twice the plasma volume of 3000 ml. Normally, most of these secretions are absorbed. A simple method of assessing gastro-intestinal losses is to estimate the urine volume and specific gravity, blood urea and haematocrit [1].

A healthy, well nourished individual undergoing surgery can tolerate several days of post-operative starvation with adequate intake of water, electrolytes and 100 g glucose daily. However, chronically malnourished patients with oral or oesophageal carcinoma, pyloric obstruction or intestinal fistula may require replacement of amino acids and fats. Intravenous protein hydrolysate and fat supplements help the proper healing of anastomosis and abdominal wounds, and prevent a burst abdomen (see Intravenous Feeding).

Patients with Digestive Complications

If the appetite is poor or digestion is impaired as is usual with pyloric obstruction, gastric carcinoma, diseases of the gall-bladder, caecum, or colon, then the desirable investigations necessary from the nutritional view-point are estimation of: (1) blood haemoglobin; (2) serum proteins, mainly albumin; (3) blood electrolytes; and (4) prothrombin time.

The patient is advised the following:

1. High protein diet consisting of milk, skimmed milk, eggs and meat as adequate protein stores in the body aid the healing of wounds.

2. In order to ensure an adequate level of potassium, vegetables, vegetable soup and fruit juices are given. Common salt is liberally

allowed in the diet in order to counteract sodium deficiency.

3. Supplements of vitamin C, 100 mg three times a day and a supplement of vitamin B complex tablets.

4. Iron as ferrous sulphate, 300 mg (5 gr) twice a day.

5. Oral antibiotics inhibit the growth of bacteria and diminish the synthesis of vitamin K. If oral antibiotics are given for a prolonged period prior to surgery, oral administration of vitamin K tablets correct this deficiency as the diminished bacterial flora does not prevent the absorption of preformed vitamin K. In patients with diseases of the liver, vitamin K, 10 mg a day, is administered orally. In patients with jaundice vitamin K, 10 mg a day, is administered parenterally.

Three Days Prior to the Operation. A fluid intake and output chart maintained 3 days prior to the operation, helps in ensuring an adequate fluid balance. Excretion of over 1200 ml of urine suggests that the patient is well hydrated. The patient should not be starved. He can have light meals and usual fluid till the evening of the operation. Three days before the operation, fried food, pulses (*dal*), cabbage or cauliflower, which tend to produce flatulence, should be stopped and a low residue diet prescribed. This reduces the tendency to post-operative flatulence which makes many patients extremely uncomfortable. Drastic purgatives should be particularly avoided as they reduce the body stores of fluids and electrolytes. It is advisable to open the bowel by a low enema or a suppository prior to the operation.

Fluid and Electrolytes after Surgery

An understanding of the changes in water, sodium and potassium balance in the body following a surgical operation is necessary. A person taking his usual oral feeds, with normally functioning kidneys, does not show an electrolyte disturbance. A slight excess of fluids and electrolytes even when given by the intravenous route is efficiently dealt with by the healthy kidneys but if the patient is kept on intravenous fluids for a few days then overloading or deficiency of fluids and electrolytes may occur.

Water. For the first 24–48 hours following surgery there is retention of fluid in the body. This is often ascribed to secretion of the anti-diuretic hormone by the posterior pituitary. The urine secreted during this period is scanty and has a high specific gravity. The tendency to retain water in the body occurs despite good functional capacity of the kidneys. During the 48 hours following an operation, fluids should not be given indiscriminately just because there is no free flow of urine.

Surgery in the hot humid climate of the Persian gulf entails a daily sweat and respiratory loss that may amount to 2–4 litres [2].

Sodium. For the first 24–48 hours after an operation there is also a tendency to retain sodium. The excretion of sodium in the urine is minimal. The lowered sodium excretion is probably due to the increased output of adrenocortical hormone following a surgical trauma. An alternative explanation to the retention of sodium is that the retention of water after surgery produces hypotonicity of the blood and sodium is retained in order to maintain osmolarity. Despite the retention of sodium the serum sodium level drops due to water retention.

Potassium. There is an increased loss of potassium in the urine due to breakdown of tissues as a consequence of the operation. Biopsies during the operation have shown that muscles near the site of operation lose 50 per cent of their potassium while the other muscles of the body lose only 10 per cent [3]. It is probable that some of the potassium loss is also due to the increased secretion of adrenocorticoids because if potassium is lost due to breakdown of tissues alone, as occurs during starvation, the ratio of the urinary loss of potassium to nitrogen is three to one but after surgery the proportion of potassium to nitrogen is greater.

The secretions of the intestinal tract contain appreciable amounts of potassium. Twenty-four hours' fluid loss through choledochostomy may contain 100 mEq of potassium. The loss through ileostomy is usually less than 11 mEq. per day.

Over-replacement

There is a tremendous misguided enthusiasm to over-replace the fluids with saline solutions. 'The objective of care is restoration to normal physiology and normal function of organs with a normal blood volume, functional body water and electrolytes' [4]. 'During the 5-year period there has been a progressive increase in the salt and water loading in patients so that those operated upon for cholecystectomy in 1967 received twice the amount of water and eleven times the amount of sodium ion, as those operated on in 1963' [5]. A patient dehydrated over the course of weeks with pyloric obstruction is likely to get pulmonary oedema when an attempt is made to replace all the fluid deficit within a course of 24 or 48 hours only.

MANAGEMENT ON THE DAY OF OPERATION

On the day of the operation usually 1500 to 2000 ml of 0.45 per cent saline is administered by slow high rectal drip, but if the patient had been malnourished prior to surgery an intravenous drip is given containing:

Glucose 5 per cent	1500 ml⎫ Total fluid
Glucose 5 per cent with saline 0·85 per cent	500 ml⎭ 2000 ml
Vitamin B complex (for intravenous use)	2 ml
Vitamin C	200 ml/g (100 mg in the first and the last pint of fluid).

Oliguria with a high specific gravity of urine on the first day is caused by retention of water by the kidneys and more than 2000 ml of intravenous fluids is not usually necessary. *Glucose* is added in order to supply 400 Calories as readily available carbohydrate for reducing the endogenous breakdown of proteins and also for the prevention of ketosis. Isotonic *saline,* 500 ml (4·5 g sodium chloride) is supplied despite the tendency to salt retention since water retention leads to hypotonicity. *Potassium* is not given on the day of operation because of oliguria. *Vitamin* B complex is administered to help the metabolism of glucose; *vitamin* C is given as it helps to promote tissue healing.

Fluid Chart
A properly maintained fluid intake and output chart up to the time when the patient can be restored to his usual oral feeds is an indispensable guide to management.

Alimentary Tract Motility after Surgery
In a normal stomach the proximal part shows less activity compared to the antral region which shows stronger peristaltic waves which

mix the food and allow its gradual passage through the pylorus. In the small intestine there is a gradient of diminishing activity from the duodenum to the ileum. With resumption of active peristaltic movement the patient passes flatus, there is absence of apparent abdominal distension and, on auscultation over the abdomen, peristaltic sounds are heard.

After abdominal operations including vagotomy, the peristaltic activity of the stomach and colon are considerably diminished but the small intestinal activity remains unaffected. The post-operative absence of bowel sounds is not always due to intestinal paralysis but probably due to emptiness of the bowel [6]. If the food can be made to enter the duodenum by nasoduodenal intubation then fluids can be started immediately after operation which may obviate the necessity for intravenous therapy.

It is not necessary even after partial gastrectomy or vagotomy combined with pyloroplasty to have a nasogastric tube, and hourly 28 ml (1 oz) water by mouth may be commenced from the day of operation [7].

Conclusion. On the day of the abdominal operation nasogastric or nasoduodenal tubes are not indispensable. Hourly oral intake of 28 ml. (1 oz) water can be tolerated. Alternatively 0.45 per cent saline may be given rectally. Intravenous therapy may be reserved only for a comparatively dehydrated or malnourished patient.

MANAGEMENT ON THE SECOND AND SUBSEQUENT DAYS

The following intravenous drip is planned on the second and subsequent days after operation:

Glucose 5 per cent   2000 ml ⎫ Total fluids
Glucose 5 per cent with   500 ml ⎭ 2500 ml
    saline 0·85 per cent
Potassium chloride 4·5 G
(To be administered only if necessary as described in the subsequent text. 1·5 G potassium chloride ampoules should be kept available and not more than one ampoule to be added to 500 ml of glucose or saline).
Vitamin B complex   2 ml
(for intravenous use)

Vitamin C   200 mg (100 mg in the first and the last pint).

The above recommendations require modifications as follows:

Aspiration and Drainage

The amount of fluid aspirated or drained should be added to the volume of fluid planned to be given for the day.

Oral Fluid

Orally or if necessary through the indwelling nasogastric tube, every hour or two, about 50–100 ml of water, tea, coffee, barley water or vegetable soup are administered. *The total volume of oral fluids given should be subtracted from the total daily requirement of 2500 ml of fluids planned to be administered intravenously.* It is necessary to emphasize that the patient should be induced to take as much fluid as possible by mouth or through the nasogastric tube, thereby reducing the needs for intravenous therapy to a minimum.

Sodium

Excess or deficiency of fluids and electrolytes may prove dangerous. If electrolyte studies are not feasible it is usually safe to give daily one pint of isotonic saline (4·5 g sodium chloride) intravenously.

Potassium

It is not necessary to give potassium chloride intravenously if the patient can take oral feeds of fruit juices and vegetable soup, unless the loss through the alimentary tract is appreciable. If pre-operatively the diet has not been adequate, then in order to avoid a tendency to post-operative distension of the intestine, potassium citrate should be given orally. Administration of potassium is necessary after operations in which the natural digestive secretions are drained out as in ileostomy or drainage of bile. The following mixture is advised:

Potassium citrate	2 G
Syrup of lemon	4 ml
Water	to make 30 ml

The mixture should be given orally or through an indwelling naso-gastric tube, 3 or 4 times a day.

Intravenous potassium chloride is indicated if there is marked gastric retention which may preclude oral absorption of food or marked loss of gastro-intestinal secretion as a consequence of vomiting, fistula, drainage or diarrhoea. Clinically there is lassitude, hypotonia and absent deep reflexes. Potassium deficiency is confirmed by: (1) depressed or inverted T wave and prolonged QT interval in the electrocardiogram; (2) low serum potassium level observed by electrolyte study. (Also see p. 169, for treatment of potassium deficiency.)

Replacement of Gastro-intestinal Aspirates

Gastro-intestinal aspiration is a common pre-operative and post-operative procedure in abdominal perforation, intestinal obstruction, paralytic ileus, etc. Different types of replacement solutions have been advocated in the past according to whether the aspirate is from the stomach, small intestine or bile. However, in practice such a clear distinction is not feasible, as usually the aspirated material is a mixture from these sources. The usual practice of replacement of fluid with normal saline, that is 154 mEq sodium with 154 mEq chloride, provides a higher concentration than aspirated fluid. This may account for the oedema and stiffness of the bowel noted when the abdomen has to be re-opened. The oedema may explain the delay in return of normal intestinal peristalsis.

The *average concentration of electrolytes* in these aspirates in routine surgical practice is approximately: *sodium* 100 mEq, *potassium* 12 mEq, and *chloride* 122 mEq. The gastro-intestinal solution suggested for *intravenous* use has the following concentration per litre [8].

Water	1000 ml	
Sodium chloride	5·9 g	
Potassium chloride	0·9 g	One litre of this solution
Ammonium chloride	0·53 g	provides sodium 100 mEq,
Dextrose	50·00 g	potassium 12 mEq, chloride
or		122 mEq.
Fructose	100·00 g	

Ammonium chloride is added to supply additional chloride. Glucose or fructose is added to provide calories.

The *volume* of above replacement fluid given intravenously equals the volume of aspirated fluid. The replacement is made every 6 hours.

BOWELS

Prior to an operation, and subsequently to relieve post-operative pain, it is usual to give drugs like morphine or pethidine. These have a tendency to produce nausea, vomiting and constipation which may limit the ingestion of food and fluids. The side-effects of these drugs are avoided if pain is relieved as far as possible by the parenteral administration of analgesics like *Novalgin*. Constipation results in flatulence, discomfort and tension at the site of the incision. If an anastomosis has been performed then flatulence stretches the suture line. In order to avoid flatulence the bowels should be moved with a glycerin suppository or by a low enema. The reluctance on the part of some surgeons to order a low enema to relieve the flatulence and discomfort of the patient the day following surgery is difficult to understand.

DIET

The aim of the clinician should be to resort to oral feeds at the earliest opportunity. We must realize that there is a profound ignorance on our part in the understanding of many physiological processes in the body. The great importance of fluid and salt for our body was recognized just prior to the Second World War and subsequently followed the realization of the role of potassium. It is only during the last few years that we have started considering the role of magnesium. We are probably quite ignorant about many other essential nutrients necessary for life. Parenteral therapy with glucose, fluids and electrolytes therefore should be given only during an emergency to tide over the crisis. Oral feeding after an operation should be resorted to as soon as there is evidence of intestinal activity. A nasogastric tube may be needed for tube feeding.

Early Post-operative Diet

After a nasogastric tube or intravenous therapy is dispensed with the patient can take the following diet:

Breakfast	Fruit juice, porridge
11·00 a.m.	Buttermilk
1·00 p.m.	Vegetable soup
	Half-boiled egg
	Mashed potato
	Banana

3·00 p.m.	Tea with biscuit
5·00 p.m.	Custard
7·00 p.m.	Vegetable soup
	Mashed potato
	Jelly

Half to one cup of water to be given every two hours.

After two days of the above diet the patient can gradually revert to his normal diet.

Principle of Diet

Easily digestible, low residue foods, should be commenced as early as feasible with supplements of vitamins B and C.

REFERENCES

[1] LEQUESNE, L.P. (1967) Fluid and electrolyte balance, *Brit. J. Surg.,* **54,** 449.
[2] TINCKLER, L.F. (1966) Fluid and electrolyte observations in tropical surgical practice, *Brit. med. J.,* **1,** 1263.
[3] WINFIELD, J.M., FOX, C.L., and MERSHEIMER, W.L. (1951) Etiologic factors in post-operative salt retention and its prevention, *Ann. Surg.,* **134,** 626.
[4] MOORE, F.D., and SHIRES, G.T. (1967) Moderation, Editorial, *Ann. Surg.,* **166,** 300.
[5] ROTH, E., LAX, L.C., and MALONEY, J.V. (1969) Ringer's lactate solution and extracellular fluid volume in the surgical patient: a critical analysis, *Ann. Surg.,* **169,** 149.
[6] ROTHNIE, N.G., HARPER, R.A.K., and CATCHPOLE, B.N. (1963) Early post-operative gastrointestinal activity, *Lancet,* **ii,** 64.
[7] HENDRY, W.G. (1962) Tubeless gastric surgery, *Brit. med. J.,* **1,** 1736.
[8] BADOE, R.A. (1970) Gastrointestinal replacement solution, *Brit. med. J.,* **3,** 622.

52. PEPTIC ULCER

In no disease does dietetic treatment give such symptomatic relief as in peptic ulcer. In the majority of uncomplicated cases drugs play only a secondary role.

A chronic ulcer formed in those regions of the gastro-intestinal tract where gastric juice comes in direct contact with the mucous membrane is known as a peptic ulcer. Such ulcers usually occur in the duodenum proximal to the ampulla of Vater and in the stomach. They sometimes occur in the lower oesophagus, in the jejunum after gastro-enterostomy or partial gastrectomy, and rarely adjacent to aberrant gastric mucosa in a Meckel's diverticulum.

Duodenal Ulcer. In Great Britain the incidence of duodenal ulcer is equally distributed among all the classes. About 10 per cent of men between the age of 45 and 54 have either had inactive or active peptic ulcer [1] which suggests that it is one of the most commonly encountered conditions. The problem of duodenal ulcer in the tropics is considerable. In India, too, it is seen to an appreciable extent amongst the poor who form the majority of general hospital patients, the maximum prevalence being in South India where the diet is low in proteins and highly spiced. Duodenal ulcer may sometimes occur in childhood. A chronic duodenal ulcer does not turn malignant.

Gastric Ulcer. In spite of the highly spiced diet in India, gastric ulcer is very infrequent in contrast to its incidence in Western countries. Data collected in Bombay showed that an ulcer of the stomach is more likely to be malignant than benign [2]. A gastric ulcer in an Indian should therefore always be considered malignant unless proved to the contrary.

Aetiology

There are many factors in the aetiology of peptic ulcer of which the following play a dominant role:

Heredity. A careful history may reveal that some of the blood relations of the patient have suffered from peptic ulcer.

Blood group. Group 0 subjects are more liable to have duodenal ulcer and a tendency to bleed than individuals of other blood groups.

Mental Stress. It is noteworthy that symptoms of peptic ulcer always increase during periods of mental stress and emotional upset. In a patient with a gastric fistula the gastric mucous membrane has been observed to become turgid, engorged and red when mental irritation or resentment was produced. Congested mucosa is easily traumatized to produce erosions and it is possible that such an erosion, bathed with acid gastric juice secreted during the interdigestive period, may become a chronic ulcer.

Season. The tendency to recurrence of peptic ulcer is greater during the monsoon and even during the mild winter season of Bombay.

Gastric Hypersecretion. Patients with *duodenal ulcers* have increased numbers of parietal cells in the stomach; consequently in an augmented histamine test the maximum acid output (MAO) is above average. There is hypersecretion of hydrochloric acid and pepsin, not only during the digestion of food but also when the stomach is empty. This hypersecretion during the interdigestive period is probably an important factor in perpetuating the ulcer. Therapy should therefore be aimed at neutralizing or diminishing the gastric secretion during the interval between the principal meals. A diagnosis of benign peptic ulcer should not be made with persistent histamine-fast achlorhydria.

Raised serum calcium enhances gastric acid and pepsin secretion [3]. This may explain the association of duodenal ulcer and hyperparathyroidism in some cases.

The gastric secretion is increased by:

Mental stress	Meat soups and extractives	Strong tea or coffee
Diminished blood sugar during fasting	Chillies and spices	Alcohol
	Protein-rich foods	Smoking

Gastric ulcers are not associated with hyperacidity and the parietal cell mass is not increased.

Fasting. Peptic ulcer is more likely to occur in individuals who have long periods of fasting between meals. The habit of some Indians of having only one or two big meals a day predisposes to peptic ulcer.

DIETETIC MANAGEMENT

The dietetic control of peptic ulcer is the sheet-anchor of medical management. The physician should not merely give oral instructions but should hand over to the patient a diet menu specifying the time to take food to suit his occupation and food habits. It is easier to prescribe a diet for a man who has fixed hours of work. For patients whose hours of work are variable the menu should be so adjusted as to suit his occupation.

Sippy's Diet. Some patients refrain from taking food despite having a peptic ulcer with a belief that rest to the stomach is the best remedy for an abdominal pain. Sippy's diet has served to focus the attention of the medical profession on frequent feeds rather than starvation. Sippy's diet is neither adequate nor practicable in the majority of the patients. Even during the acute phase of the disease many patients have not shown improvement when kept only on a milk diet but pain was rapidly relieved when a more liberal bland diet was given. Prolonged milk diet for peptic ulcer in older age group increases the incidence of coronary heart disease.

For the dietetic management of peptic ulcer the following considerations are necessary:

Calories

Adequate calories for the person according to his age, sex and occuption are to be prescribed.

Proteins

An adequate supply of proteins, about 1·2 g per kg is necessary. Milk proteins are best for this purpose. Meat soups and extractives, which are powerful stimulants to gastric secretion, are avoided. The common practice of taking meat soups an hour or two before meals 'for strength' is harmful in a patient with peptic ulcer.

Foods which Stimulate Gastric Secretion. There are certain foods which stimulate gastric secretion more than others. Meat, fish and dairy products (including milk) produce higher secretion than fruit and fruit juices, green peas and fried potatoes. The gastric secretory response is thus related to the protein content of food [4]. Despite the increased secretion of gastric juice the protein-rich foods should be given because not only do they act as a buffer but also an adequate intake of protein is beneficial for the healing of the ulcer.

Fats

Fats are useful in ulcer patients as they delay the emptying of the stomach. The products of digestion of fat in the small intestine produce enterogastrone which inhibits the secretion of gastric juice. Fats like cream, butter and olive oil can be particularly helpful in a thin patient. Fried foods are not advised as they are difficult to digest and often aggravate the symptoms.

Carbohydrates

Raw vegetables and coarse cooked vegetables are excluded as they may possibly traumatize the mucous membrane. Cooked tender vegetables, potatoes, cereals and cereal products are suitable for a patient with ulcer.

Vitamins

Vitamin C is claimed to be helpful in peptic ulcer as it promotes healing. Vitamin C deficiency is common in patients bleeding from peptic ulcer [5].

Condiments and Spices

In clinical practice, exclusion of condiments and spices and particularly chillies promotes rapid relief of symptoms.

Beverages

Caffeine increases gastric acid and pepsin secretion [6]. Repeated intake of caffeine-containing drinks may aggravate peptic ulcer. Therefore intake of tea or coffee is restricted to two cups daily. *Acid beverages* stimulate pepsin secretion. During the acute stage of ulcer, citrus fruits, pineapple, grape and carbonated beverages should be excluded [7].

Alcohol

Alcohol is avoided during the acute stage. Later, if permitted, it should be well diluted and sipped with meals.

Heavy wines and strong beers are best avoided as they aggravate symptoms.

Foods to be Avoided

1. Spices, pickles, chutney, vinegar.
2. Meat soups and extractives.
3. Course vegetables like raw onions.

4. *Pan,* betel nut (areca nut), tobacco chewing.
5. Very hot or very cold food or drink.

Frequency of Meals

Many ulcer patients are in the habit of taking their meals at long intervals. Patients with duodenal ulcer have a tendency to gastric hypersecretion during the interdigestive period. The stomach usually empties in two or three hours after a meal so that frequent feeds at two- or three-hourly intervals should be advised in order to neutralize the gastric juice. Ever since the benefit of the diet suggested by Sippy was recognized, some clinics have advised their patients twelve or even more gradations of diet. This has resulted in a great deal of confusion in the minds of medical students and patients. A simple dietetic regimen begets better co-operation from patients than the complicated graded diets. In our clinic, no particular benefit has been noted with complicated regimens. Two types of diet are recommended during the course of treatment of ulcer symptoms and the third type is recommended to be followed during remission:

Diet I is given during the period of acute pain due to peptic ulcer. The same diet is also recommended for haematemesis and melaena or pyloric obstruction. (See Diet I, p. 343).

Diet II is given when the pain of ulcer is relieved or is only occasionally present and while the patient is kept under observation. (See Diet II p. 344).

Diet III consists of general insturctions when the patient is declared cured of the current attack (see p. 345).

For an uncomplicated peptic ulcer the above diet regimens are quite effective. Patients whose symptoms are more severe or who do not respond to ambulatory treatment should be confined to bed and advised Diet I.

Is Liberal Bland Feeding Justified?

Many physicians are still afraid to advise anything but milk during the active stage of peptic ulcer. Liberal bland diet, however, has proved to be highly effective in the treatment of peptic ulcer. Meulengracht treated 1031 cases of bleeding peptic ulcer with liberal feeding of bland foods and had an overall mortality of 2·5 per cent. When cases in which death was entirely or mainly due to causes other than bleeding, as well as those who died within 24 hours of admission, and who had no chance to receive proper dietetic treatment, were excluded, the mortality was only 1·5 per cent. These results leave no doubts about the benefits of liberal bland feeds. Peptic ulcer is considered to be most active during bleeding, and if even during the episode of bleeding liberal bland diet is proved to be beneficial, then no fears should be entertained about permitting the same diet for the cure of an active ulcer without a complication.

It has also been pointed out that a special peptic ulcer diet is not necessary and consuming the routine hospital diet does not alter the rate of healing of peptic ulcer [8,9]. The routine hospital diet in Western countries is not different from the usual bland diet. In India the routine hospital diet is well spiced and definitely impedes the relief of pain and the time taken for the healing of an ulcer. Completely avoiding all spices particularly chillies, is of definite help.

DRUGS

The number of existing drugs on the market and the daily announcement of newer drugs is ample evidence that a specific drug which can cure peptic ulcer is not yet discovered. The natural history of peptic ulcer is characterized by symptom-free periods and hence credit for the remission always goes to the last drug used. Any system of medicine if persisted with for a period of time will appear to show temporary benefit, as after a period of pain from the peptic ulcer, natural remission is usual.

Drugs are indicated in the treatment of peptic ulcer in order to: (1) sedate the patients; (2) diminish secretion of gastric juice; (3) neutralize the secreted gastric juice; (4) relieve muscle spasm with antispasmodics.

In an uncomplicated case with mild peptic ulcer symptoms the neutralization of gastric juice and relief of pain is usually achieved by diet. It may be necessary to neutralize the acid with drugs in an uncomplicated case if: (1) the ulcer does not respond to diet alone within three days; (2) it is difficult for the patient to take food regularly during working hours; (3) peptic ulcer is associated with complications; and (4) associated obesity and diabetes necessitates the restriction of calories.

Antacids. The practice of administering antacids immediately after food is of no use in neutralizing the interdigestive hypersecretion.

Ulcer pain usually occurs when the stomach is empty, hence antacids are most effective if advised 2–3 hours after meals rather than immediately after meals.

Non-absorbable magnesium and aluminium hydroxide antacids administered in large doses may result in hypophosphataemia [10].

Milk Alkali Syndrome. Calcium is precipitated in the substance of the kidney in patients with peptic ulcer treated with frequent milk feeds together with soluble alkalies like sodium bicarbonate. This may result in damaged kidney function. Therefore, only the unabsorbable antacids should be used. Some of these cases may actually be due to hyperparathyroidism with associated duodenal ulcer. Increased vitamin D intake from milk may also be a contributary factor in the production of milk alkali syndrome.

Drugs Contra-indicated

Aspirin, Cortisone and Butazolidine. In a patient with peptic ulcer irritant drugs like aspirin, may precipitate haematemesis and are best avoided. In unavoidable circumstances if aspirin is advised it should be administered after food or with milk (paracetamol, codeine or *Novalgin* are analgesics which are probably harmless to the stomach). *Cortisone* or *Butazolidin* are also avoided as they may activate an ulcer.

The probable mechanisms by which these drugs cause bleeding are local irritation, altered character of mucous secretion, acid hypersecretion, or altered blood coagulation.

Rest and Relaxation

Rest and relaxation are valuable adjuncts to diet therapy. Peptic ulcer is a recurring disease and it is not practicable to confine to bed or hospitalize the patient during every *uncomplicated* attack of pain from peptic ulcer. Frequent absence from work becomes a source of great annoyance and mental tension, so it is best to allow these patients to continue their daily routine and they should be taught the art of slowing down the tempo of their work. The hours of sleep should be regulated and they should rest for an hour after lunch. They should train themselves to work during office hours only. Their office files or business worries should not come home. If they go to bed with problems on their minds they will only wake up with ulcer pain at midnight. They should not work on week-ends, if feasible.

Complete rest in bed or hospitalization is advised if the ulcer symptoms persist despite ambulatory treatment or if complications are present.

Mental Stress. Those who are under great emotional stress also require *hospitalization.* A sympathetic quiet talk by the physician goes a long way to help the patients. Those who can be helped should be taught to work for the solution of their problems without resentment. If there is no solution to their problem then teaching the patient to accept the situation philosophically will achieve results.

Teach to Live with Ulcer. There is always a tendency for duodenal ulcer to recur. The patient may feel greatly irritated and frustrated when the trouble recurs. The more the mind is focused on the ulcer the longer it takes to heal. It is essential to have mental diversion from the trouble which can best be accomplished by a hobby. Every effort should be made to prevent a recurrence (see below). The mental outlook should be so changed that the ulcer is accepted philosophically without resentment as a periodic ailment like a common cold.

FAILURE OF PHYSICIAN, PATIENT OR TREATMENT?

Despite clear written therapeutic instructions to a patient, he may not report satisfactory improvement at the next visit and it may be wrongly labelled as a failure of medical treatment. It is my experience that even an intelligent patient has often failed to fully appreciate the significance of the instructions. Careful questioning may bring forth an admission that the meals were either not taken at the *specified time* due to pressure of work or that he was induced to take spiced and irritant foods by his wife or a friend. The failure of the patient to follow dietetic regimen is either due to the failure of the physician to sufficiently impress upon the patient the necessity to follow instructions or due to the patient's indiscipline. Medical treatment should be regarded as a failure only if the patient has been *in hospital* and *definitely observed* to be taking his prescribed treatment for at least one week and still fails to show satisfactory progress. Those with *mental stress* do not improve unless hospitalized.

PREVENTION OF RECURRENCE OF PEPTIC ULCER

A neglected peptic ulcer may lead to serious complications like haematemesis and perforation or it may result in pyloric obstruction requiring major surgery. It must always be borne in mind that once an ulcer has developed the recurrence of symptoms after a few weeks or months or years is likely unless adequate care is taken. Symptomatic relief even for a few years should not lull the patient into a false assurance that the ulcer is permanently cured. Simple dietetic precautions will considerably reduce the chances of recurrence.

Individuals with a history of peptic ulcer or those whose blood relations have peptic ulcer should observe the meal pattern given in Diet III on page 345.

During periods of tension and overwork, people are inclined to skip their principal meals or take snacks instead. In fact more care is needed to follow a strict dietetic regimen during a period of mental stress.

Patients with periodic recurrence during monsoon or winter should be particularly careful to observe the dietetic pattern during those seasons.

Spices

Avoidance of spiced food is very important in tropical countries for the prevention of recurrence. Local irritation due to spiced foods prevents cure or causes a recurrence of ulcer. The extent to which diet in the tropics is spiced with chillies cannot be conceived by persons who eat European food.

Beverages

Tea or coffee is taken in excess by some patients. Frequently it is taken to 'keep company' when offered to business associates. Excessively strong tea and coffee produce irritation of the mucous membrane. Coffee should be limited to two cups a day. Weak tea with plenty of milk is permitted.

Alcohol

Excess of alcohol is an irritant to the stomach as it produces nausea, vomiting and gastritis. If taken on an empty stomach it irritates the mucous membrane. A small quantity, such as a half to one peg of whisky well diluted and taken with meals, is unlikely to cause any damage as alcohol is one of the best tranquillizers known to man [11].

Smoking

Smoking has shown an adverse effect on the healing of peptic ulcer [12]. Smoking 4–6 cigarettes in an hour markedly stimulates gastric secretion. It is best to prohibit smoking but if the patient is unwilling to stop smoking altogether, then he is permitted a cigarette after meals.

SURGERY FOR PEPTIC ULCER

Unless the patient realizes the natural exacerbations and remissions of an ulcer he is likely to be impatient and willing to submit to surgery. The surgeon should not advise an operation merely because the patient consults him. Surgery for peptic ulcer is indicated with the failure of medical treatment or with the presence of complications. Experienced surgeons are less inclined to operate on duodenal ulcers without specific indications. The operative mortality for chronic duodenal ulcer at the Mayo Clinic was over 1 per cent [13]. There are also chances of developing post-operative dumping syndrome, malnutrition, anaemia and malabsorption.

Malnutrition after gastric surgery in India is partly explained by the low intake of proteins. If the expensive 'first class' protein-rich foods cannot be taken because of cost, then an adequate intake of inexpensive vegetable proteins to supply all the amino acids needs is difficult with the small capacity of the stomach. A combination of small quantities of potatoes, pulses, cereals and half a cup of milk or milk products at *each* meal ensures simultaneous supply of all the amino acids needed for protein synthesis.

HAEMATEMESIS AND MELAENA

Haematemesis is vomiting of blood which may be derived from the mouth, oesophagus, stomach or duodenum. The commonest causes of haematemesis that are seen in the hospital wards are:

1. *Petic ulcer.* The commonest cause of haematemesis is duodenal ulcer. Benign and malignant gastric ulcers also produce haematemesis.

2. *Ruptured oesophageal varices* secondary to cirrhosis of the liver can produce severe bleeding.

3. *Acute gastritis* is a frequent cause of haematemesis. This may follow ingestion of excessive chillies and spices together with alcohol.

4. *Drugs* like aspirin and other coal-tar derivatives have been noted

to produce haematemesis. A careful history sometimes reveals ingestion of such drugs a few hours prior to the bleeding episode. Chronic arthritics usually take large amounts of aspirin which is often responsible for bleeding from the stomach.

5. *Hiatus hernia* can cause bleeding possibly due to oesophagitis.

Melaena is the passage of altered blood in the stool. Blood passed from the mouth, oesophagus, stomach, duodenum or small intestine is digested and when present in an appreciable amount, is excreted as black, tarry stools. When only a small quantity of blood is passed, the colour of the stool may not be altered but its presence as occult (hidden) blood is detected by chemical tests.

Surgery

Emergency surgery for bleeding peptic ulcer is life saving. However, a most careful clinical evaluation is necessary prior to surgery, as the site and cause of bleeding sometimes may not be found even at operation. Those with a tendency to bleed are likely to have recurrence. Evan a drastic operation, like subtotal gastrectomy, results in recurrence of bleeding during the subsequent 5–10 years [14].

Dietetic Management for Haematemesis and Melaena

It was customary to starve the peptic ulcer patient with haematemesis till Meulengracht showed excellent results with early feeding. Unless the patient is markedly nauseated or is continuously vomiting, it is best to start oral feeds. The patient is given 2-hourly small feeds as described in Diet I (p. 343).

Patients with *bleeding oesophageal varices* also require small frequent feeds. The bleeding produces anoxia of the liver and if the liver is not adequately provided with glycogen then the damage is likely to be aggravated. Repeated bland carbohydrate feeds should be given till the bleeding stops. *Hepatic coma* following bleeding from oesophageal varices in hepatic cirrhosis occurs as the products of metabolism accumulate and reach the brain due to: (1) poor hepatic function and anoxia of liver cells; (2) intra and extra-hepatic shunts due to portal hypertension; and (3) absorption of nitrogenous products produced due to digestion of the blood in the alimentary tract, and bacterial activity. It is logical to assume that the acid and pepsin of gastric juice coming in contact with the ruptured oesophageal varies interfere with clot formation. Frequent soft bland feeds for neutralizing the gastric juice are more likely to be helpful than any possible mechani-

cal harm produced during swallowing. Raising the head of the bed by
about 25 cm is also advisable to prevent a reflux of gastric juice in
the lower oesophagus.

PEPTIC ULCER

Foods	Remarks
Bread or *chappatis* of wheat, rice, maize, *jowar, bajra* or *ragi*	Permitted
Breakfast cereal of wheat, rice, oatmeal or maize	Permitted
Rice, cooked	Permitted
Pulses (*dal*) or beans	Permitted
Meat, fish or chicken	Permitted
Eggs	Permitted
Milk and milk products	Permitted
Soups	Vegetable soups permitted; exclude meat or chicken soup
Vegetable salad	Excluded
Vegetables, cooked	Permitted; exclude vegetables with coarse fibres or over-ripe seeds
Potato, sweet potato or yam	Permitted
Fat for cooking or butter	Permitted; exclude fried foods
Sugar, jaggery or honey	Permitted
Jam or *murabba*	Permitted
Pastries	Permitted as biscuits or soft cakes
Desserts	Permitted as custard, pudding or jelly
Sweets or sweetmeats	Excluded
Fruits, fresh	Permitted
Fruits, dried	Permitted
Nuts	Permitted
Condiments and spices	Excluded
Papad, chutney or pickles	Excluded
Beverages	Permitted as light tea or coffee
Water	As desired

PEPTIC ULCER
DIET I
IN HAEMATEMESIS AND MELAENA,
SUBACUTE PYLORIC OBSTRUCTION,
OR
DURING PAIN OF PEPTIC ULCER

Mixed Diet	*Vegetarian Diet*
On rising	
Milk, 1 glass	Milk, 1 glass
8 a.m.	
Orange juice, ¾ cup	Orange juice, ¾ cup
Porridge, ¾ cup with milk and sugar	Porridge, ¾ cup with milk and sugar
10 a.m.	
Eggs, 2 half boiled or poached, bread or *chappatis*	Cream or butter, 1 tablespoon with bread or *chappatis*
12 noon	
Minced meat	Cottage cheese
Boiled potato	Mashed potato
Bread or *chappatis*	Bread or *chappatis*
Apple	Banana
2 p.m.	
Custard or curd, ¾ cup	Custard or curd, ¾ cup
4 p.m.	
Milk, 1 cup with biscuits	Milk, 1 cup with biscuits
6 p.m.	
Custard or curd, 1 cup or bread with butter	Custard or curd, 1 cup or bread with butter
8 p.m.	
Minced chicken	Curd, 1 cup
Baked potato	Boiled potato
Bread or *chappatis* with butter	Bread or *chappatis* with butter
Jelly, 1 cup	Jelly, 1 cup
Before retiring	
Milk, 1 glass	Milk, 1 glass

PEPTIC ULCER
DIET II
DURING REMISSION FROM PAIN

Mixed Diet	Vegetarian Diet

On rising

Tea or coffee with biscuits or chappatis	Tea or coffee with chappatis or biscuits

Breakfast 8.30 a.m.

Orange juice	Orange juice
Porridge with milk and sugar	Porridge with milk and sugar
Eggs, 2 scrambled in milk	Khakhra or toast with butter
Toast or khakhra with butter	Banana

11 a.m.

Biscuits or buttermilk or milk, 1 cup	Biscuits or buttermilk or milk, 1 cup

Lunch 1 p.m.

Roast chicken	Curd, 1 cup
Baked potato and french beans	Mashed potato and carrots
Bread or chappatis	Rice with dal
Sweet lime	Chappatis or bread
	Orange

3.30 p.m.

Tea with biscuits, khakhra or bread and butter	Tea with biscuits, khakhra or bread and butter

5.30 p.m.

Toast or chappatis with butter or egg sandwiches	Toast or chappatis with butter, biscuits, or tomato sandwiches

Dinner

Roast mutton or boiled fish	Buttermilk, 1 cup
Mashed potato and green peas	Boiled potato and pumpkin
Bread or chappatis	Dal, 1 cup
Boiled custard	Bread or chappatis
	Jelly or ice cream

Before retiring

Milk, 1 glass with biscuits, khakhra or bread and butter	Milk, 1 glass with biscuits, khakhra or bread and butter

PEPTIC ULCER
DIET III
AFTER CURE

BREAKFAST	SNACKS	LUNCH	SNACKS	DINNER	BEFORE RETIRING
8 to 9 a.m.	10.30 to 11.30 a.m.	12.30 to 1.30 p.m.	4 to 5 p.m.	8 to 9.30 p.m.	A glass of milk

Snacks consist of biscuits, toasts or *chappatis* with or without butter; sandwiches, light cake, curd, buttermilk, milk, ice cream, custard or pudding.

REFERENCES

[1] DOLL, R., JONES, F.A., and BUCKATZSCH, M.M. (1951) Occupational factors in the aetiology of gastric and duodenal ulcers (with an estimate of their incidence in the general population), *Spec. Rep. Ser. med. Res. Coun.* (*Lond.*), No. 276, London, H.M.S.O.

[2] ANTIA, F.P., BHATNAGAR, S.M., and VYAS, M.C. (1959) Incidence of peptic ulcer and gastric cancer in Bombay, in *World Congress of Gastroentrology, Washington, D.C.* (1958), Vol. 1, Baltimore, p. 379.

[3] SMALLWOOD, R.A. (1967) Effect of intravenous calcium adminstration on gastric secretion of acid and pepsin in man, *Gut,* 8, 592.

[4] SAINT-HILAIRE, S., LAVERS, M.K., KENNEDY, J., and CODE, C.F. (1960) Gastric acid secretory value of different foods, *Gastroenterology,* 39, 1.

[5] SINGH, D., and GODBOLE, A.G. (1968) A study of plasma and gastric juice and ascorbic acid in peptic ulcer, *J. Ass. Phycns India,* 6, 833.

[6] DEBAS, H.T., COHEN, M.M., HOLUBITSKY, I.B., and HARRISON, R.C. (1971) Caffeine-stimulated acid and pepsin secretion: dose-response studies, *Scand. J. Gastroent.,* 6, 453.

[7] FLICK, A.L., (1970) Acid content of common beverages, *Amer. J. dig. Dis.,* 15, 317.

[8] DOLL, R., FRIEDLANDER, P., and PYGOTT, F. (1956) Dietetic treatment of peptic ulcer, *Lancet,* i, 5.

[9] TRUELOVE, S.C. (1960) Stilboestrol, phenobarbitone, and diet in chronic duodenal ulcer. A factorial therapeutic trial, *Brit. med. J.,* 2, 559.

[10] LOTZ, M., ZIMAN, E., and BARTTER, F.C. (1968) Evidence for a phosphorus-depletion syndrome in man, *New Engl. J. Med.,* 278, 409.

[11] JONES, F.A. (1970) A commentary on peptic ulcer, *London Clin. med. J.,* 11, 13.

[12] JONES, F.A. (1959) Epidemiology of peptic ulcer in Great Britain, with special reference to smoking, in *World Congress of Gastroenterology, Washington,* D.C. (1958), Vol. 1, Baltimore, p. 19.

[13] PRIESTLEY, J.T. (1965) Operative risk for patients with duodenal ulcer, *Mayo Clin. Proc.*, **40**, 737.

[14] SEREBRO, H.A., and MENDELOFF, A.I. (1966) Late results of medical and surgical treatment of bleeding peptic ulcer, *Lancet*, **ii**, 505.

53. FLATULENCE

Flatulence is a common abdominal symptom but there is a great deal of ignorance in understanding its mechanism. The available information on this subject is not usually based on sound evidence.

Flatulence is abdominal discomfort due to the presence of air or gas in the stomach or intestine associated with a motility disorder. It is a common complaint in the tropics, due to the high residue, spiced, vegetarian diet and the high incidence of infestation with intestinal parasites. Amongst certain sections of society a loud belch heralds the end of a hearty meal and is often an expression of thanks to the host and a tribute to the cook!

Gas can be expelled from the digestive tract either as : (1) belching from the stomach; or (2) flatus from the rectum.

Belching

Gas in the stomach is usually due to *sucking* or *swallowing* air or consuming food or drinks containing gas (aerated waters). It is only in pyloric obstruction that gas is *produced* in the stomach due to fermentation of food.

Air Swallowing (Aerophagy). An underlying nervous disturbance is the most common cause of excessive air swallowing which produces the frequently encountered symptom of aerophagia [1]. All of us swallow unconsciously a variable quantity of air with food or drink but excessive air may be swallowed by eating or drinking in various odd ways. For example a considerable amount of air is swallowed when food and fluid are sucked with a hissing noise, when betel leaves (*pan*) are chewed and during smoking.

Air Sucking. The champion belcher seen in the office practice who boasts that he can 'belch at any time with an audible noise that could

rattle the neighbourhood' is an air sucker. The air is unconsciously
sucked by elevating the chin, extending the neck, pulling the larynx
forward and with closed glottis making inspiratory effort. The negative
intrathoracic pressure during inspiration thus sucks air into the
oesophagus, since the glottis is closed. The air is then immediately
brought out with a loud belch. That this is not air swallowing but only
air sucking can be concluded from the observations that: (1) the
amount of repeatedly belched out air is out of proportion to that which
can be swallowed during that period of time; (2) there are no peristaltic
waves in the oesophagus as would occur if air was swallowed when
the patient is repeatedly belching; (3) under fluoroscopy the gastric
air bubble during belching can be seen to distend suddenly, while if
air is swallowed it should produce a gradual distension. The sucked
air may not reach the stomach but may be brought out immediately
from the oesophagus.

The diagnosis of air sucking is not difficult if: (1) there is a history
of belching in the early morning when the stomach is empty; (2) with
a little coaxing and persuasion the patient obliges by belching; and
(3) when observed under the fluoroscope the gas bubble in the stomach
increases in size just before belching and diminishes soon after.

Aerophagy associated with organic disease.   Aerophagy can mask the
symptoms of organic diseases like peptic ulcer, gastric cancer, colonic
and gall-bladder disease. The primary organic condition requires to
be diagnosed and treated.

Fermentation.   Three hours after ingestion of food the stomach is
usually empty. With pyloric obstruction, food remains in the stomach
for a long period and fermentation occurs. Pyloric obstruction is easily
excluded by radiology.

Intestinal Gases

Gas absorbed by the intestinal mucosa is removed by the portal
blood. Abdominal distension occurs with poor gas absorption following mucosal atrophy in coeliac syndrome or portal vein obstruction
in portal hypertension. The volume of normal flatus passed is 400–
1200 ml a day, greatly increased with relatively indigestible foods
such as beans. The intestinal gas contains hydrogen, methane, carbon
dioxide and nitrogen [2].

Hydrogen (H_2) production is entirely limited to the bacterial action
on the unabsorbed carbohydrates. Analysis of H_2 excretion in breath

forms a test of carbohydrate malabsorption [3]. *Disaccharidase deficiency* of *lactase* or *maltase* results in malabsorption of lactose and maltose that are fermented by the intestinal bacteria and produce H_2.

Methane (CH_4) is due to a high concentration of methane-producing bacteria. For unknown reasons higher concentrations of these bacteria occur in about one third of the population and appear to be a familial trait. Respiratory methane estimation is a simple reliable indicator of intestinal methane production [4].

Carbon dioxide in the intestine may result from: (1) diffusion from the blood into the intestine; (2) production by the intestinal bacterial fermentation of sugars; and (3) acids formed by the intestinal bacteria that react with bicarbonate.

Nitrogen may be derived from the blood by diffusion or from the swallowed air.

Halitosis

Halitosis (bad breath) may be due to the absorbed gases in the intestine that are excreted by the lungs. The treatment then consists of regulation of diet and bowel movements.

Flatus

The presence of air in the intestine is due to:

Swallowed Air. Eighty per cent of air is composed of nitrogen which is not absorbed. Swallowed air in the stomach, if not brought up, may pass through the small intestine to reach the caecum in 10–15 minutes, and be passed as flatus in 30 minutes [5, 6].

Diffusion from the Blood Stream. About 20 per cent of the gas in the intestine is due to diffusion from the blood stream.

Action of Bacteria upon Undigested Food. In the colon, unabsorbed carbohydrate as cereals, pulses and leafy vegetables rich in cellulose, are acted upon by the colonic bacteria to produce carbon dioxide and methane.

Protein putrefaction occurs when undigested proteins passing into the colon are putrefied by the anaerobic bacterial flora producing hydrogen sulphide and ammonia. Pulses and beans contain an antitryptic factor which prevents digestion. This factor can be destroyed if pulses are well cooked. Inadequately cooked pulses, eaten in a large quantity, produce marked flatulence.

Fried food is not easily digested. Undigested carbohydrates and proteins thus pass in the colon where they are acted upon by the bacterial flora producing gas.

Drastic purgatives produce intestinal hurry and propel undigested food into the colon where fermentation and putrefaction occur.

Constipation with stasis of the colonic contents always increases flatulence by promoting growth of bacteria. Instead of advising purgatives or laxatives which perpetuate constipation, a correct diet would relieve both the constipation and the flatulence [see CHAPTER 54].

Changing Intestinal Bacterial Flora

Cultures of lactic acid bacilli are sometimes advised with an aim to change the bacterial flora of the colon and diminish flatulence. However, it is not possible to alter the flora of the intestinal tract merely by administering bacterial cultures. The growth of intestinal bacteria depends upon the culture medium, which is the ingested food. Diet plays a dominant role in the growth of intestinal bacteria. Food containing lactose (milk) is more likely to promote the growth of lactic acid bacilli but the administration of milk or milk products not infrequently aggravates flatulence. Lactulose helps to change intestinal flora.

Intestinal infestations with *amoebae, flagellates* and *helminths* aggravate flatulence, particularly with the ingestion of pulses (*dal*), milk and milk products, spices and fibrous vegetables.

Pseudo-flatulence

A condition of pseudo-flatulence has been described by Sir Arthur Hurst and later by Alvarez [7]. It is produced by an undue protuberance of the abdominal wall by unconscious contraction of the diaphragm. Since there is no gas in the intestine it is called 'pseudo-flatulence'. This condition is usually seen in women, occurring as distension lasting from a few hours to a few weeks, and sometimes leading to a diagnosis of intestinal obstruction and subsequent laparotomy. Some patients may be lucky enough to escape surgery as the distension disappears without passage of gas when anaesthesia is induced.

Treatment

1. Aerophagy is treated by explaining the mechanism of air

swallowing and correcting faulty food habits.

2. The patient should be advised to chew food well as unmasticated food cannot be well digested by the intestinal enzymes.

3. Organic diseases like peptic ulcer should be treated. Colonic infestations with amoebae and *Giardia lamblia* should be eradicated with drugs.

4. Gas production by pulses and beans can be inhibited by decreasing the bacterial flora with antibiotics and bacteriostatic agents [8].

Diet. Constipation should be corrected by diet. Exclude foods that are known to the patient to produce flatulence.

Calories. Obese persons who take excessive food often suffer from flatulence. Their total calorie intake should be curtailed in order to reduce flatulence and body weight.

Proteins and Carbohydrates. If flatus is foul smelling due to protein putrefaction, meat products and eggs should be reduced to a minimum. Pulses are best excluded. Rice and potatoes are allowed in small quantities but fibrous vegetables like cabbage are prohibited.

Fats. Fried food should be avoided.

Spices. Irritant spiced food should be avoided.

Garlic is usually added to a tropical diet for taste. It also has the property of inhibiting the growth of bacteria in the colon thus reducing flatulence. Medical preparations containing garlic are also available.

Fluids. About 8–10 glasses of fluid a day help in regular bowel movement. Water should not be taken with meals as it may aggravate distension. Sucking fluid through a straw or drinking directly from a bottle leads to air swallowing.

Planning of Meals. A habit of taking only two meals per day should be changed to three or four smaller meals. Dinner should be light and eaten at least two hours before retiring.

FLATULENCE

Foods	*Remarks*
Bread or *chappatis* of wheat, rice, maize, *jowar, bajra* or *ragi*	Permitted
Breakfast cereal of wheat, rice, oatmeal or maize	Permitted
Rice, cooked	Permitted; to be excluded if carbohydrate dyspepsia
Pulses (*dal*) or beans	Excluded
Meat or fish or chicken	Permitted
Eggs	Permitted 2 per day
Milk or milk products	Permitted. Those suffering from giardiasis and amoebiasis are allowed only with tea or coffee
Soup	Permitted; thick soup excluded
Vegetable salad	Excluded
Vegetables, cooked	Permitted, beans, peas and fibrous vegetables like cabbage and cauliflower excluded
Potato, sweet potato or yam	Permitted, but excluded in carbohydrate dyspepsia
Fat for cooking or butter	Permitted; fried food excluded
Sugar, jaggery or honey	Permitted
Jam or *murabba*	Permitted
Pastry	Biscuits and light cakes permitted; fried pastries excluded
Dessert	Permitted
Sweets or sweetmeat	Excluded
Fruit, fresh	Permitted
Fruit, dried	Excluded
Nuts	Excluded
Condiments and spices	Excluded
Papad, chutney or pickles	Excluded
Water	Permitted liberally

FLATULENCE
SAMPLE MENU

Mixed Diet	*Vegetarian Diet*

Early morning

Tea, 1 cup	Tea, 1 cup

Breakfast

Cornflakes, 1 cup with skimmed milk, ½ cup and sugar, 2 teaspoons	Porridge, ¾ cup with skimmed milk, 1 cup and sugar, 2 teaspoons
Eggs, poached	
Toast with butter	Toast or *khakhra* with butter
Tea or coffee, 1 cup	Tea or coffee, 1 cup
Papaya, ½ or sweet lime	Orange

Lunch

Grilled mutton with french beans	Curd, 1 cup
Baked macaroni	Cooked turiya (*ridge gourd*)
Bread or *chappatis*	Bread or *chappatis* with *ghee* or butter, 2 teaspoons
Orange or sweet lime	Banana

4 p.m.

Tea, 1 cup	Tea, 1 cup
Biscuits and sandwiches	Biscuits and sandwiches

Dinner

Meat soup, 1 cup	Tomato soup, 1 cup
Steamed fish with boiled carrots	Butter milk, 1 cup
Baked potato	Cooked brinjals
Bread or *chappatis*	Boiled potato
Ice cream	Bread or *chappatis*
	Sago pudding

REFERENCES

[1] ROTH, J.L.A., and BOCKUS, H.L. (1957) Aerophagia: its etiology, syndromes and management, *Med. Clin. N. Amer.*, p. 1673.
[2] LEVITT, M.D., and BOND, J.H. (1970) Volume, composition and source of intestinal gas, *Gastroenterology*, **59**, 921.

[3] LEVITT, M.D., and DONALDSON, R.M. (1970) Use of respiratory hydrogen (H_2) excretion to detect carbohydrate malabsorption, *J. Lab. clin. Med.*, **75**, 937.

[4] BOND, J.H., ENGEL, R.R., and LEVITT, M.D. (1970) Methane production in man, *Gastroenterology*, **58**, 1035.

[5] MADDOCK, W.G., BELL, J.L., and TREMAINE, M.J. (1949) Gastrointestinal gas-observations on belching during anesthesia, operation and pyelography; and rapid passage of gas, *Ann. Surg.*, **130**, 512.

[6] MADDOCK, W.G. (1952) The importance of air in gastrointestinal distention, *Surg. Clin. N. Amer.*, **32**, 71.

[7] LANCET (1959) Pseudo-flatulence, Editorial, *Lancet*, **ii**, 168.

[8] RICHARDS, E.A., STEGGERDA, F.R., and MURATA, A. (1968) Relationship of bean substrates and certain intestinal bacteria to gas production in the dog, *Gastroenterology*, **55**, 502.

54. CONSTIPATION

Constipation (constipate = press together) is the commonest physiological disorder of the alimentary tract. It is characterized by infrequent, incomplete evacuation of hard, dried stools.

Normal Bowel Habit

The normal bowel movement of an individual depends upon the autonomic nervous system and the type of diet. As the former functions automatically, any therapeutic interference with it is undesirable. A vegetarian diet with its increased roughage content, produces bulkier stools. For most individuals one stool a day is necessary for good health and a feeling of well-being. Some may evacuate twice a day while a few, despite being in perfect health, may move every second or third day.

Bowel Evacuation

Inactivity and fasting produce constipation while bowel evacuation is stimulated by *physical activity* and *ingestion of food*. When a person moves about on rising in the morning, there is a propulsive mass movement of the colonic content with bowel evacuation [1]. This explains the morning evacuation of most normal individuals. Patients with diarrhoea and ulcerative colitis have maximum frequency on moving about in the morning and they benefit from rest. Entry of food into the upper small intestine increases colonic pressure activity. This explains the tendency of some normal persons to evacuate after breakfast, and in patients with diarrhoea, gastro-enterostomy and partial gastrectomy to evacuate after each meal. My experience with sigmoidoscopy confirms that the colon and rectum are empty for several hours if the patient fasts after morning defaecation, but the colon may be loaded within a short time after taking a meal or tea.

Complications of Constipation

Neglected constipation results in passage of hard stools. Straining during evacuation may lead to fissures, piles, prolapse of the rectum or inguinal hernia. It is dangerous for a patient with coronary heart disease to strain during defaecation. Distension of the bowel due to accumulated faeces may produce malaise, headache and apathy. These symptoms cannot be due to auto-intoxication as they immediately disappear on evacuation of the bowel with a suppository.

Bowel Neurosis

It is a good practice to train infants in regular toilet habits but an over-enthusiastic scrutiny of the frequency, quantity, colour and consistency of the stool by an anxious mother lays the foundation of a bowel neurosis which persists throughout life. Many of our lay intelligentsia in their thirst for medical knowledge read unauthenticated literature or consult colon quacks, who believe that the large intestine is a cesspool harbouring the germs and toxins of every conceivable disease and therefore the colon should be 'emptied' and 'cleaned' with either purgatives, enemas or bowel washes. The normal intestinal bacteria are indispensable for health. They aid in bowel function, produce vitamins and inhibit the growth of other pathogenic organisms. This can be observed during prolonged and indiscriminate use of oral antibiotics which kill the normal intestinal flora and result in vitamin deficiency and sometimes proliferation of lethal pathogenic organisms. Similarly, if bowel washes are given with the idea of rendering the colon 'clean' they will ultimately be harmful. Many colon-conscious patients' daily ritual begins with a purgative, enema or a bowel wash, without which their mind remains fixed on the bowel, with a miserable day and a sleepless night. Nature has designed the lower part of the colon for the storage of the waste products of digestion prior to evacuation. This does not produce ill health. Happy is the man who lets his bowel function automatically without interference.

Not infrequently a misguided patient complains about irregularity of bowel habit because his stool is not liquid or he does not pass a stool after every meal. When the bowel function is normal, the stools are neither liquid nor is there an evacuation after every meal.

A liquid stool is the result of hurried passage of unabsorbed food and digestive juices. With liquid stools there is loss of fluids and the electrolytes sodium and potassium. Excessive loss of fluids in a susceptible person may even precipitate thrombosis in the heart or in the brain. Drastic purgatives should, therefore, be avoided.

Straining at Stool

Many bowel-conscious patients strain after defaecation in order to 'clean the bowel'. This results in rubbing of the mucosal surfaces, inflammation and a foreign body sensation. The resultant mucous exudate increases mental agony and induces further straining to 'remove mucus'. Repeated attempts at straining produce piles and prolapse that may require surgery.

Purgatives

The habit of taking castor oil periodically has unfortunately killed many, but cured none of constipation. A purgative should never be given for undiagnosed abdominal pain as it may lead to perforation of an acute appendicitis or diverticulitis or aggravate the symptoms of intussusception or volvulus. The daily habit of purgation requires an increasing dosage to produce results. One patient had been in the habit of taking twelve to sixteen tablespoons of milk of magnesia often reinforced with half a dozen purgative tablets to have one gratifying stool!

Exacerbation of Pyelitis. In pyelitis not infrequently there is a relapse soon after a purgative. The irritation of the bowel caused by the purgative facilitates the absorption of bacteria which are then excreted by the kidneys, flaring up a latent infection of the urinary tract.

Bowel Inflammation. The habitual use of purgatives may produce clinical and radiological appearance suggestive of ulcerative colitis [2]. Damage to the myenteric plexus occurs by continued purgation [3].

Occasional Indications for Purgatives. A purgative is advised by a pathologist before a stool examination because a fresh liquid stool is likely to show trophozoites. However, a purgative is unnecessary [4] as all types of ova and cysts are more readily detected on examining a natural evacuation by the concentration method. Prior to a radiological study of the abdominal organs a purgative may be necessary to expel faeces. In gall-bladder disease, about a teaspoon of concentrated Epsom salts not only drains the gall-bladder but also helps to evacuate the bowel. Purgatives after a vermifuge may help to expel the paralysed worms.

Enema and Bowel Washes

• It is a fallacious popular notion that enemas and bowel washes are harmless. Some of the progressive individuals of our atomic age start the day with an enema and occasionally a bowel wash with an idea of achieving 'inner cleanliness'. The habitual use of enema or bowel wash leads to increasing constipation as the natural reflexes are not allowed to act. The stool after an enema contains increased amount of mucus and direct observation of the colon through a sigmoidoscope shows marked congestion and mucous secretion. A highly calculative businessman developed the habit of accurately weighing himself before and after an enema. When the weight showed an increase immediately after an enema, the rest of the day was spent on finding ways and means to get rid of the excess water his dishonest colon had retained.

Occasional Use of Enema. The occasional use of an enema is not harmful. A low enema may be necessary to initiate an excretory reflex during an acute illness, or before and after an operation. Similarly a bowel wash is sometimes indicated as a preparation for surgery on the colon or for removal of ingested poisons.

Fluid and Electrolyte Disturbance with Purges and Enemas

After purgation excessive loss of sodium and potassium is noted with radioisotope studies [5] and a low potassium syndrome may develop. Muscle biopsy may reveal diminished potassium [6]. A drastic purge or a high enema before surgery may deplete a patient of fluids and electrolytes particularly when the food intake is also reduced.

Water and Salt Intoxication. With a *plain* or *soap* water enema or bowel wash, water under pressure is spread over the entire mucous surface of the colon; excessive water absorption and intoxication may follow. Infants with megacolon who are being prepared with repeated enemas for investigations like barium enema or sigmoidoscopy may show drowsiness, apathy, weakness, excitement, convulsions and even coma and death due to the lowered osmolarity of the extracellular fluid [7] following excessive water absorption. On the other hand, *saline enemas* may lead to over-hydration and pulmonary congestion.

Causes of Constipation

There are three main types of constipation, (1) atonic; (2) spastic; and (3) obstructive.

1. Atonic constipation is most commonly due to: (a) *Lack of fluids.* In the tropics where perspiration is profuse and an adequate amount of fluid is not taken, water from the colon is more completely absorbed. This leaves a small quantity of hard dry faeces which does not produce enough distension of the lower bowel to initiate a reflex for its evacuation. (b) *Lack of roughage.* Faulty food habits which include irregular hours of meals, taking inadequate bulk, due to fasting or avoiding foods containing unabsorbable cellulose in the form of vegetables, leaves little residue for evacuation. (c) *Vitamin B deficiency.* Deficient intake of vitamin B also produces loss of tone of the bowel wall. (d) *Lack of potassium.* Deficient intake of potassium or excessive loss, as occurs with purgatives, may result in loss of bowel tone. Extreme lack of potassium produces atonic ileus. (e) *Irregular habit.* Irregular bowel habits may be due to getting up late in the morning and trying to rush through the morning rituals and breakfast, leaving very little time for the visit to the toilet before going to the office. Those living in *chawls,* sharing a bathroom amongst many, also have difficulty as the bathroom may not be available whenever there is an urge to evacuate or the unhygienic condition prevailing may make a visit to the bathroom undesirable. (f) *Purgation or enema.* The constant use of artificial aids for evacuating the bowels results in the loss of natural reflexes and tone of the bowel.

2. Spastic constipation results from excessive tone of the colonic muscles. This is due to: (a) *irritating foods;* (b) *excessive use of purgatives* which produce spasm of the intestinal tract; or (c) *mental stress.* Our colon is the image of our emotions, mental tension produces spasm of the colon and this is seen in tense, highly-strung, apprehensive individuals.

3. Obstructive constipation is usually due to malignancy or stricture of the colon.

Constipation in Children. The weekly ritual of administering castor oil or other purgatives to infants and children to 'clean' the bowels affects the tone of the intestines and ultimately leads to constipation which persists throughout life. Normal healthy children should never be given purgatives as a routine measure; instead, extra water, prune juice or fruits like banana or apricot may help.

Dietetic Management

Calories. Usual calories according to age, sex and occupation are advised.

Proteins. About 60–80 g protein are advised.

Fats. Fats stimulate the flow of bile and also lubricate the bowel. Butter, *ghee* and cooking oils are beneficial for lean patients. Fried foods should be avoided.

Carbohydrates. Adequate bulk even in an obese patient on a reducing diet can be supplied in the form of vegetables and whole fruits which are rich in unabsorbable cellulose. Bulk can also be provided by unrefined cereals which contain bran. In lean people, bananas, dried fruits like figs, raisins, dates and apricots are useful adjuncts.

Vitamins. Vitamins of the B group, preferably as brewer's yeast, help some patients to regulate the bowel function.

Minerals. Acutely ill or bed-ridden semi-starved patients require potassium in the form of vegetable soup, fruit juice or oral potassium salts to prevent constipation.

Fluids. A liberal amount of fluids, about 10 glasses or more in hot humid weather, is advised. Warm fluid taken in the early morning on an empty stomach, such as hot water or weak tea, helps some people to evacuate the bowel.

Principles of Diet. A bulk-producing diet with liberal fluids and adequate vitamins are needed for atonic constipation. High roughage and irritating foods are to be avoided in spastic constipation.

Additional Measures

In chronic constipation which does not respond to diet the following additional measures are also advised.

Exercise. Daily exercise such as a game of golf or a brisk walk is helpful.

Abdominal Massage. Talcum powder is sprinkled on the hands and abdomen. Firm pressure with the fist is applied beginning over the caecum and continuing along the ascending, transverse and descending colon up to the symphysis pubis. This movement should be repeated 20–30 times in the early morning.

Roughage. If roughage provided by green vegetables and whole fresh fruits does not relieve constipation, extra wheat bran can be added to *chappatis* or bread to produce bulk.

Hydrophilic Colloids. These are vegetable substances like *isphgul* and china grass (agar agar) which absorb a considerable amount of water thereby producing a non-irritating bulk which stimulates peristalsis. Before retiring about two or three teaspoons of *isphgul* is put on the tongue and washed down with one or two glasses of water. Commercial preparations such as *Isogel* are also available.

Lactose. One tablespoon of lactose, two or three times a day, added to fruit juice or tea is advisable for spastic constipation.

Suppository. During an acute illness, after a surgical operation or when travelling, the use of a suppository produces a quick result.

Liquid Paraffin. Non-absorbable liquid paraffin is a lubricant and provides bulk, about 30 ml is taken at bed time. The disadvantages are that it leaks through the anus soiling the clothes, and it prevents the absorption of the fat-soluble vitamins A, D, E and K. If administered two to three hours after meals, it does not interfere with vitamin absorption.

Milk of Magnesia. Constipation due to the habitual use of drastic purgatives may not respond to the above regimen alone. Under these circumstances a mild laxative like milk of magnesia may be required for a few days. The dosage should be so adjusted that one well formed stool is passed daily.

Conclusion

Constipation is not treated by a single measure alone but by a combination of measures. In most people a regular bowel habit can be formed without extra aids.

CONSTIPATION

Foods	*Remarks*
Bread or *chappatis* of wheat, rice, maize, *jowar, bajra* or *ragi*	Permitted, preferably made from whole grain with extra bran added
Breakfast cereals of wheat, rice, oatmeal or maize	Permitted
Rice	Permitted
Pulses (*dal*) or beans	Permitted
Meat, fish or chicken	Permitted
Eggs	Permitted
Milk or milk products	Permitted
Soup	Permitted
Vegetable salad	Permitted
Vegetables, cooked	Permitted
Potato, sweet potato or yam	Permitted
Cooking fat or butter	Permitted
Sugar, jaggery or honey	Permitted, lactose, 1–2 tablespoons is added for persistent constipation
Jam or *murabba*	Permitted
Pastry	Permitted as cake or biscuits
Dessert	Permitted; rich desserts excluded
Sweets or sweetmeat	Permitted
Fruits, fresh	Permitted
Fruits, dried	Prunes, apricots and figs are helpful
Nuts	Permitted
Condiments and spices	Permitted in moderation

Foods	*Remarks*
Papad, chutney, pickles	Permitted in moderation
Beverages	Permitted, only 2 cups a day; strong tea or coffee excluded
Fluid	10 glasses or more

CONSTIPATION
SAMPLE MENU

Mixed Diet	*Vegetarian Diet*

On Rising

Glass of warm water	Glass of warm water
Tea	Tea

Breakfast

Stewed figs, 4, or apricots or prunes, 8 to 10	Stewed figs, 4, or apricots or prunes, 8 to 10
Porridge with milk and sugar	Cornflakes with milk and sugar
Eggs, scrambled	Toasts or *chappatis*
Toasts or *chappatis*	Butter
Butter	Honey
Marmalade	Banana
Orange	

Lunch

Meat soup	Tomato soup
Salad from radish, lettuce, tomato, carrot, beetroot, served with dressing	Butter milk
	Salad from radish, lettuce, tomato, carrot, beetroot, served with dressing
Baked fish and french beans or	Pumpkin, cooked
Rice and fish curry	Rice with curry or *dal*
Bread or *chappatis*	Bread or *chappatis*
Banana or papaya	Grapes

4 p.m.

Tea with biscuits	Tea with biscuits

Mixed Diet	Vegetarian Diet

Dinner

Mixed Diet	Vegetarian Diet
Soup	Mixed vegetable soup
Chicken, roast with green peas	Curd
Baked potato	*dal*
Bread or *chappatis*	French beans and boiled potato
Baked custard	Bread or *chappatis*
	Murabba or jelly

At least 10 glasses of water during the course of the day.

REFERENCES

[1] HOLDSTOCK, D.J., MISIEWICZ, J.J., SMITH, T., and ROWLANDS, E.N. (1970) Propulsion (mass movements) in the human colon and its relationship to meals and somatic activity, *Gut,* **11,** 91.

[2] MARSHAK, R.H., and GERSON, A. (1960) Cathartic colon, *Amer. J. dig. Dis.,* **5,** 724.

[3] SMITH, B. (1968) Effect of irritant purgative on the myenteric plexus in man and mouse, *Gut,* **9,** 139.

[4] ANTIA, F.P., DESAI, H.G., JEEJEEBHOY, K.N., and BORKAR, A.V. (1965) Problems in the diagnosis of intestinal amoebiasis, *J. trop. Med. Hyg.,* **68,** 53.

[5] COGHILL, N.F., McALLEN, P.M., and EDWARDS, F. (1959) Electrolyte losses associated with the taking of purges investigated with aid of sodium and potassium radioisotopes, *Brit. med. J.,* **1,** 14.

[6] LITCHFIELD, J.A. (1959) Low potassium syndrome resulting from the use of purgative drugs, *Gastroenterology,* **37,** 483.

[7] HIATT, R.B. (1951) The pathologic physiology of congenital megacolon, *Ann. Surg.,* **133,** 313.

55. DIARRHOEA AND DYSENTERY

By diarrhoea is meant the passage of unformed stools. When unformed stools are accompanied by the passage of blood and mucus the illness is called dysentery. The causative organism in diarrhoea and dysentery can be isolated in many patients but in others no pathogen may be discovered in spite of a careful search [1]. It is possible that a virus may be the aetiological agent in some instances.

Dysentery

The passage of blood and mucus in the stool, as in dysentery, suggests disease of the colon. Amoebic and bacillary infections of the colon are the commonest causes of dysentery [1]. Ulcerative colitis, or non-specific chronic colonic inflammation, is not an uncommon disease even in the tropics, and gives rise to intermittent blood and mucus in the stools.

Acute Diarrhoea

Acute diarrhoea generally follows the ingestion of unhygienically handled, irritating, decomposed or stale food. In the tropics, if freshly killed meat is not immediately deep frozen but is allowed to remain for a few hours at room temperature before being frozen, decomposition occurs. Eating such meat may result in acute diarrhoea.

Traveller's Diarrhoea (Turista)

Traveller's diarrhoea usually occurs within 3 or 4 days up to a fortnight in new arrivals in a foreign country. Although many aetiologic agents are blamed, the cause remains unknown. It is usually labelled 'amoebic' or 'bacillary' dysentery, when a tourist arrives in a tropical country. However, traveller's diarrhoea occurs with great frequency even when an individual travels from one temperate zone to another, and then the condition is labelled 'virus' infection though no virus is isolated. Clinically, there is abdominal colic with nausea, vomiting and frequent stools, usually *without* blood or mucus. It frequently subsides within 1–3 days. The treatment is symptomatic. *Prophylactic* use of Entero-Vioform, one tablet 3 times, or triple sulpha one tablet twice a day, is claimed to reduce the incidence.

Chronic Diarrhoea

After an acute attack of dysentery, diarrhoea is common whenever spiced, irritant or stale food is eaten. Periodic attacks of diarrhoea in people living in the tropics may improve in the temperate climate of Europe. This improvement is due both to the cooler climate and to a change in the dietary habits, especially a reduction in the intake of spiced foods. Infestation with *Giardia lamblia* is a common cause of diarrhoea in the tropics and the symptoms are aggravated by spiced food, pulses, milk and milk products.

Nervous Diarrhoea. In some tense people, the fear of taking an examination or an interview produces diarrhoea. Recurrent diarrhoea in such people accompanies mental stress.

Hydrochloric Acid. Lack of hydrochloric acid in the stomach has been blamed for diarrhoea. In pernicious anaemia, with histamine-fast achlorhydria, diarrhoea is not a presenting feature, and therefore it can be assumed that deficiency of hydrochloric acid is not an important cause of diarrhoea.

Diseases of the Small Intestine. Diseases of the small intestine like tuberculosis produce chronic diarrhoea. Regional enteritis is a rarity in the tropics.

Fatty Diarrhoea. The causes of fatty diarrhoea are described in Chapter 56.

Malnutrition. The intestinal epithelium is constantly being shed and regenerated. With marked protein deficiency, regeneration may become deficient and diarrhoea occurs. *Vitamin deficiency* may cause diarrhoea; examples are, niacin deficiency in pellagra and vitamin A deficiency [2]. If sigmoidoscopy is performed without prior enema in a malnourished patient with diarrhoea the mucous membrane of the colon appears dry, shiny and reddish.

Carcinoma of the Colon. The presence of blood and mucus in the stool may be the earliest indication of carcinoma of the colon. All cases of dysentery should, therefore, be thoroughly investigated. Over 80 per cent of cancers of the colon occur in the distal 30 cm, which can be visualized by sigmoidoscopy even in the early stage. Pathogenic organisms thrive well in a malignant ulcer so the presence of such organisms in the stool, especially in elderly patients, must alert the physician to search for an underlying carcinoma.

Purgatives in Diarrhoea. The practice of administering purgatives during acute diarrhoea to 'flush the intestine of the irritant' is not advisable. Irritation of the bowel by the purgative may produce further depletion of fluid and electrolytes and prove disastrous.

Dietetic Management

Calories. In acute diarrhoea over 1500 Calories daily, and in chronic diarrhoea about 2500 Calories, are advised.

Proteins. Easily assimilable protein-rich foods like minced meat, egg, skimmed milk and skimmed milk preparations may be given, if tolerated. In some patients, sensitive to milk and unknowingly taking large quantities, the diarrhoea comes under control only when milk and its products are excluded from the diet.

Fats. Fats are restricted as they are not always absorbed with intestinal hurry and may aggravate diarrhoea.

Carbohydrates. Easily assimilable carbohydrate such as vegetable puree, fruit juices, or *kanjee* are given liberally.

Vitamins. Oral or parenteral vitamins, particularly water-soluble B and C, are necessary during the management of persistent diarrhoea.

Minerals. With severe diarrhoea, electrolyte balance may be markedly disturbed.

Fluids. Many patients with diarrhoea resort to self-imposed starvation which may be harmful. In all cases of diarrhoea, whether medical facilities are available or not, it is best to start with liberal amounts of fluid as water, fruit juice, vegetable or meat soups with added salt, and fresh lemon squash with sugar, jaggery or honey, in order to ensure an adequate intake of fluid and electrolytes.

Avoid
Spices, pulses, fried foods and fibrous vegetables are excluded.

Principles of Diet
The low residue diet should be non-irritating, consisting of soup, banana, biscuits, sago, arrowroot, skimmed milk, potato, eggs and minced meat. Green vegetables with a high residue should be restricted, except as purees. Fruit juices, and especially apples, pomegranate, and bael fruit are helpful.

Vomiting with Diarrhoea
When vomiting accompanies acute diarrhoea it is best to withhold

food. Intravenous saline with 5 per cent glucose may be necessary as an emergency measure. With severe vomiting and diarrhoea the loss of gastric and intestinal juices may cause such profound changes in the fluid and electrolyte balance as to be fatal. Parenteral replacement of sodium and potassium, with glucose and vitamins B and C may be needed.

It is best to start oral feeds as early as feasible.

DIARRHOEA AND DYSENTERY

Food	Remarks
Bread or *chappatis* of wheat, rice, maize, *jowar, bajra* or *ragi*	Permitted
Breakfast cereals of wheat, rice, oatmeal or maize	Permitted, arrowroot and sago *kanjee* also recommended
Rice, cooked	Permitted
Pulses (*dal*) or beans	Excluded
Meat, fish or chicken	Permitted
Eggs	Permitted, avoid fried eggs
Milk and milk products	Permitted only as skimmed milk or its products
Soup	Permitted, thick soup excluded
Vegetable salad	Excluded
Vegetables, cooked	Permitted, fibrous or over-ripe vegetables excluded
Potato, sweet potato, or yam	Permitted
Fat for cooking and butter	Excluded
Sugar, jaggery or honey	Permitted
Jam or *murabba*	Permitted, all jams with seeds excluded
Pastry	Permitted as biscuits
Dessert	Permitted as light custard
Sweets or sweetmeats	Excluded
Fruits, fresh	Permitted as juice, pomegranate or apple juice recommended: exclude berries
Fruits, dried	Excluded
Nuts	Excluded

Food	*Remarks*
Condiments and spices	Excluded
Papad, chutney and pickles	Excluded
Beverage	Permitted
Water	Permitted liberally

DIARRHOEA AND DYSENTERY
SAMPLE MENU

Mixed Diet	*Vegetarian Diet*
Tea, 1 cup	Tea, 1 cup

Breakfast

Arrowroot porridge (*kanjee*) with sugar or honey	Sago porridge (*kanjee*) with skimmed milk and sugar
Egg, 1 poached	Toast or *chappatis* with jam
Toast with apricot jam	

11 a.m.

Pomegranate or orange juice, 1 cup	Pomegranate or sweet lime juice, 1 cup

Lunch

Chicken soup, 1 cup	Vegetable puree
Minced meat with mashed potato and boiled french beans	Potato, boiled
	Skimmed milk curd, 1 cup
Bread or *chappatis*	Bread or *chappatis*
Orange	Papaya, ½

4 p.m.

Tea with biscuits	Tea with biscuits

6 p.m.

Apple or sweet lime juice, 1 cup	Apple or orange juice, 1 cup

Dinner

Mutton soup, 1 cup	Tomato soup, 1 cup
Chicken, roast	Potato mashed
Potato, baked	Pumpkin
Bread or *chappatis*	Skimmed milk, 1 cup
	Bread or *chappatis*

Before retiring

Baked apple with sugar	China grass jelly, 1 cup

REFERENCES

[1] ANTIA, F. P., CHAPHEKAR, P. M., CHHABRA, R. H., SWAMI, G. A., and BORKAR, A. V. (1961) The incidence of bacteria and parasites in dysenteric and non-dysenteric diarrhoea. A study in 800 cases, *J. Ass. Phycns India,* **9,** 723.

[2] RAMALINGASWAMI, V. (1948) Nutritional diarrhoea due to vitamin A deficiency, *Indian J. med. Sci.,* **2,** 665.

56. MALABSORPTION SYNDROME

The term malabsorption syndrome is not used to describe deficient absorption of a single nutrient like vitamin B_{12} or vitamin D, but describes lack of digestion or absorption to a variable degree of a number of substances such as *fats, proteins, carbohydrates, vitamins, minerals* and *water.* The basic *clinical features* of malabsorption are: (1) chronic ill-health, (2) anaemia; and (3) steatorrhoea, i.e. an average daily excretion of over 6 g of faecal fat. Radiologically, there may be non-specific changes, segmentation and dilatation of small intestine, or stricture and fistula formation due to an organic disease.

AETIOLOGY

Malabsorption syndrome can occur as a result of the following conditions :

Diffuse Small Bowel Mucosal Injury

Mucosal injury occurs as a result of *gluten sensitivity,* producing *coeliac disease* in children and *idiopathic steatorrhoea* in adults. In *tropical sprue* the injury has an uncertain aetiology. (Isolated *disaccharidase deficiency* may also occur due to the mucosal injury.)

Diseases Involving the Wall of the Small Bowel

Malabsorption may be produced by diverticulosis of the small intestine, tuberculosis, ileojejunitis, regional enteritis, sarcoidosis, scleroderma, Whipple's disease (intestinal lipodystrophy), malignant lymphoma or small intestinal neoplasm.

Anatomical Abnormalities of the Bowels

Intestinal resection, partial gastrectomy, and gastro-enterostomy can produce malabsorption.

Deficiency of Digestive Secretions

Pancreatic Diseases. Deficiency of the secretion of pancreatic juices occurs in: (1) *carcinoma* of the head of the pancreas; (2) *chronic pancreatitis;* (3) *pancreatic lithiasis;* (4) *fibrocytic* disease of the pancreas (mucoviscidosis). Unless there is a marked reduction in pancreatic secretion, malabsorption does not occur. In fact, malabsorption is found in only about 30 per cent of patients with chronic pancreatitis. Oil droplets in the stool on microscopic examination are a feature of pancreatic steatorrhoea. *Zollinger-Ellison* syndrome, due to a gastrin-secreting tumour of the islets of Langerhans, may result in steatorrhoea because excessive gastric acid secretion results in low intestinal pH of 2 or 3 (normal 6 or 7). Acid medium in the intestine does not allow normal bile emulsification of fat and digestion by the pancreatic lipase.

Decreased Bile Salts. Decreased bile salt *formation, excretion, bacterial deconjugation* or *hydroxylation,* and *diminished ileal reabsorption* occur with: cirrhosis, hepatitis, intrahepatic cholestasis; ductal obstruction with stone, carcinoma, stricture; small intestinal bacterial overgrowth, ileal inflammation, tuberculosis, Crohn's disease or ileal resection.

Effect of Drugs

Malabsorption may occur during prolonged use of neomycin, *Dindevan,* colchicine and phenytoin (*Dilantin*).

Blood and Lymphatics

Arterial or venous insufficiency, intestinal lymphangiectasia and lymphatic obstruction produce malabsorption.

Miscellaneous

Giardiasis, protein malnutrition (kwashiorkor), and protein-losing gastro-enteropathy may produce malabsorption.

Coeliac Disease

Coeliac disease, coeliac sprue, adult coeliac disease, idiopathic steatorrhoea, and *non-tropical sprue,* are all different names for the same disease with: (1) characteristic *flat mucosa* on intestinal biopsy; (2) dramatic clinical and histological improvement on *gluten-free diet*. *Adult coeliac disease* is the term used when the disease continues from childhood into adulthood. *Idiopathic steatorrhoea* is the term sometimes used if the disease is first discovered in adulthood in the temperate zones.

Tropical Sprue

'Tropical sprue' is a most confusing term, which has never been defined [1]. People with laboratory tests showing 'malabsorption' without identifiable cause have been labelled 'tropical sprue'. These patients are usually grossly malnourished and underweight. During their absorption tests the same loading dose as that recommended for the heavier Western populations is administered and then it is doubtful whether deficient absorption noted is really 'malabsorption'. 'Acute sprue' and 'epidemic sprue' have added to the confusion, as patients with frequency of stools with blood, mucus and even fever are included in this category [2]. Since this description denotes inflammation of the colonic mucosa it is better to segregate them by the old-fashioned term 'dysentery'.

Protein malnutrition, folic acid deficiency, intestinal parasitic infestation, increased small bowel bacterial flora or *bile salt deficiencies* are also known to exhibit a clinical and laboratory picture of malabsorption. It is therefore about time that the above known aetiological factors were distinguished from tropical sprue. Tropical sprue may be defined as 'intermittent or continuous fatty diarrhoea (steatorrhoea) due to the *primary* (unknown) absorptive defect in the *small intestine*' [1].

ABSORPTION OF NUTRIENTS IN MALABSORPTION SYNDROME

In the malabsorption syndrome there may be deficient absorption of: (1) fats; (2) proteins; (3) carbohydrates; (4) vitamins, particularly folic acid and vitamin B_{12}; (5) minerals, particularly iron, calcium and potassium; and (6) water.

Fats

Excessive excretion of fat in the stools (steatorrhoea) has drawn the most attention. *Naked eye examination* of the stool is most necessary. The stools have an offensive odour and are pale, mushy, bulky and float on water. On a regular diet, simple *microscopic examination* of the stool for fat, and staining with Sudan III may give a reasonable idea of steatorrhoea and for practical purposes may replace cumbersome stool analysis.

The total quantity of faecal fats excreted in 24 hours forms the basic investigation. With the usual daily consumption of 50–150 g fats, the average daily faecal excretion in a normal person (estimated over a period of 3–4 days), is less than 6 g. A better concept of steatorrhoea is obtained by studying faecal fat excretion over a few weeks rather than a few days. In the malabsorption syndrome the average daily faecal excretion exceeds 6 g and is usually between 10 and 30 g.

For the *estimation* of faecal fat excretion, a special diet kitchen to measure and control the intake of fats is unnecessary, as long as the patient takes his usual diet without excess fats. Analysis of stool for the estimation of split and unsplit fats is also unnecessary, if estimation of total fatty acids is made by the method of van de Kamer *et al.* [3].

The Source of Faecal Fat. The faecal fatty acids consist of: (1) *short chain fatty acids* derived by fermentation of carbohydrates. Daily excretion of these in a normal person is less than 1 g. They do not contribute to the fatty appearance of the stool but are partly responsible for the offensive odour. (2) *Long chain fatty acids*, when in excess, appear on microscopic examination as liquid fat globules. The total daily excretion normally does not exceed 5 g.

Faecal fats may *originate* from unabsorbed dietary fat, fat excreted in the biliary secretion, and synthesis from carbohydrates by the intestinal bacteria or synthesis by the intestinal cells.

Absorption Studies with Labelled Fat. If labelled I^{131} fat is given orally its absorption can be measured by the estimation of radioactivity in the blood or by the subsequent excretion of radio-iodine in the urine. In idiopathic steatorrhoea both I^{131} labelled triolein as well as labelled oleic acid are poorly absorbed. On the other hand, in pancreatic steatorrhoea triolein is poorly absorbed due to lack of pancreatic digestion while oleic acid, which does not require digestion, is well absorbed.

Proteins

Faecal excretion in excess of 3 g of nitrogen per day is termed *azotorrhoea,* but the estimation of faecal nitrogen is of little assistance.

Deficient protein *intake* produces clinical and histological changes that resemble sprue [4, 5]. This is not surprising as the intestinal mucosal turnover is very rapid (3–5 days) and protein is required for the regeneration of mucosa. Protein-deficient patients have fatty liver and their *pancreatic enzyme formation* is deficient, resulting in pancreatic steatorrhoea and deficiency of fat-soluble vitamins. With adequate protein intake there is marked clinical as well as histological improvement in the liver and the small intestine [5], and the exocrine pancreatic secretions revert to normal [6].

Peptidases [7]

Intestinal peptidases, like disaccharidases, are located in the brush border of the intestinal mucosa. Pancreatic trypsin and chymotrypsin have also been shown to bind to the intestinal brush border [8].

There are apparently several peptidases acting on different proteins. Two distinct peptidase deficiencies are recognized: (1) *peptide hydrolase* deficiency in the small intestinal mucosa results in failure to digest the protein gluten in wheat, which produces coeliac disease. Treatment with a gluten-free diet or corticosteroids restores normal digestion [9]; (2) *pteroylpolyglutamate hydrolase* (PPH: folate conjugase) deficiency in the small intestinal mucosa results in the failure of digestion of dietary folates that exist mainly as polyglutamates. For absorption the polyglutamates should be broken down into monoglutamates by folate conjugase, which is found in intestinal mucosal lysosomes [10]. Folate conjugase deficiency therefore results in folate malabsorption and deficiency.

Carbohydrates

The absorption of carbohydrates may be diminished in malabsorption syndrome. The fasting blood sugar has been found to be lower than 80 mg and the maximum rise of sugar after 50 g of glucose is only 22·6 mg per 100 ml compared to 44·6 mg in the control group. Thus, the low fasting blood sugar and a maximum rise of blood sugar of less than 40 mg after the oral administration of glucose constitutes one of the tests for the diagnosis of malabsorption.

The glucose tolerance is a relatively simple test for distinguishing the causes of malabsorption. In coeliac disease or tropical sprue there is diminished absorption and a 'flat' curve is obtained. In pancreatic disease, on the other hand, a diabetic curve is produced.

Disaccharidases

Disaccharidase, maltase, sucrase, lactase, etc., are enzymes on the brush border of the intestinal mucosa that break down disaccharides for absorption.

DISACCHARIDE	ENZYME	MONOSACCHARIDES
Maltose (starch digestion)	Maltase	glucose + glucose
Sucrose (household sugar)	Sucrase	glucose + fructose
Lactose (milk sugar)	Lactase	glucose + galactose

Causes. (1) *Primary* disaccharidase deficiency is a single enzyme deficiency. (2) *Secondary* disaccharidase deficiencies are associated with malabsorption of other nutrients also, and are seen in *mucosal diseases* (gluten enteropathies), starvation (kwashiorkor), intestinal bypass surgery; *drugs,* neomycin, colchicine; *diseases:* regional enteritis, Whipple's disease, mucoviscidosis, giardiasis, and even in ulcerative colitis.

Sucrase-Isomaltase Deficiency. These enzymes usually coexist. Infants, when started on foods including household sugar, may exhibit diarrhoea due to the primary mucosal deficiency of sucrase and isomaltase. The symptoms may sometimes be apparent only in adult life. The stool may impart a characteristic 'cheesy' smell.

Lactase Deficiency. Lactase deficiency is probably the *commonest* intestinal enzyme deficiency. Normal lactase activity is least in the duodenum, highest in the jejunum, and gradually decreases towards the distal ileum. The activity is normal at birth, but in certain races it may decrease with age. Lactase deficiency is common in Eastern countries, in Africa and among American Negroes. Reduced intestinal lactase is perhaps a genetic defect. Members of the family of a lactase-deficient patient also exhibit the deficiency [11]. It is not due to decreased milk intake because deprivation for 6 weeks does not affect the activity, nor does feeding 150 g lactose to lactase-intolerant subjects for varying lengths of time increase jejunal lactase level. *Starvation* produces generalized decrease in the intestinal enzymes which improves with parenteral feeding.

Clinically, lactase deficiency is suspected from the history. Depending upon the extent of deficiency, after taking a small or large amount of milk or milk products there is abdominal discomfort, colic, flatulence and diarrhoea. This effect is similar to that of oral mannitol since unabsorbed lactose produces osmosis and effects outpouring of fluids in the intestines. There is also retention of fluids in the small and large bowel. Bacterial fermentation in the colon of undigested lactose results in acid stools, which also causes diarrhoea [12].

Diagnosis of Lactase Deficiency. *Mucosal biopsy lactase activity* can be estimated. The results may be unreliable, however, since the lactase activity is in the brush border, and the proportion of brush border included in the homogenate depends upon the depth of the tissue removed. The activity also varies in different parts of the small intestine, hence the standard point for biopsy must be the ligament of Treitz. (1) *Lactose tolerance test.* In a normal individual after overnight fast 50 g lactose in a glass of water shows a peak blood sugar rise of 20 mg over the fasting level. Venous blood samples show false flat curves in about a quarter of the people with normal intestinal lactase, but capillary blood examination eliminates this error [13]. Flat lactose tolerance may occur even with normal mucosal lactase if stomach emptying is slow. (2) *Radiological* demonstration entails administration of barium with 25 g lactose; a flat plate taken 45 minutes later shows dilated small intestinal coils and rapid transit. (3) *Breath analysis* for hydrogen has also been suggested as a test for lactose absorption, as intestinal bacteria break down carbohydrate to liberate hydrogen which is absorbed and exhaled [14]. (4) *Clinical test* is the simplest, physiological, reliable and easily reproducible. To an overnight fasting patient 25 g lactose dissolved in a glass of water is administered orally. This amount of lactose is equivalent to that contained in 500 ml milk (1 large glass), i.e. the amount an average adult is expected to digest. In a lactase-deficient patient, within 30 to 60 minutes of lactose administration, there is abdominal discomfort or colic, borborygmi and diarrhoea lasting for 2–3 hours.

The *management* consists of permitting only the amount of milk and milk products that can be tolerated. Since the degree of deficiency is variable, many may tolerate milk that is mixed with cereals, cocoa, Horlicks, etc., which allows gradual lactose breakdown. Fermented milk products, *curd* and *butter milk* may also be tolerated to an appreciable extent since about half the lactose in milk is fermented to lactic acid. Cooked milk as a custard or pudding may also be tolerated. In some constipated lactase-deficient patients, an adequate amount of milk may not only provide healthy food but help relieve constipation.

d-Xylose Absorption Test. D-xylose is a pentose found in plants. It is absorbed mainly from the jejunum and unlike glucose it is little metabolized, so in the absence of kidney damage the amount appearing in the urine after an oral dose provides a good index of absorption. To an overnight fasting patient 25 g *d*-xylose is given orally in a glass of water in the morning. During the next 2 hours another three glasses of water are given to ensure free flow of urine. All the samples of urine for 5 hours after administering *d*-xylose are collected and the total xylose excretion measured. A healthy person below the age of 65 years excretes on an average 7·2 g *d*-xylose. Excretion of less than 4·2 g denotes deficient absorption from the jejunum, as occurs with idiopathic steatorrhoea and tropical sprue. Pancreatic diseases are not characterized by primary deficiency of absorption, hence *a*-xylose shows normal urinary excretion.

Most people tolerate oral 25 g *d*-xylose but some experience borborygmi, abdominal cramps and diarrhoea. Therefore a 5 g test dose of *d*-xylose has been proposed with urinary excretion of 1·2 g over a 5-hour period in normal subjects. This dose is not generally accepted for the diagnosis of malabsorption [15].

Xylose absorption is a simple screening test. However, *d*-xylose is metabolized by the intestinal bacteria. Overgrowth of upper intestinal bacteria produces false low *d*-xylose excretion [16]. Xylose excretion decreases with advancing age due to the deterioration of renal function [17]. Oral aspirin and indomethacin also decrease intestinal xylose absorption.

Vitamins

In malabsorption syndromes there may be diminished absorption of all vitamins. Poor absorption of folic acid and vitamin B_{12} are of importance in the production of anaemia.

Folic Acid. Dietary folates are mainly polyglutamates. For absorption they are hydrolysed by the upper intestinal mucosal enzyme *pteroyl-polyglutamate hydrolase* (PPH: *folic acid conjugase*). Deficiency of this enzyme due to mucosal damage results in non-absorption of naturally occurring dietary polyglutamates, while a routine *crystalline* folic acid (monoglutamate) absorption test may be normal. Hence, a normal folic acid absorption test does not necessarily denote absorption of natural dietary polyglutamates.

Vitamin B$_{12}$. Vitamin B$_{12}$ is absorbed from the distal part of the small intestine. Deficiency is manifested as anaemia and glossitis. Vitamin B$_{12}$ malabsorption occurs in *stagnant loop syndrome* due to stricture, fistula, anastomosis or diverticulosis. The small intestinal proliferating bacteria bind vitamin B$_{12}$ and prevent its absorption. Since the absorption improves merely on oral administration of tetracyclines or lincomycin, which destroy the bacteria, there is no primary defect in the absorption of vitamin B$_{12}$. In tropical sprue and coeliac disease the lack of absorption of vitamin B$_{12}$ is due to mucosal atrophy, so no improvement is noted with the administration of either intrinsic factor or antibiotics. Lack of vitamin B$_{12}$ absorption may be partly ascribed to the lack of *ionizable calcium*. Oral calcium lactate improves vitamin B$_{12}$ absorption.

Vitamin B Group. The other vitamins of the B group may not be absorbed and may produce evidence of deficiency.

Vitamin A and Carotene. The absorption of vitamin A and carotene is defective, hence estimation of blood levels after an oral dose is sometimes used as a test of malabsorption.

Vitamin D. Poor absorption of vitamin D in infants with coeliac disease leads to *rickets*, while in adults with idiopathic steatorrhoea it may produce *osteomalacia*. *Tetany* may occur with the low serum calcium. For treatment, oral administration of vitamin D is not effective unless high doses (e.g. 50,000 IU) are administered with a calcium supplement.

High parenteral doses of vitamin D together with a high oral intake of calcium may produce vitamin D poisoning because a gluten-free diet, usually prescribed in coeliac disease, is low in phytate which allows better absorption of calcium [18].

Vitamin K. There is deficient absorption of vitamin K which may lead to low prothrombin activity in the plasma and produce bleeding.

Minerals

Iron. In coeliac disease, deficient absorption of iron has been demonstrated by radioactive studies. Absorption improves with corticosteroids or a gluten-free diet. In tropical sprue absorption of elemental iron may be normal or greater than normal. Steatorrhoea *per se* does not result in malabsorption of elemental iron. Iron loss through gastro-intestinal cell loss may also occur.

Calcium. Deficient absorption of calcium results from: (1) atrophy of villi; (2) unabsorbed fatty acids which combine with calcium to form insoluble soaps; (3) poor absorption of vitamin D from the intestine; and (4) lactase-deficient patients who avoid milk. The serum calcium level in malabsorption may be low.

Parathyroids. The lowered serum calcium in some cases stimulates the parathyroid glands. When the deficiency of vitamin D and calcium produces diminished calcium in the bone (osteomalacia) the bony matrix is unaffected. Associated hyperactivity of the parathyroid glands leads to absorption of bony matrix. Excessive stimulation of the parathyroids may produce secondary hyperparathyroidism, and parathyroid adenomata have required surgical removal. When the parathyroids are stimulated, tetany, if previously present, may disappear as calcium is mobilized from the bones.

Potassium. A large amount of potassium may be lost in the stools. Potassium depletion used to be one of the most important complications of malabsorption syndromes, and it was responsible for many deaths before its importance was realized. Deficiency of potassium produces muscular weakness and even muscular paralysis. Atony of the bowel due to potassium deficiency aggravates intestinal distension. Potassium deficiency may mask tetany due to a lowered serum calcium level, but when potassium is administered the muscle weakness disappears and tetany becomes manifest.

Water

There is a delayed excretion of a water load in patients with steatorrhoea. This delay could be due to two causes, slow absorption or impaired excretion. Both factors are responsible for the delayed excretion seen in patients with steatorrhoea. The delayed absorption may cause nocturnal frequency of urine.

SMALL INTESTINAL BACTERIA
(Stagnant loop syndrome) [19]

The normal human upper small intestinal bacteria rarely exceed 10^3–10^4 per ml. They reside on the mucus layer of the mucosa. Normally the gastric hydrochloric acid and intestinal peristaltic movements prevent bacterial overgrowth. The aerobic and anaerobic *bacterial overgrowth* occurs with *stagnant loop syndrome* due to surgery, intestinal strictures or small intestinal diverticulosis, neuromuscular abnormality as in diabetic neuropathy, or *invasion* of colonic bacteria by means of the incompetent ileocaecal valve due to disease or surgery. Increased upper intestinal bacterial flora is common in *tropical sprue* [20]. Broad-spectrum antibiotics help to produce remission.

Overgrowth of small intestinal bacteria results in disturbed *bile salt metabolism* and *malabsorption of fat, vitamin B_{12}, protein* and *xylose*.

Steatorrhoea occurs as a result of bacterial proliferation that deconjugates bile salts. *Vitamin B_{12}* absorption is decreased as the bacteria bind the vitamin and make it unavailable for absorption [21]. *Folic acid* absorption is *normal*. Bacteria synthesize folic acid and since it is absorbed preponderantly from the jejunum, the blood level of folic acid is normal or sometimes even higher with stagnant loop of the duodenum or the jejunum but not with that of the ileum.

Bacteria also synthesize thiamine, riboflavine, biotin and vitamin K, which are all absorbed.

Hypoproteinaemia may occur due to protein *loss* in the stagnant loop. The protein *synthesis* is diminished with bacterial breakdown of amino acids in the intestine, which can be seen from the increase in urinary excretion of indoles on administration of tryptophan. Ammonia produced from the bacterial breakdown of other amino acids is converted to urea. *Xylose* excretion test may show a low value with bacterial metabolism of xylose [16].

Treatment. Oral tetracyclines, 250 mg four times daily, or lincomycin (which acts mainly on the anaerobic bacteria), 500 mg 8-hourly, correct malabsorption [22] within a few days of therapy.

BILE

The *primary bile acids*, (1) cholic acid; and (2) *chenodeoxycholic acid*, are formed in the liver from cholesterol. With the amino acids glycine or taurine they conjugate to form glycocholic and glycochenodeoxycholic; or taurocholic and taurochenodeoxycholic acid. Glycine conjugates are three times more than taurine. These conjugates combine with a base (sodium) to form *bile salts*. The bile salts are reabsorbed from the *ileum* to maintain enterohepatic circulation and normal bile concentration.

Intestinal bacteria act on bile salts to: (1) *deconjugate* them to form free bile acids again—cholic acid or chenodeoxycholic acid and further split them to form (2) *secondary bile acids*: (a) *deoxycholic* acid from cholic acid; and (b) *lithocholic acid* from chenodeoxycholic acid. These are also absorbed and enter the enterohepatic circulation. Deoxycholic acid is known to be toxic to the intestinal mucosa and to interfere with absorption of fat and glucose.

Bile Salts and Steatorrhoea

The total *bile salt pool* in the body is about 2·5–4 g. These acids keep the cholesterol of bile in solution but cholesterol precipitates and gall-stones form when the body pool is decreased. Conjugated bile salts: (1) emulsify fats; (2) activate lipase to split fat into fatty acids and monoglycerides; and (3) form mixed micelles which aid fat absorption.

Fat digestion and absorption proceed satisfactorily when the intestinal bile salt concentration is 5 to 15 millimols per litre, but when it drops below 4 millimols per litre this results in steatorrhoea. Bile salt concentration is decreased with: (1) (?) *deficient formation* in hepatic cirrhosis; (2) *diminished reabsorption* from the ileum with diseases such as Crohn's disease, tuberculosis, or ileal resection; (3) *increased bacterial deconjugation* with stagnant loop syndrome after surgery, strictures or jejunal diverticulosis. Decreasing the bacterial growth with antibiotics eliminates steatorrhoea. Bile salt deconjugation was not a factor in tropical sprue seen in South India [23].

Oral administration of isotopically labelled carbon in glycocholic acid is excreted in the breath as $C^{14}O_2$. Bacterial overgrowth in the small intestine increases bile acid deconjugation and excretion of $C^{14}O_2$ in the breath. Breath test is therefore suggested as a rapid, simple, tubeless out-patient procedure for detecting increased deconjugation of bile acids in intestinal diseases [24].

HISTOLOGY OF SMALL INTESTINE

Devices allowing suction biopsy of the small intestinal mucosa are of considerable use. Atrophy of the intestinal villi is the principal change which reduces the absorptive area of the intestine. Whether the changes in the intestinal mucous membrane are primary or secondary to malabsorption is not satisfactorily established. The fundamental physiological defect in coeliac disease, and possibly tropical sprue, is ascribed to atrophy of the intestinal mucous membrane which does not absorb food.

The dissecting microscope in a *normal* biopsy displays digitate (finger-like) villi of an average length (430 μ) and three times the width (130 μ). The grades of abnormality are: grade I, ridges; grade II, convolutions; and grade III, flat mucosa.

Microscopic examination of specimens obtained from different areas of the small intestine shows variations. Therefore, the standard site for obtaining biopsy is the duodenojejunal junction (ligament of Treitz). There are also pitfalls in the random microscopic examination as tangential sections display flat mucosa even in a normal person, hence correlation with the biopsy under the dissecting microscope helps better assessment. In coeliac disease the proximal small intestine is more markedly affected than the distal. On a gluten-free diet the recovery is first noted in the distal intestine. The extent, the degree and the site of mucosal involvement determine the clinical picture and the results of the malabsorption tests, e.g. marked vitamin B_{12} malabsorption with distal small intestinal damage.

Histochemically there is deficiency of the mucosal enzymes in coeliac disease, which rapidly recovers within a week of gluten-free diet.

Flat intestinal mucosa is not exclusively noted in coeliac disease but is also known to occur in tropical sprue, protein starvation, kwashiorkor, dermatitis herpetiformis, hypogammaglobulinaemia, Whipple's disease, Zollinger-Ellison syndrome, eosinophilic gastro-enteritis, and primary intestinal lymphoma. The mucosal changes in tropical sprue are similar to but less severe than those in coeliac disease. The clinical, biochemical and histological findings may have no correlation [25].

CLINICAL MANIFESTATIONS

The symptomatology of coeliac disease, tropical sprue and idiopathic steatorrhoea is about the same. A composite description of the syndromes follows below.

The symptoms may begin at any age, including infancy, but onset after the age of 60 is uncommon. Many patients, even in adult life, may show stunting of growth suggesting that the absorption defect developed earlier in life. The commonest complaints are *weakness* and *lassitude* with loss of *weight* of over 10 lbs. The commonest gastro-intestinal disturbance is *diarrhoea*. There is also flatulence, mild abdominal pain, anorexia, nausea and vomiting. Some may complain of increased nocturnal micturition. Nutritional deficiency may manifest itself as glossitis, tetany, bone pains and paraesthesia, and convulsions (probable pyridoxine deficiency), while objective evidence of nutritional disturbance is seen as a smooth tongue, oedema, dry skin, bleeding, pigmentation, dermatitis herpetiformis, peripheral neuropathy and proximal muscle atrophy. Subacute combined degeneration of the cord may occasionally the be seen.

LABORATORY INVESTIGATIONS

The minimum investigations required for the diagnosis of malabsorption syndrome are the following: (1) The *faecal fat excretion* may be variable from day to day. Over a period of 3–4 days an average daily excretion of over 6 g suggests steatorrhoea. (2) The blood count may show iron deficiency *microcytic anaemia,* or *macrocytic anaemia* due to folic acid or vitamin B_{12} deficiency. The anaemia may be due to a combined deficiency of all the three factors. (3) The fasting *blood sugar* may be lower than 80 mg. After 50 g of glucose the normal maximum rise is over 40 mg but in malabsorption the rise is less. In malabsorption due to pancreatic disease, however, a diabetic curve may be found. (4) *Radiology of the small intestine* is necessary to diagnose tuberculous enteritis, diverticulosis of the small bowel, regional enteritis, etc. In coeliac disease and tropical sprue the small intestine shows dilatation and flocculation of barium decribed as 'deficiency pattern'. The flocculation is partly explained by increased mucus secretion. The flocculation and segmentation are nonspecific changes and may even be noted in normal individuals, depending upon the type of barium used. There is diminished motility of the small intestine. In a patient who improves with a gluten-free diet, diminished motility with barium meal may be the first change noted when gluten is reintroduced. (5) *Small intestinal biopsy.*

Immunological Aspects

The serum of some patients suffering from coeliac disease contains antibodies to gliadin and the immunoglobulin IgA is increased [26].

There is also favourable response to corticosteroids in such patients and auto-immunity is therefore also suggested as a cause of coeliac disease.

GLUTEN

Dicks, in Holland, noted that children with coeliac disease kept better health during the German occupation when nutrition was poor. Subsequently, when nutrition improved and wheat was more freely available, children actually deteriorated in health. The offending food was wheat protein, gluten, which caused malabsorption. This observation has stimulated the study of malabsorption in many parts of the world.

Gluten is a plant protein which is found in wheat, *rye* (a cereal used in Western countries to prepare bread) and barley. Oats and maize also contain a gluten which is harmless. As wheat is universally grown, most of the reported work refers to wheat gluten. If gluten is removed from wheat then the gluten-free wheat starch can be eaten without harm by patients with coeliac disease.

Gluten consists of two fractions, glutenin and gliadin. It is the gliadin fraction which is the offending substance. When partially digested gluten, as peptide, is fed, the toxicity persists. In coeliac disease too the digestion progresses to the peptide stage and hence the toxicity is manifest. Gluten completely hydrolysed to the amino acid stage, however, is not toxic. This strongly suggests that in coeliac disease there is a primary defect in the peptidase enzyme system which breaks down peptides into amino acids. Gliadin contains several peptides, but a particular peptidase as a causative factor has not yet been demonstrated [27], nor is it settled whether the peptidase deficiency is primary or secondary to mucosal atrophy. Crude papain (not crystalline) can break down gliadin which is well digested by patients with coeliac disease [28].

TREATMENT

It is with the knowledge that gluten is a toxic product that a gluten-free diet is recommended. Flatcher and McCririck [29] have given a comprehensive list of food-stuffs to be avoided on a gluten-free diet. For Indians, who generally do not eat in hotels or who do not buy ready-made foods from the market, the simple instruction to avoid wheat in any form during cooking serves the purpose.

Coeliac Disease

A gluten-free diet is without question the most effective therapy in coeliac disease, giving an immediate response. *Adult coeliac disease* responds to gluten-free diet. This favourable response in adults is *slower*, however, than in children. Long term follow-up shows that the majority of patients do well after 2 years of strict gluten-free diet. Intestinal mucosa reverts to normal but this is no guarantee against a relapse. Even those in remission may show low serum folic acid or low serum iron levels.

Pregnancy. *Relapse* is more likely in females during pregnancy and it may help to revert to gluten-free diet during this period [30]. Thirteen of 57 adults treated had to resume gluten-free diet. The remainder were normal but 19 had low serum folate and 11 had low serum iron. Childhood coeliac disease usually persists even though it is symptomless, and here it is suggested that the gluten-free diet should be lifelong. Infertile women with coeliac disease may become pregnant with gluten restriction [31]. Maternal malabsorption can produce infants presenting as congenital rickets.

Causes of Failure of a Gluten-free Diet. The usual cause of failure is incomplete exclusion of gluten from the diet. This may be due to poor co-operation by the patient or the taking of gluten in a disguised form, as for example when wheat flour has been used in sausages, baking powder, gravies, sauces, mayonnaise and canned products like soups, fish, beans and tomatoes.

Supplementary Treatment. Despite the beneficial effects of the gluten-free diet, associated conditions also require management for full therapeutic effects: (1) Avitaminosis can be corrected by the administration of *multivitamin* preparations. In some patients with tropical sprue parenteral administration of *vitamin* B_{12}, 100 micrograms on alternate days, may be necessary as an adjunct to *folic acid* therapy. (2) *Oral broad-spectrum antibiotics* may be necessary to inhibit the intestinal bacterial activity which perpetuates the malabsorption. (3) Anterior pituitary deficiency may be present and may be responsible for the deficient absorption of water and glucose. The pituitary deficiency may result in secondary suprarenal deficiency as improvement is noted on the administration of *adrenocorticoids*. *Corticosteroids* produce clinical as well as histological improvement, despite continuing gluten, but there is rapid relapse on discontinuation of corticosteroids. In some patients with coeliac disease, despite gluten-free diet, adequate improvement is not noted due to associated *lactase deficiency*. For such patients withholding milk and milk products proves useful.

Lymphoma of the jejunum is not an uncommon complication after two decades of gluten enteropathy.

Tropical Sprue

The therapy of tropical sprue may vary according to the various aetiological factors labelled as tropical sprue. In general the following, either alone or in combination, help to produce a remission and even a cure: (1) *Parenteral folic acid*, 5 mg daily, though it has had excellent results in some cases from Puerto Rico, does not produce satisfactory results in the majority of Indians. (2) *Protein malnutrition* is indistinguishable from tropical sprue which is indicated as being due to other causes. On a high protein diet alone, there is remarkable clinical, biochemical and jejunal biopsy improvement [5]. (3) Administration of bile salts sometimes helps in cases of steatorrhoea. (4) Broad-spectrum antibiotics, tetracyclines or lincomycin have also been found effective when there is intestinal bacterial overgrowth.

Medium Chain Triglycerides for Steatorrhoea

The usual dietary fats are mostly *long chain triglycerides* (LCT) of fatty acids of over 14 carbon atoms. LCT, for absorption, require healthy small intestinal mucosa and bile to form chylomicron, with absorption taking place via the *lymphatics*. In diseases of the small intestinal mucosa and lymphatics, the LCT are not absorbed, with consequent steatorrhoea.

Medium chain triglycerides (MCT) are mixed triglycerides of 6–10 carbon atoms which are easily broken down by pancreatic as well as intestinal mucosal lipase [32] and do not form chylomicrons. MCT are therefore absorbed even with pancreatic and bile salt deficiencies or lymphatic obstruction. Being water-soluble, MCT are mostly absorbed via the *portal vein*.

Uses. MCT foods are used during steatorrhoea in: (1) premature infants; (2) massive intestinal resection (short bowel syndrome); (3) bile deficiency with biliary atresia, cholestasis, cirrhosis, and stagnant loop syndrome (where bacterial deconjugation of bile salts occur); (4) pancreatic diseases: chronic pancreatitis, cystic fibrosis (muco-viscidosis); (5) *small intestinal* diseases, coeliac disease, regional enteritis, Whipple's disease; (6) *lymphatic disorders,* chyluria, chylo-thorax, intestinal lymphangiectasia; (7) familial hypercholesterolaemia.

Portagen and MCT Oil (Mead Johnson) are commercial products. The powder contains skimmed milk, sucrose, cornstarch, coconut oil, safflower oil (to prevent essential fatty acid deficiency), vitamins and minerals.

Side-effects may be minor, and include nausea, vomiting, and borborygmi. Diarrhoea in lactase-deficient patients may occur due to the high lactose in skimmed milk. In partial gastrectomy sudden hyperosmolar solution in the gut produces diarrhoea. MCT with carbohydrate feeding does not produce ketosis in normal individuals, but this is a possibility in severe diabetics. In cirrhotics with portal systemic shunts, MCT can be detected in the spinal fluid in hepatic coma [33].

GLUTEN-FREE DIET

Permissible foods	*Foods excluded*
Cereals: rice, oatmeal, *jowar, bajra, ragi, maize* (corn)	All preparations made from *wheat* like *chappatis,* bread and biscuits, cakes, flakes, soups, sauces and gravies. All commercial foods must be most carefully scrutinized to discover whether they contain wheat. When no definite information is available, the food product must be completely excluded
All pulses (*dal*) All fruits All vegetables Potatoes Meat, fish, poultry, eggs	

Permissible foods	*Foods excluded*
Milk and milk products	With associated lactase deficiency they aggravate diarrhoea and may have to be restricted or stopped
Soups	
Beverages: tea, coffee, aerated waters	
Seasoning in moderation and dressings of garlic, ginger, vinegar	
Sweet and sweetmeats	Without wheat

GLUTEN-FREE DIET
SAMPLE MENU

Mixed	*Vegetarian*

Breakfast

Mixed	Vegetarian
Cornflakes with milk, sugar or honey	Sweet lime juice
Fried eggs, 2	Curd, 1 cup
Corn bread or bread made with gluten-free wheat flour or rice *chappatis*	*Bajra chappatis*
Tea or coffee	Tea or coffee
Orange	Banana

Lunch

Mixed	Vegetarian
Fried fish, chips and french beans	Butter milk, 1 cup
Chicken cutlet, tomato and beetroot salad	Radish and cucumber salad
	Rice with *dal*
	Jowar or *bajra chappatis*
	Papaya

or

Rice and meat curry
Corn bread, *jowar,* or *bajra chappatis,* or bread made with gluten-free wheat flour
Apple

Mixed	*Vegetarian*

4 p.m.

Mixed	Vegetarian
Corn bread or *bajra chappati* with butter or cake or biscuits made with gluten-free wheat flour Cashew nuts Tea	*Bajra chappatis* with butter Ground nuts Tea

Dinner

Mixed	Vegetarian
Chicken soup Roast mutton Baked potato Pumpkin Corn bread or *bajra* or *jowar chappatis* or bread made with gluten-free wheat flour Brown custard	Tomato soup Curd, 1 cup Boiled potato Spinach Rice *chappatis* Ice-cream

REFERENCES

[1] ANTIA, F. P., *et al.* (1971) Panel discussion, tropical sprue, *Indian Practitioner*, **24,** 87.

[2] MATHAN, V. I., and BAKER, S. J. (1968) Epidemic tropical sprue and other epidemics of diarrhoea in South Indian villages. A comparative study, *Amer. J. clin. Nutr.*, **21,** 1077.

[3] KAMER, J. H. VAN DE, HUININK, H. TEN B., and WEYERS, H. A. (1949) Rapid method for the determination of fat in feces, *J. biol. Chem.*, **177,** 347.

[4] CHUTTANI, H. K., MEHRA, M. L., and MISRA, R. C. (1968) Small bowel in hypoproteinemic states, *Scand. J. Gastroent.*, **3,** 529.

[5] TANDON, B. N., MAGOTRA, M. L., SARAYA, A. K., and RAMALINGASWAMI, V. (1968) Small intestine in protein malnutrition, *Amer. J. clin. Nutr.*, **21,** 813.

[6] TANDON, B. N., *et al.* (1970) Recovery of pancreatic function in adult protein-calorie malnutrition, *Gastroenterology*, **58,** 358.

[7] PETERS, T. J. (1970) Intestinal peptidases, *Gut*, **11,** 720.

[8] GOLDBERG, D. M., CAMPBELL, R., and ROY, A. D. (1969) Binding of trypsin and chymotrypsin in human intestinal mucosa, *Scand. J. Gastroent.*, **4,** 217.

[9] DOUGLAS, A. P., and BOOTH, C. C. (1970) Digestion of gluten peptides by normal human jejunal mucosa from patients with adult coeliac disease, *Clin. Sci.*, **38,** 11.

[10] BERNSTEIN, L. H., GUTSTEIN, S., WEINER, S., and EFRON, G. (1970) The absorption and malabsorption of folic acid and its polyglutamates, *Amer. J. Med.*, **48,** 570.

[11] DESAI, H. G., *et al.* (1970) Incidence of lactase deficiency in control subjects from India. Role of hereditary factors, *Indian J. med. Sci.*, **24,** 729.

[12] CHRISTOPHER, N. L., and BAYLESS, T. M. (1971) Role of small bowel and colon in lactose-induced diarrhoea, *Gastroenterology,* **60,** 845.

[13] McGILL, D. B., and NEWCOMER, A. D. (1967) Comparison of venous and capillary blood samples in lactose tolerance testing, *Gastroenterology,* **53,** 371.

[14] CALLOWAY, D. H., MURPHY, E. L., and BAUER, D. (1969) Determination of lactose intolerance by breath analysis, *Amer. J. dig. Dis.,* **14,** 811.

[15] RINALDO, J. A., and GLUCKMANN, R. F. (1964) Maximal absorption capacity for xylose in non-tropical sprue, *Gastroenterology,* **47,** 248.

[16] GOLDSTEIN, F., et al. (1970) Intraluminal small intestinal utilization of *d*-xylose by bacteria. A limitation of the *d*-xylose absorption test, *Gastroenterology,* **59,** 380.

[17] KENDALL, M. J. (1970) The influence of age in the xylose absorption test, *Gut,* **11,** 498.

[18] DAVIS, P. (1960) Vitamin D poisoning: a report of two cases, *Ann. intern. Med.,* **53,** 1250.

[19] TABAQCHALI, S. (1970) The pathophysiologic role of small intestinal bacterial flora, *Scand. J. Gastroent.,* **5; 6** (Suppl.), 139.

[20] GORBACH, S. L., et al. (1970) Tropical sprue and malnutrition in West Bengal. I. Intestinal microflora and absorption, *Amer. J. clin. Nutr.,* **23,** 1545.

[21] SCHJONSBY, H., PETERS, T. J., HOFFBRAND, A. V., and TABAQCHALI, S. (1970) The mechanism of vitamin B_{12} malabsorption in the blind loop syndrome, *Gut,* **11,** 371.

[22] GORBACH, S. L., and TABAQCHALI, S. (1969) Bacteria, bile, and the small bowel, *Gut,* **10,** 963.

[23] KAPADIA, C. R., RADHAKRISHNAN, A. N., MATHAN, V. I., and BAKER, S. J. (1971) Studies on bile salt deconjugation in patients with tropical sprue, *Scand. J. Gastroent.,* **6,** 29.

[24] FROMM, H., and HOFMANN, A. F. (1971) Breath, test for altered bile-acid metabolism, *Lancet,* **ii,** 621.

[25] MISRA, R. C., KASTHURI, D., and CHUTTANI, H. K. (1967) Correlation of clinical, biochemical, radiological and histological findings in tropical sprue, *J. trop. Med. Hyg.,* **70,** 6.

[26] KENRICK, K. G., and WALKER-SMITH, J. A. (1970) Immunoglobulins and dietary protein antibodies in childhood coeliac disease, *Gut,* **11,** 635.

[27] BERG, N. O., DAHLQVIST, A., LINDBERG, T., and BORDEN, A. (1970) Intestinal dipeptidases and disaccharidases in coeliac disease in adults, *Gastroenterology,* **59,** 582.

[28] MESSER, M., ANDERSON, C. M., and HUBBARD, L. (1964) Studies on the mechanism of destruction of the toxic action of wheat gluten in coeliac disease by crude papain, *Gut,* **5,** 295.

[29] FLETCHER, R. F., and McCRIRICK, M. Y. (1958) Gluten-free diets, *Brit. med. J.,* **2,** 299.

[30] SHELDON, W. (1969) Prognosis in early adult life of coeliac children treated with a gluten-free diet, *Brit. med. J.,* **2,** 401.

[31] MORRIS, J. S., AJDUKIEWICZ, A. B., and READ, A. E. (1970) Coeliac infertility: an indication for dietary gluten restriction, *Lancet,* **i,** 213.

[32] PLAYOUST, M. R., and ISSELBACHER, K. J. (1964) Studies on the intestinal

absorption and intramucosal lipolysis of medium chain triglycerides, *J. clin. Invest.*, **43**, 878.

[33] LINSCHER, W. G., BLUM, A. L., and RYAN PLATT, R. (1970) Transfer of medium chain fatty acids from blood to spinal fluid in patients with cirrhosis, *Gastroenterology*, **58**, 509.

57. ULCERATIVE COLITIS

Ulcerative colitis is a disease of unknown aetiology characterized by inflammation and ulceration of the colon resulting in the frequent passage of stools with blood and mucus. The onset resembles an attack of dysentery in the tropics but the failure to isolate any pathogenic organism, the failure to respond to the usual therapeutic measures and the tendency to exacerbations and remissions draws attention to the fact that the disease is ulcerative colitis. The lesion commonly involves the proctosigmoid alone, or with more extensive involvement, the entire colon.

There is now increasing awareness that some cases labelled as ulcerative colitis are in fact granulomatous colitis (Crohn's disease).

The disease is seen in both Western and Eastern countries. Those practising general medicine may see only occasional cases, but because of the highly disturbing nature of this recurring disease the patients tend to collect at centres where physicians have a special interest in the management of this disease. In Bombay, it is uncommon among poorer patients, but it is relatively more frequent in the middle class families. Among patients referred for gastro-intestinal investigations in charitable hospitals the incidence is 0·1 per cent, while in private gastro-enterology practice the incidence is 1·5 per cent. The disease is more common in females. During pregnancy there may be an exacerbation of symptoms in some patients while in others there may be remarkable remission.

The primary aetiological factor is not yet established. Exacerbations are more likely during mental conflicts and emotional stress. *Allergy* to certain foods may be a factor in precipitating the disease, and exclusion of the offending foods may prove rewarding.

Milk is one of the foods which is not well tolerated by patients who suffer from colonic disease and its exclusion may be of help. In some cases, recurrence of symptoms coincident with the reintroduction of milk has been demonstrated [1]. High titre antibodies to cow's milk in the sera of the patients suffering from ulcerative colitis have been found. However, this does not prove milk allergy, as the antibodies may only be the consequence of protein absorption from the inflamed colon. It is worth trying a regime consisting of a milk-free diet for all patients. Not infrequently, diarrhoea on taking milk is due to small intestinal lactase deficiency. A long-term milk exclusion is liable to drastically reduce calcium intake [2].

DIETETIC MANAGEMENT

Malnutrition in ulcerative colitis may be the result of insufficient food consumption, excessive nitrogen loss through blood, mucus and necrotic colonic mucosa, and electrolyte loss in the faeces. Liver damage is not unusual in ulcerative colitis impairing proper synthesis of proteins and storage of fat-soluble vitamins. The metabolic rate is increased due to associated pyrexia. Frequent hospitalization and absence from work may also lead to loss of income and inability to afford nutritious food. A strict low residue diet is not necessary, and indeed in some patients may lead to faecal stasis [3].

Calories
An adequate supply, about 2000–2500 Calories, should be aimed at.

Proteins
Patients with ulcerative colitis lose about 4–8 g faecal nitrogen compared to the normal excretion of 2 g. In severe ulcerative colitis 20 g nitrogen (equivalent of 125 g protein) may be lost daily. The serum albumin is low. More protein, i.e. 100–150 g per day should be supplied. This can be achieved in a person taking a mixed diet. In a vegetarian it is a difficult task, particularly when exclusion of milk is also tried in the hope of producing a remission. Parenteral amino acid replacement may have to be resorted to (See Intravenous Feeding).

Fats
Usual foods which contain fats are permitted. Fat in cooking is permitted if the patient tolerates extra fat. Fried foods are not easily digested.

Carbohydrates

They form the easily absorbable source of energy. Bulk-producing vegetables are restricted so as to allow better intake of more nourishing foods. When there is excessive nausea and diarrhoea a 5 per cent intravenous glucose drip with supplements of vitamins and replacement of mineral loss is necessary.

Vitamins

Commercial multivitamin preparations should be administered orally. If diarrhoea is profuse, parenteral administration may be necessary.

Minerals

Mineral loss may be marked and unless replaced may contribute to a fatal outcome.

Sodium. A patient with moderately advanced ulcerative colitis passes a large volume, over 400 ml of faeces per day and may lose considerable sodium and potassium [4]. The sodium loss is proportionate to the amount of faeces [5]. When the oral sodium intake is increased both the sodium content and the volume of faeces also increase. Sodium loss is approximately 100 mEq (6 g expressed as sodium chloride) per litre of stool. The loss can be replaced either by giving extra salt in food or by saline infusion if necessary.

Potassium. Potassium loss also can be estimated as 30 mEq (2·2 g expressed as potassium chloride) per litre. Unusually high excretion of potassium, even 167 mEq per day, may sometimes be encountered [5].

Manifestations of potassium deficiency such as weakness, hypotonia, abdominal distension and even electrocardiographic changes occur. Oral administration of potassium salts as potassium citrate is helpful. Intravenous administration of potassium chloride requires careful management.

Iron. Iron by the oral route is usually not well tolerated. If anaemia is marked then blood transfusions or a few intramuscular injections of 100 mg each of iron-dextran complex may be given. Iron given parenterally is stored in the body and utilized when necessary. The serum iron level is usually low in ulcerative colitis and iron is needed even in the absence of anaemia.

Fluids

A liberal intake of fluids should be ensured to prevent dehydration. The passage of at least 1200 ml of urine indicates that a patient is well hydrated.

Spices

All forms of irritant and stale foods should be strictly avoided.

SUPPLEMENTARY FEEDING

Supplementary feeding of preparations made from commercial protein concentrate may help in supplying high proteins. The Central Middlesex Hospital, London, prepares such a supplement from *Complan* (Glaxo). Eight level tablespoons of *Complan* is mixed with 500 ml of water or milk. The powder is rigorously stirred and then strained to remove lumps. Two pints of the mixture provides:

	Complan in water	*Complan in milk*
Calories	1000	1720
Proteins (g)	70	106
Sodium (g)	0·9	1·5
Potassium (g)	2·4	4·2

The supplement is suitably flavoured with cocoa, chocolate, coffee essence or orange juice and chilled before serving in frequent small quantities.

If the patient has no appetite then a thin nasogastric tube may be passed and 2 litres of the prepared supplement be given by drip.

Intravenous Feeding

Intravenous feeding is of great help in the medical management of severe cases of ulcerative colitis [6]. However, most patients with ulcerative colitis may recover without any special intravenous feeding programme.

ULCERATIVE COLITIS

Foods	*Remarks*
Bread or *chappatis* of wheat, rice, maize, *jowar, bajra* or *ragi*	Permitted, should be made from finely ground flour

Foods	Remarks
Breakfast cereals of wheat, rice, oatmeal or maize	Permitted
Rice, cooked	Permitted
Pulses (*dal*) and beans	Permitted as *dal* water
Meat, fish or chicken	Permitted
Eggs	Permitted
Milk and milk products*	Permitted
Soups	Permitted
Vegetable salad	Excluded
Vegetables, cooked	Permitted if tender
Potato, sweet potato or yam	Permitted
Fat for cooking and butter	Permitted, fried foods not permitted
Sugar, jaggery and honey	Permitted
Jam or *murabba*	Permitted
Pastry	Permitted as biscuits only
Desserts*	Permitted
Sweet and sweetmeats*	Permitted
Fruits, fresh	Permitted
Fruits, dried	Excluded
Nuts	Excluded
Condiments and spices	Excluded
Papad, chutney or pickles	Excluded
Beverages	Permitted in moderation
Water	Liberal

ULCERATIVE COLITIS
SAMPLE MENU

Mixed Diet	*Vegetarian Diet*
Breakfast	
Cornflakes, 1 cup with milk* and sugar	Quaker Oats, ¾ cup with milk* and sugar
Eggs, 2 half-boiled or poached	Toasts or *chappatis*
Toast with apricot jam	Honey
Tea* or coffee*	Orange
Banana, 1	

Mixed Diet	*Vegetarian Diet*

11 a.m.

Arrowroot porridge* (*kanji*), 1 cup	Sago porridge* (*kanji*), 1 cup
or	or
Supplementary feed**	Supplementary feed**

Lunch

Minced meat with boiled potato and carrots	Rice with *dal* water
Baked macaroni	Baked potato
Bread or *chappatis*	Mashed pumpkin
Banana	Curd*, 1 cup
	Bread or *chappatis*
	Apple

4 p.m.

Tea*	Tea*
Biscuits, 4	Biscuits, 4

6 p.m.

Sago or Quaker Oats porridge* (*kanji*), 1 cup	Arrowroot porridge (*kanji*), 1 cup
or	or
Supplementary feed*	Supplementary feed**

Dinner

Baked fish	Rice with *dal* water
Roast leg of chicken with boiled potato and french beans	Mashed potato
Bread or *chappatis*	Vegetable puree
Custard*, ½ cup	Buttermilk*, 1 cup
	Bread or *chappatis*
	China grass jelly*

* Milk or milk products permitted only if tolerated by the patient.
** See page 392 (Complan)

REFERENCES

[1] TRUELOVE, S. C. (1961) Ulcerative colitis provoked by milk, *Brit. med. J.*, **1**, 154.
[2] JONES, F. A. (1966) Comments on colitis, *Proc. roy. Soc. Med.*, **59**, 369.
[3] LENNARD-JONES, J. E., LANGMAN, M. J. S., and JONES, F. A. (1962) Faecal stasis in proctocolitis, *Gut*, **3**, 301.
[4] COGHILL, N. F., *et al.* (1956) Sodium and potassium absorption and excretion in patients with ulcerative colitis before and after colectomy, *Gastroenterologia*, **86**, 724.

[5] SMIDDY, F. G., SMITH, I. B., GREGORY, S. D., and GOLIGHER, J. C. (1960) Faecal loss of fluid, electrolytes and nitrogen in colitis before and after ileostomy, *Lancet*, **i**, 14.

[6] DUDRICK, S. J., LONG, J. M., STREIGER, E., and RHOADS, J. E. (1970) Intravenous hyperalimentation, *Med. Clin. N. Amer.*, **54**, 577.

58. LIVER DISEASES

The liver is a very important organ in which many metabolic processes occur. Toxins and bacteria absorbed from the intestine may directly reach the liver and produce injury. Dietary deficiencies by themselves have been shown not only to produce morphologic changes in the liver but also to make the organ susceptible to the injurious effects of infections and toxins.

NUTRITION AND LIVER DISEASES

Proteins

Protein deficiency has produced fatty change and even necrosis of the liver in animals. The liver can be protected from these changes by certain amino acids. The occurrence of similar changes in man from isolated protein deficiency is debatable.

Choline contains a methyl group and can be formed in the body from methionine. Administration of choline prevents *fatty changes* in the liver in experimental animals and mobilizes fat already present.

Cystine is an amino acid containing sulphur. In the body, cystine can be formed from methionine. Deficiency of cystine in animals produces *necrosis* of the liver cells.

Methionine is another amino acid which prevents the liver damage caused by experimental dietary deficiency. Its sulphur can be used in the synthesis of cystine, while from its methyl radical choline can be synthesized. Caseinogen of milk and animal proteins are rich in methionine and, therefore, the administration of milk or animal foods may prevent necrosis of the liver cells or deposition of fat within them both of which may lead to cirrhosis.

In summary the morphologic changes produced in experimental animals by protein deficiency are: (1) fatty changes; (2) hepatic necrosis; (3) cirrhosis of the liver.

Proteins and Amino Acids in 'Acute' Liver Failure. Although amino acids are useful in preventing liver damage and in supplying the building material for the regeneration of the liver, their administration *during acute hepatic failure and hepatic coma* is harmful. In these circumstances the liver is so badly damaged that it cannot properly metabolize them and toxic products of metabolism accumulate in the blood precipitating coma. Intravenous administration of amino acids or protein hydrolysates and the enthusiastic feeding of proteins, should be avoided when the liver is severely damaged.

Fats

Deposition of fat in the liver cells is a manifestation of dietary deficiency of proteins or of toxic injury. This knowledge has led many clinicians to drastically reduce dietary fat during the treatment of liver damage. Fatty changes in the liver do not occur when usual amounts of fat are administered, as long as proteins, mainly of animal origin, containing adequate choline and methionine are given also. The amount of protein needed to prevent fatty liver is in proportion to the total calorie intake. If the basic protein requirements are met then calories can be supplied in large amounts in the form of carbohydrates or fats[1] without producing fatty liver. *In chronic liver* diseases, where a high calorie diet is indicated for a prolonged period, unnecessary restriction of fats make the food unpalatable to the patient. *In hepatic precoma and coma* fats should be withheld from the diet as they are not metabolized by the liver.

In experimentally-produced cirrhosis, saturated fats delay while unsaturated fats promote cirrhosis [2].

Carbohydrates

Glycogen protects the liver cells against damage. Carbohydrates can be directly metabolized by the tissues and, in severe liver damage when proteins and fats are contra-indicated, carbohydrates are useful not only for meeting the calorie requirements but also for reducing the endogenous breakdown of proteins by their 'protein sparing effect'.

Glycogen storage diseases occur due to enzyme defects. *Von Gierke's disease* occurs due to glucose-6-phosphatase deficiency resulting in excessive deposition of glycogen in the liver and kidneys.

Alcohol

In experimental animals injury to the liver by hepatotoxic agents and deficiency states is enhanced by the simultaneous administration of alcohol. Alcohol supplies calories but it cannot be stored in the liver as glycogen. When alcohol is taken there is a proportionate increase in the need for protein and vitamins of the B group. Further, the gastritis produced by alcoholic excess reduces appetite and intake of proteins. A chronic alcoholic is often deficient in proteins, carbohydrates and vitamins which makes his liver highly vulnerable to any infection or toxin.

Alcohol is also known to have direct action on the lipid metabolism in the liver by: (1) enhancing fatty acid synthesis; (2) decreasing fatty acid oxidation; and (3) producing specific stimulation to triglyceride formation [3].

In malnourished patients, acute hepatic damage and jaundice, due to consumption of alcohol is recognized [4]. The clinical picture resembles viral hepatitis.

Vitamins

Vitamin A is stored in the liver. In chronic hepatic diseases vitamin A storage is reduced and supplements should be given.

Vitamin D is also stored in the liver. No specific symptoms have been ascribed to deficient storage of vitamin D in chronic liver disease.

Vitamin E prevents hepatic necrosis in rats kept on a low protein diet [5]. The role of vitamin E in the prevention or treatment of hepatic diseases in man has not yet been assessed.

Vitamin K derivatives require the presence of bile for intestinal absorption. They are needed for the production of prothrombin by the liver cells. Unlike vitamins A and D, deficiency of vitamin K can be rapidly observed as a lowered blood prothrombin level. In early *obstructive jaundice,* although there is obstruction to bile flow and thus a reduction in the intestinal absorption of vitamin K, the liver cells are relatively healthy and produce prothrombin in response to parenteral vitamin K. In marked *hepatocellular damage,* even the parenteral injection of vitamin K may fail to restore an adequate level of blood prothrombin.

In general, vitamins of the *B group* have a beneficial effect on the liver. *Vitamin B_{12}* has been considered to have a lipotropic effect on the liver since it appears to aid in transmethylation with a possible choline sparing effect [6]. The stores of vitamin B_{12} are reduced in cirrhosis.

Minerals

Sodium. If a patient is fed by intravenous drip during *hepatic failure* it is most important to note the evidences of imbalance by observing the amount of urine excreted, oedema or ascites and blood urea level. Gross imbalance of electrolytes may occur and prove fatal. Sodium retention is a factor in the production of ascites and oedema in *cirrhosis* of the liver and sodium restriction is necessary in such patients.

Potassium. Potassium is stored in the liver during the deposition of glycogen and released with its breakdown. The serum potassium level should be watched carefully during the treatment of *acute hepatic disorders,* especially when continuous intravenous feeding has been instituted. *During diuretic therapy* in cirrhotic patients, potassium is excreted in large quantities, so oral potassium supplements in the form of fruit juice or potassium salts are necessary.

Iron. The liver stores iron. Abnormal storage of iron may occur in the liver in cirrhosis, haemosiderosis and haemochromatosis.

Chillies and Spices

The role of chillies and spiced foods in the production of liver damage has not been assessed. Many people in tropical countries are used to eating heavily spiced food, particularly chillies, a taste inconceivable to Europeans. It is likely that the active principles in spices, when absorbed from the intestine, damage liver cells and this may be a contributing factor in the development of the cirrhosis so extensively seen in tropical countries.

Bush Tea

An infusion made from various herbs known as 'bush tea' is consumed by the poor population of Jamaica. This predisposes to veno-occlusive disease and ultimately leads to hepatic cirrhosis.

REFERENCES

[1] MINDRUM, G. M., and SCHIFF, L. (1955) The use of a high-fat diet in cases of fatty liver, *Gastroenterology,* **29,** 825.

[2] GYORGY, P., GOLDBLATT, H., and GANZIN, M. (1959) Dietary fat and cirrhosis of the liver, *Gastroenterology,* **37,** 637.

[3] LIEBER, C. S. (1963) Pathogenesis of hepatic steatosis, *Gastroenterology,* **45,** 760.

[4] BACKETT, A. G., LIVINGSTONE, A. V., and HILL, K. R. (1961) Acute alcoholic hepatitis, *Brit. med. J.*, **2**, 1113.

[5] GYORGY, P., and GOLDBLATT, H. (1949) Further observations on the production and prevention of dietary hepatic injury in rats, *J. exp. Med.*, **89**, 245.

[6] STRENGTH, D. R., SCHAEFER, E. A., and SALMON, W. D. (1951) The relation of vitamin B_{12} and folacin to the utilization of choline and its precursors for lipotropism and renal protection in rats, *J. Nutr.*, **45**, 329.

59. JAUNDICE

Jaundice is the yellow discoloration of the skin and mucous membranes with bile pigments, due to rise in the serum bilirubin. Jaundice may be produced by the following mechanisms:

1. *Haemolytic,* due to excessive breakdown of red blood cells.

2. *Obstructive,* due to *intrahepatic obstruction* (cholestasis) or *extra hepatic* obstruction to bile flow. The extrahepatic obstruction may also be called 'surgical jaundice' as it is a mechanical obstruction of the hepatic or common bile-ducts, which can be relieved surgically.

3. *Hepatocellular,* due to primary damage to the parenchymal cells either by viral infection or by toxic drugs.

The commonest cause of jaundice is viral hepatitis.

VIRAL HEPATITIS

Viral jaundice is usually a self limiting disease. Most patients recover with only rest, diet and vitamins. The patient should be kept under skilled medical supervision as in a few cases, especially with poor nourishment, the disease may take a serious turn and require vigorous treatment.

There is a very low mortality amongst young army personnel of Western countries who are well nourished. The mortality and morbidity is higher in the poorly nourished population of the tropics. Some of these patients have ascites at the onset of jaundice and their liver biopsy shows a marked degree of cellular collapse. The higher mortality is due to the more severe course of the disease in chronically malnourished subjects who take highly spiced food. During recovery it is best to keep the patient under observation till liver function returns to normal. A malnourished liver, further damaged by infection, is likely to become cirrhotic.

In all cases of jaundice, especially in the elderly, the possibility of *obstruction* of biliary flow by a gall-stone or carcinoma should be borne in mind because relief of the obstruction, before the liver cells are permanently damaged, may be helpful.

DIETETIC MANAGEMENT OF VIRAL HEPATITIS

The dietary treatment of viral hepatitis has passed through various phases of evolution because of conclusions drawn from observations in small series of cases without proper controlled study. Extensive studies in army personnel [1] have shown that patients forced to eat a diet throughout hospitalization supplying 3000 Calories and 150 g of protein, supplemented with vitamins improved more rapidly than those who ate only what they chose. Viral hepatitis tends to run a more severe course in undernourished patients than in well nourished young army personnel who are admitted to the hospital at the onset of the disease. Modifications in the dietary recommendations are, therefore, necessary according to the severity of liver damage and the metabolic capacity of the liver.

Calories

In a 60 kg patient during *hepatic precoma and coma* about 1000 Calories are supplied, if necessary by nasogastric tube feeding or as intravenous glucose. *In severe or moderate jaundice* about 1600 to 2000 Calories are provided.

Proteins

The liver metabolizes the products of intestinal protein decomposition and, with marked deterioration of hepatic function, products of protein breakdown may accumulate and lead to coma. On the other hand, an adequate supply of proteins is needed for the liver cells to regenerate and thus judicious advice about the intake of proteins is necessary. (1) With *hepatic precoma or coma,* protein- containing foods are withheld and only high carbohydrate-containing foods are given. (2) With *severe jaundice* (serum bilirubin over 15 mg) an average intake of 40 g of protein daily is of help in the regeneration of the hepatic cells but a higher intake may precipitate coma (foods with a moderate protein content are cereals, porridge, rice, biscuits, bread, *khakhra* and *chappatis*). (3) When the *jaundice is less,* or on recovery from jaundice, 60–80 g proteins daily are permitted (foods with a high protein content are pulses, beans, eggs, fish and meat).

Lipotropic Factors. Chalmers *et al.* [1] have shown that patients given supplements of choline did not have a shorter duration of illness than those given placebos. The practice of administering methionine and choline or other amino acids is not only unnecessary but even harmful as they may precipitate hepatic coma. The lipotropic factors only help in preventing deposition or removal of fat if present in excess. Deposition of fat in liver cells is not a feature of viral hepatitis and with an adequate supply of protein, fatty changes in the liver do not occur.

Fats

The observation in animals that a high-fat, low-protein diet produces fatty liver has sometimes led to the false assumption that fats should be prohibited in viral hepatitis. There is no evidence that when the usual amount of protein is taken, the average consumption of fat is harmful. Fats make the food more palatable and increase the calorie intake. During *hepatic precoma and coma,* due to the severe hepatocellular failure, fats are not metabolized by the liver and should not be given. In *severe jaundice* about 30 g of fat daily is permissible. In *moderate to mild jaundice* about 50–60 g of fat daily may be given.

Carbohydrates

Carbohydrates are necessary to provide calories and reduce the endogenous breakdown of proteins to a minimum. *Intravenous glucose* is indicated in the early phase of viral hepatitis when severe nausea and vomiting prevent the patient from taking oral feeds, *or* when there is severe hepatocellular damage with depleted liver glycogen. As soon as the patient can take oral feeds, fruits, fruit juice, vegetables and vegetable juices, sugar, jaggery, and honey are given, not only to provide carbohydrates but also to supply adequate electrolytes.

Vitamins

During all stages of hepatitis, preparations of the *vitamin B group, vitamin C,* 500 mg in divided doses, and *vitamin K,* 10 mg daily, are helpful. During the early stage of hepatitis, with anorexia, nausea or vomiting, and during hepatic precoma and coma, the vitamins may be given parenterally.

Minerals

If food is not taken orally then a careful watch should be kept on the serum *sodium* and *potassium* levels. Fruit juice and vegetable and meat soups with added salt, given orally or through a nasogastric tube, help in maintaining the electrolyte balance.

Parenteral Feeding

With severe nausea and vomiting it may not be possible for the patient to take oral feeds and parenteral feeding becomes necessary. An infusion of 10 per cent glucose solution maintained at a slow rate of about 30 drops per minute, a total of 2000–2500 ml of fluid and 800–1000 Calories are supplied each day — enough calories to prevent the endogenous breakdown of protein to a minimum. Vitamin preparations as advised above should be supplied and a careful watch kept on the blood electrolytes. It is best to return to oral feeds at the earliest opportunity.

Bed Rest

The question of bed rest in viral hepatitis has also been studied by Chalmers *et al.* [1] Patients moving about in the wards improved as rapidly as did patients kept strictly in bed. Those feeling physically well become uncooperative if confined strictly to bed. On follow-up study after one year no difference was noted amongst those treated with enforced complete rest and those allowed up in the ward during the active phases of the illness. On the basis of these results the patient with mild to moderate jaundice may be allowed to go to the bathroom and to sit on the verandah in the evenings. This results in a better appetite. Normal activity should be permitted only when the serum bilirubin level is under 1·5 mg per 100 ml and the bromsulphthalein retention after a dose of 5 mg per kg, is less than 5 per cent after 45 minutes.

DIET IN SEVERE JAUNDICE
VIRAL HEPATITIS OR OBSTRUCTIVE JAUNDICE

(Total serum bilirubin *over* 15 mg)

Foods	Remarks
Bread or *chappati* of wheat, rice, maize, *jowar*, *bajra* or *ragi*	Permitted

Foods	Remarks
Breakfast cereal of wheat, rice, oatmeal or maize	Permitted
Rice	Permitted
Pulses (*dal*) or beans	Excluded
Meat, fish or chicken	Excluded
Eggs	Excluded
Milk or milk products	Permitted
Soups	Permitted, thick soups excluded
Vegetable salad	Permitted in a small quantity
Vegetables, cooked	Permitted
Potato, sweet potato or yam	Permitted
Fat for cooking, and butter	Excluded
Sugar, jaggery or honey	Permitted
Jam or *murabba*	Permitted
Pastry	Permitted as biscuits only
Desserts	Permitted as light custard or ice cream
Sweetmeat	Excluded
Fruits, fresh	Permitted
Fruits, dried	Permitted
Nuts	Excluded
Condiments and spices	Excluded
Papad, chutney or pickles	Excluded
Beverages	Permitted, strong tea or coffee excluded
Water	Liberal

DIET IN SEVERE JAUNDICE
VIRAL HEPATITIS OR OBSTRUCTIVE JAUNDICE

(Total serum bilirubin *over* 15 mg)

SAMPLE MENU

Vegetarian *and* Mixed diet

Proteins	40 g
Fats	26 g
Carbohydrates	318 g
Calories	1670

Breakfast
Cornflakes, 1 cup with skimmed milk, ½ cup, and
  honey *or* sugar, 2 teaspoons
Toast
Banana
Tea or coffee

Mid-morning
Fruit juice, 1 cup

Lunch
Mixed vegetable soup
Rice
Mashed potato
Cooked french beans
Bread or *chappatis*
Orange, 1 or dates, 4

3.30 p.m.
Tea
Biscuits

6 p.m.
Sugar-cane or orange juice, 1 cup

Dinner
Tomato soup, 1 cup
Butter milk, 1 cup
Cooked spinach
Bread, 2 slices or *khakhra,* 4
Light custard, ½ cup

DIET IN MILD TO MODERATE JAUNDICE
VIRAL HEPATITIS OR OBSTRUCTIVE JAUNDICE

(Total serum bilirubin *below* 15 mg)

Foods	*Remarks*
Bread or *chappatis* of wheat, rice, maize, *jowar, bajra* or *ragi*	Permitted
Breakfast cereal of wheat, rice, oatmeal or maize	Permitted
Rice	Permitted

Food	Remarks
Pulses (*dal*) or beans	Permitted thin *dal,* 1 cup, excess may cause flatulence
Meat or fish or chicken	Permitted
Egg	Permitted
Milk or milk products	Permitted
Soups	Permitted as thin soup, thick soups excluded
Vegetable salad	Permitted
Cooked vegetable	Permitted
Potato, sweet potato or yam	Permitted
Fat for cooking, and butter	Permitted, 2 tablespoons a day. Fried food excluded
Sugar, jaggery or honey	Permitted
Jam or *murabba*	Permitted
Pastry	Permitted as biscuits
Dessert	Permitted as light custard, jelly, ice cream
Sweetmeat	Permitted
Fruits, fresh	Permitted liberally
Fruits, dried	Permitted
Nuts	Excluded
Condiments and spices	Excluded
Papad, chutney or pickles	Excluded
Beverages	Permitted
Water	As desired

DIET IN MILD TO MODERATE JAUNDICE
VIRAL HEPATITIS OR OBSTRUCTIVE JAUNDICE

(Total serum bilirubin *below* 15 mg)

SAMPLE MENU

Mixed Diet		*Vegetarian Diet*	
Approximately		*Approximately*	
Proteins	78 g	Proteins	60 g
Fats	59 g	Fats	57 g
Carbohydrates	313 g	Carbohydrates	348 g
Calories	2100	Calories	2150

Mixed Diet	*Vegetarian Diet*

Breakfast

Cornflakes, 1 cup with skimmed milk, ½ cup and jaggery, 2 tea-spoons	Puffed rice, 1 cup with skimmed milk, 1 cup and sugar or honey, 1 tablespoon
Half-boiled eggs, 2, Toast, 1 with butter, 1 teaspoon	Toast, 2 with butter, 2 teaspoons, jam, 1 teaspoon
Fresh figs, 4 *or* orange, 1	Apple, 1
Tea or coffee	Tea or coffee

Mid-morning

Fruit juice *or* sugar-cane juice, 1 cup	Fruit juice *or* sugar-cane juice, 1 cup

Lunch

Roast mutton	Curd, 1 cup
Boiled potato	Thin *dal,* 1 cup
Mixed vegetable salad	Rice, 2 tablespoons
Cooked spinach	Cooked pumpkin, ½ cup
Bread, 1 slice or *chappatis,* 2	*Chappatis,* 4 with butter, 2 teaspoons
Guava or apple	Mango or banana

4 p.m.

Tea	Tea
Biscuits, 4 *or* cake	Biscuits, 4 to 6 or cake

Dinner

Minced meat, 3 tablespoons	Butter milk, 1 cup
Baked sweet potato	Boiled potato
Boiled french beans	Cooked cauliflower
Bread, 2 slices or *chappatis,* 4	*Khakhra,* 4 with butter, 2 teaspoons
Rice pudding, 1 cup	Grapes

Before retiring
Skimmed milk, 1 cup

REFERENCE

[1] CHALMERS, T.C. *et al.* (1955) The treatment of acute infectious hepatitis. Controlled studies of the effects of diet, rest and physical reconditioning on the acute course of the disease and on the incidence of relapses and residual abnormalities, *J. clin. Invest.,* **34,** 1163.

60. HEPATIC PRECOMA AND COMA

Hepatic precoma and coma may be defined briefly as a syndrome characterized by disordered consciousness, confusion, the general features of organic psychosis, a flapping tremor of the outstretched hands, hypertonicity with flexor responses until terminally, and fetor hepaticus.

Mechanism

Hepatic coma may be produced by: (1) *Acute hepatocellular failure* following viral hepatitis, acute alcoholic hepatitis, Weil's disease, the anaesthetic agent halothane (*Fluothane*), accidental damage to the hepatic artery, usually during biliary surgery, and drugs: hydrallazine, amine oxidase inhibitors, phenelzine (*Nardil*). (2) *Chronic portosystemic* encephalopathy with or without gross liver damage occurs following *natural* intrahepatic and extrahepatic shunts, with cirrhosis or portal vein obstruction or *surgical* portacaval shunt.

Normally *ammonia* is formed by bacterial decomposition in the intestine and is transported to the liver where it is converted into urea and excreted by the kidneys. In patients with hepatic coma this process of ammonia detoxication may not occur and increased blood ammonia levels are frequently noted. The blood ammonia in such patients increases especially with: (1) upper intestinal bleeding, due to absorption of digested blood; (2) a high protein diet; or (3) the administration of ammonium salts, particularly ammonium chloride used as a diuretic for the treatment of ascites.

Indoles and *phenols* which are normally absorbed from the intestine may similarly enter the general circulation without detoxication due to severe hepatocellular damage or intra- and extra-hepatic shunts. Since the liver is the key organ for such detoxification it is likely that a *combination of toxic products* of metabolism, rather than a single factor, produces hepatic coma.

Precipitating Causes

1. *Viral hepatitis* may rarely follow a fulminating course with coma at the onset, or it may produce progressive liver damage and precipitate coma after a few weeks.

2. *In cirrhosis of the liver* coma may be precipitated by rapid abdominal paracentesis, gastro-intestinal haemorrhage or by the ad-

ministration of ammonium chloride as a diuretic. Mental deterioration is sometimes noted after chlorothiazide therapy particularly if the diuretic response is brisk. Excessive urinary loss of potassium and hypokalemia may be partly responsible for the neuropsychiatric state as it may improve with potassium supplements. In advanced hepatic cirrhosis the administration of a high protein diet or of amino acids may also precipitate coma.

3. *Surgery* performed in patients with severe hepatocellular damage, due to viral hepatitis, cirrhosis or prolonged obstructive jaundice, may precipitate coma. Anaesthesia, anoxia, blood loss, tissue breakdown and the administration of drugs like morphine and pethidine are all contributory factors in the production of coma after operation.

Jaundice may not be a prominent feature in coma occurring at the *onset* of viral hepatitis, or in portosystemic encephalopathy, but it is marked with progressive hepatocellular failure.

Haemorrhages

During acute hepatic necrosis there is increased *intravascular coagulation* due to release of coagulating factors from necrosed liver cells. The associated reduced synthesis of clotting factors due to hepatitis enhances bleeding tendency. The coagulation defect is difficult to combat. Stored blood supplies prothrombin factors VII, X and XI, while fresh blood supplies factors V and platelets also. Transfusions of blood containing citrates lowers ionized serum calcium and aggravates bleeding tendency. This is combated by adding 10 ml 10 per cent calcium gluconate in each litre of blood transfused.

Hepatorenal Syndrome

With increasing coma there may also be suppression of urine, which in turn causes an accumulation of the excretory products of metabolism and a disturbance of fluid and electrolyte balance. The reason for the suppression of urine is not known and the kidneys do not show gross histological damage. The hepatorenal failure is the result of renal vasoconstriction [2] and reduced blood flow to the renal cortex [5]. *Tubular damage* occurs following a marked rise in bilirubin, secondary infection or bleeding tendency.

In obstructive jaundice renal failure is common after surgery. Administration of intravenous mannitol pre- and post-operatively decreases the incidence of renal failure [3].

In *acute hepatocellular failure* exchange transfusions, human-cross-circulation between man and baboon, and extracorporeal pig liver perfusion, are experimental procedures undertaken only in organized institutions and not done as an occasional experiment. The survival rate even after such procedures is not much better than for those treated conservatively. 'Blunderbuss meddling with nature does more harm than good' [1].

DIETETIC MANAGEMENT

Calories
The minimum intake should be about 1000 Calories.

Proteins
Since nitrogenous products of protein metabolism appear to cause coma, no protein should be given. The *endogenous* breakdown of proteins is prevented as far as possible by a high carbohydrate diet (protein sparing effect). The *bacterial* breakdown of protein in the gastrointestinal tract *is inhibited* by the oral administration of broad-spectrum antibiotics, preferably neomycin, 1 G 6-hourly. If neomycin is not available streptomycin, 1 G 6-hourly by mouth, may be given instead. A regular bowel action should be obtained with an enema or bowel wash. Over-enthusiastic bowel washes may contribute to potassium loss.

After the patient recovers from coma, protein-containing foods such as cereals, biscuits and milk are gradually resumed.

Fats
With gross liver damage fats are not metabolized and should not be given.

Carbohydrates
Carbohydrates are used by the tissues for energy even when the liver cells are badly damaged. If over 600 Calories daily are provided by carbohydrates the endogenous breakdown of protein is reduced to a minimum. Glycogen-depleted liver cells are also very susceptible to injury. For these reasons, carbohydrate-rich foods should be given liberally during hepatic precoma and coma.

Continuous *intragastric drip* is preferred to the intravenous method. Dextrimaltose 10–15 per cent solutions, because of its gradual breakdown to glucose and its absorption along the intestinal tract, is better tolerated than 10–15 per cent solution of glucose.

Hypoglycaemia is common as the hepatic glycogen stores are depleted and there may perhaps be prolongation of action of endogenous insulin due to its reduced degradation by the failing liver. Hypoglycaemia may not occur during administration of continuous intravenous glucose which is routinely given to a comatosed patient. In an alcoholic, hypoglycaemic coma may be mistaken for alcoholic intoxication.

Continuous carbohydrate feeding through the nasogastric tube or intravenously prevents hypoglycaemic attacks in hepatic coma.

Vitamins

Vitamins of the B group, necessary for the metabolism of carbohydrates, vitamin C, 500 mg, and vitamin K, 10 mg, a day, are administered parenterally.

Minerals

Electrolyte balance is disturbed in liver failure due to the altered diet, the destruction of liver cells and the diminished excretion of urine. Correction of fluid or electrolyte imbalance requires the most urgent and careful attention. High serum *potassium* values are common with acute tissue breakdown and associated diminished urine formation. Infusion of glucose reduces tissue catabolism and prevents the rise of serum potassium.

Parenteral Feeds

Gross electrolyte disturbances are more likely with parenteral feeding than oral or nasogastric tube feeding. If parenteral feeding becomes essential, an intravenous infusion of 2000–2500 ml of 10 per cent glucose daily provides 800–1000 Calories. Higher concentrations of glucose tend to produce thrombosis of the vein. Vitamins of the B group, and vitamins C and K are also administered parenterally, preferably in divided doses.

Altering colonic bacteria: colonic *proteolytic* bacteria break down proteins to nitrogenous toxic products and ammonia. This proteolytic bacterial growth is reduced by promoting the growth of acid-forming *lactobacilli* in the colon following the feeding of cultures of *lactobacilli* or lactulose.

Lactulose is a non-absorbable *synthetic* disaccharide. It is composed of one molecule each of galactose and fructose. It is not broken down by the intestinal enzymes, but by the colonic bacterial enzymes to produce carbon dioxide, lactic and acetic acid. These acids reduce colonic pH, which not only decreases ammonia absorption from the gut, but may actually aid ammonia excretion from the blood *into* the gut. The daily dose of lactulose is about 100 to 150 ml divided into 3 or 4 doses. The side-effect is diarrhoea. Lactulose administered over prolonged periods reduces the episodes of chronic portosystemic encephalopathy associated with raised ammonia. The effect of lactulose in fulminant hepatitis is not proved [4].

HEPATIC PRECOMA AND COMA
SAMPLE MENU

150 ml of the following with nasogastric tube:

6·0 a.m.	Fruit juice
8·0 a.m.	Mixed vegetable soup
10·0 a.m.	Lemon squash with honey, 2 tablespoons
12·0 noon	Barley water with sugar, 2 tablespoons
2·0 p.m.	Fruit juice
4·0 p.m.	Tomato juice
6·0 p.m.	Sugar-cane juice
8·0 p.m.	Mixed vegetable soup
10·0 p.m.	Fruit juice
12·0 midnight	Lemon squash with sugar or jaggery, 2 tablespoons

REFERENCES

[1] SHERLOCK, S. (1969) The management of acute hepatocellular failure, *Brit. J. hosp. Med.,* July, 1257.

[2] EPSTEIN, M.D., *et al.* (1970) Renal failure in the patient with cirrhosis, *Amer. J. Med.,* **49,** 175.

[3] DAWSON, J.L. (1968) Acute postoperative renal failure, in obstructive jaundice, *Ann. roy. Coll. Surg. Engl.,* **42,** 163.

[4] ZEEGEN, R., *et al.* (1970) Some observations on the effects of treatment with lactulose on patients with chronic hepatic encephalopathy, *Quart. J. Med.,* **39,** 245.

[5] KEW, M. C., *et al.* (1971) Renal and intrarenal blood-flow in cirrhosis of the Liver, *Lancet,* **ii,** 504.

61. HEPATIC CIRRHOSIS

Hepatic cirrhosis is common both in the tropics and in temperate zones. In South East Asia it is frequently associated with a primary malignant tumour of the liver.

The diagnosis of cirrhosis of the liver in its early stages is difficult. The cirrhotic process may commence many years before it becomes clinically obvious, and usually the patient is first seen at a late stage with complications, such as ascites, ruptured oesophageal varices or hepatic coma. Liver function tests are not always abnormal in the early stages. In my experience, the material obtained from a cirrhotic liver by needle biopsy may not always be adequate and thus the morphological changes may not give a certain diagnosis. Peritoneoscopy has been a very helpful diagnostic aid in such cases [1].

Formerly such diverse opinions were held about the clinical and pathological features of cirrhosis that it was necessary to develop a universal working concept about its diagnosis. At the Fifth Pan American Congress of Gastroenterology held at Havana, Cuba in 1955 the diagnostic features of cirrhosis were defined and its classification and nomenclature worked out. The primary change in cirrhosis is *widespread* liver cell *necrosis* due to viral hepatitis, alcohol, etc. This necrosis results in *collapse* of liver cells and intrahepatic *shunts*, due to the proximity of the hepatic artery and portal vein to the central vein. The necrosis and collapse also stimulate *nodular regeneration* and *fibrosis*.

It is helpful to look upon cirrhosis of the liver as an end result of liver injury. Scar tissue on the skin reveals the end result of a cut, burn or infection. Similarly, cirrhosis of the liver is the structural and functional end result of nutritional, infective or toxic changes in the liver, Experimentally, the liver is found to be more susceptible to any injury when there is associated malnutrition and therefore adequate nutrition appears to safeguard the liver against cirrhosis.

The healthy liver has a remarkable capacity to regenerate with adequate nutrition, but a grossly damaged cirrhotic liver may not be able to regenerate because normal hepatic circulation is disorganized by intrahepatic shunts.

Aetiology

The aetiology of cirrhosis is probably multiple. The role of some factors suggested by clinical studies are discussed below.

Hepatitis. Twenty-seven per cent of proved cirrhotics at the B.Y.L. Nair Charitable Hospital, Bombay, gave a history suggestive of a previous attack of viral hepatitis. It is also assumed that a significant number have anicteric hepatitis.

Alcohol. It has been frequently stated that alcohol is not a factor in the production of cirrhosis in Eastern countries. Twenty-five per cent of patients with cirrhosis at the B.Y.L. Nair Charitable Hospital, Bombay, gave a history of heavy alcohol consumption for several years. The proportion of patients who were heavy drinkers can be assumed to have been even higher because some patients would deny such a history from fear of the 'dry laws' currently prevalent in the State.

Nutrition. Any injury to the liver is aggravated when the nutrition is poor and thus under-nutrition has always been blamed as a cause of cirrhosis. Necrosis due to injurious agents more readily occurs in cases of malnourished liver.

Fatty Liver. Fatty liver is an expression of poor nutrition. In experimental studies unsaturated fats promote the development of cirrhosis whereas saturated fats retard this process [2].

Toxins of Food. 'Bush tea' has a toxic effect on the liver. *Aflatoxin* is also blamed as a cause of cirrhosis. *Chillies* and *spices* are frequently taken in inordinate amounts by many Indians. These irritant foods when absorbed are likely to damage the liver cells. However, the effect of such substances on the liver is as yet unknown.

Types
Some of the unusual types of cirrhosis in tropical countries are:

Veno-occlusive Disease (V.O.D.) [3]. A condition of veno-occlusive disease occurring in undernourished infants, children and adults in Jamaica, has been described. The disease has been ascribed to the consumption of 'bush tea' which is an infusion made from various types of herbs taken by the local population for medicinal or other purposes. Experimentally, infusions made from *Crotalaria fulva* and *senecio* produced veno-occlusive changes in cattle [4]. The earliest *morphological* change in human veno-occlusive disease is subendothelial thickening of hepatic venous branches which progresses to obliteration of the lumen with the subsequent development of cirrhosis.

Clinically the patients present with evidence of cirrhosis such as hepatomegaly, ascites and sometimes haematemesis from oesophageal varices.

Indian Childhood Cirrhosis. Cirrhosis of the liver in infants is a common disease in Eastern countries. The clinical and histological features are similar to those of adult cirrhosis. Usually they are seen between the ages of 1 and 3 but even babies less than a year old may show an advanced stage of the disease [5]. Histologically, veno-occlusive changes seen in Jamaica are not noted. On critical analysis, race, sex, place in the family, malnutrition, Rh incompatibility, ABO blood groups, syphilis and age of weaning had no aetiological significance. Clinically there is ascites, enlargement of the liver and spleen; jaundice may occur in the terminal stages. The prognosis depends on the histological appearance of the liver. Milder cases survive for long periods but in advanced cases there is fibrous constriction of the individual liver cells and death occurs within a month [5].

Cirrhosis of the Liver in South Africa. In South Africa, especially in children of the low income group, excessive iron deposits in the cirrhotic liver have been reported [6]. This seems to occur as a result of an excessive intake and absorption of iron. Cooking food in iron vessels may provide as much as 100 mg of iron a day while a low phosphorus diet of maize allows increased absorption of iron from the intestine.

DIETETIC MANAGEMENT

Calories

The patients are usually emaciated by the time cirrhosis of the liver is diagnosed. A high calorie diet is necessary but, due to anorexia and ascites, it is difficult for the patient to take more than 2000–2500 Calories.

Proteins

The serum albumin, which is exclusively synthesized by liver cells, is low in cirrhosis and the hypo-albuminaemia is further aggravated by the loss of a considerable amount of albumin into ascitic fluid. A high protein diet is helpful for regeneration of the liver. In the absence of hepatic coma a high intake of proteins, about 2 g per kg body weight, is advisable. If the patient is in precoma or coma, proteins should be withheld till the patient is tided over the crisis.

The parenteral or oral administration of *choline* or *methionine* is not indicated, if sufficient protein is taken in the diet. In non-alcoholic cirrhotics where fatty changes are not observed they do not serve any useful purpose. Even when fatty changes are seen in the liver, regression occurs with the administration of adequate dietary protein and without the use of lipotropic factors.

Fats

One gramme of fat per kilogram of body weight is given. Even if fatty changes are present in the liver there should be no hesitation in supplying fats provided adequate amounts of proteins are also given.

Carbohydrates

Carbohydrates should be supplied liberally so that the liver may store glycogen. Liver function improves when an adequate store of glycogen is present in the hepatic cells.

Minerals

Sodium is restricted only when there is ascites and oedema. Allowing a normal salt intake makes the food more appetizing if there is no ascites. *Dilutional hyponatraemia* with serum sodium even below 110 mEq/1 may occur in patients with ascites. It is due to water retention and is treated with water restriction. During the administration of diuretics for the treatment of ascites, *potassium* salts have to be given in order to prevent hypokalaemia. *Iron* may be required for the correction of anaemia. Radioactive iron absorption in alcoholic cirrhotics is *decreased* by the *oral* administration of pancreatin. This suggests pancreatic deficiency as a factor in increased iron absorption [7] and possible haemochromatosis. Iron absorption is also increased after shunt operations.

Principles of Dietetics

A high calorie, high protein, high carbohydrate and high vitamin diet helps the regeneration of the liver and helps to prevent the formation of ascites.

HEPATIC CIRRHOSIS

Foods	Remarks
Bread or *chappatis* of wheat, rice, maize, *jowar, bajra* or *ragi*	Permitted
Breakfast cereal of wheat, rice, oatmeal or maize	Permitted
Rice	Permitted
Pulses (*dal*) and beans	Permitted
Meat, fish or chicken	Permitted
Eggs	Permitted
Milk or milk products	Permitted. Vegetarians should have liberal helpings of skimmed milk
Soup	Permitted*
Vegetable salad	Permitted*
Vegetables, cooked	Permitted*
Potato, sweet potato or yam	Permitted
Fat for cooking, or butter	Permitted
Sugar, jaggery or honey	Permitted
Jam or *murabba*	Permitted
Pastries	Permitted
Dessert	Permitted
Sweetmeats	Permitted
Fruits, fresh	Permitted
Fruits, dried	Permitted
Nuts	Permitted
Condiments and spices	Permitted in the minimum quantity to encourage better food intake
Papad, chutney or pickles	Excluded
Beverage	Permitted
Water	As desired

N.B.—Salt intake to be prohibited during ascites.

* Quantity to be restricted in order to permit better intake of other protein-rich foods.

HEPATIC CIRRHOSIS
SAMPLE MENU

Mixed Diet

Approximately

Proteins	112 g
Fats	67 g
Carbohydrates	240 g
Calories	2010

Vegetarian Diet

Approximately

Proteins	110 g
Fats	52 g
Carbohydrates	286 g
Calories	2050

Breakfast

Mixed Diet

Cornflakes, 1 cup with skimmed milk, 1 cup and sugar, 2 teaspoons
Eggs, 2 scrambled with 2 teaspoons butter or *ghee*
Toast, 2
Tea or coffee, 1 cup
Sweet lime or *chiku*, 1

Vegetarian Diet

Porridge, ¾ cup with skimmed milk, 1 cup and sugar, 2 teaspoons
Cottage cheese, 3 tablespoons
Khakhra, 4 or toast, 2
Butter, 2 teaspoons
Tea or coffee
Orange

Mid-morning

Skimmed milk, 1 cup

Skimmed milk, 1 cup

Lunch

Steamed fish
Yoghurt or milk, 1 cup
Sliced tomatoes
Boiled peas
Bread, 2 slices or *chappatis*, 4
Groundnuts, 16

Curd prepared from skimmed milk, 1 cup
Beetroot salad
Cooked brinjals, ¾ cup
Rice, 2 tablespoons
Dal, 1 cup
Bread, 2 slices or *chappatis*, 4
Sweet lime or orange

4 p.m.

Tea with bread and butter

Tea
Almonds, 8 or
Groundnuts, 20

Dinner

Roast chicken
Baked potato
Boiled cabbage
Bread, 2 slices or *chappatis*, 4

Cottage cheese, 3 tablespoons
Skimmed milk curd, 1 cup
Boiled potato, 1
Cooked spinach, 1 cup

| *Mixed Diet* | *Vegetarian Diet* |
| Baked custard, 1 cup | *Dal*, 1 cup
Bread, 2 slices or *chappatis*, 4 |

Before retiring
Skimmed milk, 1 cup with skimmed milk powder, 2 tablespoons.

REFERENCES

[1] ANTIA, F.P., DESAI, H.G., and DESHPANDE, C.K. (1966) Peritoneoscopy and liver biopsy in hepatic cirrhosis, in *Proceedings of the First Congress of the International Society of Endoscopy*, Tokyo, p. 494.

[2] GYORGY, P., GOLDBLATT, H., and GANZIN, M. (1959) Dietary fat and cirrhosis of the liver, *Gastroenterology*, 37, 637.

[3] BRAS, G., JELLIFFE, D.B., and STUART, K.L. (1954) Veno-occlusive disease of liver with nonportal type of cirrhosis, occurring in Jamaica, *Arch. Path.* 57, 285.

[4] BRAS, G., BERRY, D.M., and GYORGY, P. (1957) Plants as aetiological factor in veno-occulsive disease of the liver, *Lancet*, i, 960.

[5] ANTIA, F.P., and BHARADWAJ, T.P. (1956) Infantile cirrhosis, *Gastroenterologia*, 86, 406.

[6] GILLMAN, J., and GILLMAN, T. (1945) Structure of the liver in pellagra, *Arch. Path.*, 40, 239.

[7] DELLER, D.J. (1965) Iron[59] absorption measurements by whole body counting studies in alcoholic cirrhosis, haemochromatosis and pancreatitis, *Amer. J. dig. Dis.*, 10, 249.

62.   FATTY LIVER

Normal fat content of the liver is less than 10 per cent but when it exceeds this amount it is called 'fatty liver'. In experimental animals protein deficiency or deficient intake of lipotropic factors, methionine and choline produce fatty liver. Most of the lipids that accumulate in fatty liver are triglycerides [1].

Normally fatty acid in the liver is metabolized as (1) esterification to form triglycerides; (2) combination with proteins synthesized by the liver to form soluble lipoprotein for transport to other sites; (3) esterification with cholesterol; (4) incorporation into phospholipids; and

(5) oxidation to carbon dioxide or ketone bodies.

Fatty liver occurs when: (1) *excess fatty acids* are brought to the liver from absorbed dietary fat or on release from adipose tissue; (2) fatty acid synthesis is increased; (3) fat oxidation is decreased; or (4) with deficient protein formation, lipoproteins are not formed, resulting in decreased fat removal.

The pathological conditions predisposing to fatty liver are *alcoholism* which increases the rate of synthesis of fatty acids and the conversion to triglycerides, while reducing the rate of oxidation of fatty acids and release of lipoprotein from the liver. Even in casual drinkers fat accumulates in the liver [2]. Other pathological conditions with fatty liver are protein-calorie malnutrition (kwashiorkor), starvation, obesity, malabsorption syndrome, ulcerative colitis, regional enteritis, jejuno-ileal bypass for gross obesity, chronic pancreatitis, or drugs such as carbon tetrachloride or massive tetracycline therapy administered along with kidney damage, particularly during pregnancy.

FATTY LIVER IN INFANTS AND CHILDREN

A deficient intake of proteins may result in a fatty liver. In infants and children the liver is laden with fat in various conditions as: (1) in kwashiorkor seen mostly in infants and children. Kwashiorkor has been also described in adults but the available descriptions are few. (2) In the West Indies, fatty liver disease has been described in infants. The presenting symptoms are oedema and vomiting. These infants do not show evidence of changes in the skin and hair due to protein deficiency as seen in kwashiorkor. (3) In South Africa, fatty liver has been described in association with deposits of iron in the liver.

FATTY LIVER IN ADULTS

(1) Fatty liver is described among alcoholics in Western countries. This liver is more likely to be firm to the touch, and shows deranged liver function. (2) In India, fatty liver is seen in adults and is due to malnutrition. These adults are seen with diarrhoea, underweight, ascites, oedema of the legs, dry scaly skin and a palpable liver that is usually very soft. They are markedly anaemic, with a low serum albumin. Other liver function tests fail to show gross abnormality. These patients improve on a hospital diet of 2000 Calories containing 75–100 g

proteins, but lipotropic factors are not necessary. It is likely that the dramatic permanent improvement claimed by some physicians in cases of hepatic cirrhosis in children and adults, diagnosed clinically without adequate biopsy studies, was in reality that of cases of fatty liver and not cirrhosis.

REFERENCES

[1] ISSELBACHER, K. J. (1964) Alcohol, hyperlipaemia and the fatty liver, *Abbottempo*, **2**, 9.

[2] RUBIN, E., and LIEBER, C. S. (1968) Alcohol induced hepatic injury in non-alcoholic volunteers, *New Engl. J. Med.*, **278**, 869.

63.　KWASHIORKOR

(Protein-calorie malnutrition)

Kwashiorkor (red boy) is a clinical syndrome seen in the poorer people of Asia and Africa. The manifestations do not occur when there is combined deficiency of calories and protein. It occurs when adequate calories are derived from carbohydrates but the protein intake is low. Kwashiorkor is usually seen in infants between 1 and 3 years of age, as it is at this period of life after weaning that the demand for proteins for growth is greatest.

It is a mistake to consider *marasmus* as due to pure calorie deficiency and *kwashiorkor* as isolated protein deficiency; there is no difference in the diets of children with marasmus or kwashiorkor. Moreover, initially marasmic children may subsequently develop kwashiorkor, while those with kwashiorkor on shedding oedema may appear marasmic [1]. *Mental development* is retarded but this may well be related to the environment rather than to malnutrition. *Stunting* of growth does not necessarily follow a period of severe malnutrition, as with successful treatment these children may outgrow their siblings [2].

Clinically, the syndrome consists of the following features. There is retarded growth. Gastro-intestinal disturbances occur with anorexia, nausea and frequent diarrhoea. Normal intestinal epithelium regenerates every 3–5 days, but with protein deficiency the regeneration is poor and consequent *mucosal atrophy* resembles coeliac disease. There is asso-

ciated *lactase deficiency* and *diminished pancreatic digestive secretion.*
All the factors lead to diarrhoea. There is generalized oedema of the
body. The hair may be light coloured or markedly depigmented. The
skin shows localized jet black patches on the pressure sites, flexure
aspects and genital region. These patches exfoliate and leave a hypo-
pigmented area surrounded by a hyperpigmented zone.

On examination the liver may be palpable and soft. Stomatitis and
ulcers in the mouth occur due to *vitamin B* deficiency. Deficiency of
vitamin A produces night blindness and xerophthalmia. The *heart* is
affected by anaemia and malnutrition, and radiologically it appears
small. The electrocardiogram shows tachycardia, low voltage complexes,
and changes due to hypopotassaemia [3].

Anaemia is normocytic or macrocytic. The serum *proteins* are low,
particularly the serum *albumin,* which may even be less than 1 g per
cent. The serum *potassium* values may be markedly lowered, and a
value as low as 1·4 mEq per litre has been noted. The serum *calcium*
level may also be low. *Magnesium* deficiency may be noted on muscle
biopsy [4]. *Moderate fasting hypoglycaemia* with sugar 20 mg per 100
ml, and profound hypoglycaemia with coma and hypothermia, occur
with associated severe parasitic or bacterial infection [5].

Amino acid absorption is decreased after calorie and protein starvation [6].

Liver biopsy shows fatty changes, more in the periphery than in the
centre of the lobules, and fatty cysts are usually seen. Reduced synthesis
of lipoprotein, which normally helps fat removal from the liver, may
be the cause of fatty liver rather than deficiency of lipotropic factors.
There is also cellular infiltration and evidence of fibrosis.

Serum Transferrin (Siderophillin).   No biochemical test, including
serum protein values, is a good guide to the severity or clinical progress
of protein-calorie malnutrition. Estimation of serum transferrin, however, is claimed to be a good indication of kwashiorkor [7]. The normal
serum transferrin in Europeans is 2 mg per ml. Serum transferrin levels
below 0·45 mg per ml are diagnostic of severe protein-calorie malnutrition, and values below 0·3 mg per ml carry a grave prognosis [8].
Therapy with a high protein diet with rising serum transferrin is a sign
of good progress, while a falling serum transferrin denotes a grave
outcome. After one week of treatment the serum transferrin may
sometimes rise tenfold [7].

The *mortality* depends upon the degree of fatty infiltration of the liver, the degree of malnutrition and the available medical care. Jaundice is ominous. The usual causes of death are intercurrent infection, hepatic coma, low serum potassium, or cardiac failure.

DIETETIC MANAGEMENT

Kwashiorkor is primarily a disease of absolute as well as relative protein deficiency. The treatment consists of supplying adequate proteins and of eradicating any intercurrent infection that may be present.

Calories

The daily requirement for a child is 90–100 Calories per kilogram of expected body weight. A child of 2 years requires 1000 Calories daily.

Proteins

Adequate *milk* for infants and children is important both for prophylaxis against kwashiorkor and for its treatment. A protein intake supplying 20 per cent of the total calories is necessary. Thus a child of 2 years requiring 1000 Calories should have 200 Calories supplied by 50 g of protein. Administration of *skimmed milk powder* has proved to be most valuable. Bengal gram (*chana*), as it is relatively cheap, is a very good source of protein [9]. As milk is expensive, an alternative vegetable protein mixture, 6 g per kg body weight with small quantities of skimmed milk, is also suggested.

DIETS IN KWASHIORKOR*

1 MILK PROTEIN	g/kg body weight	cals/kg body weight	2 VEGETABLE PROTEIN MIXTURE	g/kg body weight	cals/kg body weight
Skimmed milk	9	36	Wheat flour	18	63
Bread	20	70	Cotton-seed flour	6	24
Butter	7	63	Sugar	10	40
Sugar	7	28	Ghee	7	63
Bananas	2		Skimmed milk	3	12

*Gopalan, C. (1967) Malnutrition in childhood in the tropics, *Brit. med. J.*, 2, 603.

Fats

As long as adequate proteins are supplied the usual dietary fat is helpful in making the food palatable and increasing calorie intake.

Vitamins

Multivitamin preparations are helpful.

Minerals

The serum *potassium* level may be markedly low [3]. The oral administration of potassium salts is advisable, for example potassium citrate, 300 mg four times a day. *Calcium* salts as calcium lactate, 300 mg three times a day, are also useful. *Iron* therapy with a low serum transferrin may increase free circulating iron and may be a cause of death [10]. Iron therapy is therefore advised after a week of high protein diet. *Magnesium sulphate heptahydrate* 50 per cent in a dose of 1 ml for a child under 9 kg and 1·5 ml for a child over 9·5 kg, given every 12 hours for the first 3 days then once daily, improves ECG and there is a remarkable clinical improvement with adequate dosage. [11].

Parenteral Therapy

As the fluid and electrolyte disturbance may be marked, parenteral therapy can be dangerous. It is therefore best to administer all nutrients orally.

REFERENCES

[1] GOPALAN, C. (1970) Some recent studies in the Nutrition Research Laboratories, Hyderabad, *Amer. J. clin. Nutr.*, **23**, 35.

[2] GARROW, J.S., and PIKE, M.C. (1967) The long-term prognosis of severe infantile malnutrition, *Lancet*, **i**, 1.

[3] SMYTHE, P.M., SWANEPOEL, A., and CAMPBELL, J.A.H. (1962) The heart in kwashiorkor, *Brit. med. J.*, **1**, 67.

[4] MONTGOMERY, R.D. (1960) Magnesium metabolism in infantile protein malnutrition, *Lancet*, **ii**, 74.

[5] WHARTON, B. (1970) Hypoglycaemia in children with kwashiorkor, *Lancet*, **i**, 171.

[6] ADIBI, S.A. ALLEN, E., and RAWORTH, R. (1970) Impaired jejunal absorption rates of essential amino acids induced by either dietary caloric or protein deprivation in man, *Gastroenterology*, **59**, 404.

[7] ANTIA, A.U., McFARLANE, H., and SOOTHILL, J.F. (1968) Serum siderophyllin in kwashiorkor, *Arch. Dis. Child.*, **43**, 459.

[8] McFARLANE, H., *et al.* (1969) Biochemical assessment of protein-calorie malnutrition, *Lancet*, **i**, 392.

[9] VENKATACHALAM, P.S., SRIKANTIA, S.G., MEHTA, G., and GOPALAN, C. (1956) Treatment of nutritional oedema syndrome (kwashiorkor) with vegetable protein diets, *Indian J. med. Res.*, **44**, 539.

[10] MCFARLANE, H., *et al.* (1970) Immunity, transferrin and survival in kwashiorkor, *Brit. med. J.*, **4**, 268.

[11] CADDELL, J.L. (1967) Studies of protein-calorie malnutrition II. A double blind clinical trial to assess magnesium therapy, *New Engl. J. Med.*, **276**, 535.

64. GALL-BLADDER DISEASE

The gall-bladder is a thin-walled reservoir situated on the under-surface of the liver. It can store about 40–50 ml of bile. The liver secretes about 700 ml of bile a day, which, when not required for digestion, is concentrated and stored in the gall-bladder. Acute and chronic cholecystitis, usually associated with gall-stones, are the commonest diseases of the gall-bladder.

The incidence of gall-stones is very high in Western countries, being present in at least 20 per cent of women over the age of 40 and in 20 per cent of men over 70 [1]. The overall incidence of gall-stones in Oriental countries is low, but varies in different regions. Among the Chinese in Singapore the higher incidence of stones in the gall-bladder as well as the biliary ducts is attributed to opium-eating which produces spasm of the sphincter of Oddi and causes stagnation of bile [2].

The gall-stones formed in the gall-bladder, and sometimes in the common or hepatic ducts, are predominantly cholesterol, mixed with some bile pigments, calcium carbonate and phosphate. Sometimes pure cholesterol or pure pigment stones may occur with haemolytic jaundice.

Cholesterol Stones

The gall-stones are formed when cholesterol precipitates in bile. Cholesterol, bile salts and phospholipid in their normal proportions keep bile liquid. The bile salts and phospholipid (lecithin) exist as micelles that solubilize cholesterol. Cholesterol in bile is precipitated by: (1) *Increased concentration (supersaturation) of cholesterol.* The *liver* of patients with gall-stones secretes supersaturated bile [3]. High calorie consumption enhances high hepatic cholesterol secretion, which favours gall-stone formation. (2) Decreased concentration of hepatic secretion of *bile salts* and *phospholipids* precipitates cholesterol. Normal subjects have a bile acid pool of 2·4 g and daily cholic acid production of 0·36 g. In *cholesterol gall-stone patients* the bile acid pool is reduced to 1·3 g while daily cholic acid production is 0·2 g [4]. Bile acids are normally absorbed from the terminal ileum. Increased small intestinal bacterial activity deconjugates bile salts that are poorly absorbed. The bile acid pool is therefore reduced with: (a) diminished hepatic formation; (b) increased intestinal bacterial deconjugation (malabsorption syndrome); (c) inflammation of small bowel (regional enteritis) [5], tuberculosis; or (d) increased excretion (ileostomy).

Cholesterol. The higher intake of cholesterol is not now considered to cause gall-stone, since the capacity of the human intestine to absorb dietary cholesterol is limited [6]. The ingestion of cholesterol does not influence concentration of biliary cholesterol. However, the cholesterol concentration of *hepatic bile* is higher in patients with gall-stones who also consume high calorie diet [7].

Phospholipids (Lecithin). These assist in increasing the micellar size to keep cholesterol in solution. Diminished bile acid pool also reduces phospholipid secretion [8] and precipitates cholesterol.

The gall-bladder bile of the Masai of East Africa has a high ratio of phospholipid to cholesterol and of bile acid to cholesterol. This creates an enormous reserve capacity to dissolve cholesterol and protects these people from cholesterol gall-stones [9].

Stasis, during the last months of pregnancy or with opium-eating, predisposes to stone formation [2].

The *gall-bladder* is not the prime cause of cholesterol gall-stone formation, except that stasis of bile in the gall-bladder during fasting periods and at nights allows precipitation of supersaturated cholesterol.

Inflammation of the gall-bladder, due either to bacterial or chemical factors, favours bile salt absorption and consequent cholesterol precipitation.

Conclusion. Cholesterol is precipitated as a result of supersaturated *hepatic* cholesterol secretion with high calories and increased intake of proteins, fats and carbohydrates. However, cholesterol in the bile does not precipitate without *decrease* in the relative concentrations of bile acids and lecithin which solubilize cholesterol [10].

Pigment Stones

Haemolytic jaundice may be associated with pigment stones. The liver conjugates bile pigments with glucuronic acid to make water-soluble bilirubin glucuronide. Liver damage by virus etc., results in disturbed conjugation and insoluble pigments precipitate in the intrahepatic or larger ducts. Patients with only *bilirubin stones* do not show cholesterol saturation in the hepatic or gall-bladder bile [11].

Spontaneous Disappearance of Gall-stones

In rare cases gall-stones detected on X-ray may not be seen on subsequent X-ray examination or exploration. The disappearance of stones may be due to their passage through the common bile-duct, if the stones are relatively small, or by the formation of a fistula between the gall-bladder or bile-duct and the intestinal tract (usually duodenum), when large stones can be passed without much pain or discomfort. [12] In the present state of our knowledge there is no drug or diet which can definitely dissolve gall-stones. Oral administration of over 6 months of chenodeoxycholic acid is reported to decrease the size of cholesterol stones. [13] Since chenodeoxycholic acid can be converted to secondary bile acid (lithocholic acid) the effect of long term follow up of chenodeoxycholic acid are awaited.

Spurious excretion of gall-stones has been noted even in the early part of the last century (and many such hoaxes are continued even today) as seen from this letter of William Babington to Sir Everard Home. [14]

17, Aldermanbury,
Feb. 2, 1813.

Dear Sir,

The following are the circumstances relating to the change produced upon olive oil, by passing through the stomach and intestines of the elderly person, whose case I mentioned to you at the last meeting of our Animal Chemistry Society. The lady, in question, had for several years past suffered from severe affections of the stomach, which, from the attendant symptoms, were considered as occasioned by the irritation of biliary concretions. Many remedies having been resorted to without affording her other than temporary benefit, she has been advised to try the effects of olive oil, taken to the quantity of two or three ounces at a time, and to be repeated as circumstances might require. From this she experienced most immediate relief, and, on the subsequent examination of what passed from the bowels, globular concretions were uniformly observed, which by the persons about her were considered as the gall-stones, which had previously been productive of so much distress. ....In a few days I was summoned to make my proposed visit, and, upon examining the substances collected, I found their appearance to be much as I have already described to you, namely, that of distinct globules, varying in size from that of a large pea to the bulk of a moderate grape, of a cream colour, and slightly translucent, of sufficient consistence to preserve their form, and to bear being cut by a knife, like soft wax, but at the points of their contact disposed to cohere. When exposed to heat, they readily melted, and then at once exhibited their original oily character. The change, which they have since experienced, has taken place in the water in which they have been kept.

I am, dear Sir,
Yours always, very faithfully,
Sd/- Wm. Babington.

To Sir Everard Home, Bart.

DIETETIC MANAGEMENT

Cholelithiasis, associated with attacks of biliary colic, obstructive jaundice or recurrent cholangitis, is to be treated by surgery. The mere presence of *asymptomatic* gall-stones in the elderly, however, is not an indication for surgery. Dietetic management is necessary to *prevent* gall-stone formation.

Calories

Gall-bladder disease is prevalent among those communities *consuming significantly more calories* than others, though the relative proportions of protein, fat and carbohydrate are the same as those in people without gall-stones [7]. The minimum number of calories to maintain normal body weight is therefore advised.

Protein

Higher protein intake also increases biliary cholesterol concentration [7]. A normal 60–80 g protein intake is permitted.

Fats

Symptoms of bloating, belching and dyspepsia usually ascribed to gall-bladder disease are as common even in those with normal gall-bladder function. The intolerance of fatty foods may not have been present but may follow the advice of the physician to avoid fried food, which may create a phobia. Those complaining of dyspepsia with fried food, when fed with fat so disguised as not to be recognizable, did not complain that the adverse symptoms were produced [15].

Fats Advised. For patients in whom fats do not produce symptoms, administration of vegetable oils like olive oil and unhydrogenated groundnut or *til* oil are helpful in draining the gall-bladder. Digestion of fat is a powerful stimulus for the contraction and evacuation of the gall-bladder, so preventing stasis.

Fats Contra-indicated. If there are adhesions to the gall-bladder or there is obstruction to the biliary flow, gall-bladder contraction may produce discomfort. In such patients a low fat diet is advised. Tolerance to fat should be determined by trial.

Fried foods are excluded if they produce discomfort.

Carbohydrates

Since biliary cholesterol increases with higher calorie intake and since carbohydrates contribute to excess calories, a high carbohydrate diet should be avoided.

Vitamins

If a low fat diet is prescribed fat-soluble vitamins A, D, E and K should be given as supplements.

A high fluid intake should be encouraged.

Principles of Diet

Adequate calories to bring the body weight to the ideal level. If fats are tolerated then unsaturated vegetable fats should be given. If fats are not tolerated, a low fat diet is advised. Fried foods should be avoided.

GALL-BLADDER DISEASE

Foods	Remarks
Bread or *chappatis* from wheat, rice, maize, *jowar, bajra* or *ragi*	Permitted
Breakfast cereals of wheat, rice, oatmeal or maize	Permitted
Rice, cooked	Permitted
Pulses (*dal*) or beans	Permitted as thin *dal*
Meat, fish or chicken	Permitted; brain, liver, kidney and fatty meats like duck and bacon excluded
Eggs	Permitted if no discomfort
Milk or milk products	Permitted with cream removed
Soup	Permitted, thick soups excluded
Vegetable salad	Permitted
Vegetables, cooked	Permitted
Potato, sweet potato or yam	Permitted
Fat for cooking, or butter	Permitted if no symptoms. Fried foods excluded
Sugar, jaggery or honey	Permitted
Jam or *murabba*	Permitted
Pastry	Permitted only as biscuits or light cakes
Dessert	Permitted as light custard or ice cream
Sweets or sweetmeat	Excluded
Fruits, fresh	Permitted
Fruits, dried	Excluded
Nuts	Excluded
Condiments and spices	Excluded
Papad, chutney or pickles	Excluded
Beverage	Permitted
Fluid	Liberal

GALL-BLADDER DISEASE
SAMPLE MENU

Mixed Diet	*Vegetarian Diet*

Morning

Tea	Tea

Breakfast

Cornflakes with skimmed milk and sugar	Porridge with skimmed milk and sugar
Egg, 1 poached*	Toast with guava jam
Toast with apricot jam	Tea or coffee
Tea or coffee	Banana
Orange	

Lunch

Clear soup, 1 cup	Mixed vegetable soup
Minced meat with boiled potato and french beans	Thin *dal*, ½ cup
Beetroot and lettuce salad	Cooked carrots and pumpkin
Bread or *chappatis*	Tomato and cucumber salad
Apple	Bread or *chappatis*
	Papaya

4 p.m.

Tea with biscuits	Tea with biscuits

Dinner

Chicken soup	Tomato soup
Roast leg of chicken with cooked spinach and mashed potato	Thin *dal* ½ cup
	Baked potato and cooked pumpkin
	Butter milk (prepared from skimmed milk)
Bread or *chappatis*	Bread or *chappatis*
Jelly	Sago pudding

* excluded if produces discomfort

REFERENCES

[1] RAINS, A.J.H. (1968) Gall stone disease, *Brit. med. J.,* **1,** 295.
[2] HWANG, W.S. (1970) Cholelithiasis in Singapore, *Gut,* **11,** 141, 148.
[3] SMALL, D.M., and RAPO, S. (1970) Sources of abnormal bile in patients with cholesterol gallstones, *New Engl. J. Med.,* **283,** 53.

[4] VLAHCEVIC, Z.R., *et al.* (1970) Diminished bile acid pool size in patients with gallstones, *Gastroenterology,* **59,** 165.

[5] COHEN, S., KAPLAN, M., GOTTLIEB, L., and PATTERSON, J. (1971) Liver disease and gallstones in regional enterits, *Gastroenterology,* **60,** 237.

[6] WILSON, J.D., and LINDSEY, C.A. (1965) Studies on the influence of dietary cholesterol on cholesterol metabolism in the isotopic steady state in man, *J. clin. Invest.,* **44,** 1805.

[7] SARLES, H., *et al.* (1970) Diet cholesterol gallstones and composition of the bile, *Amer. J. dig. Dis.,* **15,** 251.

[8] SWELL, L., and BELL, C.C. (1968) Influence of bile acids on biliary lipid excretion in man, *Amer. J. dig. Dis.,* **13,** 1077.

[9] BISS, K., *et al.* (1971) Some unique biologic characteristics of the Masai of East Africa, *New Engl. J. Med.,* **284,** 694.

[10] THISTLE, J.L. (1970) Letter to the Editor, *Amer. J. dig. Dis.,* **15,** 779.

[11] VLAHCEVIC, Z.R., BELL, C.C., and SWELL, L. (1970) Significance of the liver in the production of lithogenic bile in man, *Gastroenterology,* **59,** 62.

[12] GARDNER, A.M.N., HOLDEN, W.S., and MONKS, P.J.W. (1966) Disappearing gallstones, *Brit. J. Surg.,* **53,** 114.

[13] DANZINGER, R.G., HOFFMAN, A.F., SCHOENFIELD, L.J., and THISTLE, J.L. (1972) Dissolution of cholesterol gallstones by chenodeoxycholic acid, *New Engl. J. Med.,* **286,** 1.

[14] HOME, E. (1813-14) On the formation of fat in the intestines of living animals, *Phil. Trans. B.,* **103,** 146.

[15] TAGGERT, D., and BILLINGTON, B.P. (1966) Fatty foods and dyspepsia, *Lancet,* **ii,** 464.

65. ANAEMIA

Anaemia is a condition in which there is a diminished oxygen carrying capacity of the blood as a result of a reduction in total circulating haemoglobin and/or a reduction in red cell mass. Anaemias can be broadly classified as: (1) *Dyshaemopoietic,* where there is insufficient blood formation which may be due to an inadequate intake, absorption or utilization of factors essential for erythropoiesis. The factors essential for the formation of red blood cells are: (a) minerals of which iron is the most important but traces of cobalt as vitamin B_{12} are also necessary—the role of copper is as yet uncertain; (b) proteins; (c) vitamins of the B group, particularly B_{12}. folic acid and vitamin C; (d) hormones; (e) pigments. (2) *Haemorrhagic,* due to extravascular blood loss. The common causes of blood loss are bleeding piles, excessive menstruation and pregnancy. Peptic ulcer, oesophageal varices and hiatal hernia are common causes of blood loss from the gastro-intestinal tract. Aspirin causes gastric irritation and oozing and is a common cause of unexplained anaemia in aged arthritic patients. Hookworm infestation is a common cause of anaemia in the rural areas of tropical countries but the infestation is infrequent amongst urban population [1]. (3) *Haemolytic,* due to excessive intravascular blood destruction. These anaemias can be regarded as due either to defects in the red cells or to circulating haemolytic agents.

Anaemic women are known to shed hair. Sudden hair loss is noted in blood donors whose serum iron falls below normal [2].

Anaemias in the Tropics [3]

About 15 per cent of patients studied have megaloblastic anaemia and such cases are found at high altitudes and in cool regions. This anaemia responds to vitamin B_{12} and folic acid, but some cases also require iron for a complete cure. The other 85 per cent of the patients from hot humid areas have iron deficiency anaemia.

Iron Deficiency Anaemia

Iron deficiency is the most common cause of anaemia. Deficiency of iron may occur as a result of: (1) diminished intake; (2) deficient absorption; or (3) loss.

Intake. Iron intake is adequate in the tropics because the staple diet, consisting of cereals, has a high iron content of about 5–8 mg per 100 g. The iron intake in the tropics is therefore probably greater than the average intake of 12–15 mg a day in Western countries.

Absorption. Usually only 10 per cent of ingested iron is absorbed but the absorption of iron under the dietary conditions prevailing in tropical countries is probably lower. This is because cereals, the staple diet in the tropics, besides having a high iron content, also have a high content of *phytate* which forms insoluble and non-absorbable iron phytate in the intestine. Other factors in a tropical diet which may inhibit iron absorption are the relatively high *phosphate* and low *calcium* content; the excess phosphate may bind iron and prevent its absorption. The habit of eating betel leaves with lime (calcium carbonate) provides calcium which combines with the free phosphate in the intestine so increasing the uncombined iron available for absorption.

Vitamin C increases absorption of iron. Fruits and vegetables are relatively expensive in underdeveloped countries and only small quantities are available to the poorer people. It is likely that an insufficient intake of vitamin C is a factor in the poor absorption of iron from cereals. Sour lime juice squeezed on food may be a way of correcting this deficiency and thus of enhancing iron absorption.

Loss. *Parasites* associated with iron deficiency anaemia are those causing chronic blood loss either from the gastro-intestinal or urinary tract. These include *hookworms* (*Ankylostoma duodenale, Necator americanus*), the *whipworm* and *schistosomes*.

Hookworm. Each *Ankylostoma duodenale* worm may cause a daily 0·2 ml blood loss, that is 10 times more than *Necator americanus*. Heavy hookworm infestation can cause a daily blood loss of up to 250 ml, equivalent to a daily 29 mg iron loss as shown by the isotope technique [4]. About 3 ml plasma is lost per 100 *Necator americanus*. This loss can lead to marked hypo-albuminaemia and oedema in a severely malnourished individual.

Whipworm. *Trichuris trichiura* infestation with over 800 parasites leads to anaemia. The daily blood loss measured in heavy infestation was up to 8·6 ml [5].
Fifteen mg oral elemental iron daily as ferrous sulphate tablets or enrichment of staple foods is effective in overcoming frank anaemia in school children with heavy parasitic infestation [6].

Schistosoma mansoni and Schistosoma haematobium. These are common in Egypt. They can produce a daily blood loss of up to 26 and 126 ml respectively. [7] *Malarial parasites* cause anaemia with haemolysis. *Diphyllobothrium latum* produces megaloblastic anaemia due to vitamin B_{12} deficiency.
Sweat contains variable amounts of iron, the content being related to desquamation of the skin. Depending upon the amount of perspiration, iron losses through sweating vary between 0·3 and 2·3 mg a day. People in the hot tropical plains may lose 3–10 litres of fluid as sweat each day and there is a greater prevalence of iron deficiency among them than among those who live in the cooler hills.
Iron loss in females occurs during the child-bearing period. During each menstrual period an average of 15–20 mg of iron is lost. There is a continuous drain of iron during pregnancy and this affects mothers

below the age of 20 more than older women because below the age of 20 growth continues and the blood volume is still increasing. It is estimated that with each pregnancy and childbirth the iron loss may be about 500 mg. Added to this, the daily loss through lactation averages 1 mg. Most women from among the poor class thus have an iron deficiency anaemia and it is not rare to see a patient admitted to the hospital with a haemoglobin level of less than 10 per cent.

Protein-calorie malnutrition causes anaemia with hypoplasia of the bone marrow. This improves with protein feeding and daily 25 micrograms folic acid. Only occasionally is vitamin B_{12} or vitamin E required. Glucose-6-phosphate dehydrogenase deficiency may contribute to haemolytic anaemia following infections or drugs [8].

Anaemia in the Temperate Zone

Even in temperate countries where standards of nutrition are better, iron deficiency anaemia frequently occurs and accounts for 92 per cent of all anaemias [9]. Eating clay and sometimes laundry starch (possibly as a source of calories) is also responsible for anaemia [10] as these substances decrease iron absorption.

Nutritional anaemias due to deficiency of folic acid, vitamin B_{12} and pyridoxine have been described in the respective chapters.

DIET

In every case of anaemia the cause should be discovered and treated. In clinical practice nutritional anaemia is commonly associated with over-all undernutrition and an all-round balanced diet should be given. Usually, diet alone is not adequate and therapy with specific supplements are also needed. In patients with a very poor diet or malabsorption, vitamin B_{12} deficiency may be the cause of anaemia. A nursing mother with such an anaemia secretes little vitamin B_{12} in the milk and so her breast-fed infant may also become deficient.

A list of foods suitable for anaemia patients is given below:

Vegetarian

Cereals, milk, pulses, lettuce, spinach, beans, tomato, citrus fruit (orange), figs, prunes, resins, apricots, almonds, walnuts, pistachios. Sour lemon squeezed on food is the most inexpensive and palatable form of taking vitamin C.

Non-vegetarian
Mutton, beef, liver, kidney, eggs.

Prevention
Supplements of 10 mg iron prevent iron deficiency anaemia [11]. Most authorities agree that more expensive iron preparations or quick or slow release preparations have no advantage over ferrous sulphate. Ferrous sulphate, 100 mg tablets, hardly cost *even 1 paise* per day, yet effectively prevent anaemia in women.

ANAEMIA

Foods	Remarks
Bread or *chappatis* of wheat, rice, maize, *jowar, bajra* or *ragi*	Permitted
Breakfast: cereals of wheat, rice, oatmeal or maize	Permitted
Rice, cooked	Permitted
Pulses, *dal* or beans	Permitted
Meat, fish, chicken	Permitted, specially liver, kidney and bone marrow
Eggs	Permitted
Milk and milk products	Permitted
Soup	Permitted, specially liver soup
Vegetable salad	Permitted
Vegetables, cooked	Permitted
Potato, sweet potato or yam	Permitted
Fat for cooking, and butter	Permitted
Sugar, jaggery or honey	Permitted
Jam or *murabba*	Permitted
Pastries	Permitted
Desserts	Permitted
Sweets or sweetmeats	Permitted
Fruits, fresh	Permitted
Fruits, dried	Permitted, specially raisins, currants, dried figs, prunes
Nuts	Permitted
Condiments and spices	Permitted in moderation
Papad, chutney or pickles	Permitted in moderation
Beverages	Permitted
Fluids	Liberal

ANAEMIA
SAMPLE MENU

Mixed Diet	*Vegetarian Diet*

Breakfast

Cornflakes with milk and sugar	Stewed prunes
Eggs, 2 scrambled with butter or *ghee*	Porridge with milk and sugar or honey
Toasts or *chappatis* with butter	Toast or *chappatis* with butter
Tea or coffee	Tea or coffee
Fresh figs	Orange

Lunch

Chicken soup	Cottage cheese with lettuce salad
Grilled liver, tomato and potato chips	Cooked brinjals
Cooked spinach with sour lime	Rice with *dal*
Bread or *chappatis*	Buttermilk
Papaya or orange	Bread or *chappatis*
Groundnuts	Banana

4 p.m.

Tea, 1 cup	Tea, 1 cup
Cake or biscuits	Raisin cake

Dinner

Meat soup	Tomato soup
Fried fish	Curd
Roast chicken with green peas and boiled potato	Cooked carrots and potato
Bread or *chappatis*	*Dal*
Ice-cream	Bread or *chappatis*
	Jallebi or pudding

REFERENCES

[1] ANTIA, F.P., DESAI, H.G., JEEJEEBHOY, K.N., and BORKAR, A.V. (1964) Incidence of intestinal helminths in Bombay, *Indian J. med. Sci.,* **18,** 635.

[2] SANDERSON, K.V. (1967) Hair-fall in blood-donors, *Lancet,* **i,** 681.

[3] FOY, H., KONDI, A., and SARMA, B. (1958) Anaemias of the tropics, India and Ceylon, *J. trop. Med. Hyg.,* **61,** 27.

[4] ROCHE, M., PEREZ-GIMENEZ, M.E., LAYRISSE, M., and DI PRISCO, E. (1957) Study of urinary and faecal excretion of radioactive chromium C^{51} in

man. Its loss associated with hookworm infestation, *J. clin. Invest.*, **36**, 1183.

[5] LAYRISSE, M., APARCEDO, L., MARTINES-TORRES, C., and ROCHE, M. (1967) Blood loss due to infection with *Trichuris trichiura*, *Amer. J. trop. Med. Hyg.*, **16**, 613.

[6] BRADIFIELD, R.B., *et al.* (1968) Effect of low levels of iron and trace elements on haematological values of parasitized school children, *Amer. J. clin. Nutr.*, **21**, 68.

[7] FARID, Z., PATWARDHAN, V.N., and DARBY, W.J. (1969) Parasitism and anaemia, *Amer. J. clin. Nutr.*, **22**, 498.

[8] WATSON-WILLIAMS, E.J. (1968) Anaemia in the tropics, *Brit. med. J.*, **4**, 34.

[9] FRY, J. (1961) Clinical patterns and course of anaemias in general practice, *Brit. med. J.*, **2**, 1732.

[10] ROSELLE, H.A. (1970) Association of laundry starch and clay ingestion with anaemia in New York City, *Arch. intern. Med.*, **125**, 57.

[11] ELWOOD, P.C., WATERS, W.E., and GREENE, W.J.W. (1970) Evaluation of iron supplements in prevention of iron-deficiency anaemia, *Lancet*, **ii**, 175.

66. UNDERWEIGHT

In Western countries obesity is common while in the tropics people are often underweight due to poverty or lack of dietetic knowledge. Sometimes poor physique is due to debilitating diseases like tuberculosis, the malabsorption syndrome, diabetes or cancer. A person who is underweight is specially liable to tuberculosis and acute infectious diseases, though some sturdy hill tribes, despite being underweight, have amazing stamina.

Tonics

A large sum of money is spent in every country on tonics, vitamins and chicken extracts for increasing weight. With a limited budget the same money could more wisely be spent on nourishing, high caloric foods. Tonics are only helpful to improve the appetite in debilitating diseases. Vitamins are indispensable for life but they do not increase weight. Expensive extracts of chicken do not supply appreciable calories.

Hypoglycaemic Drugs

Insulin reduces the blood sugar and increases the secretion of gastric juice and peristalsis. Plain insulin may be injected subcutaneously 20–30 minutes before the principal meals in sufficient dosage (about 7 Units) to produce a feeling of hunger, care being taken that the meals are taken at regular intervals. Injections of long-acting insulin once a day have also been used. Oral hypoglycaemic agents are more convenient than insulin and may be tried for a short period [1].

It is more difficult to increase weight than to lose it and perseverance is essential. If the thin individual is very active then adequate rest should be advised.

Cyproheptadine hydrochloride, an anti-allergic drug, increases the electrical activity of the hypothalamic feeding centre [2] and in underweight subjects produces weight gain [3], but also tends to produce drowsiness.

Calories

For increasing weight the total calorie intake should be in excess of energy requirements. If an individual needs 2000 Calories for his normal activity then a diet containing 2500 Calories should be prescribed. The increase should be gradual over the course of one or two weeks otherwise digestive disturbances may occur.

Proteins

A liberal supply of protein, over 1·2 g per kg, is necessary for tissue building.

Fats

High-calorie fatty foods such as cream, butter, margarine and oils help to increase the weight. Fatty foods should not be taken at the beginning of a meal as they reduce appetite. A sudden increase in fatty foods may produce diarrhoea.

Carbohydrates

Leafy vegetables with a low carbohydrate content should be restricted and preference given to those with a high calorie equivalent like potato and yam. Cereals and cereal products such as bread and biscuits, supply many calories at low cost.

Vitamins and Minerals

With a liberal diet there is no necessity for extra vitamin and mineral supplements.

Fluids

Fluids should not be taken before or with a meal but only after a meal so that food intake is not reduced.

Exercise and Bowels

Regular outdoor exercise helps to stimulate the appetite. Constipation may reduce the appetite so the bowel movements should be regulated with adequate fluids, exercise and fruits like stewed figs, apricots or prunes.

Principle of Diet

High-calorie, high-protein, high-fat and high-carbohydrate diet. (High-calorie foods are cereal and cereal products, pulses including *chana,* groundnuts, potato, yam, fats and oils, desserts, sweets, nuts, dried fruits).

UNDERWEIGHT

Foods	*Remarks*
Bread or *chappatis** of wheat, rice, maize, *bajra, ragi* or *jowar*	Permitted
Breakfast cereal of wheat, rice, oatmeal or maize	Permitted
Rice*, cooked	Permitted
Pulses (*dal*) or beans*	Permitted
Meat or fish or chicken	Permitted
Eggs	Permitted
Milk or milk products*	Permitted
Soup	Permitted
Vegetable salad	Permitted in smaller quantity to allow intake of other high calorie foods
Vegetables, cooked	Permitted
Potato, sweet potato or yam*	Permitted
Fat for cooking*	Permitted
Sugar, jaggery, or honey*	Permitted
Jam or *murabba**	Permitted
Pastry*	Permitted
Dessert*	Permitted
Sweets or sweetmeat*	Permitted

Foods	*Remarks*
Fruits, fresh	Permitted
Fruits, dried*	Permitted
Nuts*	Permitted
Condiments	In moderation
Papad, chutney, pickles	In moderation
Beverages	Permitted, preferably with extra milk
Fluid	Liberal but not before or during meals

N.B.—Brisk walk or exercise or outdoor games morning and evening.
* Foods which when taken in larger quantity provide high calories.

UNDERWEIGHT
SAMPLE MENU

Mixed Diet	*Vegetarian Diet*

Breakfast

Stewed prunes	Stewed figs or apricots
Cornflakes, 1 cup with milk and sugar	Porridge with milk and honey
Eggs, fried	Toast, 3 to 4 or *chappatis* with butter and jam
Toast, 3 to 4 with butter and jam	Banana
Banana	Tea
Tea or coffee	

11 a.m.

Cocoa in milk, 1 cup	Milk, 1 cup
	Biscuits

Lunch

Meat cutlets, 2 with fried potatoes and peas	Curd, 1 cup
Macaroni and cheese or rice with curry	Potato mashed in butter
	French beans
	Rice with *dal*
Bread and butter	Bread and butter or *chappatis* with *ghee*
Fruit salad with cream	Groundnuts
Walnuts	

Mixed Diet	*Vegetarian Diet*

4.30 p.m.

Tea	Tea
Biscuits or sandwiches	Cake or coconut water and kernel or milk, 1 cup

Dinner

Fried fish	Buttermilk, 1 cup
Roast chicken with baked potato and fried lady's fingers	*Dal,* 1 cup
	Brinjals fried
Bread with butter	Bread with butter or *chappati* with *ghee*
Pudding	Ice cream

Before retiring

Glass of milk	Glass of milk with honey, 1 tablespoon.

N.B.—The quantity of food should be increased gradually.

REFERENCE

[1] HOENIG, J., and GITTLESON, N.L. (1961) Weight gaining: a therapeutic trial with tolbutamide, *Brit. med. J.,* **2,** 1403.
[2] CHAKRAVARTY, A.S., PILLAI, R.V., ANAND, B.K., and SINGH, R.V. (1967) Effect of cyproheptadine on the electrical activity of the hypothalamus feeding centre, *Brain Res.,* **6,** 561.
[3] SARDESAI, H.V., *et al.* (1970) Weight gain with cyproheptadine hydrochloride ('Periactin'). A double blind trial in underweight medical students, *Indian. J. med. Sci.,* **24,** 716.

67. OBESITY

Obesity is a weighty problem. Obesity can be defined as the generalized accumulation of excess fat in the body. It invites disability, diseases and premature death. Excess fat is as much a physical hindrance as carrying a load of the same weight day and night. It gives rise to breathlessness on moderate exertion such as climbing stairs. Obesity predisposes to diseases like angina pectoris, coronary thrombosis,

high blood pressure, stroke, diabetes, gall-bladder disease and osteo-
arthritis of weight-bearing joints. Surgical operations and pregnancy
carry an increased risk in the obese.

Life expectancy diminishes with excess weight. Life insurance statistics
bear out the fact that 'an extra inch at the waist line is a year less of
life line'. The mortality of men who are 10 per cent overweight is
about one-fifth higher than average and in those who are more than
20 per cent overweight the excess mortality is about one-third [1].

Obesity is due either to : (1) excess calorie consumption, or
(2) decreased energy output and lack of exercise. *Excess weight* compared to the average weight does not necessarily mean obesity. For
the extra weight may be due to body fluid, bone or muscles. The tradi-
tional height-weight-age tables do not give a valid measure of leanness
or fatness of an individual. The triceps and subscapular *skin-fold
measurements* give better assessment. Their standards for British children
are available [2]. In routine medical practice only a glance at the bulging abdomen in males and unduly prominent hips in females, is
adequate for the diagnosis of obesity.

Fatty Tissue in Obesity.   Excessive weight gain during the first 6 months
of life usually tends to obesity in later life [3]. The *number* of fat cells are
apparently determined early in life. With increasing age the fatty
tissues loose the ability to grow in number, hence after adulthood
the fat cells increase only in *size* but not in number. Conversely, reduction in the weight of an adult, reduces only the fat cell size but not
the number [4]. The increase in the number of fat cells may be due to
endocrine, behavioural, genetic factors or a mixture of these factors [5].
The knowledge that the *number of adipose cells is increased at juvenile
onset of obesity* explains lifelong struggle of some people to reduce
weight. Thus over-nutrition in childhood by the doting mother has
to be guarded against.

The larger the adipose cell size, the less sensitive they are to *insulin*.
After weight reduction, the decrease in size of the fat cells permits
glucose entry into the cells and the insulin sensitivity returns to
normal [6]. The improved carbohydrate tolerance after reducing weight
is because enough room has been created to allow glucose to be deposited
in the cell by the action of insulin.

Appetite.   In the hypothalamus there are two pairs of nuclei, median
and lateral, which regulate appetite. Experimentally, a lesion of the

median nuclei increases appetite while a lesion of the lateral nuclei results in loss of appetite. The functions of these nuclei are regulated by the higher cortical centres in the brain. Thus, a happy frame of mind and pleasant surroundings, as during a picnic, will stimulate the appetite. A decrease in the blood sugar level stimulates the vagal centres in the medulla, thereby causing hunger contractions of the stomach and increasing secretion of gastric juice.

Aetiology

Overeating. Overeating is the prime factor in obesity. Any excess of ingested calories over energy expenditure is stored as fat. Obesity is like a bank account. If a person takes in 2500 Calories daily and his calorie output is 2300, then he saves 200 Calories which are stored as fat. An extra slice of bread or a banana provides 50–100 Calories and such slight excess amounts to a considerable accumulation in the course of time. *Dietary habit* also plays a part in determining body weight. From a variety of foods, a fat person usually chooses fried potatoes while a thin person prefers vegetable salad.

Obesity does not depend upon the quantity of food eaten but on its calorie equivalent. Cucumber provides 16 Calories per 100 g but the same weight of roasted groundnuts (peanuts) is equivalent to 600 Calories. Usually an obese person solemnly declares that he eats very little, which may be true if his diet consists mainly of butter, bread, cheese and sweets. His food has a higher calorie equivalent but quantitatively he takes much less than his lean brother who prefers fruit and vegetables.

Psychology of Eating. In some cases overeating is a compensatory mechanism to attain self-satisfaction when there has been failure or frustration in life. Obese individuals eat more if excess food is *served on the table* but are unlikely to make even a small effort to open a near-at-hand refrigerator to get more food [7]. *Not bringing more food to the table* is the best method for avoiding temptation to over-eat. A housewife with children is more exposed to food and more likely to be obese than a woman working in an office.

Frequency of Meals. Those taking three meals showed a greater tendency to overweight, to increased serum cholesterol, and to diminished glucose tolerance than those taking five meals [8]. However, on a low calorie diet the weight loss was the same regardless of the frequency of meals [9]. People with insomnia and in the habit of eating when awake at night will definitely increase in weight due to the enhanced calorie intake. *It is the total intake of calories rather than the frequency of meals* that determines the weight change. With the constant calorie intake, whether to advise three or more frequent meals is best judged from the convenience and habit of the individual.

Sedentary Habits. Obesity is most common after the age of 35. Most of us do more physical work and also take more exercise before this age than in later life. With the approach of middle age, promotion to executive jobs involves longer hours at the desk with less physical work. Food consumption either remains the same or may even increase with the improved economic status.

Hormones. Dysfunction of the *thyroid, pituitary* or *suprarenals* may result in obesity. The female sex hormones also play a role as obesity may occur after pregnancy, after removal of the ovaries or uterus, or at menopause. If there is an underlying endocrine cause, its treatment results in more encouraging response to diet. *Insulin,* as stated above, plays a contributory role in obesity.

Smoking. Cessation of smoking increases weight not only by increased food intake but also due to reduced metabolism and oxygen consumption [10]

Heredity. The role of heredity in obesity is not well understood. It is possible that abnormal genes may be responsible for excessive hunger or an imbalance of the endocrine glands or a tendency to deposit fat. However, the dietetic habit of a family rather than hereditary factors may be responsible for obesity. The children of a family who eat fried foods, cereals, milk products and sweets will be heavier than their neighbours who relish green vegetables, fruits and meat.

Metabolism in Obesity

The excess calories consumed are not all converted into an increase in weight, but are also disposed of by excess heat production. The expenditure of energy by healthy subjects under basal conditions, or on sitting or standing up show appreciable variations. The *basal* metabolic rate (BMR) may not rise but the metabolism is increased immediately after a meal and during exercise [11]. In the obese the blood sugar, triglycerides as well as insulin levels are high, suggesting insulin resistance. Insulin enhances the deposition of glucose and triglycerides in the normal cells but not in enlarged fat cells. A high carbohydrate diet increases blood sugar and further stimulates *beta* cells, which after a course of time may be exhausted, resulting in diabetes. The increased triglycerides in the blood may also partly be due to increased synthesis in the obese.

Fads of the Fat

Every fat individual has his own theories as to the cause and treatment of obesity. He sincerely believes that some mechanism other than his high calorie diet has caused his obesity. Similarly, for treatment he tries everything else but a low calorie diet. Some believe they are fat because they drink too much water in between meals or during the day. If it were possible for water to provide calories and be stored as fat the greatest problem in the world, that of feeding the population would immediately disappear. The frustrated obese patient in his never ending search for a new method of losing weight may try sour lime in the early morning which may erode the enamel and destroy his teeth. A kindly friend may advise him to take a particular food-stuff having a 'specific reducing property'. This food-stuff, if it is in excess of his total calorie requirement, merely increases his waist line. Some purists try to avoid mixing proteins, fats or carbohydrates at a meal. This needs special foods as all our commonly used natural foods are combinations of proteins, fat and carbohydrates, except sugar which is pure carbohydrate, and oils and animal fats which provide pure fat. The juices of our alimentary canal are designed by nature for the digestion of mixed food. All types of 'mono diet' like the meat diet, egg diet and buttermilk diet usually result in monotony and this may reduce appetite.

Some clinics have advocated a highly effective, extremely low calorie diet by which the patient loses 2–4 kg in a week or two. These drastic measures can only be enthusiastically undertaken for a short period and then the patient reverts to his usual diet or may even eat excessively with a result that he may become fatter than before. It has been observed that after a period of low food intake during a prolonged fever like typhoid, a thin individual puts on weight when he resumes his usual food. Thus the enthusiast who loses 4 kg in two weeks by drastic diets, may, on resumption of his usual food, gain 10 kg by the end of 20 weeks.

Massage

Massage only helps the masseur to reduce his own weight. For the patient the massage is a passive activity which hardly utilizes any calories. When weight is lost on a low calorie diet the skin becomes lax and wrinkled and this can be prevented by massage. Massage therefore does not reduce weight but during appreciable reduction helps in maintaining the elasticity of the skin. Massage can also help to break painful fatty lumps.

Steam Baths

What patient would not prefer to 'sweat out' 1–2 kg within an hour, in a steam chamber, rather than achieve the same weight loss by two to four weeks of 'tears and toil' on a reducing diet? Unfortunately he sweats in vain. After sudden profuse sweating the sole craving of an exhausted and weak patient is to drink water which the dehydrated tissues retain. The original weight is thus restored. Dehydration also predisposes to renal calculi and even coronary thrombosis. A steam bath may help jockeys or prize fighters who are a few pounds overweight to lose weight for the 'weigh in' but it has no place in the treatment of obesity.

WEIGHT REDUCTION AND MAINTENANCE

1. *A determination to follow a low calorie diet* is the basic requirement before any reducing programme is started. Only a mentally well adjusted individual can succeed in losing weight, for diet and exercise must be pursued with devout zeal. No amount of mere wishing has ever shed even a gramme of weight. Those who have no determination are always talking to their friends or doctors in the hope of finding out about some 'secret' pills or food instead of taking a low calorie diet.

2. A medical check is necessary before commencing a reducing programme.

3. The dietetic programme consists of: (a) a low calorie diet designed to reduce the weight by 3–4 kg per month till the ideal body weight is reached; (b) a moderate calorie diet to maintain the ideal weight for three to six months; (c) a reversion to the usual diet with such a mental reorientation that foods of high calorie value are taken in small judicious helpings.

The patient is checked every week while on a reducing diet and a loss in weight of 3–4 kg is expected by the end of the month. The weight loss is more rapid during the first month than during the subsequent months. If there is no loss of weight the patient may not be following the instructions rigidly and details of all foods taken by the patient should be reviewed. It is not unusual to find that extra bread, nuts or cream are the cause of trouble. Obese people tend to find loopholes in the instructions and take prohibited foods because no clear statement has been made about them. A written dietetic prescription should always be given with definite instructions *to exclude all other foods not mentioned*.

4. Not taking breakfast may sharply increase the appetite at lunch. Three regular meals should, therefore, be taken.

5. With a low food and fluid intake, constipation may occur. This can usually be avoided by ensuring that the diet contains adequate fluids and bulk-producing vegetables and fruits. If necessary, milk of magnesia is advised.

6. Exercise according to the capacity of the patient is recommended.

Exercise. The claim of some fat people that they eat less than average may in fact be true if they have less energy expenditure due to sedentary habits and complete lack of exercise. Self-consciousness prevents the obese from taking part in sports, particularly those where scanty clothing reveals their anatomy. Avoiding open-air sports or swimming exercises enhances obesity. Cinematographic studies have demonstrated that even though the obese participate in sports, they are relatively less active on the field compared to others [12]. We do not require scientifically planned experiments to observe that those who take regular moderate exercise are seldom obese. Thus, if a fat person takes moderate exercise with a low calorie diet he will almost always lose weight.

Metabolism during Weight Reduction

Calories. The initial weight loss in the obese is of salt and water. The subsequent loss of adipose tissue depends upon a *low calorie intake* regardless of whether it is derived from carbohydrate, fat or proteins. It is not possible to calculate mathematically the weight loss from the calories advised, because on chronic caloric restriction the *body reduces* metabolic oxidation and energy expenditure [13]. Though counting calories is the fundamental concept in sustained weight reduction, exercise and physical activities are very important adjuvants.

Carbohydrates. With constant calorie intake, a low carbohydrate and high fat diet was claimed to reduce more weight than high carbohydrate diet, but this is not so [14]. On a 400 calorie diet ketosis increases with fat diet and decreases with a carbohydrate diet, while calories from proteins and fats result in raised blood urea, uric acid and lipids, particularly cholesterol. Thus, a low carbohydrate diet may be hazardous [15].

Drugs

To eat and yet reduce weight with a pill is the perpetual hope of all fat people who are an easy prey to the advertisement of reducing tablets. Drugs are utterly useless in a reducing regimen except in specific glandular deficiencies or occasionally for reducing the appetite. The commonly used drugs are:

Thyroid. The most grateful patients are those with hypothyroidism who improve after adequate treatment with thyroid extract. Unless thyroid deficiency is proved, the routine administration of thyroid to obese persons is not desirable.

Appetite Reducing Drugs. The anorectic drugs are amphetamine, fenfluramine (*Ponderex*), diethylpropion (*Tenvate*), phenmetrazine (*Preludin*), etc. These drugs are not substitutes for low calorie diet and exercise. They are not safe without medical supervision, and, unless the diet is regulated, weight reduction does not occur.

Diuretics and Purgatives. Diuretics and purgatives have the same temporary effect as a steam bath, and, unless definitely indicated, they may be harmful.

Formula Diets. Expensive canned formula diets, with added vitamins, which supply less than 1000 Calories per tin are available commercially. They contain hydrophilic substances which absorb water in the stomach and produce a sense of satiety. Such foods are readily taken by obese patients for a few days and they are satisfied by noting some reduction in weight. However, with the resumption of their ususal diet the original weight is quickly restored. It is difficult to understand the psychology of those who, like experimental laboratory animals, feed themselves on processed formulae. These formulae have the disadvantage that they do not permit the patient to get any knowledge of what foods to eat and what foods to avoid when the usual diet is resumed.

Summary. There are no drugs which can be used with advantage in the treatment of obesity. Unless the patient really desires to lose weight, no reduction occurs without an unshakable will to follow the low calorie diets. The obese person who wants to rely on drugs has no real will to reduce and never succeeds in losing his excess weight and maintaining it.

Fasting

Total fasting, allowing only water and multivitamins, for a prolonged period is the quickest method of losing weight. The average weight loss of 7–8 kg during the first 10–12 days is subsequently more gradual. Prolonged fasting up to 249 days is reported [16]. Such a regimen has only been followed under hospital conditions.

The *dangers* of fasting include electrolyte imbalance, loss of hair, fatty liver, abnormal electrocardiogram, lapse in memory, gouty attack in a susceptible patient, and even death with the post-mortem finding of fragmentation of heart muscle fibres [17]. Therapeutic fasting is hazardous and no more efficacious than caloric restriction in the obese [18], and follow-up studies after a few months may show regain of the weight lost [19].

Jejuno-ileal Shunt

In the markedly obese, the proximal 35 cm of jejunum is anastomosed to the terminal 10 cm of the ileum to reduce small intestinal food absorption. The initial rapid decline in weight after a time stabilizes at a lower level. The resultant loose skin requires plastic surgery. The adverse metabolic effects of jejuno-ileal shunt have not yet been fully assessed. There is diarrhoea, water, electrolyte and vitamin deficiency, hernia, liver dysfunction and fatty liver. Jejunal shunts in morbid obesity must be considered an *experimental procedure* which cannot be commended for wide application [20]. 'Obesity is a risk undertaken voluntarily, like smoking or pregnancy or oral contraception. As long as the patient understands the risks, and in this instance is given every encouragement to reduce food intake and increase activity, the doctor has performed his proper function. It is not his job to increase the risks of the obese's life with drastic cures' [21] such as fasting or jejuno-ileal shunt.

Dangers of Rapid Reduction

Very rapid weight reduction may prove harmful. Drastic reduction may follow a self-administered diet or an extremely low calorie diet published in a popular magazine.

1. *Hernia.* A latent umbilical or inguinal hernia may become manifest or a hernia may develop due to diminution of fat in the hernial sac and to straining during defaecation. To prevent the development of a hernia, light abdominal exercise should be taken regularly and constipation avoided.

2. *Gall-bladder disease.* Drastic weight reduction can cause gall-bladder disease [22]. This effect may be due to an increase in blood lipids, particularly cholesterol. Drastic reducing diets do not contain fat and it is also possible that the stimulus to gall-bladder contraction is therefore lacking and is responsible for biliary stagnation and resultant cholecystitis.

3. *Peptic ulcer, haematemesis and melaena.* Starvation may cause bleeding from a peptic ulcer. This may be due to lack of neutralization of gastric juice by food.

DIETETIC MANAGEMENT

Calories

The guiding principle of all reducing diets is to provide few calories. It is not the quantity of food but the low calorie equivalent that produces weight loss. Unless there are special indications, the patient is allowed to continue with his routine work. About 20 Calories per kilogram of ideal body weight are prescribed for a sedentary worker and 25 Calories for a moderately active worker.

Proteins

Proteins are necessary for tissue repair and have a high specific dynamic action. About 1 g of protein per kg bodyweight may be given.

Fats

Since fats are a concentrated source of energy they should be restricted. It is best to supply the quota of fats as vegetable oils (except coconut and palm) so that enough essential fatty acids are supplied for proper nutrition.

Carbohydrates

To produce a feeling of satiety, and regular bowel movements, bulk-producing carbohydrates like green vegetables and fruits are liberally prescribed. Starches with a high carbohydrate content like potatoes and rice, are restricted.

Weight Loss with Various Foods

The weight loss is proportionate to the intake of calories as long as proteins, fats and carbohydrates are taken in the usual proportions. Experimentally, if 1000 Calories are supplied for a short period as a diet containing a disproportionate amount of fat or carbohydrate, then with a high fat diet the weight reduction is more rapid than with a high carbohydrate diet. The weight loss with a constant calorie intake therefore varies with the composition of diet. The insensible loss of water rises with a high fat and a high protein diet and falls with a high carbohydrate diet [23]. The advantage of a high fat low calorie diet is short-lived, however, and the rate of weight loss over a prolonged period is no greater than from an isocaloric diet consisting mainly of carbohydrate [24].

Vitamins

With prolonged restriction of fats there is likely to be a deficiency of fat-soluble vitamins A and D, which may be supplemented.

Minerals

Restriction of sodium as common salt is helpful in a weight reducing diet. Excess sodium in the body predisposes to the retention of fluid.

Fluids

If salt is restricted then fluids can be taken liberally as extra fluids are excreted by the healthy kidneys. A glass of water taken before meals may help to cut down the intake of food.

MANAGEMENT AFTER REDUCTION

During weight reduction and *after* achieving normal weight a follow-up is necessary. Not infrequently the patient loses weight to show his self-control and please the doctor. Advising patients to carefully note the time, quantity and type of food taken, makes them conscious of the value of foods and guides them for the future control of obesity. A personal diary and a weighing scale therefore play a great part in the actions of a motivated patient.

Many people, having achieved the goal of reduction to a desired weight, want to celebrate. They crave for the foods they have been denied. This impulse should be checked as otherwise months of effort will be in vain. They should, however, feel free to eat foods which they were used to taking and should have the privilege of enjoying themselves at parties. This can be only achieved if there is an honest attempt to follow the following instructions.

1. Take all foods as desired but avoid snacks between meals and *restrict helpings* of: (a) cereal products, mainly bread and *chappatis* or *puris;* (b) fried foods and foods to which fat is added liberally for cooking; (c) milk products prepared from cream or butter; (d) nuts; and (e) desserts.

2. Check the weight at least every week on a reliable scale. A serious view should be taken of even a kilogram of excess weight. Foods mentioned in the above paragraph should be completely stopped till the ideal weight is regained.

3. Daily exercise should be taken with the same enthusiasm and zeal as during the reducing programme. After the excess weight has been lost, the enthusiasm for daily exercise should be maintained.

OBESITY

Daily Ration

	Mixed Diet	Vegetarian Diet
Bread or *chappati* of wheat, rice, maize, *jowar, bajra* or *ragi*	3 slices of bread or 6 thin *chappatis* of wheat or 3 small *chappatis* of other cereal	3 slices of bread or 6 thin *chappatis* of wheat or 3 small *chappatis* of other cereal
Breakfast cereal of w h e a t, r i c e, oatmeal or maize	Excluded	Excluded

Daily Ration

	Mixed Diet	Vegetarian Diet
Rice	Excluded	Excluded
Pulses (*dal*) or beans	¾ cup thin *dal*	1½ cup thin *dal*
Meat, fish or chicken	2 small helpings	—
Eggs	2	—
Milk or milk products	1 cup skimmed milk (cow's or buffalo's)	2 cups skimmed milk (cow's or buffalo's)
Soup	2 cups thin soup	2 or 3 cups thin soup
Vegetable salad	Permitted	Permitted
Vegetables, cooked (tender)	Permitted	Permitted
Potato, sweet potato yam	Excluded	Excluded
Sugar, jaggery or honey	3 teaspoons	3 teaspoons
Jam or *murabba*	Excluded	Excluded
Pastry	Excluded	Excluded
Dessert	Permitted from the above ration of milk and sugar	Permitted from the above ration of milk and sugar
Sweet or sweetmeat	Excluded	Excluded
Fruit, fresh	3 average helpings	3 average helpings
Fruit, dried	Excluded	Excluded
Nuts	Excluded	Excluded
Condiments and spices	Moderation	Moderation
Papad, chutney and pickles	Moderation, exclude pickle in oil	Moderation, exclude pickle in oil
Beverages	Tea or coffee from daily ration of milk and sugar mentioned above	Tea or coffee from daily ration of milk and sugar mentioned above
Fluids	Liberal	Liberal

OBESITY
SAMPLE MENU

Mixed Diet	*Vegetarian Diet*

Morning

Tea, 1 cup with milk*, 2 table-spoons, sugar, 1 teaspoon**

Tea, 1 cup with milk*, 2 table-spoons, sugar**, 1 teaspoon

Breakfast

Eggs, 2 half-boiled or poached or scrambled in milk*
Toast, 1
Orange or grape fruit

Skimmed milk*, 1 cup
Toast, 1 or *khakhra*, 2
Sweet lime

Lunch

Meat soup, 1 cup
Boiled fish or roast mutton
Vegetable salad from radish, tomato, cucumber, lettuce with dressing of vinegar, pepper and sour lime
Cooked french beans
Bread, 1 slice or *chappatis*, 2
Papaya, ½ or pear, 1

Mixed vegetable soup, 1 cup
Thin *dal*, ¾ cup
Vegetable salad from radish, tomato, cucumber, lettuce with dressing of vinegar, pepper and sour lime
Cooked pumpkin
Bread, 1 slice or *chappatis*, 2
Custard apple

4 p.m.

Tea with 2 tablespoons milk*, sugar, 1 teaspoon**

Tea with 2 tablespoons milk*, and sugar**, 1 teaspoon

6 p.m.

Apple, 1

Orange

Dinner

Chicken soup, 1 cup
Chicken, roast
Cooked brinjals
Bread, 1 slice or *chappatis*, 2
Brown custard prepared with the remainder of ration of milk* and sugar**

Tomato soup, 1 cup
Skimmed milk* curd, ½ cup
Cooked carrots
Thin *dal*, ¾ cup
Bread, 1 slice or *chappatis*, 2
Ice cream prepared from the remainder of ration of milk* and sugar**

Daily ration
  * Milk, skimmed (cow's or buffalo's), 1 cup
  ** Sugar, 3 teaspoons

Daily ration
  * Milk, skimmed (cow's or buffalo's), 2 cups
  ** Sugar, 3 teaspoons

REFERENCES

[1] BRITISH MEDICAL JOURNAL (1970) The overweight child, *Brit. med. J.*, **2**, 64.

[2] TANNER, J.M., and WHITEHOUSE, R.H. (1962) Standards for subcutaneous fat in British children: percentiles for thickness of skin-folds over triceps and below scapula, *Brit. med. J.*, **4**, 46.

[3] EID, E.E. (1970) Follow-up study on physical growth of children who have excessive weight gain in first six months of life, *Brit. med. J.*, **2**, 74.

[4] BRAY, G.A. (1970) Measurement of subcutaneous fat cells from obese patients, *Ann. intern. Med.*, **73**, 565.

[5] HIRSCH, J., and KNITTLE, J.L. (1970) Cellularity of obese and non-obese adipose tissue, *Fed. Proc.*, **29**, 1516.

[6] SALANS, L.B., KNITTLE, J.L., and HIRSCH, J. (1968) Role of adipose cell size and adipose tissue insulin sensitivity in the carbohydrate intolerance in human obesity, *J. clin. Invest.*, **47**, 153.

[7] NISBETT, R.E. (1968) Determinants of food intake in obesity, *Science*, **159**, 1254.

[8] FABRY, P., *et al.* (1964) Frequency of meals. Its relation to overweight, hypercholesterolaemia, and decreased glucose tolerance, *Lancet*, **ii**, 614.

[9] BORTZ, W.M., *et al.* (1966) Weight loss and frequency of feeding, *New Engl. J. Med.*, **274**, 376.

[10] GLAUSER, S.C., *et al.* (1970) Metabolic changes associated with the cessation of cigarette smoking, *Arch. environm. Hlth*, **20**, 377.

[11] MILLER, D.S., MUMFORD, P., and STOCK, M.J. (1967) Gluttony. 2. Thermogenesis in overeating man, *Amer. J. clin.Nutr.*, **20**, 1223.

[12] BULLEN, B.A., REED, R.B., and MAYER, J. (1964) Physical activity of obese and non-obese adolescent girls appraised by motion picture sampling, *Amer. J. clin. Nutr.*, **14**, 211.

[13] BRAY, G.A. (1969) Effect of caloric restriction on energy expenditure in obese patients, *Lancet*, **ii**, 397.

[14] BORTZ, W.M., WROLDSON, A., MORRIS, P., and ISSEKUTZ, B. (1967) Fat, carbohydrate, salt and weight loss, *Amer. J. clin. Nutr.*, **20**, 1104.

[15] KREHL, W.A., LOPEZ, S.A., GOOD, E.I., and HODGES, R.E. (1967) Some metabolic changes induced by low carbohydrate diet, *Amer. J. clin. Nutr.*, **20**, 139.

[16] THOMPSON, T.J., RUNCIE, J., and MILLER, V. (1966) Treatment of obesity by total fasting for up to 249 days, *Lancet*, **ii**, 992.

[17] GARNETT, E.S., *et al.* (1969) Gross fragmentation of cardiac myofibrils after therapeutic starvation for obesity, *Lancet*, **i**, 914.

[18] ROOTH, G., and CARLSTROM, S. (1970) Therapeutic fasting, *Acta med. scand.*, **187**, 455.

[19] MACCUISH, A.C., MUNRO, J.F., and DUNCAN, L.J.P. (1968) Follow-up study of refractory obesity treated by fasting, *Brit. med. J.*, **1**, 91.

[20] SCOTT, H.W., *et al.* (1970) Jejunoileal shunt in surgical treatment of morbid obesity, *Ann. Surg.*, **171**, 770.

[21] LANCET (1970) Drastic cures for obese, *Lancet*, **i**, 1094.

[22] CROHN, B.B. (1959) Some effects of too rapid weight reduction, in *World*

Congress of Gastroenterology, Washington, D.C. 1958, Vol. I, Baltimore, p. 478.

[23] KEKWICH, A., and PAWAN, G.L.S. (1956) Caloric intake in relation to body-weight changes in the obese, *Lancet,* ii, 155.

[24] PILKINGTON, T.R.E., GAINSBOROUGH, H., ROSENOER, V.M., and CAREY, M. (1960) Diet and weight-reduction in the obese, *Lancet,* i, 856.

68. DIABETES MELLITUS

There is no disease which provokes greater thought on diet than diabetes. Many unfortunate diabetics, dreading a strict dietetic regimen for the rest of their life, try pills, herbs and infusions, strongly recommended by friends and relatives, who claim to have tried them and appear symptom-free without a diet. These specifics are claimed to be so potent and effective that urine or blood examinations for sugar are declared unnecessary. This happy state continues till suddenly they wake up one night with a complication of diabetes like a paralytic stroke, coronary thrombosis or blindness. Others may not wake up, and pass into coma.

Diabetes mellitus (diabetes = flow through, mel = honey) is a chronic metabolic disorder, with a strong hereditary basis, with high blood sugar and is usually associated with passage of sugar in the urine.

Diabetes is no more a dreaded disease. *A well managed* diabetic has a good expectancy of life. *Neglect* of the condition produces irreparable damage to the arteries during the course of years. Most of the complications of diabetes are due to gradual and irreversible arterial damage, which may ultimately lead to gangrene, apoplexy, coronary infarction, kidney disease or blindness. Diet is the sheet-anchor of treatment in obese elderly diabetics and a useful supplement to insulin therapy in younger ones.

Unfortunately diabetes in the earlier stages can be symptomless and patients tend to neglect the disease. Cases are usually discovered at a routine life insurance examination, or a physical check up in industry or when urine is examined pre-operatively or for ailments like sciatica, boils or carbuncles.

Insulin

Insulin, produced by the *beta* cells of the islets of Langerhans in the pancreas, is necessary for the proper metabolism of glucose. The usually accepted view is that diabetes is due to a deficiency of insulin in young thin subjects but not necessarily so in the elderly obese diabetics.

Normal Insulin Requirement. The approximate daily insulin requirement in a non-diabetic whose pancreas is removed is 40 Units daily. It should not be concluded from this that the normal pancreas secretes about 40 Units of insulin per day. With removal of the pancreas the insulin requirement is reduced as food is not absorbed so well. Furthermore, the *alpha* cells, which produce the hyperglycaemic substance, glucagon, are removed together with the *beta* cells. It has been estimated that even 10 per cent of functioning pancreatic tissue is enough to prevent diabetes.

Patients with pancreatitis are also more sensitive to insulin due to decreased glucagon secretion. After a hypoglycaemic attack, and following insulin therapy, the patient may develop *insulin resistance*.

One milligram of pure insulin measures 24 International Units. Serum insulin measured by the immunological method is known as *immunoreactive insulin* (IRI). Serum, rather than plasma, insulin should be assayed since the addition of heparin shows a higher plasma insulin level [1].

'Little' insulin is the hitherto known, usual normal insulin released from the *beta* cells of the pancreas. *Proinsulin ('big' insulin)* has a larger molecule and is the precursor of the smaller molecule (*'little'* insulin). During pancreatic stimulation with glucose, after a couple of hours the newly formed 'big' insulin is prematurely released and found circulating in the blood [2]. Epinephrine and norepinephrine inhibit insulin release.

Action. Insulin regulates carbohydrate, fat and protein metabolism. Insulin allows: (1) glucose penetration into the cell membrane; (2) synthesis of fatty acids from carbohydrates; and (3) amino acid transport into the cell for the formation of tissue proteins. In the *absence* of insulin: (a) the blood sugar is raised and liver glycogen is depleted; (b) serum lipids increase and ketone bodies accumulate in the blood; (c) the liver converts amino acids to glucose (gluconeogenesis) with increased nitrogen excretion. This reduces protein synthesis. Insulin is the only hormone that promotes storage of fatty acids in the cells against about 11 hormones which tend to release cellular fatty acids.

Glucagon.

Alpha cells of the pancreas secrete *pancreatic glucagon. Enteroglucagon* is secreted by the intestine and its action is identical to that of pancreatic glucagon. Apparently the action of insulin is the opposite of that of glucagon, but paradoxically glucagon promotes insulin secretion. Oral glucose increases plasma glucagon, which stimulates insulin release [3]. Glucagon stimulates: (1) secretion of insulin; (2) hepatic glucose formation from amino acid (gluconeogenesis); and (3) the breakdown of hepatic glycogen to release glucose (glycogenolysis). Glucagon is an essential hormone in blood sugar homeostasis and helps to raise the blood sugar level. *Decreased* glucagon secretion produces hypoglycaemic attacks. *Therapeutically,* intramuscular or subcutaneous 1 mg glucagon is used during hypoglycaemic attacks. Glucagon also increases the strength of the heart muscle contraction, and unlike digitalis does not irritate the heart muscle. Glucagon is therefore sometimes used in heart failure as a continuous intravenous drip. Glucagon decreases appetite and gastric secretion.

Endocrine

Some hormones, secreted by the pituitary, suprarenal and the thyroid gland are antagonistic to the action of insulin.

AETIOLOGY

Predisposing Factors

Heredity. Heredity plays the most important role in conferring susceptibility to diabetes. The closer the blood relationship of a person to a diabetic the greater are his chances of developing the disease. When both parents are diabetic the chances of the children getting diabetes are considerably increased. Anybody with a family history of diabetes should take more than usual care to prevent the disease and detect it in its earliest stages.

Obesity. A strong predisposing factor in middle aged diabetes is obesity. Increasing weight is always a danger signal. Middle aged obestity is due to increase in the size of fat cells and not the number. Obese people on glucose load secrete more than the normal amount of insulin [4] but there is no room for glucose deposition in the cells, hence the glucose tolerance test exhibits a diabetic curve. With weight reduction the fat cells reduce in size and the glucose tolerance test may then show normal results [5].

The amount of insulin extracted from the pancreas of an obese diabetic at post-mortem is as much as in a normal person, while in a juvenile diabetic it is considerably less [6]. This suggests that the secretion of insulin in an obese diabetic is about normal but with the increase in weight the same amount of insulin is not sufficient to meet the increased demand. When diabetes occurs in an obese person it is usually a *relative deficiency* of insulin secretion as the same amount may be adequate to maintain normal carbohydrate metabolism if the weight is normal.

DETECTION OF EARLY DIABETES

All adults should have their urine examined for sugar twice a year, and more often if: (1) diabetes has occurred in any blood relation; (2) there is a sudden increase in weight; (3) unexplained loss of weight occurs; (4) nocturia develops; (5) recurrent skin infections occur; (6) a wound does not heal; or (7) children have been over-weight at birth.

Urine Examination

Examination of an early morning sample of urine may fail to detect early diabetes mellitus. It is necessary to observe the following proce-dure to detect early diabetes:

1. Urine is voided just before a meal.

2. Breakfast or lunch is taken with the usual helpings of carbo-hydrate-rich foods such as bread, *chappatis,* rice, fruits and sweets.

3. Three hours after the meal urine is voided and examined for sugar.

If a reducing substance is found in the urine it may be glucose or some other substance. If the reducing substance is glucose then it may be due to diabetes mellitus, alimentary or renal glycosuria. Blood sugar over 120 mg per 100 ml either in a fasting state or 2 hours after a meal denotes diabetes mellitus. A glucose tolerance curve may be necessary for the diagnosis of diabetes mellitus and its differentiation from alimentary and renal glycosuria.

Glucose oxidase tablets (*Clinitest*) and strips (*Clinistix*; *Tes-tape*), used for detection of glucose in the urine, depend upon the specificity of glucose oxidase to reduce when glucose is oxidized. They deteriorate with age and exposure to air, particularly in conditions of tropical humidity. False negative test may occur with vitamin C, and false positive from contaminated glassware or pus in the urine [7].

Glucose Tolerance Curve

The above method of urine examination has great practical value as a secreening test in detecting early diabetes mellitus. If there is sugar in the urine a glucose tolerance test is then performed. If diabetes mellitus is discovered it may be primary, secondary to endocrine disturbance of the thyroid, suprarenal, or pituitary.

There is neither unanimity on the correct loading dose for glucose tolerance test, nor are the criteria defined for the early diagnosis of borderline diabetes mellitus. A dose of 40 g glucose per square metre of body surface is recommended by the American Diabetes Association [8]. The commonly employed loading doses of glucose are 50 g; 100 g; 1 g per kg body weight; or 1·75 g per kg ideal body weight. In obesity a higher amount of glucose is given which does not take into account the ideal weight. After a loading dose the values of venous blood considered to be the upper limit of normal are 160 mg at 1 hour, 140 mg at 1½ hours and 120 mg at 2 hours. Capillary blood obtained by pricking the finger tip approximates to arterial blood. In the fasting state capillary blood sugar is 2–3 mg higher than venous blood. After a glucose load the capillary blood may even be 50–70 mg higher.

Prolonged fasting tends to produce a diabetic curve (decreased sugar tolerance) because fasting raises the glucagon level, which inhibits liver glycogen deposition and increases endogenous glucose production (gluconeogenesis). Therefore, prior to the glucose tolerance test a *minimum* of 150 g or preferably 250 g carbohydrate should be given for 3 days and an ambulatory state adopted, as bed rest produces a diabetic curve [8]. *Potassium depletion* during fasting produces a diabetic curve while potassium therapy increases the ability of the pancreas to secrete insulin [9]. *Drugs* tending to produce diabetic curve are *oral contraceptives, salicylates, nicotinic acid* and *benzothiazides.*

Decreased blood sugar levels are noted with antibiotic drugs and monoamine oxidase inhibitors.

Posture. Thin subjects may have the lower border of the stomach in the pelvis when sitting up. During a glucose tolerance test they show lower blood sugar values during sitting, when stomach emptying is delayed, than when lying on the right side with rapid stomach emptying [10]. *During menstruation* lower values are noted with oral glucose tolerance test than in the middle of the menstrual cycle, when the stomach probably empties more rapidly [11].

A *screening test* for diabetes with only *one blood sample,* is to administer to the overnight fasting patient 1 g glucose per kg body weight; *at 2 hours* the sample of blood collected is estimated for true glucose (glucose oxidase method). Values of over 110 mg of venous blood are highly suspicious of diabetes and require a glucose tolerance curve. The *urine* collected *at 2 hours* is also examined for sugar.

Mental stress has a marked effect on blood sugar fluctuations that produce difficulty in evaluation of diabetic therapy.

CLINICAL TYPES OF DIABETES

From the dietetic point of view the most practical classification of diabetes is by age:

1. Juvenile diabetic.
2. Adult diabetic.
3. Senile diabetic.

Juvenile Diabetics

Juvenile diabetics are primarily deficient in insulin. They are thin and have a tendency to lapse into ketosis due to marked deficiency of insulin. They require a high calorie diet to maintain their body weight and the necessary amount of insulin to maintain the blood sugar level.

Adult Diabetics

Adult diabetics are usually obese. They are comparatively resistant to insulin and require relatively more insulin to bring down the blood sugar than thin juvenile diabetics.

Insulin is necessary to convert glucose into glycogen and the excess glucose is stored as fat. It has been suggested that in an obese diabetic the body cells are fully laden with fat. There being no space in these fat-laden cells for further deposition of glycogen, hyperglycaemia and glycosuria result. If the fat is removed from the body cells by weight reduction then room becomes available for the deposition of glycogen and diabetes disappears. In clinical practice *most obese diabetics are cured by reduction of weight.*

Senile Diabetics

In elderly people there is a tendency for the pancreas to undergo fibrosis. This results in diminished insulin production. These patients require normal calories and a small amount of insulin.

Insulin-sensitive diabetes while commonest in the young may occur at all ages, even in the elderly.

METABOLISM OF THE DIABETIC

Calories

Weight of a diabetic. The total intake of calories is more important for a diabetic than the exact proportions of proteins, fats and carbohydrates in his diet. A personal weighing scale is as indispensable to a diabetic as examination of the urine for sugar. It is best to keep a diabetic on a well-balanced diet providing the lowest number of calories which will maintain his body weight at 5 per cent below his ideal weight. The ideal body weight depends upon age, sex, height and body frame. Many diabetics consume more calories than they need. These additional calories require extra insulin. The calorie requirements are:

1. In an *obese* diabetic the calories should be restricted to *reduce* the body weight and then maintain the weight at 5 per cent below the ideal weight.
2. In a diabetic of *normal weight* enough calories should be given to *maintain* the weight.
3. In an *underweight* diabetic enough calories should be given to *increase* the weight and maintain it at 5 per cent below the ideal weight.

Example. A forty-year-old male, height 165 cm (65 inches), should have an ideal body weight of 60 kg (132 lbs). If he is obese and weighs 75 kg his weight should be reduced to 56 kg by the low calorie diet advised for obese diabetics. If he is thin and weighs 50 kg his weight should be increased to 57 kg by the diet recommended for thin diabetics.

In the tropics the calories needed to maintain body weight are 10 per cent less than in temperate regions. The calorie requirements for maintaining the body weight are:

Occupation	Calories per kg per day	
	Tropics	*Temperate zone*
Sedentary	30	33
Moderate activity	40	44
Heavy manual work	50	55

Carbohydrates

There is a derangement of carbohydrate metabolism in diabetes as manifested by hyperglycaemia and glycosuria. The assumption that regulation of carbohydrates alone can effectively control diabetes is erroneous. The ingested food goes into the metabolic pool where it is reconverted to carbohydrates and fats. Thus even on a diet exclusively of meat and fats with a negligible amount of carbohydrate, as in Eskimos, carbohydrates are continuously formed in the body. The digestive enzymes reduce ingested carbohydrates to monosaccharides (glucose) which are absorbed into the blood stream and deposited as glycogen in the muscles and liver by the action of insulin. In diabetes due to deficiency of insulin the metabolism of carbohydrates is disturbed. This does not imply that the carbohydrate intake should be drastically curtailed in order to bring down the blood sugar. Even in a normal person marked diminution in the intake of carbohydrates for a few days produces a sugar tolerance curve resembling that of a diabetic. Therefore, a sugar tolerance test should not be performed unless the patient has had 250 g of carbohydrates per day for at least three days prior to the test. In a diabetic, drastic restriction of carbohydrates should not be advised as this further lowers the sugar tolerance. If adequate carbohydrates are given there is a reduction in fat metabolism and consequently less ketone bodies are formed. About 175–250 g of carbohydrates should be given to a diabetic of normal weight. This amount is decreased in an obese and increased in a thin diabetic.

Sorbitol. Hydrogenation of sugar produces an alcohol derivative, sorbitol, which is less sweet. Unlike other sugars, sorbitol is absorbed very slowly by the intestinal tract and so it does not appreciably alter the blood sugar level during absorption though it supplies as many calories as sugar. Because of this sorbitol is used in the preparation of chocolate, jams, marmalade, food preserves and other canned products manufactured specially for diabetics in Western countries. Absorbed sorbitol is first converted by the liver into fructose and then into glucose.

Proteins

A diet high in protein is good for the health of diabetics because: (1) it supplies the essential amino acids needed for tissue repair; (2) protein does not raise the blood sugar during absorption as do carbohydrates; (3) it does not supply as many calories as fats.

One gramme of protein per kilogram body weight is adequate but more may be given and the amount of fats and carbohydrates proportionately reduced.

Fats

Fats are metabolized in the body to provide heat and energy. Fats, however, cannot be oxidized as readily as carbohydrates. The normal end products of oxidation of fats are carbon dioxide and water.

Ketone Bodies. Beta-hydroxybutyric acid, acetoacetic acid and acetone are collectively known as the ketone (acetone) bodies. The accumulation of these products results in diabetic *coma*. Acetone is a volatile substance which is excreted by the lungs and gives a characteristic sweet odour to the breath, which is helpful in suggesting diabetes as a cause of coma.

Ketone bodies are intermediate products of normal fat metabolism. They are produced in the liver and utilized by the tissues to provide energy. When carbohydrate metabolism is normal, fats are metabolized to a relatively small extent, and the small quantity of ketone bodies produced is completely utilized by the tissues to supply energy, no excess being left for excretion in the urine. In a *neglected diabetic,* carbohydrates cannot be utilized for energy because of the deficiency of insulin, and so the energy requirements have to be met with fats. The excessive breakdown of fats in an attempt to provide energy results in an accumulation of ketone bodies which the tissues are not able to utilize rapidly. Ketone bodies thus accumulate in the blood and are excreted in the urine. Daily metabolism of about 100 g carbohydrates prevents ketosis.

Metabolic acidosis (ketosis) occurs with: (1) diabetes mellitus, with excess endogenous fat breakdown to supply the body needs; (2) decreased calorie intake; or (3) excessive demand; and (4) trauma.

Diabetic Coma

The four types of coma associated with diabetes are: (1) ketosis with high blood sugar; (2) hypoglycaemic; (3) hyperosmolar hyperglycaemic non-ketotic; (4) lactic acidosis.

Hyperosmolar Hyperglycaemic Non-ketotic Diabetic Coma (HHNK). In middle aged diabetics, acute dehydration following gastro-enteritis or pancreatitis, or drugs that enhance diabetes (corticosteriods, thiazides or diphenylhydantoin) or severe diuresis, may result in fever, hypovolaemia, shock and coma. There is glycosuria, raised blood sugar (as much as 1000 mg per 100 ml and over), leucocytosis, haemoconcentration exhibiting as raised haemoglobin, haematocrit, serum proteins, urea nitrogen, but low serum potassium. There is no ketosis, and consequently there is absence of Kussmaul breathing. The initial treatment is of hypovolaemic shock with isotonic saline and plasma volume expanders.

Lactic Acidosis: Non-ketotic Diabetic Acidosis [12]. *Accelerated anaerobic glycolysis* secondary to decreased oxygen supply and peripheral circulatory shock results in lactic acidosis with raised blood lactate and reduced arterial pH. It may occur with the normal blood levels of ketone bodies and is often known as *non-ketotic diabetic acidosis.* Lactic acidosis occurs with diabetes mellitus, alcoholism, arteriosclerosis, bacterial infection, heart disease, liver disease, glycogen storage disease, leukaemia, starvation and severe anaemia. Phenformin therapy for diabetes is usually stated to be a cause of lactic acidosis but the above-mentioned associated factors also contribute to it. The usual therapy is intravenous glucose, insulin and bicarbonate.

Summary. When carbohydrates are not utilized for energy as in diabetes, or are not available as in starvation, the excessive breakdown of fats produces ketone bodies at a more rapid rate than the tissues are able to utilize them. Under these circumstances they accumulate in the blood and are excreted in the urine.

Vitamins
Carbohydrates are not completely metabolized when there is a deficiency of vitamin B. It is postulated that products of partial carbohydrate metabolism, like pyruvic acid, accumulate due to the deficiency of vitamin B and damage to nerves results in peripheral neuropathy. A diabetic requires supplements of vitamin B. It is also advisable to supply vitamin A, as the liver, which is the storehouse of this vitamin, may be damaged in diabetes.

Fluids
A liberal fluid intake is allowed.

TREATMENT OF DIABETES

The principles of treatment of diabetes are:
Diet.
Exercise.
Insulin.
Oral drugs (sulphonylurea and guanide compounds).

Diet

1. Weighing scales are an indispensable guide for a diabetic. The body weight should be brought and maintained at 5 per cent less than the ideal body weight as assessed from height, sex and age.

2. The most important consideration is the amount of total calories ingested. For an individual taking his usual well-balanced diet, a precise brain-racking mathematical calculation of protein, fat and carbohydrate intake is unnecessary. The diet varies according to whether the patient is obese, of normal weight, or underweight.

Diet for an Obese Diabetic. 1. Restrict calories to bring down the weight to 5 per cent below normal. For an *uncomplicated* obese diabetic insulin should not be considered. *The treatment is with a reducing diet alone in the first instance.*

2. If sugar is still present in the urine after a few days on the reducing diet the dietetic treatment has not failed. Persist with the diet till the weight is brought down to the desired level.

3. When the weight is reduced to the desired level give enough calories to maintain the body weight at 5 per cent below the ideal weight.

4. If an untreated obese diabetic loses weight because of excessive loss of sugar in the urine then a valuable opportunity of treatment has been lost as the pancreas *now* shows signs of exhaustion.

5. Most obese diabetics could be made sugar-free, and even regain normal sugar tolerance, with systematic weight reduction by diet alone, and without the use of insulin or antidiabetic tablets.

6. The ideal time to consider insulin or oral tablets is when the weight has been brought down to 5 per cent below ideal weight and sugar still persists in the urine.

Diet for Normal Weight Diabetic. A well-balanced diet with the minimum calories needed to maintain weight. If sugar still persists in the urine then insulin or oral antidiabetic drugs are indicated.

Diet for Underweight Diabetic. Enough calories should be provided to increase the weight to normal. Enough calories are needed thereafter to maintain this weight. Underweight diabetics always require insulin and/or oral antidiabetic drugs to regulate their blood sugar.

A diabetic benefits from a high protein, moderate carbohydrate and low fat diet. Extra vitamins of the B group are beneficial.

Exercise

Exercise is a very useful measure in the management of diabetes. It utilizes carbohydrate (or energy) and reduces the requirement for insulin or antidiabetic tablets if these are being taken. Uniform and regulated exercise like a brisk walk, swimming or a game of golf are best suited for the middle-aged patient. Some moderately severe diabetics have been able to play even the most rigorous games. A world tennis champion had moderately severe diabetes which was controlled with treatment.

Insulin

Insulin is indicated in an underweight diabetic or in a normal weight diabetic who despite proper diet has hyperglycaemia and glycosuria. A long-acting insulin requiring a single daily injection is generally used. The initial dose is injection of 5–10 Units before breakfast. A chart is kept of the amount of sugar excreted in the sample of urine voided about 2 or 3 hours after breakfast, lunch and dinner. The dose of insulin is then gradually increased by 2–5 Units every third day till the maintenance dose is determined. The maintenance dose is the minimum amount of insulin required to keep urine sugar free. If any of the samples of urine show sugar or there are clinical symptoms of hypoglycaemia manifest as nervousness, tremors, palpitations or sweating then the intake of carbohydrate at each meal is balanced with the insulin dose. Decreasing or increasing the amount of carbohydrate-rich food as bread, *chappatis* or fruit at a particular meal may serve the purpose.

Oral Drugs

The only oral drugs which have proved of value are sulphonylurea and guanide compounds. Some clarification is required regarding diet and the use of these compounds. These drugs are not the panacea for all diabetics because: (1) they are usually ineffective in juvenile diabetics; (2) they are not recommended for patients with any complication of diabetes; (3) their long-term deleterious side-effects have not yet been fully assessed; (4) dietetic control is still essential even with the tablets. Sulphonylureas are most effective in obese diabetics and when the pancreas is at least partially functioning. These fat diabetics are those who with a weight-reducing diet could not only rid their urine of sugar but could regain near-normal glucose tolerance. The diabetic's prayer to be able to eat what he likes without harm remains unanswered despite the introduction of oral antidiabetic drugs.

The oral antidiabetics commonly used are: (1) *Sulphonylureas* (*tolbutamide* with a half life of 4–5 hours, *chlorpropamide* with a half life of about 36 hours and glybenclamide with a half life of 6-8 hours); they act through pancreatic insulin, by means of secretion of endogenous insulin by the pancreas. (2) *Biguanides* (with timed disintegration (T-D) the half life is 12–14 hours). They act by means of utilization of glucose by the peripheral tissues and *not* through endogenous insulin.

Weight Change with Oral Antidiabetics

Suphonylureas stimulate secretion of pancreatic insulin. Fat synthesis is promoted by insulin and as a result there is sometimes increase in weight in diabetics treated with sulphonylureas. *Biguanides*, on the other hand, may produce weight loss probably due to: (1) anorexic effect; (2) breakdown of fat (lipolytic effect) of biguanide on adipose tissue; (3) malabsorption, as there is decreased intestinal absorption of glucose [13]. In obese *non-diabetics* phenformin does not decrease weight [14].

Remissions

Remission in obese diabetics with weight loss is quite common but natural remissions are also noted even in juvenile diabetes [15].

THE DIABETIC DIET

Dietary instructions for a diabetic must be simple. As there is considerable variation in the quality, and therefore the chemical composition of food and in modes of cooking, precise calculations for balancing calories, protein, fat and carbohydrates are impossible. All that can be achieved is an approximation. Weighing all foodstuffs is a formidable prospect, because a patient has to follow a diet for the rest of his life. A dining table is not a grocer's counter with a balance and weights. It is easier to express quantities in terms of household measures than to advise accurate scientific calculations which are resented by the patient and usually not practised. The greater the flexibility offered to the patient in his choice of foods the easier it is for him to follow the instructions.

The following is a useful practical guide constructed at some sacrifice of 'scientific accuracy.' The word 'meal' denotes breakfast, lunch or dinner. Unless otherwise stated all foods mentioned are as cooked and served.

Bread or 'Chappati'

A slice of bread refers to a medium slice weighing about 30g while a *chappati* (unleavened bread) refers to a thin one made from 15g of *wheat flour*. An average *small chappati* of *bajra* or *jowar* is made from 30 g of flour, thus one of these can be taken instead of a slice of bread or 2 thin wheat *chappatis*. Bread and *chappatis* usually form the principal source of calories in the lower income groups. The number of slices of bread or of *chappatis* eaten at each meal should therefore be regulated by the calorie requirement.

	Slice of bread or small *chappatis* of *bajra* or *jowar*	Wheat *chappatis*, thin
Thin diabetic (at each meal)	2	4
Normal weight diabetic (at each meal)	1	2
Obese diabetic (only allowed for breakfast)	1	2

Some patients have a notion that brown bread or *chappatis* made of millets (*bajra* or *jowar*) can be eaten in any quantity without harm. This is a mistaken idea as all types of cereals and millets provide about 100 Calories per 30 g (1 oz) of dry flour.

An average slice of bread provides 75 Calories while a thin wheat *chappati* provides 40 Calories.

Breakfast Cereals

These are only prescribed for a thin diabetic. A diabetic of average weight can take breakfast cereal in exchange for 1 slice of bread or 2 wheat *chappatis*. Milk and sugar taken with breakfast cereals are added from the daily ration.

Average helping of breakfast cereal = 100 Calories.

Rice

An occasional helping of rice is allowed to a diabetic of normal weight. A thin diabetic may have it every day. Those who are particularly fond of rice can exchange their ration of 2 wheat *chappatis* or 1 slice of bread for 4 tablespoons of rice.

Four tablespoons of cooked rice = 100 Calories.

Pulses (dal), Dried Peas and Beans

Pulses are important in Indian dietetics. They supply a fair quantity of protein in a vegetarian diet. The following recommendations are for cooked thin *dal* as served.

	Mixed diet	*Vegetarian diet*
Thin diabetic ⎫	1 cup per meal al-	
Normal weight diabetic ⎬	lowed as exchange	
Obese diabetic ⎭	for dish of egg, meat	1 cup twice a day
	chicken, fish or one	
	cup of milk or its	
	products	

1 cup thin *dal* = 100 Calories.

Dried peas and beans also could be made into same consistency as thin *dal* and provide 100 Calories per cup.

Meat (Mutton, Beef, Pork, Fish, Chicken, Liver, Kidney, Brain)

These are protein-rich foods. An average helping of lean meat, fish, chicken, liver, kidney or brain, each weighs approximately 100 g before cooking. When cooked the weight may be reduced considerably but the calorie equivalent remains the same. The fat in meat provides extra calories.

An average helping of lean meat, fish, chicken, liver, kidney or brain = 100 Calories.

Egg

Eggs are excellent food. They may be taken as such or cooked with a ration of fat or milk or incorporated into dishes.

1 average European hen's egg = 80 Calories

1 average Indian hen's egg = 50 Calories

One helping of meat or fish or chicken or 1 European or 2 Indian eggs are allowed at each meal for all diabetics taking a mixed diet.

Milk and Milk Products

These are the main source of protein for the vegetarians. Milk is served as such or as buttermilk or curd. The calorie value of buttermilk or curd is the same as the milk from which it was made.

Daily ration of milk in cups

	Skimmed milk (cow's or buffalo's)	Cow's whole milk	Buffalo's whole milk
1. Thin			
Mixed diet	3	2	$1\frac{1}{2}$
Vegetarian diet	5	$3\frac{1}{2}$	$2\frac{3}{4}$
2. Normal weight			
Mixed diet	$2\frac{1}{2}$	2	$1\frac{1}{2}$
Vegetarian diet	4	3	2
3. Obese			
Mixed diet	1	–	–
Vegetarian diet	3	2	$1\frac{1}{2}$

Cow's whole milk, $\frac{3}{4}$ cup = 100 Calories.
Buffalo's whole milk, $\frac{1}{2}$ cup = 100 Calories.
Cow's or buffalo's skimmed
    milk, about $1\frac{1}{4}$ cup = 100 Calories.

Skimmed milk powder. Skimmed milk powder is advised in a vegetarian diet to provide protein without appreciably increasing the calorie content of the diet. It is relatively cheap yet easily digestible. The other inexpensive protein-rich foods like pulses (*dal*), gram (*chana*), and groundnut, are rather difficult to digest and add considerably to the calorie content of the diet. Skimmed milk powder can be added to any drink or food preparation. One tablespoon of skimmed milk powder added to 3 tablespoons of wheat flour makes delicious *chappatis* (unleavened bread) Skimmed milk powder contains the same number of calories whether derived from cow's or buffalo's milk.

Two tablespoons of skimmed milk powder = 100 Calories.

Soup

Thin soups made either from meat or vegetables have a low calorie content and can be taken *ad lib*. It is best for a thin diabetic to have a small helping of soup so that other foods with adequate calories can be taken. Conversely, if an obese diabetic takes a big helping of soup at meal times it gives him a sense of satiety without increasing his calorie intake.

Thick soups usually contain flour, peas, potato, nuts, etc., which have a high calorie equivalent. To keep the diet simple, thick soups are best avoided.

Vegetables

Vegetables are the best sources of bulk with few calories in the form of carbohydrate. An obese diabetic who requires much bulk with few calories should be advised to take a good quantity of vegetables. A thin diabetic should take less vegetables to leave room for other more nourishing foods.

Five and Ten per cent Vegetables. Most books on dietetics confuse patients by emphasizing the carbohydrate content of vegetables. The calorie content of both '5 and 10 per cent' vegetables is so low that they do not appreciably increase the total intake of calories however much is taken.

Leafy Vegetables. All leafy vegetables like spinach and cabbage are of such low calorie value that they can be eaten freely by all diabetics.

Other Green Vegetables. Other green vegetables, such as pumpkin, brinjals, lady's fingers, french beans, etc., if tender can be eaten freely. An exception is over-ripe beans, which have a high calorie equivalent. French beans when tender have a low calorie equivalent but when the beans are ripe the calorie value increases appreciably.

Root Vegetables (except potato and sweet potato). Root vegetables like carrots, radish, onion, and turnip also provide few calories and can be taken as desired.

One or two helpings of the leafy, or root vegetables mentioned above can be taken at each meal.

Peas and Beans. Peas and beans have a high calorie equivalent and are already considered together with pulses. They can be taken as a substitute for pulses.

Vegetable Salad. Vegetables used for salad are cucumber, lettuce, onion, radish, and tomato. All can be taken liberally by all diabetics, especially the obese. Vinegar, dried pepper, green pepper, mustard and sour lime may be used as a dressing. Since the aim in an obese diabetic is to reduce the calorie intake, any dressing containing oil is avoided.

Average helping of salad vegetable plus one or two cooked vegetables (mentioned above under leafy vegetables, other vegetables or root vegetables) at a meal = 100 Calories.

Potato and Sweet Potato

Potatoes and sweet potatoes supply an appreciable number of calories so their quantity is restricted. An average medium size potato weighs 100 g. It is advisable for the patient to weigh a 100 g potato or sweet potato in order to get an idea of the size. Potatoes are advised as follows:

Thin diabetic   One medium size potato at lunch *or* dinner.
Normal weight diabetic ⎫ One medium size potato occasionally allow-
                        ⎬ ed in exchange for any other 100 Calorie
Obese diabetic   ⎭ food item mentioned, e.g. 1 slice of bread or
                          2 *chappatis* or 1 cup skimmed milk.

Medium size potato or sweet potato weighing 100 g = 100 Calories.

Fat for Cooking

Ghee, butter, oil, margarine or *vanaspati* are used for cooking. They contain concentrated calories hence their intake should be regulated. The total quantity of fat advised should be taken partly as seed oil (unsaturated).

The measured daily ration of fat can be used for any purpose—even for frying. The amount allowed varies with the caloric content of the diet. The ration of fat is:

Thin diabetic   1 tablespoon per meal
Normal weight diabetic   2 teaspoons per meal
Obese diabetic   1 teaspoon per meal

One tablespoon butter, *ghee,* oil, margarine or *vanaspati* = 100 Calories.

Sugar, Jaggery (gur) or Honey

These are almost pure carbohydrate foods. Some diabetics feel that the only dieting necessary is to stop taking sugar. It is best for patients to know the daily ration of sugar. The daily ration should not be taken at one time but reasonably distributed through the day. Sugar may be taken either with tea or, if desired, with the ration of milk for the preparation of sweets, custard or ice cream.

	Daily ration (Sugar, *gur* or honey)
Thin diabetic	4 teaspoons
Normal weight diabetic	3 teaspoons
Obese diabetic	Exclude, saccharin may be substituted

One teaspoon sugar, jaggery (*gur*) or honey = 20 Calories.

Jam (murabba)

These are best avoided by a diabetic. If a patient is fond of them then only *one level teaspoon* of jam or *murabba* may be substituted for one teaspoon of the sugar ration.

Pastries, Biscuits

All pastries should be avoided because of the variable content of sugar and fat. Three average size thin unsweetened biscuits can be substituted for a slice of bread or potato.

Dessert

China grass jelly is permitted. If a patient wants to have his dessert from his daily ration of milk, sugar and egg, he can do so.

Fruits

Fruits supply carbohydrate and are also good sources of vitamin C. One of the following fruits of an average size is allowed 2 or 3 times a day: tangerine, orange, sweet lime, apple, guava, $\frac{1}{2}$ small papaya, $\frac{1}{2}$ melon, $\frac{1}{4}$ small water melon, a bunch of 24 grapes, 10 strawberries or gooseberries. An average banana or mango contains more calories and is usually best avoided. If a patient wishes, one banana or one mango may be allowed two or three times a week, instead of the regular quota of fruit.

An average helping of fresh fruit supplies 50–100 Calories.

Dried Fruits

Dried fruits are not permitted.

Nuts

These are allowed as an exchange food, the equivalent of 100 Calories being substituted for 1 cup skimmed milk, 1 slice of bread or 2 thin wheat *chappatis* at a meal time.

12–15 almonds or 16–20 groundnuts or 30 pistachios or 8 cashew nuts or 3 walnuts = 100 Calories.

Papad, Chutney and Pickles

These are allowed in moderation. Pickles made in oil are not permitted.

Beverages

Beverages like tea and coffee are permitted, with milk and sugar taken from the daily ration. Unsweetened drinks such as soda water and barley water need not be restricted.

Foods which Provide High Calories

If the food habit conforms to the conventional menu then, with a constant calorie intake, the amount of sugar passed in the urine is about the same after that meal every day. If there are wide fluctuations in the sugar passed in the urine, e.g. no sugar in the urine passed 3 hours after breakfast one day but a brick red precipitate the next day at the same time then changes in the diet should be strongly suspected. The common foods which cause these fluctuations are *chappatis,* bread, rice, potato, pulses, banana, mangoes, nuts and sweets. The quantity of these foods taken should be strictly regulated.

Locker Food. If a patient on a diet regimen shows gross fluctuations in the urinary sugar excretion from day to day, it can be assumed that the patient is taking extra food. Mere denial of this is unreliable. The ungentlemanly act of opening the bedside-locker of the in-patient usually reveals a stock of biscuits or sweets which 'are just brought by the relatives but have never been touched'.

THIN DIABETIC
SAMPLE MENU

Diet till the body weight is increased to 5 per cent below ideal weight

Mixed Diet		Vegetarian Diet	
Approximately		*Approximately*	
Proteins	100 g	Proteins	90 g
Fats	90 g	Fats	70 g

DAILY RATION

GROUP	FOODS	THIN DIABETIC	
		Mixed Diet	*Vegetarian Diet*
I.	1 helping of breakfast cereal (30 g) 1 slice of bread 2 thin wheat *chappatis* or *khakhra*	Cereal and 2 slices of bread *or* 4 thin *chappatis* at breakfast	Cereal and 2 slices of bread *or* 3 thin *chappatis* at breakfast
	1 small *chappati* of *bajra, jowar* or *ragi* 4 tablespoons cooked rice 1 medium potato 3 biscuits	Any *two* of these at *each* lunch and dinner	Any *three* of these at *each* lunch and dinner
II.	*Pulses (dal)* dried peas and beans	1 cup per meal allowed as exchange for: an item of non-vegetarian food in Group III *or* 1 cup milk or products prepared from it.	2 cups thin *dal* per day
III.	*Non-vegetarian foods* 2 eggs Average helping (about 100 g before cooking) of chicken, lean meat, fish, pork, ham, liver, kidney, brain or sweetbread	Any *one* at each meal	
IV.	*Salad* All vegetables used for salad as cucumber, cabbage, lettuce, onion, radish, tomato etc.	Small quantity	Small quantity
V.	*Cooked tender vegetables*	—do—	—do—
VI.	*Soups* Thin soup of vegetable, meat or chicken	—do—	—do—
VII.	*Milk* *Daily ration* of milk, cow's or buffalo's (any milk preparation like curd, buttermilk or dessert may be prepared from the rationed amount)	3 cups skimmed milk (cow's or buffalo's) or 2 cups cow's whole milk or $1\frac{1}{2}$ cups buffalo's whole milk	5 cups skimmed milk (cow's or buffalo's) or $3\frac{1}{2}$ cups cow's whole milk or $2\frac{3}{4}$ cups buffalo's whole milk

OF DIABETIC (MEAL refers to breakfast, lunch or dinner).

NORMAL WEIGHT DIABETIC		OBESE DIABETIC	
Mixed Diet	*Vegetarian Diet*	*Mixed Diet*	*Vegetarian Diet*
Any *one* of these at *each* meal	Any *one* of these at breakfast	Any *one* of these at *each* meal	Any *one* of these at *each* meal
	Any *two* of these at *each* lunch and dinner		
1 cup per meal allowed as exchange for: an item of non-vegetarian food in Group III *or* 1 cup of milk or products prepared from it	2 cups thin *dal* per day	1 cup per meal allowed as exchange for: non-vegetarian food in Group III *or* 1 cup skimmed milk or products prepared from it	2 cups thin *dal* per day
Any *one* at each meal	—	Any *one* at each meal	—
Allowed liberally	Allowed liberally	Allowed liberally	Allowed liberally
—do— —do—	—do— —do—	—do— —do—	—do— —do—
$2\frac{1}{2}$ cups skimmed milk (cow's or buffalo's) *or* 2 cups cow's whole milk *or* $1\frac{1}{2}$ cups buffalo's whole milk	4 cups skimmed milk (cow's or buffalo's) *or* 3 cups cow's whole milk *or* 2 cups buffalo's whole milk	milk 1 cup skimmed milk (cow's or buffalo's)	3 cups skimmed milk (cow's or buffalo's) *or* 2 cups cow's whole milk or $1\frac{1}{2}$ cups buffalo's whole milk

DAILY RATION

GROUP	FOODS	THIN DIABETIC	
		Mixed Diet	Vegetarian Diet
VIII.	*Sugar* Daily ration of sugar, honey, jaggery (may be used in beverages or in the preparation of desserts)	4 teaspoons per day	4 teaspoons per day
IX.	*Dessert* Prepared from the daily ration of milk and sugar as given above	Permitted	Permitted
X.	*Beverages* Coffee and tea (with milk and sugar from daily ration mentioned above), barley water and aerated water (with saccharin but without sugar)	Permitted	Permitted
XI.	*Fruits* 1 orange, 1 sweet lime, 1 apple, 1 pear, $\frac{1}{4}$ melon, $\frac{1}{2}$ papaya, 24 grapes, 8 strawberries or gooseberries	Any *one* item, 2 or 3 times a day	Any *one* item, 2 or 3 times a day
XII.	*Nuts* 3 walnuts 30 pistachios 8 cashew nuts 12–15 almonds 16–20 groundnuts 4 dates	Permitted as exchange for any	
XIII.	*Fat for cooking* or *butter*	3 tablespoons per day	3 tablespoons per day
XIV.	*Papad,* chutney or pickles without oil	In moderation	In moderation

OF DIABETIC (MEAL refers to breakfast, lunch or dinner).

	NORMAL WEIGHT DIABETIC		OBESE DIABETIC	
	Mixed Diet	*Vegetarian Diet*	*Mixed Diet*	*Vegetarian Diet*
	3 teaspoons per day	3 teaspoons per day	Not permitted	Not permitted
	Permitted	Permitted	Permitted	Permitted
	Permitted	Permitted	Permitted	Permitted
	Any *one* item, 2 or 3 times a day	Any *one* item, 2 or 3 times a day	Any *one* item, 2 or 3 times a day	Any *one* item, 2 or 3 times a day

one item of the above Group I, II or III

	Mixed Diet	*Vegetarian Diet*	*Mixed Diet*	*Vegetarian Diet*
	6 teaspoons per day	6 teaspoons per day	3 teaspoons per day	3 teaspoons per day
	In moderation	In moderation	In moderation	In moderation

Mixed Diet		*Vegetarian Diet*	
Carbohydrates	290 g	Carbohydrates	340 g
Calories	2400	Calories	2400

Morning

Tea, 1 cup with milk, and sugar from ration

Tea, 1 cup with milk and sugar from ration

Breakfast

Cornflakes† with milk, 1 cup and sugar from ration
Eggs, 2 half-boiled*
Toast, 2††
Orange**

Porridge, 1 cup† with milk, 1 cup and sugar from ration
Chappatis, 4††
Butter, 2 teaspoons
Apple, 1**

Lunch

Fish, baked, average piece*
Cooked carrots
Bread, 2 slices††
Curd, 1 cup*
papaya, ½**

Cooked french beans
Rice, 4 tablespoons†
Dal, 1 cup*
Chappatis, 4††
Curd, 1 cup*
Sweet lime, 1**
Groundnuts, 16

4 p.m.

Tea, 1 cup with milk, 2 tablespoons and sugar from ration
Biscuits, 3†

Milk, 1 cup with biscuits, 3†

Dinner

Mutton, roast*
Boiled potato, 1†
Cooked cauliflower
Bread, 2 slices††
Ice cream from the remainder of ration of milk and sugar

Cooked pumpkin
Baked potato, 1†
Dal, 1 cup*
Chappatis, 4††
Curd, 1 cup*
Pudding from the remainder of ration of milk and sugar

Daily ration

Skimmed milk, 3 cups
Sugar, 4 teaspoons

Skimmed milk, 5 cups
Sugar, 4 teaspoons

Fat for cooking (preferably as oil) and butter, 3 tablespoons

(†)   Any *one* other item from Group A ⎫
(††)   Any *two* other items from Group A ⎪   from TABLE 27 [pp. 483–4] may
(*)   Any *one* other item from Group B ⎬   be substituted
(**)   Any *one* other item from Group C ⎭

NORMAL WEIGHT DIABETIC
SAMPLE MENU

Mixed Diet		*Vegetarian Diet*	
Approximately		*Approximately*	
Proteins	90 g	Proteins	65 a
Fats	60 g	Fats	50 g
Carbohydrates	180 g	Carbohydrates	225 g
Calories	1700	Calories	1700 g

Morning

Tea, 1 cup with sugar from ration   Tea, 1 cup with milk, 2 table-
                                     spoons and sugar from ration

Breakfast

Eggs, 2 half-boiled or poached*   Milk, 1 cup*
Toast, 1†   *Khakhra,* 4
Butter, 1 teaspoon   Butter, 2 teaspoons
Orange**   Orange, 1**

Lunch

Mutton soup, 1 cup   Mixed vegetable soup, 1 cup
Roast mutton, 1 average helping*   Cooked cauliflower
Boiled peas, 4 tablespoons*   *Dal,* 1 cup*
Cooked cabbage   Sliced tomato and cucumber
                                       salad
Vegetable salad with vinegar   *Chappatis,* 2†
  dressing   Curd, 1 cup*
Bread, 1 slice†   Grapes, bunch of 24**
Papaya, ½**

4 p.m.

Tea, 1 cup with milk, 2 table-   Skimmed milk, 1 cup*
  spoons and sugar from ration
Apple, 1**

Dinner

Chicken soup, 1 cup   Tomato soup, 1 cup

Mixed Diet	*Vegetarian Diet*
Baked fish, average helping*	Cooked cabbage
Cooked french beans	Potato, baked, 1†
Skimmed milk, 1 cup*	*Dal,* 1 cup*
Bread, 1 slice†	*Chappatis,* 2
Pudding from the remainder of	Buttermilk, 1 cup*
ration of milk and sugar	Pudding from the remainder of
	ration of milk and sugar

Daily ration

Skimmed milk, 2½ cups	Skimmed milk, 4 cups
Sugar, 3 teaspoons	Sugar, 3 teaspoons

Fat for cooking (preferably as oil) and butter, 6 teaspoons

(†)   Any *one* other item from Group A ⎫
(*)   Any *one* other item from Group B ⎬ from TABLE 27 [pp. 483–4] may
(**)   Any *one* other item from Group C ⎭ be substituted

OBESE DIABETIC
SAMPLE MENU

Diet till body weight is reduced to 5 per cent below ideal body weight

Mixed Diet		*Vegetarian Diet*	
Approximately		*Approximately*	
Proteins	80 g	Proteins	65 g
Fats	45 g	Fats	30 g
Carbohydrates	165 g	Carbohydrates	220 g
Calories	1400	Calories	1400

Morning

Tea, 1 cup with milk, 2 table-spoons	Tea, 1 cup with milk, 2 table-spoons

Breakfast

Eggs, 2 half-boiled or poached*	Skimmed milk, 1 cup*
Toast, 1†	*Khakhra,* 2†
Orange**	Sweet lime**

Lunch

Meat soup, 1 cup	Tomato soup, 1 cup
Boiled fish, average helping*	Cooked cauliflower
Cooked pumpkin	*Dal,* 1 cup*
Vegetable salad from cabbage,	Vegetable salad from cabbage,

Mixed Diet	*Vegetarian Diet*
celery, cucumber, lettuce, onions, radish or tomato with vinegar and pepper	celery, cucumber, lettuce, onions, radish or tomato with vinegar and pepper
Bread, 1 slice†	*Chappatis,* 2†
Bunch of 24 grapes**	Buttermilk, 1 cup
	Papaya, $\frac{1}{2}$**

4 p.m.

Tea, 1 cup with milk, 2 tablespoons	Tea, 1 cup with milk, 2 tablespoons
Apple, 1**	Apple, 1**

Dinner

Soup, 1 cup	Mixed vegetable soup
Mutton, lean roast, 1 helping*	Cooked carrots
Cooked brinjal	Thin *dal,* 1 cup*
Bread, 1 slice†	*Khakhra,* 2
	Skimmed milk, 1 cup*

Daily ration

Skimmed milk, 1 cup	Skimmed milk, 3 cups
Sugar not permitted	Sugar not permitted

Fat for cooking (preferably as oil) and butter, 3 teaspoons

(†)	Any *one* other item from Group A	⎫
(*)	Any *one* other item from Group B	⎬ from TABLE 27 (see below) may
(**)	Any *one* other item from Group C	⎭ be substituted

TABLE 27

FOODS OF APPROXIMATELY THE SAME CALORIE AND PROTEIN VALUES

So that the patient can vary his diet, make it more attractive, and suit his purse, foods have been divided into Groups A, B and C. From the sample menu any other items of food listed in the same Group can be substituted.

Except for over-ripe vegetables with seeds, potato, sweet potato, yam or green peas, other vegetables can be freely taken as mentioned in the text.

GROUP A		GROUP B	
Biscuits	3	*Dal,* thin	1 cup
Breakfast cereals	One helping	Peas or beans	4 tablespoons or as
Banana	1		1 cup of thin *dal*
Chappatis	2	Eggs	2 small or 1 large

(Wheat, thin)		Milk, cow's	¾ cup
Chappatis (jowar		buffalo's	½ cup
bajra or ragi)	1	skimmed	1 cup
Khakhra	2	Skimmed milk	
Potato (medium)	1	powder	2 tablespoons
Rice	4 tablespoons	Meat	Average helping
		Fish	Average helping
		Chicken	Average helping
		Almonds	12–15
		Cashew nuts	8
		Groundnuts	16
		Pistachios	30
		Walnuts	3

GROUP C

Apple	1	Guava	1
Figs	3	Papaya	½
Grapes	24	Water-melon	¼
Orange	1	Melon	½
Sweet lime	1		

REFERENCES

[1] HENDERSON, J.R. (1970) Serum insulin or plasma ?, Lancet, ii, 545.

[2] GORDON, P., and ROTH, J. (1969) Circulating insulins 'big' and 'little', Arch. intern. Med., 123, 237.

[3] SAMOLS, E., MARRI, G., and MARKS, V. (1965) Promotion of insulin secretion by glucagon, Lancet, ii, 415.

[4] PERLEY, M.J., and KIPNIS, D.M. (1967) Plasma insulin responses to oral and intravenous glucose: studies in normal and diabetic subjects, J. clin. Invest., 46, 1954.

[5] SALANS, L.B., KNITTLE, J.L., and HIRSCH, J. (1968) The role of adipose cell size and adipose tissue insulin sensitivity in carbohydrate intolerance in human obesity, J. clin. Invest., 47, 153.

[6] WRENSHALL, G.A., and BEST, C.H. (1956) Extractable insulin of the pancreas and effectiveness of oral hypoglycaemic sulfonylureas in the treatment of diabetes in man. A comparison, Canad. med. Ass. J., 74, 968.

[7] SUTHERLAND, H.W., STOWERS, J.M., and CHRISTIE, R.J. (1970) Factors affecting sensitivity of glucose-oxidase strips used in test for glycosuria, Lancet, i, 1071.

[8] AMERICAN DIABETES ASSOCIATION (1969) Standardization of the oral glucose tolerance test. Report of the Committee on Statistics of the American Diabetes Association, Diabetes, 18, 299.

[9] ANDERSON, J.W., HERMAN, R.H., and NEWCOMER, K.L. (1969) Improvement in glucose tolerance of fasting obese patients given oral potassium, Amer. J. clin. Nutr., 22, 1589.

[10] DESAI, H.G., and ANTIA, F.P. (1968) Effect of posture on glucose tolerance curve, in *Diabetes in the Tropics, 20–22 January*. Diabetic Association of India, Bombay, p. 191.

[11] MACDONALD, I., and CROSSLEY, J.N. (1970) Glucose tolerance during the menstrual cycle, *Diabetes*, **19**, 450.

[12] BRITISH MEDICAL JOURNAL (1970) Lactic acidosis, *Brit. med. J.*, **4**, 258.

[13] HOLLOBAUGH, S.L., RAO, M.B., and KRUGER, F.A. (1970) Studies on the site and mechanism of action of phenformin. Evidence for significant 'non-peripheral' effects of phenformin in glucose metabolism in normal subjects, *Diabetes*, **19**, 45.

[14] HART, A., and COHEN, H. (1970) Treatment of obese non-diabetic patients with phenformin: a double-blind cross-over trial, *Brit. med. J.*, **1**, 22.

[15] BRITISH MEDICAL JOURNAL (1970) Remissions in diabetes mellitus, *Brit. med. J.*, **3**, 539.

69. GOUT

Gout is an inherited disease preponderantly occurring in males and is due to an abnormal uric acid metabolism. There is a raised serum uric acid and deposition of urate (uric acid salt) in the cartilages and articular cartilages of the joints. There are recurrent attacks of pain and swelling of the joints, frequently the metatarsophalangeal joint of the big toe but other joints may also be affected. Joints subject to trauma are most liable to be involved.

Only 5–10 per cent of gouty patients are females. In such cases gout seldom manifests before menopause. Gouty patients tend to have more intellectual capacity and drive [1], hence hyperuricaemia and gout are sometimes considered to be status symbols.

URIC ACID METABOLISM

Source

The source of uric acid is: (1) *Exogenous*. The exogenous source of uric acid is food with a high purine content such as meat and glandular meat like liver, pancreas and kidney. About 200–500 mg of uric acid is derived from this source in a person who eats animal food. (2) *Endogenous*. Purines, present as nucleoproteins in the nuclei of the cells, when broken down yield uric acid. On a purine-free diet between 300 and 600 mg uric acid derived from this endogenous source is excreted daily in the urine.

Serum Uric Acid

The upper limit of normal serum uric acid is less than 6 mg per 100 ml in men and 5 mg per 100 in women. Uric acid is a waste product serving no useful purpose. The biochemical pathway for its formation is complex. It is formed from substances like glutamine, glycine and formic acid to inosinic acid and uric acid. The enzyme hypoxanthine guanine phosphoribosyltransferase (HG-PRTase) allows a major portion of inosinic acid to be reconverted to purines (guanine and hypoxanthine), for the formation of useful metabolic products including protein synthesis, and thus to reduce uric acid formation.

Uric acid estimation may be fallacious. It should be made in serum or plasma and not the whole blood. The enzymatic uricase method with ultraviolet spectrophotometry is the most accurate [2]. Routine uric acid estimation in hospital-admitted male patients showed serum urate values over 7·0 mg per 100 ml in 13 per cent, due to azotaemia, acidosis or diuretic therapy. Only about 20 per cent of these patients had gout requiring therapy, hence clinical assessment is more helpful than diagnosis by serum uric acid [3[.

Excretion

Uric Acid in the Urine. The urates are completely filtered through the glomeruli and totally reabsorbed by the tubules. Tubular *secretion* accounts for almost the entire urinary uric acid excretion [4]. The total daily excretion of uric acid in the urine on a mixed diet is about 1 g. If a routine microscopic examination of urine shows uric acid crystals it does not necessarily mean a high uric acid excretion as even on a purine-free diet the daily excretion of 300–600 mg endogenous uric acid can precipitate as crystals if the urine is strongly acid. Estimation of the total 24-hour excretion of uric acid in the urine also has no significance in assessing uric acid metabolism unless the total dietetic intake of purines is also known.

Intestinal bacteria degrade about one third of the uric acid formed daily by normal subjects and convert it into carbon dioxide and ammonia. This degradation decreases by intestinal bacteriostatic drugs. In *gouty subjects* as well as during *renal insufficiency* the urinary urate excretion is decreased and intestinal bacterial disposal is therefore increased [5]. However, intestinal degradation plays no role in the mechanism of gout.

A small amount of urate is destroyed by peroxidase destruction by the *leucocytes* and a little is excreted through sweat.

URIC ACID METABOLISM IN GOUT

Heredity. Gout is a hereditary disorder of uric acid metabolism. Studies of the serum of gouty patients and also members of their families show high serum uric acid levels. They have a tendency to synthesize more uric acid than normal persons, and also have a greater tendency to hypertension, toxaemia of pregnancy, renal infection and renal damage. The renal damage is secondary to persistently raised serum uric acid levels over several years.

Primary and Secondary Gout. When gout is due to a hereditary abnormality of uric acid metabolism it is known as 'primary' gout. When gout is due to a raised serum uric acid level resulting from the excessive breakdown of cell nuclei as in blood diseases like leukaemia, pernicious anaemia, polycythaemia and haemolytic anaemias, it is known as 'secondary' gout.

Serum Uric Acid Level in Gout. In primary as well as secondary gout the serum uric acid level is high for several years before an attack occurs. The critical level of serum uric acid below which gout does not occur is 6 mg per cent in males and 5 mg per cent in females.

Body Pool. The total miscible pool of uric acid in the body estimated by isotope studies in a normal person is about 1 g . In a gouty patient the miscible pool of uric acid may be even 15 times greater.

Mechanism of Increased Uric Acid in Gouty Patients

Hypoxanthine Guanine Phosphoribosyltransferase (HG-PRTase) Deficiency. The enzyme hypoxanthine guanine phosphoribosyltransferase (HG-PRTase) recycles a considerable amount of the precursors of uric acid, hypoxanthine and guanine, and thus reduces uric acid production and urinary excretion. Complete or partial deficiency of HG-PRTase results in some cases of gout.

1. *Complete deficiency of HG-PRTase* (*Lesch-Nyhan syndrome*) [6].

Lesch-Nyhan syndrome is characterized by involuntary choreo-athetoid movements, spasticity, mental retardation and a compulsive self-mutilatation by chewing lips and fingers. There is excessive urinary uric acid excretion due to a complete deficiency of HG-PRTase [7].

Partial deficiency of HG-PRTase explains some patients with familial gout and in these cases allopurinol does not decrease excretion of purine catabolite hypoxanthine and xanthine [8].

2. *Excessive breakdown* of cellular nucleoproteins occurs in secondary gout as in polycythaemia and the leukaemias. In these diseases administration of N^{15} labelled glycine shows an increased uric acid excretion reaching a maximum in 10 days because the glycine is first incorporated into the cell nuclei to form nucleoproteins and subsequently broken down before excretion.

3. *Diminished urinary uric acid excretion:* raised serum lactate, fasting and alcohol decrease urinary urate excretion and raise serum uric acid.

Organic Acids (Lactic and Keto Acids). Organic acids compete with uric acids for urinary excretion. Administration of lactate results in decreased urinary urate excretion and raised serum uric acid. Alcohol ingestion increases serum lactate because a greater amount of pyruvates is converted to lactate [9]. Severe muscular exercise and respiratory acidosis raise the serum lactate level and may precipitate gouty attack. In *glycogen storage disease* raised serum lactate and gout are probably associated with hypoglycaemia and ketonaemia [10], and increased purine biosynthesis.

Gouty tophi are frequent in avascular cartilagenous areas, as anaerobic glycolysis produces lactic acid and lowered pH facilitates deposition of urate crystals.

Fasting. Fasting increases the serum uric acid level in the normal as well as gouty individual, since increase in beta-hydroxybutyric acid and acetoacetic acid decreases renal excretion of urate, although acetone has no such effect [11]. In gouty patients, fasting raises serum uric acid by 1·1 mg per 100 ml in 24 hours and by 2·0 mg after 48 hours [12]. Obese patients starving for a week on an average have a serum uric acid increase of 14·7 mg per 100 ml [13].

Alcohol. Sixty to 100 g alcohol with low purine diet produce minor changes in serum urate levels, but larger doses of alcohol increase serum uric acid by decreasing urinary urate excretion. Serum uric acid is higher when a patient is intoxicated than when sober, due to increased blood lactate [14]. Alcohol, along with fasting, raises serum uric acid more than fasting alone [12], and fluctuations of uric acid, either a rise or fall are associated with an attack of gout [12].

Drugs. *Thiazides* decrease tubular excretion of urate and raise serum uric acid. Thiazides may thus precipitate gouty attacks in susceptible individuals. In such cases the simultaneous administration of allopurinol is advocated as a prophylaxis [15]. *Salicylate in low dosage* blocks only renal tubular secretion of urate to cause a rise in the blood uric acid. (In *high doses* of over 5 g, salicylate blocks both the tubular secretion and reabsorption, and thus enhances uric acid excretion; the blood uric acid level is decreased, but the action of salicylate is antagonistic to uricosuric drugs such as probenecid. The cause of this is unknown.)

The causes of gout are multiple and operate severally, e.g. a man with inherited enzyme defect may also be an alcoholic, and may develop renal diseases or take thiazide which reduces uric acid excretion.

Gout in Vegetarians

It has been generally believed that gout is less common amongst vegetarians than among meat eating people. In India gout appears to be a relatively uncommon disease but is sometimes seen amongst the vegetarians.

GOUTY ARTHRITIS

The *pathogenesis* of acute gouty arthritis is not clearly understood. *Monosodium urate monohydrate* crystals recovered from the synovial aspiration are specially noted inside the phagocytes during attacks of gout. Precipitation of urate crystals and leucocytic activity is presumed to be responsible for an attack of gouty arthritis. Acute gouty arthritis occurs during *increase* or *decrease* in the serum uric acid by 1 mg [12]. Thus attacks of gout may be precipitated when serum uric acid is: (1) *rising* with fasting, high fat diet or treatment with thiazide; or (2) *falling* with allopurinol or haemodialysis. The gouty *tophi* of monosodium urate monohydrate are precipitated when serum uric acid is over 7 mg, hence the necessity to reduce serum uric acid. The precipitation is more likely in avascular tissue as cartilage, where anaerobic glycolysis producing lactic acid decreases the pH.

Pseudogout mostly effects the knee joints. Synovial fluid aspiration from an arthritic joint reveals calcium pyrophosphate crystals. On radiology there is articular calcification and plasma uric acid is normal.

KIDNEY DISEASE AND KIDNEY STONES

The incidence of *renal disease* in gouty patients is very high. The kidney diseases follow persistent high blood uric acid. *Monosodium urate monohydrate* and *uric acid crystals* are precipitated in the collecting ducts. Though gout is rarely fatal, death from gout is a result of kidney disease or its sequelae.

Kidney stones in gouty patients and members of their family are a common occurrence. The stones are mostly of uric acid with oxalate and phosphate. They are usually non-opaque, but with sufficient calcium a shadow may be cast.

At alkaline pH of urine (7·35–7·40) uric acid remains as *soluble sodium salt,* while at acid pH 5·0 approximately 75 per cent of uric acid exists in a *free state* which because it is insoluble precipitates in the urine. This highly *concentrated acid* urine is responsible for 15–20 per cent of gouty patients developing uric acid stones. *Ileostomy patients* also, because of loss of fluid and base from the ileostomy opening, have a high incidence of uric acid stones [16].

Prevention of urate stones entails ensuring daily excretion of 2000–3000 ml urine to prevent urinary concentration and acidification. Patients with chronic renal calculus disease associated with high blood uric acid show diminished tendency to stone formation when treated with allopurinol to reduce serum uric acid to less than 5 mg per 100 ml [17].

DIETETIC MANAGEMENT

The dietetic treatment of gout has undergone a great deal of re-orientation due to the changing concept of the disease. The high purine diet alone used to be blamed. In a gouty patient the recent demonstration of: (1) direct synthesis of uric acid from the normal products of metabolism; and (2) an abnormality of excretion of uric acid either due to excessive tubular reabsorption or a defect in tubular secretion has focussed more attention on the hereditary defect of uric acid metabolism and less on the high purine intake. However, in a susceptible person an acute attack of gout is likely to be precipitated by purine-rich foods.

I. FOODS OF HIGH PURINE CONTENT

Always to be excluded

Fish roe
Fish like herring, salmon, sardine
Liver
Kidney
Sweetbread
Meat extracts and soups

II. FOOD OF MODERATE PURINE CONTENT

Permitted *only* during quiescent stage

Meat	Asparagus	*Chickoo*
Fish like pomfret, shell-fish like prawns, lobster	Beans	Custard apple
	Brinjals	
Chicken	Cauliflower	
	French beans	
	Green peas	
	Mushroom	
	Spinach	
	Pulses	

III. FOODS OF NEGLIGIBLE PURINE CONTENT

Always permitted

All vegetables except in II
All fruits except in II
Milk and milk products
Eggs
Fats and oils
Sugar and sweets
Cereals

Calories

Obese persons may be more prone to gout. The body weight should be reduced to normal not only to prevent recurrence of gout but also to prevent changes in the weight-bearing joints which occur in the obese. A heavy meal supplying high calories should be avoided as it tends to precipitate an attack.

Proteins and Purines
Meats having a high purine content such as roe of fish, sweetbread, liver, kidney; fish like herring, salmon, and sardines; meat extracts and meat soups are always excluded. Flesh in the form of meat, fish and fowl are excluded during an acute attack but allowed as an average helping during quiescent periods. About 60 g protein a day is adequate, preferably supplied as vegetable or milk proteins.

Fats
Fat consumption is restricted partly because its ingestion tends to cause retention of urates by the kidney, and partly to prevent obesity.

Carbohydrates
During an attack of gout the main source of calories should be from carbohydrate for its 'protein sparing effect' which reduces the endogenous protein breakdown.

Fluids
Liberal fluids should be advised to ensure a daily excretion of about 2000 ml of urine.

Beverages
Tea or coffee contain methyl purines which are not converted by the body into uric acid. About 2 or 3 cups a day are permitted.

Alcohol
There appears to be an individual susceptibility to an attack of gout after ingestion of alcohol. Usually gouty patients tolerate a couple of ounces of white wine or whisky, but not beer, stout or red wines.

Principles of Dietetics
Low purine, low protein, easily digestible diet with a liberal fluid intake.

GOUT

Foods	Remarks
Bread or *chappatis* of wheat, rice, maize, *jowar, bajra* or *ragi*	Permitted*
Breakfast cereals of wheat, rice, oat, or maize	Permitted*
Rice cooked	Permitted*
Pulses (*dal*) or beans	½ cup thin *dal* twice a day. Exclude during an acute attack
Meat, fish or chicken	Average helping 100 g per meal. Exclude during acute attack. Always exclude sweetbread, kidney, liver, fish roe, herring.
Egg	Permitted
Milk or milk products	Permitted*
Soup	Excluded; vegetable soup permitted
Vegetable salad	Permitted
Vegetables, cooked	Permitted. Exclude asparagus, brinjals, cauliflower, french beans, green peas, mushrooms and spinach during acute attack and only one of these twice a week during remission.
Potato, sweet potato or yam	Permitted*
Cooking fat or butter	2 tablespoons a day
Sugar, jaggery or honey	Permitted*
Jam or *murabba*	Permitted* Exclude jam with seeds
Pastry	Permitted
Dessert	Permitted as light custard and pudding*
Sweet or sweetmeats	Permitted*
Fruits, fresh	Permitted. Exclude berries
Fruits, dried	Permitted*
Nuts	Permitted*
Condiments and spices	Restricted. Exclude during acute attack
Papad, chutney, pickles	Restricted during acute attack

Foods	*Remarks*
Beverages	Permitted, 2 cups a day
Fluids	Liberal

* To be restricted for the obese.

GOUT
SAMPLE MENU

Mixed Diet	*Vegetarian Diet*

Breakfast

Porridge, ¾ cup with milk, ½ cup and sugar, 1 tablespoon	Cornflakes, 1 cup with milk, 1 cup and sugar, 1 tablespoon
Poached eggs, 2	Toast or *khakhra* with honey
Toast or *chappatis* with marmalade	Orange
Apple	Tea or coffee
Tea or coffee	

Lunch

Chicken, roast	Mixed vegetable salad
Cucumber, radish, beetroot and lettuce salad	Ridge gourd (*turiya*) cooked
Carrots, cooked	Rice with *dal*, ½ cup
Baked macaroni	Buttermilk, ½ cup
or	Bread or *chappatis*
Rice with curd	Banana
Bread or *chappatis*	

4 p.m.

Tea	Tea
Biscuits	Biscuits

Dinner

Mixed vegetable soup, 1 cup	Tomato soup, 1 cup
Eggs, 2 scrambled	Mashed potato and lady's fingers
Pumpkin, cooked	Curd, 1 cup
Bread or *chappatis*	Bread or *chappatis*
Custard, boiled	*Jallebi*

REFERENCES

[1] BROOKE, G.W., and MUELLER, E. (1966) Serum urate concentration among University Professors, *J. Amer. med. Ass.*, **195**, 415.

[2] LIDDLE, L., SEEGMILLER, J.E., and LASTER, L. (1959) Enzymatic spectrophotometric method for determination of uric acid, *J. lab. Clin. Med.*, **54**, 903.

[3] PAULLUS, H.E., COUTTS, A., CALABRO, J.J., and KLINENBERG, J.R. (1970) Clinical significance of hyperuricemia in routinely screened hospitalized men, *J. Amer. med. Ass.*, **211**, 277.

[4] GUTMAN, A.B., and Yü, T.F. (1968) Uric acid nephrolithiasis, *Amer. J. Med.*, **45**, 756.

[5] SORENSEN, L.B. (1965) Role of intestinal tract in the elimination of uric acid, *Arthr. and Rheum.*, **8**, 694.

[6] LESCH, M., and NYHAN, W.L. (1964) A familial disorder of uric acid metabolism and central nervous system function, *Amer. J. Med.*, **36**, 561.

[7] SEEGMILLER, J.E., ROSENBLOOM, F.M., and KELLEY, W.N. (1967) Enzyme defect associated with sex-linked human neurological disorder and excessive purine synthesis, *Science*, **155**, 1682.

[8] KELLEY, W.N., ROSENBLOOM, F.M., MILLER, J., and SEEGMILLER, J.E. (1968) An enzymatic basis for variation in response to allopurinol. Hypoxanthine guanine phosphoribosyltransferase deficiency, *New Engl. J. Med.*, **278**, 287.

[9] ISSELBACHER, K.J., and GREENBERGER, N.J. (1964) Metabolic effects of alcohol on the liver, *New Engl. J. Med.*, **270**. 351, 402.

[10] ALEPA, F.P., HOWELL, R.R., KLINENBERG, J.R., and SEEGMILLER, J.E. [1967) Relationship between glycogen storage disease and tophaceous gout, *Amer. J. Med.*, **42**, 58.

[11] GOLDFINGER, S., KLINENBERG, J.R., and SEEGMILLER, J.E. (1965) Renal retention of uric acid induced by infusion of beta-hydroxy-butyrate and acetoacetate, *New Engl. J. Med.*, **272**, 351.

[12] MACLACHLAN, M.J., and RODNAN, G.P. (1967) Effects of food, fast and alcohol on serum uric acid and acute attacks of gout, *Amer. J. Med.*, **42**, 38.

[13] ALDERMANN, M.H., and DAVIS, R.P. (1965) Hyperuricaemia in starvation, *Proc. Soc., exp. Biol. (N.Y.)*, **118**, 790.

[14] LIEBER, C.S., JONES, D.P., LOSOWSKY, M.S., and DAVIDSON, C.S. (1962) Interrelation of uric acid and ethanol metabolism in man, *J. clin. Invest.*, **41**, 1863.

[15] NICOTERO, J.A., *et al.* (1970) Prevention of hyperuricemia by allopurinol in hypertensive patients treated with chlorothiazide, *New Engl. J. Med.*, **282**, 133.

[16] CLARKE, A.M., and McKENZIE, R.G. (1969) Ileostomy and the risk of urinary uric acid stones, *Lancet*, **ii**, 395.

[17] SMITH, M.J.V., and BOYCE, W.H. (1969) Allopurinol and urolithiasis, *J. Urol. (Baltimore)*, **102**, 750.

70. KIDNEY DISEASES

The kidneys excrete waste products of the body in general and the end products of protein metabolism in particular. These excretory products of metabolism are retained if the quantity of urine or its concentration is inadequate. *Urea* is one of these end products of protein metabolism. The normal daily excretion is about 30 g which is more than any other solid excreted in the urine. Urinary urea is derived from ingested food and the breakdown of body tissues. On a mixed diet about half is derived from the ingested food, and the rest from the breakdown of tissue proteins. The maximum capacity of the kidneys to concentrate urea is 4 per cent. In order to excrete 30 g of urea at the maximum concentration (4 per cent) at least 750 ml of urine should be voided daily.

At the onset of acute nephritis the excretion of urine is markedly diminished. Urea and other end products of protein metabolism are retained. The formation of urea and other waste products can be considerably diminished by restricting the intake of exogenous dietary proteins and diminishing the endogenous breakdown of tissue proteins by supplying 'protein sparers' like carbohydrates and fats. The intake of proteins cannot be restricted indiscriminately, however. Urea clearance is diminished on a low protein vegetarian diet and the function of the kidney improves on a high protein diet [1]. Adequate proteins should be supplied as soon as the kidneys recover and normal urinary flow is resumed.

Kidney diseases may present themselves as either:

1. *Nephritic syndrome* is characterized by haematuria, oliguria, oedema and hypertension. The commonest cause of this is acute nephritis (Ellis Type I) which is possibly an allergic reaction in the kidney to streptococcal infection with complete recovery in 80 per cent of cases. Other causes are acute pyelonephritis, acute metallic poisoning and renal infarction.

2. *Nephrotic syndrome* (Type II nephritis) is characterized by a gradual onset of oedema with massive proteinuria and a lowered plasma albumin and gamma globulin level; complete recovery is infrequent. Other causes are Kimmelstiel-Wilson syndrome, disseminated lupus, bilateral renal vein thrombosis especially secondary to amyloid disease, amyloidosis, malaria and syphilis.

3. *Chronic renal failure* characterized by polyuria with low specific

gravity, hypertension and cardiac failure, mental confusion and dehydration.

ACUTE NEPHRITIS:
DIETETIC MANAGEMENT

Calories
The total intake should be about 1700 Calories.

Proteins
The intake of proteins is reduced to a minimum by excluding protein-rich foods. During the acute phase if anuria develops then proteins should be stopped and 10–20 per cent glucose or fructose can either be given orally or through intragastric drip. When urine flow re-commences the protein intake is increased. If the urine passed is 500–700 ml, about 0·5 g proteins per kg body weight is allowed. With free flow of urine the daily intake is then increased to the usual of about 60 g. Prolonged restriction of proteins leads to asthenia and anaemia.

Fats
The end products of metabolism of fats do not depend upon the kidneys for their excretion so fats can be administered even during anuria. Pure fats, however, are unpalatable.

Carbohydrates
The main source of energy for patients with acute nephritis is carbohydrate.

Vitamins
Vitamin C, 100 mg three times a day, should be given as deficiency has been noted in acute nephritis. Vitamin B complex is also useful.

Minerals
Normal kidneys under hormonal control automatically regulate the sodium and potassium needs of the body. In acute nephritis the kidneys are unable to excrete sodium and potassium and so body electrolyte balance is disturbed. Mineral intake, therefore, has to be restricted or given according to the needs, as judged by electrolyte

studies if feasible. *Sodium* is restricted as long as oedema persists. When oedema subsides the intake of sodium as common salt is gradually increased. *Potassium* should also be restricted when there is scanty flow of urine. Only two helpings daily of either fruit juice or vegetable soup are permitted.

Fluids

Apart from the water excreted in the urine, about 1000 ml is also lost daily through respiration, invisible perspiration and defaeca-tion. The daily intake of fluids and output of urine should be charted. Daily fluid replacement should be 1000 ml plus daily amount ex-creted in the urine. If the urine excreted is 500 ml then the fluid requirement is 1000 + 500 = 1500 ml. Fluids supplied with liquid foods as fruit juice, milk, tea and soups should be measured and taken into account in the estimation of total fluid allowance.

Principles of Diet

Low protein, high carbohydrate, low sodium with restricted fluids. For foods and sample menu, see pages 500–1.

NEPHROTIC SYNDROME

This is characterized by a varying degree of proteinuria and oedema. Massive proteinuria results in lowering of serum albumin and decreased colloid osmotic pressure which leads to oedema. Serum cholesterol values are raised. There is usually no retention of nitrogenous waste products in the early stages The total quantity of urine excreted may be normal.

DIETETIC MANAGEMENT

Calories

About 2000 Calories are supplied.

Proteins

There is loss of albumin in the urine leading to lowered serum al-bumin and protein depletion of the tissues. A high protein diet con-taining at least 1·5–2 g protein per kg body weight is advised. A relatively cheap source of proteins is skimmed milk powder which can be taken with fruit juice or mixed with flour to make *chappatis*.

Concentrated protein foods are also available in the market. Groundnuts and pulses (*dal*) including Bengal gram (*chana : futana*) are palatable inexpensive protein-rich foods.

Fats

The usual quantity of fats, 1 g per kg, is advised. Whether the high blood cholesterol seen in Type II nephritis is a compensatory mechanism or some metabolic defect is not yet known. A controlled clinical trial alone should decide whether it is advantageous to attempt reduction of the serum cholesterol level by supplying unsaturated fats.

Carbohydrates

After the daily needs of proteins and fats are satisfied the remaining calories are supplied by carbohydrates.

Vitamins

Vitamin C, 100 mg three times a day and vitamins of B group may be given as suppleme 's.

Minerals

Sodium retained in the body maintains oedema. A low sodium diet is helpful during the oedematous stage. A convenient method of restricting sodium is to avoid salt in cooking and also at the table. Foods to which salt has been added as salted butter, biscuits, preserved meat and fish are excluded. Prolonged deprivation of sodium leads to electrolyte imbalance which impairs kidney function and aggravates oedema. If the oedema persists despite sodium restriction, the blood electrolytes should be estimated, and salt allowed if the sodium level is low. When the oedema subsides a moderate intake of salt is permitted. (For foods and sample menu, see pp. 502–3.)

PYELONEPHRITIS
(Pyelitis)

Pyelonephritis is commonly caused by *B. coli* infection. In pregnant women it may occur as an ascending urinary infection.

The factors which precipitate or reactivate a dormant infection are: (1) obstruction in the urinary tract due to inflammation, stone or new growth; (2) purgatives or bowel washes in some patients precipitate an acute attack of pyelitis which probably is due to absorption of bacteria due to bowel irritation.

The advent of chemotherapy and antibiotics has made drastic dietetic treatment of pyelitis obsolete. A *ketogenic* diet, high in fat and low in carbohydrate, evolved to make the urine acid was formerly advocated because *B. coli* do not thrive in an acid medium. This diet was unbalanced and highly unpalatable. Similarly an acid ash diet has limited use [see Chapter 77]. Constipation should be treated by diet [see Chapter 54]. Purgatives should be avoided.

DIETETIC MANAGEMENT
(Pyelonephritis, Cystitis and Urethritis)

Calories

About 1800–2200 Calories are permitted.

Proteins

During acute infection only about 30 g of protein are allowed and the amount is gradually increased with improvement.

Fats

There is no restriction to the fat intake.

Carbohydrates

Adequate carbohydrates are advised to supply caloric needs.

Fluids

Adequate amount of fluids are given to ensure passage of 1500 ml of urine.

Alcohol, Condiments and Spices are Strictly Prohibited

ACUTE NEPHRITIS

Foods	Remarks
Bread or *chappatis* of wheat, rice, maize, *jowar, bajra, ragi*	Permitted
Breakfast cereal of wheat, rice, oatmeal or maize	Permitted
Rice, cooked	Permitted

Foods	Remarks
Pulses (*dal*) or beans	Excluded
Meat, fish or chicken	Excluded
Eggs	Excluded
Milk or milk products	3 cups
Soup	Excluded
Vegetable salad	Permitted
Vegetables, cooked	Permitted
Potato, sweet potato, or yam	Permitted
Fat for cooking, or butter	Permitted
Sugar, jaggery or honey	Permitted
Jam or *murabba*	Permitted
Pastries	Permitted, if prepared without salt
Dessert	Permitted
Sweets or sweetmeat	Permitted
Fruits, fresh	Permitted
Fruits, dried	Permitted
Nuts	Excluded
Condiments and spices	Excluded
Papad, chutney or pickles	Excluded
Beverages	Weak tea or coffee
Fluid	Total liquids including milk and tea or coffee, 5 cups

N.B.—In oedematous stage no salt is allowed in cooking or at the table. Purchased foods to which salt is added are not permitted.

ACUTE NEPHRITIS
SAMPLE MENU

Vegetarian and Mixed Diet

Approximately
Proteins 30 g: Fats 63 g: Carbohydrates 255 g: Calories 1700.

Morning
Tea or coffee, 1 cup

Breakfast
Toast, 2 or *chappatis,* 4
Butter, 2 teaspoons
Jam, 1 teaspoon

Banana, 1
Tea or coffee, 1 cup

11 a.m.

Milk, 1 cup with sugar, 1 teaspoon

Lunch

Mashed potato with butter, 2 teaspoons
Lettuce and cucumber salad
Cooked cauliflower
Rice, 4 tablespoons with tomato soup, ½ cup
Bread, 1 slice or *chappatis,* 2
Orange or papaya

4 p.m.

Tea, 1 cup
Biscuits, 3 with butter, 1 teaspoon

Dinner

Cooked pumpkin
Bread, 1 slice or *chappatis,* 2 with butter, 2 teaspoons
Baked apple with sugar, 2 teaspoons and cream, 1 tablespoon

N.B.—No salt in cooking or at the table.

NEPHROTIC SYNDROME

Foods	Remarks
Bread or *chappatis* of wheat, rice, *jowar, bajra* or *ragi*	Permitted
Breakfast cereal of wheat, rice, oatmeal or maize	Permitted
Rice, cooked	Permitted
Pulses (*dal*) or beans	Permitted
Meat, fish or chicken	Permitted liberally
Eggs	Permitted
Pulses	1–2 cups
Milk or milk products	Permitted—preferably as skimmed milk
Soup	Excluded
Vegetable salad	Permitted
Vegetables, cooked	Permitted
Potato, sweet potato or yam	Permitted

Cooking fat or butter	Permitted
Sugar, jaggery or honey	Permitted
Jam or *murabba*	Permitted
Pastries	Permitted—without salt
Dessert	Permitted
Sweets or sweetmeat	Permitted
Fruit, fresh	Permitted
Fruit, dried	Permitted
Nuts	Permitted
Condiments and spices	Excluded
Papad, chutney or pickles	Excluded
Beverages	Permitted
Water	Restricted in oedematous stage

N.B.—In oedematous stage no salt is allowed in cooking or at the table. Purchased foods to which salt is added are not permitted.

NEPHROTIC SYNDROME
SAMPLE MENU

Mixed Diet	*Approximately*	*Vegetarian Diet*	*Approximately*
Proteins	118 g	Proteins	110 g
Fats	68 g	Fats	72 g
Carbohydrates	228 g	Carbohydrates	252 g
Calories	2000	Calories	2100

Breakfast

Cornflakes, 1⅓ cup with skimmed milk, 1 cup and sugar, 2 teaspoons

Eggs, 2 poached
Toast, 1 or *chappatis,* 2
Tea or coffee, 1 cup

Porridge, ⅔ cup with milk, 1 cup and sugar, 2 teaspoons

Cottage cheese, 2 tablespoons
Bread, 1 slice or *khakhra,* 2
Tea or coffee, 1 cup

Mid-morning

Skimmed milk, 1 cup
Banana, 1

Skimmed milk, 1 cup with skimmed milk powder, 2 tablespoons

Lunch

Tomato salad

Buttermilk, 1 cup

Minced meat, 4 tablespoons	Vegetable salad
Cooked pumpkin	Cooked brinjals
Rice, 2 tablespoons	Rice, 2 tablespoons
Curd, ½ cup	*Dal,* 1 cup
Bread, 1 slice or *chappatis,* 2	Bread 2 slices or *chappatis,* 4
Walnuts, 4	Groundnuts, 15

4 p.m.

Tea or coffee, 1 cup	Tea or coffee, 1 cup

Dinner

Fish baked, 1 helping	Cottage cheese, 3 tablespoons
Roast leg of chicken	Curd, 1 cup
Potato, 1 mashed with 1 teaspoon	Cooked spinach, 2 tablespoons
butter	*Dal,* 1 cup
Cooked cauliflower	Bread, 1 slice or *khakhra,* 2
Bread, 1 slice or *chappatis,* 2	
Bread pudding, ½ cup	

Before retiring

Skimmed milk, 1 cup	Skimmed milk, 1 cup with skim-med milk powder, 2 table-spoons.

REFERENCE

[1] CHITRE, R.G., NADKARNI, D.S., and MONTEIRO, L. (1955) The effect of protein nutrition on the urea clearance in human subjects, *J. postgrad. Med.,* **1,** 79.

71· RENAL FAILURE

ACUTE RENAL FAILURE

Anuria leads to accumulation of the waste products of protein metabolism in the blood. In anuria without excessive trauma, fever or infection, the blood urea nitrogen may rise only 10–15 mg per 100 ml daily. The serum potassium level rises by 0·7 mEq per day [1]. The rise in the serum potassium is the result of its release from the breakdown of glycogen or tissue proteins in order to provide calories. The usual cause of death in anuria is not the rise in blood urea, but either potassium intoxication which occurs after about a fortnight, when the serum level rises over 10 mEq per litre, or over-zealous treatment with fluids, with a view to stimulating urinary flow resulting in water intoxication.

Most cases of anuria due to medical conditions or complicating pregnancy recover within a few days. Dialysis with the 'artificial kidney' should be left for the experts where facilities are available. In the absence of these expert facilities and of a thorough knowledge of fluids and electrolytes, the best help that can be rendered to the patient is to give the minimum of therapy and interfere with nature as little as possible. Administration of intravenous fluids without good reason may do harm. A reduction in the endogenous protein breakdown, and thus in the excretion of nitrogen, can be achieved by a diet excluding proteins but supplying carbohydrates and fats. Fluids are limited to 500–1000 ml plus the equivalent amount of daily urine excretion.

Acute renal failure implies acute suppression of kidney function. It may be: (1) prerenal; (2) renal; or (3) post-renal.

Prerenal

Prerenal failure is due to: (1) *Decreased plasma volume* (*hypovolaemia*) that reduces renal blood flow and the glomerular filtration rate. As the kidney function is normal in the early stages, there is scanty urine volume (less than 400 ml) with high specific gravity (over 1025). Decreased plasma volume occurs in *deficient fluid intake*, *excessive fluid loss* in severe vomiting and diarrhoea, or *loss of blood* with haemorrhages or loss of *plasma* in severe burns. (2) *Decreased renal blood flow and decreased glomerular perfusion rate* may occur (with or without dehydration) with trauma, surgery, anaesthesia, handling of viscera, and hepatorenal syndrome in liver failure.

Urinary sodium concentration of less than 20 mEq/1 in acute renal failure suggests that the kidneys have retained the power to reabsorb sodium and are capable of reasonable function while the scanty urine is due to decreased renal perfusion. *Prolonged shock and blood volume deficiency subsequently produce renal damage.* The kidneys then lose the ability to reabsorb sodium, resulting in urinary sodium excretion of over 20 mEq/1 with a specific gravity of less than 1022 despite scanty urine.

Renal

Renal failure occurs with: (1) *acute kidney damage* in acute glomerulonephritis, Weil's disease, acute pyelonephritis; (2) *acute tubular necrosis* with continued prerenal failure, described above, mismatched transfusion, crush injuries, sulphonamides, blood loss in pregnancy, acute ischaemic vascular damage or nephrotoxins.

Acute renal failure sometimes occurs with contrast media used for pyelography or cholecystography [2].

Post-renal

Post-renal failure occurs when there is obstruction of urinary flow due to enlarged prostate, renal calculi, stricture of the urethra or retroperitoneal fibrosis.

Kidney function is known to recover after as much as 6 weeks of acute urinary suppression if the patient is kept on peritoneal dialysis or haemodialysis with artificial kidney.

DIETETIC MANAGEMENT OF
ACUTE RENAL FAILURE

Calories

A minimum of 600–1000 Calories is necessary. A higher calorie intake of carbohydrates and fats is desirable.

Protein

All foods containing proteins are stopped if the patient is under conservative treatment and the blood urea nitrogen is rising. However, if he is on peritoneal dialysis or haemodialysis, then a daily intake of 40 g protein is desirable as it will reduce the endogenous protein breakdown and maintain health.

Fats

Calorie supply from fats is desirable and should be allowed liberally.

Carbohydrates

A daily minimum of 100 g of carbohydrate is essential to minimize the tissue protein breakdown. This would require 2 litres of 5 per cent intravenous glucose, as higher concentrations produce venous thrombosis. Since the fluid intake in acute renal failure is to be drastically limited, it is best to give *oral feeds* of glucose or fructose solution 15 per cent 700 ml made palatable with lime juice. If the patient cannot be fed by mouth, a *nasogastric tube* is passed and a minimum of 15 per cent 700 ml glucose or dextrimaltose is administered.

Fluid

The total fluid permitted is 500 ml + total losses through the urine and gastro-intestinal tract. With visible perspiration an additional 500 ml may be necessary.

Sodium

Sodium loss in the urine is measured and replaced. *Dilutional hyponatraemia* (serum sodium below 120 mEq) occurs because of water retention. Water restriction rather than salt administration is then indicated.

Potassium

Potassium intoxication (hyperkalaemia) occurs with a daily rise of 0·7 mEq serum potassium. Deleterious effects of potassium on the heart are combated by intravenous *calcium gluconate* 10 per cent 30–50 ml, while the electrocardiogram is monitored. An attempt is made to *deposit* glycogen, and thereby *potassium in the cells,* by administering intravenous 10 per cent glucose 200 ml mixed with crystalline insulin 10 Units, or a glucose solution 15–20 per cent 200 ml through a nasogastric drip with subcutaneous crystalline insulin 10–15 Units. *A bowel wash* removes 100 mEq potassium.

Cation exchange resins are subsequently useful to reduce high serum potassium. Polystyrene sodium sulphonate (Kay-exalate) is administered orally in doses of 15 g two or three times a day [3]. This resin exchanges for potassium and for its excretion from the gut calcium sorbitol is used as an osmotic cathartic. *Resonium-A,* which exchanges calcium for potassium, is used in doses of 15–30 g orally [4]. Both the above resins can also be used by means of *high rectal retention enema* to avoid nausea, vomiting and intestinal obstruction due to faecal impaction.

Aluminium resin is claimed to have an additional function of decreasing intestinal phosphate absorption by precipitating aluminium phosphate in the gut. This may help in cases of hyperphosphataemia, which carries an associated danger of metastatic calcification in chronic renal failure [5]. It was originally claimed that aluminium is not absorbed; however, absorption and raised blood aluminium level (hyperaluminaemia) are noted though the side-effects are not known [6].

Haemodialysis or peritoneal dialysis is considered in *acute renal failure* of the *low catabolic type* (average type) when the blood urea is over 200 mg per 100 ml. The diet may then be raised to 2000–3000 Calories with 40 g protein. If the patient cannot take oral feeds, intravenous fat (*Intralipid*) and amino acid solution (*Aminosol*) are given [4] (see Intravenous Feeding). *In acute renal failure of the high catabolic type* (crush injury, major surgery, sepsis) the blood urea rises more than 50 mg a day and dialysis is considered earlier, even on the second or third day.

CHRONIC RENAL FAILURE

The causes of chronic renal failure are progression of acute nephritis or nephrosis, chronic pyelonephritis, renal calculi, subacute bacterial endocarditis, polycystic kidneys, analgesic nephropathy (phenacetin), diabetes, amyloidosis and gout. The urine volume depends upon the glomerular filtration rate. The urine specific gravity is low.

The normal kidney function includes regulation of body fluids, electrolytes, pH and excretion of non-volatile metabolites. Once chronic renal failure occurs, then regardless of the cause the clinical picture is the same. The manifestations are [7]: (1) *general:* dehydration or water intoxication, sodium depletion, hyperkalaemia, acidosis, increased susceptibility to infection; (2) *cardiovascular:* oedema of the lungs and ankle, hypertension, arrhythmias and pericarditis; (3) *gastro-intestinal:* anorexia, vomiting, hiccoughs; (4) *neurological:* peripheral neuropathy, twitching, convulsions, coma; (5) *haemopoietic system:* anaemia; (6) *skin:* pigmentation, pruritus, purpura; and (7) *skeletal:* renal dystrophy, metastatic calcification and dwarfism.

Plasma Creatinine. The upper limit of *normal* serum creatinine is 1·4 mg per 100 ml for males and 1·3 mg per 100 ml for females. The production of creatinine is closely related to the muscle mass and is fairly constant in an individual, being independent of diet or exercise. Creatinine is completely excreted by the glomeruli. As there is no tubular reabsorption, estimation of serum creatinine gives a good indication of the *glomerular filtration rate.*

Glomerular Filtration Rate (GFR) [8]. GFR from plasma creatinine is calculated as:

$$\text{GFR for men} = \frac{92}{\text{plasma creatinine}}$$

$$\text{GFR for women} = \frac{70}{\text{plasma creatinine}}$$

Acidosis. The non-volatile acids are excreted by the kidneys. Chronic renal failure therefore produces acidosis that can be corrected by the administration of sodium bicarbonate. Acidosis produces calcium reabsorption from the bones, osteomalacia and renal osteodystrophies. Rapid correction of acidosis may result in calcium redeposition in the bones, and tetany.

Anaemia. *Blood loss* occurs with nose bleeding, haematuria, ecchymosis or gastro-intestinal bleeding. The bleeding episodes are due to deficient coagulatory factors and increased vascular fragility. The depression of the bone marrow is due to *decreased erythropoietin* (renal hormone that aids bone marrow in the formation of erythrocytes). Haemolysis also contributes to anaemia.

Folic acid deficiency probably produces hypersegmentation of polymorphs that disappears with folic acid supplements [9].

Anaemia of chronic renal failure is very resistant to treatment. Since anaemia is well tolerated, only *iron* and *folic acid supplements* are given and rigorous therapy is not advocated. Packed cell transfusion is sometimes necessary when the haemoglobin falls below 6 g per cent.

Nervous System. *Peripheral neuropathy,* particularly in the lower extremities, is increasingly observed with the prolongation of life by haemodialysis. Some neuropathies are related to nitrofurantoin (*Furadantin*) toxicity. Itching and tingling with calcium deposits in the skin may be confused with peripheral neuropathy. Only in a few cases is the neuropathy related to vitamin deficiency or diabetes.

Mental aberration, memory loss, lassitude, lethargy, depression, stupor and coma are associated with diminished cerebral oxygen utilization.

DIETETIC MANAGEMENT OF CHRONIC RENAL FAILURE

Calories

Thirty-five to 50 Calories per kg weight is supplied mainly from carbohydrate and fats for protein-sparing effect.

Protein

Urea is converted to ammonia by the intestinal bacteria [10]. Even orally fed urea or ammonium chloride raises the blood nitrogen level, and oral antibiotics reduce such conversion. During severe protein restriction this raised blood nitrogen is utilized for the formation of non-essential amino acids and proteins [11].

In chronic renal failure 40 g protein is permitted, but when the glomerular filtration rate is below 10 ml per minute, marked protein restriction is necessary since urea production is increased with protein intake. The *absolute minimum* protein requirement is 20 g. Patients do not usually adhere to a 20 g protein diet and for prolonged periods are more likely to follow a 40 g mixed protein diet. When the glomerular filtration rate falls below 4 ml per minute a 20 g protein diet must be insisted upon as the body then synthesizes non-essential amino acids from the body ammonia nitrogen, while essential amino acids are provided mainly from *egg* and *milk* protein. During chronic renal failure severe protein restriction reduces blood urea to 100 mg per 100 ml, which decreases uraemic symptoms. The protein and water content of foods are given in TABLE 28, page 514.

Fats

The serum triglycerides are raised partly due to excessive carbohydrate feeding or to large amounts of glucose administered for haemodialysis. For energy, fats with carbohydrates are recommended in uraemic patients.

Carbohydrate

In uraemia, carbohydrates provide the main source of energy to reduce endogenous protein breakdown. Sugars and cereals from which proteins are removed, are liberally permitted as wheat starch (hominy), and protein-free bread (phenylketonuric bread). Vegetables and fruits are suitably processed to decrease the potassium content [p. 511].

The glucose tolerance test may show: (1) a *false diabetic curve* due to raised serum creatinine and uric acid, which are reducing substances. Therefore the blood sugar should be estimated by the glucose oxidase method; (2) the *diabetic curve* noted in patients with uraemia is due to insulin resistance, which in reality is pseudo-diabetes since it reverts to normal on haemodialysis. The metabolite causing the insulin resistance is not identified but is not urea [12]. True diabetes is sometimes seen.

Fluids

In the *early stages* of chronic renal failure there is loss of ability to concentrate urine that increases urinary water excretion in an attempt to excrete the solutes, and the patient is allowed liberal fluids. *Dehydration* and a further increase in blood urea result when there is associated anorexia or vomiting which prevents fluid intake. Intravenous fluid therapy is necessary at this stage.

With progressive kidney damage the glomerular filtration rate and urine volume diminish. This results in *oedema* and *dilutional hyponatraemia* necessitating fluid restriction.

Sodium

Sodium depletion easily occurs as the kidneys lose their power of conserving sodium. Loss of appetite and deficient intake aggravate sodium deficiency, which results in contraction of the blood volume, a fall in glomerular filtration rate, and a further deterioration of kidney function. Associated water depletion may mask sodium deficiency because at that stage serum sodium estimation reveals normal values. A *therapeutic trial* with sodium is then necessary, *provided there is no clinical evidence of sodium overload,* as described below. Replacement of sodium deficiency is achieved with intravenous saline or additional oral intake of salt and fluid. The patient is then carefully watched for sodium overload.

Sodium overload is associated with water retention and is clinically detected by oedema of the legs, engorged neck veins, pulmonary congestion and hypertension. Sodium restriction is then necessary.

Potassium

Hyperkalaemia (increased serum potassium) results from tissue breakdown releasing potassium, and scanty urine decreasing urinary potassium excretion. A combination of hyperkalaemia, hypocalcaemia and hypermagnesaemia produces adverse myocardial effects exhibiting as arrhythmias and electrocardiographic changes. The management of potassium intoxication is described under acute renal failure [p. 507].

Potassium intake of foods must be reduced. Vegetables and potatoes are palatable but rich in potassium. Their potassium content is considerably lowered by slicing and rinsing in running water, subsequently placing them in a temperature of 50–60° for 2 hours and again rinsing in running water [13].

Hypokalaemia. This is less frequently noted. It occurs when diuresis takes place following removal of urinary obstruction. Oral, or if necessary intravenous, potassium is administered.

CALCIUM, PHOSPHORUS, VITAMIN D, PARATHYROID AND RENAL OSTEODYSTROPHY

The serum calcium is low, yet tetany is rare as metabolic acidosis keeps the ionized calcium level higher. Correction of acidosis may precipitate tetany.

Serum calcium is decreased with chronic renal acidosis due to: (1) loss of acid-soluble calcium carbonate from the bones; and (2) *vitamin D resistance,* probably due to defect in the conversion of vitamin D into active metabolite 25-hydroxycholecalciferol. There is also accelerated vitamin D destruction [14]. Vitamin D resistance produces: (a) decreased calcium absorption and low serum calcium; (b) impaired skeletal response to parathyroid; and (c) defective bone mineralization.

Vitamin D resistance and decreased serum calcium produces *secondary parathyroid hyperfunction.* Hyperparathyroidism results in increased bone reabsorption and *increased serum calcium.* A severe degree of hyperparathyroidism may require parathyroidectomy.

Serum phosphorus is raised due to defective phosphorus excretion with increasing renal damage. Raised serum phosphorus further stimulates parathyroid activity.

Renal osteodystrophy is the term used to describe bony changes due to calcium, phosphorus, vitamin D and parathyroid disturbances. Depending upon the relative metabolic dysfunctions, the resulting bony changes observed are retardation of bony growth (renal rickets), osteoporosis, osteomalacia, osteitis fibrosa, or osteosclerosis.

Metastatic Calcium Deposits. Hyperparathyroidism increases serum calcium level while serum phosphate is increased due to its decreased urinary excretion. Body deposits of calcium phosphate occur with raised serum level when the product $Ca \times P$ exceeds 70. The deposits in the conjunctiva produce *granular conjunctivitis* [15] (red eye), skin itching, and calcification in the lungs, kidneys, heart and peri-articular tissues.

Treatment

Hypocalcaemia is treated with 1·25 g calcium carbonate four times (5 g) daily; this improves acidosis, raises the serum calcium level and by binding dietary phosphate decreases its absorption [16]. With *severe hypocalcaemia,* large daily doses of vitamin D 25,000–400,000 Units may be required [17], but close observation should be kept on the serum calcium level to avoid over-treatment producing hypercalcaemia.

Hyperphosphataemia is avoided by giving a low phosphate diet. Aluminium hydroxide in a daily oral dose of 4–8 g decreases mineral absorption and helps to give relief in 'réd eye' and itching. Vigorous treatment may produce phosphate depletion syndrome with anorexia, nausea and weakness [18].

Dialysis

Haemodialysis is started when it is not possible to maintain the patient on diet alone, and the blood urea rises above 200 mg per cent. Dialysis contributes to loss of *ascorbic acid* and folic acid. During 4–6 hours of haemodialysis 14–16 g *amino acids are lost.*

REFERENCES

[1] FRANKLIN, S.S., and MERRILL, J.P. (1960) Acute renal failure, *New Engl. J. Med.,* **262,** 711.

[2] McEVOY, J., McGEOWN, M.G., and KUMAR, R. (1970) Renal failure after radiological contrast media, *Brit. med. J.,* **4,** 717.

[3] MERRILL, J.P. (1970) Acute renal failure, *J. Amer. med. Ass.,* **211,** 289.

[4] SHARPSTONE, P. (1970) Acute renal failure, *Brit. med. J.,* **4,** 158.

[5] CHUGH, K.S., SWALES, J.D., BROWN, C.L., and WRONG, O.M. (1968) Aluminium resin for the treatment of the hyperkalaemia of renal failure, *Lancet,* **ii,** 952.

[6] BERLYNE, G.M., *et al.* (1970) Hyperaluminaemia from aluminium resins in renal failure, *Lancet,* **ii,** 494.

[7] OGG, C. (1970) Chronic renal failure, *Brit. med. J.,* **4,** 223.

[8] TAKACS, F.J. (1969) Clinical evaluation of renal function, *Lahey Clin. Bull.,* **18,** 71.

[9] SIDDIQUI, J., FREEBURGER, R., and FREEMAN, R.M. (1970) Folic acid, hypersegmented polymorphonuclear leukocytes and the uraemic syndrome, *Amer. J. clin. Nutr.,* **23,** 11.

[10] RICHARDS, P., *et al.* (1967) Utilization of ammonia nitrogen for protein synthesis in man, and the effect of protein restriction and uraemia, *Lancet,* **ii,** 845.

[11] GIORDANO, G., *et al.* (1968) Incorporation of urea N^{15} in amino acids of patients with chronic renal failure on low nitrogen diet. *Amer. J. clin. Nutr.,* **21,** 394.

TABLE 28
FOOD VALUES*

BREAD AND CEREAL protein 2 g		VEGETABLE (unsalted) protein 1 g		FRUIT protein 0·5 g water 80 ml		DAILY SUPPLEMENTS OF PROTEINS OF HIGH BIOLOGICAL VALUE TO PROVIDE ESSENTIAL AMINO ACIDS	
water 5 ml	water 65 ml						
G	G		G		G		G
Bread 25	Corn 80	Asparagus	40	Apple	200	*Non-vegetarian*	*Vegetarian*
Crackers 25	Cooked macaroni 60	Green beans	100	Banana	59	Egg 1	Milk 250 ml
Popped corn 15	Cooked oatmeal 100	Beets	100	Canteloupe	80	Meat 30	
Popped rice 30	Peas 50	Broccoli	35	Cherry	60	Milk 100 ml	
Puffed wheat 15	Baked potato 80	Brussels sprouts	35	Fruit cocktail	100		
Shredded wheat 20	Boiled potato 100	Cabbage	100	Grapes	100		
Sugar cookies 40	French fried potato 50	Carrots	100	Grapefruit	100	LIBERALLY PERMITTED	
	Mashed potato 100	Cauliflower	50	3 Lemons (juice)	50	*Carbohydrates*	*Fats*
	Cooked rice 100	Celery	100	Orange	50	Sugar	Butter
	Cooked spaghetti 60	Cucumber	100	Peach	100	Dextrimaltose	Ghee (clarified butter)
	Cooked sweet potato 100	Lettuce	150	Pear	200	Jelly	Oil
		Onions	60	Pineapple	150	Hard sweets	
		Spinach	35	Plum	100	Honey	
		Squash	100	Strawberry	100	Aerated water	
		Tomatoes	100	Tangerine	60	Sherbets	
		Tomato puree	100	Water melon	100		

* Levin, S., Winkelstein, J.A., and Barnes, G. (1967) Modified diet and infrequent peritoneal dialysis in chronic anuric uremia, *New Engl. J. Med.*, **277**, 619.

TABLE 29

CHRONIC RENAL FAILURE

FOODS PERMITTED

20 g protein diet		40 g protein diet	
Eggs*	2	Orange juice with dextrose	4 oz
Low-protein bread	4 slices	Cream of wheat	4 oz
Salt-free butter	9 squares	Egg**	1
Jelly	6 tablespoons	Breakfast cube steak	2 oz
Salt-free string beans	½ cup	White toast	3 slices
Shredded lettuce	½ cup	Butter	10 squares
Grape juice	½ cup	Jelly	3 oz
Canned peaches	2 medium halves	Milk	8 oz
Canned apple sauce	½ cup	Steamed potato	1 medium
Low-protein pudding	2 servings	Carrots	2 oz
Danish dessert	1 serving	Lettuce	2 oz
		Oil and vinegar dressing	1 oz
		Canned pears	2 halves
		Blended juice with dextrose	4 oz
		Mashed sweet potato	3 oz
		Chopped spinach	2 oz
		Lettuce	2 oz
		French dressing	1 oz
		Canned peaches	2 halves
		Apple juice with dextrose	4 oz

* 300 ml milk for vegetarians.
** 150 ml milk for vegetarians.

TABLE 30

CHRONIC RENAL FAILURE

SAMPLE MENU*

			CAL.	PROTEIN g	NA mg	K mg
Breakfast						
Apple sauce, ½ cup	..	..	91	0·2	2	65
Wheat-starch pancakes (2)	..	..	337	0·8	80	37
1 teaspoon butter	..	..	45	0·07	123	3

Table 30 Contd.

			CAL.	PROTEIN g	NA mg	K mg
1 teaspoon jam	..	..	88	—	6	22
Lunch						
1 slice special bread with	..	..	128	0·3	18	4
1 pat butter	..	..	45	0·07	123	3
Caesar salad						
½ head lettuce	..	..	14	0·6	6	160
2 radishes	..	..	4	0·25	4	80
½ cucumber	..	..	7	0·3	3	80
1 tomato	..	..	11	0·6	1·5	122
1 hard-boiled egg	..	..	81	6·3	60	43
Dressing						
1 teaspoon oil	..	..	111	—	—	—
1 teaspoon vinegar	..	..	10	—	—	—
Cake, iced	..	..	527	1·3	22	97
7-Up, (or lemonade) 8 oz	..	..	120	—	2	—
Dinner						
Veal roast, 1 oz. salt free**	..	..	63	6·3	20	128
½ cup fresh carrots	..	..	31	0·9	33	222
¼ cup fresh green beans	..	..	12	0·6	2	75
½ cup fruit cocktail	..	..	76	0·4	5	161
Lettuce wedge, 100 g (¼ head)	..	..	14	0·6	6	160
with lemon wedge	..	..	1	0·02	0·01	5
Pineapple juice, 4 oz	..	..	35	0·4	1	75
Evening Snack						
Ginger ale, 8 oz	..	..	120	0	19	1
Special muffin	..	..	155	0·3	90	7
2 teaspoons butter	..	..	90	0·14	246	6
Totals :	..	..	2236	20·5	883	1556

*　Franklin, S.S. (1970) Uremia, newer concepts in pathogenesis and treatment, *Med. Clin. N. Amer.*, **54**, 411.
**　For vegetarians ¾ cup of milk is substituted.

[12] Spitz, U.M., *et al.* (1970) Carbohydrate metabolism in renal disease, *Quart. J. Med.,* **39**, 201.

[13] Tsaltas, T.T. (1969) Dietetic management of uremic patients: I. Extraction of potassium from foods for uremic patients, *Amer. J. clin. Nutr.,* **22**, 490.

[14] Avioli, L.V., Birge, S.J., and Slatopolsky, E. (1969) Nature of vitamin C resistance in patients with chronic renal disease, *Arch. intern. Med.,* **124**, 451.

[15] Berlyne, G.M. (1968) Microcrystalline conjunctival calcification in renal failure. A useful clinical sign, *Lancet,* **ii**, 366.

[16] Makoff, D.L., *et al.* (1969) Chronic calcium carbonate therapy in uremia, *Ann. intern. Med.,* **123**, 15.

[17] Stanbury, S.W. (1966) The treatment of renal osteodystrophy, *Ann. intern. Med.,* **65**, 1133.

[18] Lichtman, M.A., Miller, D.R., and Freeman, R.B. (1969) Erythrocyte adenosine triphosphate depletion during hypophosphatemia in a uremic subject, *New Engl. J. Med.,* **280**, 240.

72. RENAL FAILURE: SURGERY AND NUTRITION

The feeding problems during surgery in renal failure are as follows: (1) to provide only the amount of fluid adequate to replace the insensible loss; (2) to provide the minimum nitrogen that could be best utilized for protein synthesis; and (3) to provide adequate calories.

Fluids. With complete suppression of urine the quantity of *fluid* administered is *limited to 1000 ml* to replace the insensible water loss. If the patient passes urine then the volume of additional fluid administered corresponds to the volume of urine passed.

Protein. The minimum nitrogen for necessary metabolism should be provided, but any excess nitrogen accumulates in the blood to enhance the uraemic state. *Essential amino acids* in the minimal recommended quantity, with a total of 6·35 g amino acids [1] containing 1 g nitrogen, are administered intravenously. The intestinal bacteria break down urea into ammonia, which is absorbed. Nitrogen of raised blood ammonia is utilized by the liver for the synthesis of *non-essential amino acids,* which together with the intravenously administered essential amino acids, synthesize body proteins [2].

Calories. The calories should be made up with carbohydrates and fats. This non-protein source of calories is essential to reduce endogenous protein breakdown.

Since the volume of fluid is restricted, the solutions advised are: (1) *hypertonic carbohydrate* as 20 per cent *fructose* 500 ml (400 Calories) *or* up to 30 per cent *sorbitol* 500 ml (600 Calories) [3]; and (2) *fat emulsion* as *Intralipid* 20 per cent 500 ml, that provides 900 Calories. Thus, 1300–1500 Calories are provided in a minimum volume of 1 litre of fluid.

In *North America* intravenous fat emulsions are not in vogue, therefore 50–70 per cent glucose solution is used to provide the calories. The solution is infused continuously at a constant rate over 24 hours each day. *Hypertonic glucose* produces thrombosis of the veins unless administered in one of the deeper veins. The hypertonicity of fluid (3000–4000 mOsm per litre) requires the glucose solution to be delivered into the superior vena cava via the percutaneous infraclavicular sub-clavian vein catheterization [4], where dilution with a large quantity of blood prevents venous thrombosis.

Careful attention should be paid to study the serum *electrolytes* and replace them as required. *Multivitamins* are administered daily. The patients can be maintained on intravenous feeding for several weeks. This mode of feeding considerably reduces the need for dialysis, reduces blood urea nitrogen and helps restore disturbed electrolyte balance. The patient may maintain or even gain weight, and clinical symptoms of nausea, vomiting and diarrhoea disappear.

REFERENCES

[1] ROSE, W.C., WIXOM, R.L., LOCKHART, H.D., and LAMBERT, G.F. (1955) The amino acid requirement of man, XV. The valine requirement, summary and final observations, *J. biol. Chem.*, **217**, 987.

[2] RICHARDS, P., *et al.* (1967) Utilisation of ammonia nitrogen for protein synthesis in man, and the effect of protein restriction and ureamia, *Lancet*, **ii**, 845.

[3] BYE, P.A. (1969) The utilization and metabolism of intravenous sorbitol, *Brit. J. Surg.*, **56**, 653.

[4] DUDRICK, S.J., and RHOADS, J.E. (1971) New horizons for intravenous feeding, *J. Amer. med. Ass.*, **215**, 939.

TABLE 31

FORMULATION OF HYPERTONIC SOLUTION FOR RENAL FAILURE*

PREPARATION OF AMINO ACID MIXTURE		PREPARATION OF NUTRIENT SOLUTION
Essential amino acids	*Minimum daily requirement (g)*	
L—isoleucine	0·70	Glucose 50 — 70% 750 — 1000 ml
L—leucine	1·10	Essential L—amino acids 100 ml (6·35 g)
L—lysine	0·80	
L—methionine	1·10	Volume .. 850 — 1100 ml
L—phenylalanine	1·10	Calories .. 1500 — 2500 Cal
L—threonine	0·50	Glucose .. 375 — 500 g
L—tryptophan	0·25	Nitrogen .. 1 g
L—valine	0·80	
Total:	6·35 in 100 ml water	

ALTERNATIVELY

Amino acid mixture as above + Fructose 20%, 500 ml
OR
Sorbitol 20—30%, 500 ml

AND
Intralipid 20%, 500 ml

Volume 1100

Calories 1300—1500
Nitrogen 1 g

* Dudrick, S.J., Steiger, E., and Long, J.M. (1970) Renal failure in surgical patients; treatment with intravenous essential amino acids and hypertonic glucose, Surgery, **68**, 180.

73. URINARY CALCULI

The end products of metabolism, like uric acid, phosphate and oxalate from the ingested food and tissue breakdown, are excreted by the kidneys along with the minerals like sodium, calcium and magnesium. In the urine these crystalloids are in a supersaturated state. Calcium phosphate and calcium magnesium ammonium phosphate remain in solution in acid urine but precipitate in alkaline urine. Calcium oxalate is in supersaturation whether the urine is acid or alkaline. Despite supersaturation the crystalloids remain in solution due to the presence of normal colloids. If the crystals are precipitated and bound by an organic mucoid matrix then a stone is formed.

Stone Formation
The essential phase in calculus formation is condensation of the specific molecules within the collecting system. These molecules are both mucopolysaccharides and mucoproteins united by a strong chemical bond to form the *matrix* and in them deposition of crystals occurs as a secondary phenomenon.

The *mucopolysaccharides* may be derived from the bony matrix as may occur when the bone is broken down in hyperparathyroidism or may be derived from the connective tissue of the urinary tract. The origin of the *mucoproteins* is still obscure. They may be derived from the transitional epithelium.

The formation of a stone in the urinary passage is favoured by: (1) *Concentration.* A concentrated urine predisposes to stone formation, while a dilute urine diminishes the chances. (2) *Reaction.* Crystals of phosphate remain in solution while urates precipitate in an acid medium. Calcium oxalate crystals are more likely to be precipitated in acid urine. (3) *Colloids.* The exact role of colloids is not known but they help to keep the crystals in a supersaturated solution. The presence of *abnormal colloids,* however, initiates stone formation by cementing together the precipitated crystals.

Aetiology

Heredity. Detailed family history may show that some of the blood relations of a patient with renal calculi had similar trouble. There may be a hereditary defect of metabolism that predisposes to stone formation.

Climate. Those residing in hot tropical climates are prone to develop urinary calculi. The incidence of acute episodes of renal colic is noted to be higher during the hot rather than the cold weather. During the hot weather less urine is formed as more water is lost through perspiration. It is also claimed that during the hot weather, with exposure to the sun, more vitamin D is formed which increases absorption of calcium from the gut and thus leads to increased calcium excretion.

Fluids. In the tropics a lot of fluid is lost through perspiration so crystals are easily precipitated in the scanty concentrated urine. If the daily volume of urine is over 1500 ml (50 oz) stasis and concentration is avoided and the urine is not strongly acid or alkaline. A patient who has renal calculi should drink enough fluids to keep the urine volume over 2000 ml (70 oz). *An adequate fluid intake is the simplest and best safeguard against urinary stone formation.*

Vitamin B Complex. The metabolites excreted in the urine are significantly altered by the vitamin content of the diet. The administration of tryptophan increases while vitamin B_6 decreases the urinary oxalate excretion.

Vitamin A. Vitamin A is necessary for the nutrition of epithelium. Vitamin A deficiency produces roughening of the urinary tract epithelium. On this roughened epithelium it is possible that crystals precipitate and lead to stone formation. Vitamin A deficiency, however, does not appear to play a part in stone formation in India.

Vitamin D and Calcium. Excessive urinary excretion of calcium predisposes to formation of calcium stone. Vitamin D increases calcium absorption from the intestinal tract. Excessive vitamin D with calcium administered indiscriminately over a prolonged period to growing children or pregnant and lactating mothers may result in stone formation. In the areas of the tropics where the calcium content of the water is high and vitamin D is formed by exposure of the skin to sunlight a considerable amount of calcium is absorbed from the gut.

Hyperparathyroidism. In hyperparathyroidism there is excessive breakdown of the cementing matrix of bone and of inorganic calcium and phosphorus, these are concentrated in the urinary tract and may form stones.

Recumbancy. Prolonged bed rest, particularly when the patient is immobilized as during the treatment of diseases of the spine, leads to generalized decalcification of bones. The products of breakdown of the bones are excreted in the urine, and may form stones.

Congenital Malformations, Stasis and Infection. Congenital malformations of the renal pelvis, ureter or bladder; stasis due to stricture or prostatic enlargement; or urinary infection; all predispose to stone formation.

There is increased incidence of kidney stones in inflammatory bowel disease [1].

TYPES OF RENAL CALCULI

The commonest renal calculi are oxalates, urates or phosphates, combined with calcium.

Calcium

Calcium stones being radio-opaque can be seen on plain X-ray. The normal range of urinary calcium in adults taking an ordinary diet is 100–300 mg per day for men and 100–250 mg per day for women. Patients who pass calcium stones in general tend to show hypercalcinuria.

Idiopathic hypercalcinuria occurs with increased intestinal calcium absorption. A stone-former with higher calcium intake will have increased calcium absorption and urinary excretion compared to normal subjects. Hence, instead of measuring fasting serum and urinary calcium, an oral loading test with calcium citrate 100 mg per kg gives serum and urinary calcium values higher in hypercalcinuria than in normal subjects [2]. Some cases of hypercalcinuria and stone formation may have parathyroid adenoma despite normal serum calcium [3]. Glucose or sucrose ingestion in kidney stone-formers and their relatives results in higher urinary concentration of calcium [4]. Hypercalcinuria with renal stone formation occurs in hyperparathyroidism, tubular acidosis, sarcoidosis and Cushing's syndrome.

Sodium cellulose phosphate orally administered adsorbs calcium ion in the intestine and thus prevents hyperabsorption of dietary calcium, increases faecal calcium excretion and decreases urinary calcium absorption [5]. Fifteen g daily in three 5 g doses with meals is recommended in the treatment of hypercalcinuria and prevention of renal stone formation.

Oxalate

Normal urinary oxalate excretion is about 17–40 mg per day. The patient with oxalate stone may also have normal oxalate excretion. Ingestion of spinach, tomatoes, strawberries, chocolate or tea produces temporary increase in oxalates in all individuals and is known as *secondary hyperoxaluria*. It is possible to decrease the oxalate content of vegetables by using phosphorous fertilizer.

Vitamin B -deficient cats have increased urinary oxalate excretion probably due to excessive endogenous breakdown resulting in oxalate nephrocalcinosis. In humans, a daily oral dose of 200 mg magnesium oxide and 10 mg pyridoxine reduces *recurrence* of kidney stone [6].

Primary hyperoxaluria is a familial metabolic error not related to the exogenous oxalate intake but the daily urinary oxalate excretion may be 100 mg. The source of excessive urinary oxalate is probably unusual conversion of glycine to oxalate. Generalized deposition of oxalates in the body is labelled as *oxalosis*.

Clinically there may not be any signs or symptoms with primary hyperoxaluria. It may become apparent usually at 1–4 years of age only when urinary calculus formation occurs, which may produce repeated urinary colic, haematuria and urinary infection. Nephrocalcinosis is late to develop and kidney function fails. Depending upon the duration of the condition, hypertension, papilloedema, cardiac failure, and uraemia may occur with fatal termination.

Calcium Oxalate

Crystals of calcium oxalate are mostly found in acid urine but may also be present in neutral or alkaline urine. Most urinary stones seen in India and Great Britain contain calcium oxalate to a greater or lesser extent and these stones may or may not be associated with increased urinary calcium excretion.

Uric Acid

The average daily excretion of uric acid is 0·5–1·0 g. When the urine is strongly acid, uric acid crystals are precipitated and can be seen microscopically. The mere finding of uric acid crystals in the urine does not denote any abnormality in uric acid metabolism but only indicates that the urine is strongly acid. Unless uric acid excretion is estimated on a controlled diet no conclusions can be drawn about uric acid metabolism.

Uric acid stones are common in patients with gout and are also seen in the tropics.

Phosphate

The normal daily excretion of inorganic phosphate is 500–1500 mg in males and 500–900 mg in females. Phosphates remain in solution in acid urine and form a visible heavy precipitate in strongly alkaline urine of a healthy person. Samples of urine kept for several hours frequently turn strongly alkaline because of formation of ammonia by urea-splitting micro-organisms and a heavy deposit of phosphate forms which has no clinical significance.

The daily excretion of phosphate is not increased in patients with stones. Phosphate stones tend to form in the bladder when there is stasis and infection due, for example, to paraplegia or prostatic enlargement. Some infecting organisms split urea into ammonia, and phosphates precipitate in the strongly alkaline urine and are bound together by matrix.

Magnesium

Low urinary magnesium excretion and higher urinary calcium excretion (lower magnesium/calcium ratio) predispose to renal stone formation in hyperparathyroidism [7]. These people may benefit from supplements of magnesium [8].

Cystine

Cystinuria is an inherited condition which is due to defective reabsorption by the renal tubule of the amino acids cystine, lysine, arginine and ornithine. The loss of the essential amino acid lysine results in stunted growth. Cystinuric patients are at higher risk of impaired cerebral function. *Treatment* consists of increasing fluids and reducing methionine by reducing animal protein, and substituting vegetable protein. Lysine supplement promotes growth. Chlordiazepoxide (*Librium*) is claimed to reduce cystine crystalluria [9]. D-penicillamine is nephrotoxic but N-acetyl-D-penicillamine, 2–4 g daily in divided 6-hourly doses, decreases urinary cystine excretion [10] and formation of cystine stones.

DISSOLVING KIDNEY STONES

Acute renal colic manifests the ureter's attempt to expel a foreign body. A small stone will be voided in the urine sooner or later, the administration of antispasmodics makes its passage easier. Treatment during this stage consists in the relief of pain, the administration of antispasmodics and a large quantity of fluids. It is a mistake to believe that any particular drug can help in dissolving a stone. Such claims are only made by quacks. The passage of a calculus after a severe bout of pain convinces the patient and his sympathizers that a particular drug has 'dissolved the stone'. The passage of a stone with these so called 'solvents' should not lull a patient into a false sense of security that he has got rid of his disease. Renal colic should be taken as nature's warning signal to investigate the renal tract and to take precautions against future stone formation.

Cystine stones may be dissolved by a daily water intake of 2000 ml and the drugs mentioned above. *Uric acid stones* have been dissolved during a period of 6 months by liberal fluid intake and oral alkalies to maintain urinary pH between 6·4 to 7. Alkalinization above pH 7 carries the danger of phosphate stones [11]. The *recurrence* of all kidney stones is effectively prevented by ensuring at least 2000 ml urine daily.

Bladder stones (as distinct from kidney stones) are common in children in villages of South-East Asia [12], but their prevalence could not be attributed to a specific diet.

URINE EXAMINATION

During and after an attack of colic, all specimens of urine should be passed in a chamber pot and examined immediately with the naked eye for calculi. If a calculus is passed it should be analysed chemically. It is of the utmost importance to examine repeated samples of urine macroscopically and microscopically for red blood cells *during* an attack of colic. The presence of these cells gives confirmatory evidence that the acute abdominal pain is arising from the urinary tract. The absence of red cells a few days after the colic is of no help in the diagnosis.

DIETETIC MANAGEMENT

Fluids

During an attack of renal colic there is a tremendous enthusiasm for fluids and diet, which usually wanes. Calculus formation is a gradual process extending over a long period of time and once a tendency to stone formation has developed it will persist throughout life. Vigilance with fluid intake and diet is needed indefinitely.

The fundamental principle in the treatment of urinary calculi is to supply adequate fluids like water, coconut and barley water, sherbet, aerated water, fruit juice and weak tea in order to ensure the passage of over 2000 ml (70 oz) of urine per day. A heavy manual worker in a hot humid climate, to compensate for the fluid loss through perspiration, should drink more fluids than a sedentary office worker in a cooler climate. A dilute urine avoids concentration of solids and also tends to make the urine neutral, thus preventing the strong acid or alkaline reaction which predisposes to precipitation of crystals. The simplest guide to the patient is to tell him to drink enough fluids to see that the urine when voided is light in colour.

Foods

Although the role of diet in the formation of urinary stones is not well established, it is advisable to restrict foods which are rich in calcium, oxalate or uric acid, according to the type of stone formed. Thus, a person who has passed a calcium oxalate stone should avoid a diet rich in calcium and oxalate. If he cannot resist the temptation to eat strawberries or tomatoes occasionally, then he should drink additional water for the next day or two. It is also claimed that milk or cheese, if taken with food rich in oxalate, lead to the precipitation of non-absorbable calcium oxalate in the intestine.

Vitamins

Vitamin A may be helpful in a person deficient in it.

PREVENTION OF RENAL CALCULI

Urinary calculi may be due to hereditary metabolic defect and the exact role of diet is not settled. Yet people with a history of stone formation in a blood relation or those who have had renal colic can probably diminish their chances of calculus formation by the following measures:

1. By drinking enough fluid to excrete 2000 ml (70 oz) of urine a day. During hot humid weather with excessive sweating, extra fluids must be taken.

2. As calcium oxalate is the commonest constituent of stones, by restricting foods rich in oxalates as listed in TABLE 32.

3. By seeking prompt and adequate treatment for any urinary infection.

4. By moving as much as possible if confined to bed.

TABLE 32

FOODS RICH IN

CALCIUM	OXALATE	URIC ACID
Beans	Beef	Fish, herring
Cauliflower	Cashew nuts	Fish roe
Egg yolk	*Chickoo*	Salmon
Figs	Chocolates	Sardine
Milk and milk products (butter and *ghee* need not be restricted)	Cocoa Custard apple *Knush khush*	Kidney Liver Meat extracts
Molasses	Rhubarb	Soups
Potatoes	Spinach	Sweetbread
	Strawberries	
	Tea	
	Tomato	

REFERENCES

[1] GELZAYD, E.A., BREUER, R.I., and KIRSNER, J.B. (1968) Nephrolithiasis in inflammatory bowel disease, *Amer. J. dig. Dis.*, **13**, 1027.
[2] PEACOCK, M., KNOWLES, F., and NORDIN, B.E.C. (1968) Effect of calcium administration and deprivation on serum and urine calcium in stone-

forming and control subjects, *Brit. med. J., 2,* 729.

[3] ADAMS, P., CHALMERS, T.M., HILL, L.F., and TRUSCOTT, B. McN. (1970) Idiopathic hypercalciuria and hyperparathyroidism, *Brit. med. J., 4,* 582.

[4] LEMANN, J., JR., PIERING, W.F., and LENNON, E.J. (1969) Possible role of carbohydrate-induced calciuria in calcium oxalate kidney-stone formation, *New Engl. J. Med., 280,* 232.

[5] PARFITT, A.M., *et al.* (1964) Metabolic studies in patients with hypercalciuria, *Clin. Sci., 27,* 463.

[6] GERSHOFF, S.N., and PRIEN, E.L. (1967) Effect of daily MgO and vitamin B_6 administration to patients with recurring calcium oxalate kidney stones, *Amer. J. clin. Nutr., 20,* 393.

[7] SUTTON, R.A.L., and WATSON, L. (1969) Urinary excretion of calcium and magnesium in primary hyperparathyroidism, *Lancet,* **i,** 1000.

[8] OREOPOULOS, D.G., SOYANNOWO, M.A.O., and McGEOWN, M.G. (1968) Magnesium/calcium ratio in urine of patients with renal stones, *Lancet,* **ii,** 420.

[9] FARISS, B.L., and KOLB, F.O. (1968) Factors involved in crystal formation in cystinuria, *J. Amer. med. Ass., 205,* 846.

[10] STOKES, G.S., POTTS, J.T., LOTZ, M., and BARTERS, F.C. (1968) New agent in the treatment of cystinuria: N-acetyl-D-penicillamine, *Brit. med. J.,* **1,** 284.

[11] MAKERIGIANNIS, D., and GACA, A. (1970) Dissolution and prevention of recurrence of uric acid stones in kidney by oral medication, *Dtsch. med. Wschr., 95,* 1383.

[12] CHUTIKORN, C., VALYASEVI, A., and HALSTEAD, S.B. (1967) Studies of bladder stone disease in Thailand. II. Hospital experience, urolithiasis at Ubol Province Hospital, 1956–1962, *Amer. J. clin. Nutr., 20,* 1320.

74. ATHEROSCLEROSIS AND CORONARY HEART DISEASE

Contributed by R.H. Dastur

A better knowledge of nutrition, advances in preventive medicine and control of bacterial disease by antibiotics has increased life expectancy and made more prominent degenerative arterial diseases. A person is said to be 'as old as his arteries'. Indeed, when the arteries of the heart, brain and kidneys show degenerative changes, the circulation and nutrition of these organs suffer. A great deal of research has been undertaken to understand the cause of atherosclerotic change, so that effective measures may be instituted towards prevention.

Ninty-five per cent of coronary heart disease is due to coronary atheroma and atherosclerosis. The raised plasma lipid level is correlated with the production of atherosclerosis.

The following factors modify plasma lipids:

1. Heredity	11. Carbohydrates
2. Age	12. Insulin
3. Hormones	13. Vitamins
4. Total calories	14. Minerals
5. Cholesterol	15. Water
6. Triglycerides	16. Smoking
7. Lipoproteins	17. Mental stress
8. Total fat	18. Exercise
9. Saturated and unsaturated fats	19. Diet
10. Proteins	20. Drugs

Heredity

Heredity plays a part in coronary heart disease. Short, stocky and short-necked subjects are more likely to develop coronary heart disease than tall, thin people. Probably the environment, dietary habits and the mode of living of a family also predispose to coronary heart disease.

Age

Coronary heart disease usually manifests itself after the age of 50 but with a strong hereditary predisposition it occurs earlier. Indians tend to develop coronary heart disease at an earlier age than the people of Western countries. Myocardial infarction and ischaemic heart disease have also been observed in infants and children [1].

Hormones

Sex Hormones. Although atherosclerosis occurs both in males and females, males in general are more predisposed to coronary heart disease. Prior to menopause the disease is uncommon in females but later in life the incidence may be about the same as it is in males. It is possible that the female sex hormones have an inhibitory effect on coronary artery disease. However, the masculine love of rich food, alcohol and tobacco, rather than sex hormones, may be responsible for the higher incidence in the male. Oestrogens administered to males with coronary artery disease lower the plasma cholesterol level, but the large doses required for this effect result in impotence and gynaeco-mastia.

Thyroid. The total blood lipid and cholesterol level is high in hypothy-roidism and low in hyperthyroidism. Thyroid accelerates cholesterol breakdown to cholic acid.

Total Calories

The serum lipids rise with an increase in the total calorie intake. The early Yemenite immigrants to Israel were richer and consumed more calories and fats than later immigrants of the same age and sex. The total lipid level was significantly higher and mortality from athero-sclerosis four times greater in these early settlers. The obese are more prone to heart disease than those with a normal body weight. In over-weight patients with coronary heart disease, the extra weight has been shown to be due to excess of body fat as compared to the controls whose weight was mainly due to the muscle tissue. Although they have the same body weight those taking physical exercise are less likely to develop coro-nary heart disease than sedentary workers who accumulate fat. Obesity indirectly burdens the heart [see p. 441]. Obesity is the result of excess calorie intake, but the heredity and metabolism of an individual may also be responsible for the ease with which the weight is increased.

Cholesterol

In the study of atherosclerosis cholestrol has been the focus of atten-tion for two reasons: (1) cholesterol deposits are found in atheromatous patches; (2) compared to other lipids cholesterol is more easily estimated.

Source. The sources of cholesterol are: (1) *exogenous* from food [see p. 37]; (2) *endogenous synthesis* from acetate by the *liver* and the *intes-tines,* particularly the ileum.

Endogenous Cholesterol Synthesis. The endogenous synthesis of cholesterol is partly regulated by the dietary cholesterol intake. Even on a cholesterol-free diet, cholesterol for the body needs will be synthesi-zed by (1) the liver, and (2) the intestines. *Liver synthesis is reduced with high cholesterol diet, fasting* (low calorie intake), and *increased bile flow in the intestine that facilitates dietary cholesterol absorption. Intestinal cholesterol synthesis increases* with diminished bile flow to the intestine.

The intestinal synthesis is only partially suppressed with cholesterol feeding, while fasting has negligible effects. Endogenous cholesterol synthesis suppression is variable, being less in United States Caucasian than East Africans [2]. High blood cholesterol in obstructive jaundice may partly be due to decreased flow of bile in the intestine, which stimulates increased intestinal synthesis.

The cholesterol absorption capacity of the intestine is limited to only 300–500 mg a day [3]. Despite high cholesterol diet a major part of serum cholesterol is derived from endogenous synthesis [4], mainly from carbohydrate.

Sitosterol is a vegetable sterol (animal sterol is cholesterol) present in soya-bean, cotton-seed, etc. When given orally it is not absorbed by the digestive tract. Five to 10 g given orally to man over a period of months lowers the serum cholesterol level because sitosterol combines with the cholesterol of food and bile to form unabsorbable compounds. Attempts have been made to reduce serum cholesterol by daily oral administration of 5–10g sitosterol in divided doses.

Plasma Cholesterol

PLASMA CHOLESTEROL AND TRIGLYCERIDES [5]

AGE	Cholesterol	Triglyceride
0–19	120–230	10–140
20–29	120–240	10–140
30–39	140–270	10–150
40–49	150–310	10–160
50–59	160–330	10–190

The plasma cholesterol and triglycerides circulate as lipoproteins and the percentage content is as follows [6]:

LIPOPROTEIN	CHOLESTEROL %	TRIGLYCERIDE %
Chylomicron	5	5
Pre-beta: very low density lipoprotein (VLDL)	13	55
Beta: Low density lipoprotein (LDL)	70	29
Alpha: High density lipoprotein	17	11

Thus, most of the plasma cholesterol is in low density lipoprotein while most of triglyceride is in very low density lipoprotein.

The plasma cholesterol level in both men and women remains about the same until the age of 20, and then increases with age, more so in males. A single plasma cholesterol estimation is not conclusive as even with ordinary activity and diet, the level shows significant fluctuations. The plasma cholesterol level changes with the posture: on assuming an erect from a recumbent posture, within 15 minutes the plasma cholesterol values increase by 13 per cent [7]. These values are higher in blood group A than groups O or B [8]. The cholesterol in atherosclerotic arteries is in a dynamic state and exchanges with that in the blood.

North Americans consuming about 45 per cent of calories as fat have high plasma cholesterol. British subjects show no relationship between the actual fat intake and content of serum cholesterol or the incidence of coronary artery disease [9]. Indian labourers of the lower middle and working classes, who are suffering from coronary heart disease, have on the average a dietary fat content of 50·7 g, i.e. 20 per cent of the calorie intake, and only 19 per cent of these patients have serum cholesterol higher than 250 mg per cent [10]. Therefore coronary heart disease is *not necessarily related* to high fat intake or high plasma cholesterol.

Triglycerides [see p. 40]

Plasma Triglyceride Sources. (1) *Exogenous* plasma triglyceride is derived from the ingestion of *fatty acids*. The absorbed triglycerides raise the plasma level for 3–4 hours after food and circulate as *chylomicrons* that are taken up by the cells of liver, adipose tissue and other organs. In exogenous hyperlipidaemia the circulating chylomicrons are not cleared from the plasma.

2. *Endogenous.* Plasma triglycerides are derived from *carbohydrates* and synthesized into the glycerides by the *liver* and the *intestine*. The *liver* is the main organ producing triglycerides from free fatty acids (FFA), *carbohydrate* and two carbon fragments. The endogenous triglyceride level rises a few days after ingestion of carbohydrate and may persist. Sugars (sucrose, fructose and lactose) stimulate *insulin* secretion, which enhances triglyceride formation (lipogenesis) [12].

Endogenous Hypertriglyceridaemia. The majority of patients with diabetes or coronary heart disease *synthesize* triglycerides (*endogenous* *hypertriglyceridaemia*). Patients with types II, III, IV and V hyperlipoproteinaemia have endogenous hypertriglyceridaemia [11].

Lipoprotein lipase (clarifying factor) is an enzyme concentrated mainly in the capillary walls and body cells. It breaks down plasma chylomicrons and other lipoproteins into glycerol and fatty acids, to facilitate their entry into body cells. Hyperlipaemia after a meal is rapidly cleared by an intravenous injection of *heparin,* which is known as *post-heparin lipolytic activity* (PHLA). This action of heparin is probably effected through the release of lipoprotein lipase from the tissues.

Lipoproteins [5]

Lipids are insoluble but their attachment to proteins of different densities forms *soluble lipoproteins. Transport* of all lipids is achieved by the formation of soluble lipoproteins (except free fatty acids—FFA —that are derived from the breakdown of depot fats). The plasma lipoprotein estimations therefore reflect the lipid concentration. The various proteins to which lipids are attached are: (1) *alpha,* a high density protein, forming *alpha-lipoprotein;* (2) *beta,* or low density protein, forming low density lipoprotein (LDL); (3) *pre-beta,* or very low density lipoprotein (VLDL); and (4) chylomicrons.

These lipoproteins are isolated by:

1. *Ultra-centrifugation* that separates the *densities* as: (a) high (*alpha*); (b) low (*beta*); (c) very low (*pre-beta*) density lipoproteins; and (d) chylomicrons. The last contain very minute amounts of lipoprotein.

2. *Electrophoresis.* Separating these lipoproteins by electrophoresis is the commoner and easier method for identification of *alpha-, beta-,* and *pre-beta*-lipoproteins.

The *lipoproteins* consist of: (a) the specific lipoprotein, mentioned above, (b) cholesterol, and (c) phospholipid. *Beta*-lipoproteins contain more cholesterol than other lipoproteins.

Lipoproteinaemia of the following five different types have been described.

Lipoproteinaemia [13,14]

Type I Lipoproteinaemia (Exogenous Hyperlipaemia). The disease is familial. *Infants* are seen with abdominal colic, hepatosplenomegaly and lipaemia retinalis. In adults recurrent abdominal pain mimics pancreatitis. The pain is accompanied by leucocytosis. Normally, the plasma is cleared of *chylomicrons* within a few hours of food due to the *lipoprotein lipase* (clearing factor) activity. In type I lipoproteinaemia the overnight fasting plasma is creamy and on standing forms a creamy layer on top. Decreased lipoprotein lipase activity is inferred from the failure of heparin injection to clear the plasma of chylomicrons. The *treatment* consists of allowing butter and medium chain triglycerides [p. 384] in the diet, since these short and medium chain triglycerides are absorbed by the portal vein and do not form chylomicrons for absorption. The other dietary fats are excluded. *Drugs* are not necessary.

Type II (Familial Hypercholesterolaemia); Hyper-Beta-Lipoprotein-aemia. This is a familial disorder and the trait could be detectable even at birth. *Clinically* there are tendon xanthoma mainly of the tendo Achillis, and an accelerated rate of atherosclerosis and coronary heart disease at an early age. *Investigations* reveal *high serum cholesterol* and high *beta*-lipoproteinaemia on electrophoresis (LDL). The *dietary treatment* consists of restriction of carbohydrates, especially sugars, low cholesterol and 15 per cent fats used as poly-unsaturated (oils) or medium chain triglycerides [p. 384]. *Drug* therapy decreases LDL by about 15 per cent, while a further 25–35 per cent fall in LDL is achieved with daily 24 g cholestyramine.

Type III. This is common. *Clinically,* it is seen in *adults* with atherosclerosis of the coronary arteries *and* peripheral arteries. Xanthoma occurs, particularly of the palms and digital creases. *Investigations* reveal glucose *intolerance* (diabetes) and raised plasma cholesterol, and triglycerides; *electrophoresis* shows *a broad beta band* (merging of pre-beta and beta bands). The *treatment* is to *control weight* with low calorie diet and low carbohydrates. Drug therapy consists of clofibrate, *D*-thyroxine or nicotinic acid.

Type IV (Endogenous, Carbohydrate-Induced Hyperlipidaemia). This is the *commonest* type seen in adults. It is associated with coronary heart disease and excessive lipid synthesis. *Clinically,* atherosclerosis and coronary heart disease are common. *Investigations* reveal slightly elevated cholesterol but triglyceridies are markedly raised and on electrophoresis there is *pre-beta* lipoproteinaemia (VLDL). The *diet* is aimed at reducing overweight and restricting carbohydrates to 125 g. The poly-unsaturated fats (oils) are increased to constitute 40–50 per cent of the calorie intake. The *drug* therapy comprises clofibrate, *D*-thyroxine or nicotinic acid.

Type V. This is a combination of type I with high chylomicrons (*exogenous* hyperlipaemia) and type IV *pre-beta* hyperlipoproteinaemia (*endogenous* lipoproteinaemia). The patients are obese, and abdominal crisis resembling type I lipoproteinaemia may occur. Glucose *intolerance* (diabetes) is common. The treatment is weight control with low fat and low carbohydrate diet. The *drug* therapy consists of nicotinic acid or clofibrate.

Conclusion. Lipoprotein pattern analysis has helped distinguish *exogenous fat-induced* raised plasma lipids (chylomicrons) from *endogenous carbohydrate-induced* synthesis that raises plasma lipoproteins. The increased *endogenous* lipogenic activity is most common in all patients with atherosclerosis [15]. In coronary heart disease patients, lipoproteinaemia is noted in 54 per cent (29 per cent *beta*-lipoproteinaemia and 25 per cent *pre-beta*-lipoproteinaemia [16]. For *screening* the general population, electrophoresis for lipoprotein is no more helpful than estimation of cholesterol and triglycerides [17].

Total Fat

The serum cholesterol level is not necessarily dependent upon its intake. Increasing the amount of fat in the diet, without increasing the cholesterol intake, elevates the serum cholesterol level.

Saturated or Unsaturated Fats

Saturated Fats. The following fats have a higher proportion of saturated fatty acids: (1) animal fats which include fats derived from pork, beef and meat drippings; (2) fats derived from dairy products and milk products like cream, butter, *ghee* and egg yolk; (3) hydrogenated vegetable oils. Hydrogenation of unsaturated seed oils like groundnut or cotton-seed oil produces saturated fats called margarine, vegetable *ghee* or *vanaspati*. Coconut and palm oils, though vegetable products, are relatively saturated in the natural state.

Unsaturated Fats. Unsaturated fats include *vegetable oils* like groundnut or cotton-seed in their *natural form*. Marine oils derived from shark, whale, cod, halibut, etc., are also unsaturated.

A diet low in *saturated* fats (animal and hydrogenated oils and high in *unsaturated* fats (vegetable or marine oil) lowers the incidence of coronary infarction, sudden death and cerebral infarction, but not the total mortality [18]. *Vegetable oils* diminish the plasma cholesterol not only due to poly-unsaturated fatty acids but also because the plant sterol (sitosteról) content inhibits cholesterol absorption. Vegetarians have a lower plasma cholesterol which is elevated with the intake of meat, fish and fowl because of the increase in the consumption of total fat, saturated fatty acids, cholesterol and proteins.

The composition of body fat can be changed by varying the type of dietary fat. Consumption of vegetable fats results in fatty tissues containing more unsaturated fatty acids than controls [19].

Dangers of Unsaturated Fats. Caution is required with over-enthusiasm in giving only unsaturated vegetable or marine fats and completely avoiding saturated fats. For unsaturated fats are more easily oxidized and administration of oxidized fats to rats produces gastric ulcer and gastric carcinoma. In Japan and in Sweden the consumption of unsaturated fish oil may be a contributory factor in the high incidence of gastric carcinoma [20]. In experimental animals, cirrhosis is more readily produced by the administration of unsaturated fats, whereas saturated fats delay its production [21].

Proteins

Casein prevents atherosclerosis in monkeys. However, casein deficiency is unlikely to be a cause of atherosclerosis, particularly in Western countries where milk is consumed freely.

Carbohydrates

The tremendous enthusiam shown during the last two decades in blaming ingestion of cholesterol and fatty foods as a prime factor in atherogenesis has waned with the knowledge that carbohydrates play a major role in lipid *synthesis*. The body can sythesize lipids (triglycerides and cholesterol) from carbohydrates (endogenous synthesis). When 35–40 per cent calories were supplied as carbohydrate more than 90 per cent of patients with coronary heart disease showed increased serum lipids and frequent hypercholesterolaemia. This endogenous synthesis was controlled by reducing the daily carbohydrate intake to 125–150 g as starches and excluding sugars such as sucrose, fructose and lactose [15].

Sugar. Ischaemic heart disease was ascribed to increased sugar intake mainly in tea and coffee, but in Great Britain sugar intake was found not to be significantly higher in patients with myocardial infarction. Since tea and coffee drinking is frequently associated with cigarette smoking, the slightly increased sugar intake is usually associated with accompanying cigarette smoking [22].

The problem is apparently not solved as *fructose* (contained in household sugar and fruits) is more readily converted to triglycerides than glucose [23]. Sugars, which are rapidly absorbed, increase secretion of pancreatic insulin, that has a lipogenic action. Reducing sugar intake for 5 months decreased serum triglycerides. [24].

Alcohol. Alcohol increases caloric intake and stimulates the production of *beta* lipoproteins. [25].

Insulin

Atherosclerotic patients have diabetes or a tendency to hyperglycaemia and increased insulin secretion [26]. Insulin produces atherogenesis in the following ways: (1) it stimulates deposition of fat in the arterial wall [12]; and (b) it inhibits tissue lipase, thus decreasing fat removal from the arteries. Patients with myocardial infarction have relative insulin resistance and an abnormal type of insulin secretion. Excess intake of calories and carbohydrates is frequently the cause of ischaemic heart disease [15] as without overnutrition the abnormality may not be manifest. Hyperinsulinism is a result of overnutrition.

During acute myocardial infarction insulin secretion is decreased, possibly following shock which reduces pancreatic blood flow resulting in decreased sugar tolerance and increased plasma free fatty acids.

Vitamins

Nicotinic Acid. Nicotinic acid decreases serum lipids probably by decreasing endogenous synthesis. *Therapeutically* nicotinic acid is used to decrease serum lipid level.

Vitamin C. The pathology of atherosclerosis reveals dilated capillaries invading the intima from the vasa vasorum and occasionally directly from the arterial lumen. These capillaries frequently rupture and produce intimal haemorrhage that may occlude the artery by its expansion or by precipitating thrombosis. In vitamin C deficiency due to poor ground substance haemorrhage occurs more easily [27].

Minerals

Potassium, Glucose, Insulin. Glucose utilization by the heart muscle is dependent upon insulin. After myocardial infarction the majority of deaths are due to cardiac arrhythmias presumably caused by deficient myocardial potassium. Intravenous potassium, glucose and insulin treatment was advocated to facilitate potassium entry in the myocardium and to reduce immediate mortality, but this was not found to be of any value. The apparent failure of this regimen was, however, ascribed to inadequate insulin dosage [28].

Calcium supplement of 0·89 g for 21 days increased serum cholesterol and triglycerides and increased faecal lipid excretion [29]. Exposure to *sulphide* in industries is also blamed for coronary heart disease [30]. *Cadmium* produces hypertension in animals. It accumulates with age and a higher concentration is noted in the kidneys. Increased cadmium in the air may have some correlation with hypertension and arteriosclerotic heart disease [31]. Moreover, cigarette smoking increases exposure to cadmium. *Lithium* is higher in hard water and has also been suggested as being antagonistic to ischaemic heart disease risk factors such as hypertension, diabetes, tissue uric acid and serum lipid levels. Hence, the addition of lithium to drinking water has been advocated as a prevention for heart disease [32]. *Lead* from water pipes contributes to a higher lead content of the bones in people who have lived and died in soft water rather than hard water areas [33].

Water

Soft or more acid water with a lower calcium and magnesium content probably causes higher incidence of cardiac arrhythmias after coronary infarction, which leads to sudden death. *Hardness of water* is associated with higher *calcium* and a lower mortality from cardiovascular disease [34].

Smoking

In coronary heart disease, cigarette smoking produces myocardial oxygen deficiency [35]. In heavy smokers *beta* and *pre-beta* lipoproteins are increased. The serum cholesterol and phospholipid levels are more affected by smoking in women than in men [36]. Heavy cigarette smokers have a higher incidence of atherosclerosis and myocardial infarction than non-smokers [37].

Among 34,000 British physicians, atherosclerotic heart disease was 1·5 to 2·00 times higher in cigarette smokers than non-smokers [38], while the fatal and non-fatal myocardial infarction rate was 2·5 times more in smokers. Younger men and heavier smokers are more likely to be affected. If a patient with heart disease stops smoking, the adverse effect on the heart is reduced [38]. Smoking may increase platelet adhesiveness in some individuals. The relationship between smoking and sugar intake is discussed above.

Mental Stress

Ischaemic heart disease is reported to be common among business executives, lawyers and doctors who are subject to constant mental strain. However, the incidence of coronary infarction has also been noted to be fairly high among labourers admitted at the B.Y.L. Nair Charitable Hospital, Bombay. The higher incidence in recent times has been blamed on the mental stress of modern living. Blood samples for cholesterol obtained from medical students during their normal studies, when compared with those obtained during examinations, showed a rise from 191 to 235 mg per 100 ml serum [39].

Exercise

Coronary heart disease is more likely in sedentary workers than those taking moderate physical exercise which tends to open up coronary collateral vessels. Austrian military personnel with better physical fitness due to exercise had a lower incidence of myocardial infarction than corresponding servicemen in the United States [40]. Four weeks after myocardial infarction the mortality among the least active was three times higher than in the active group [41]. *After recovery* from the acute attack, physical exercise improves cardiac function [42].

Thus, physical exercise may prevent the first and subsequent attacks of coronary heart disease and is beneficial after recovery from infarction. The patient is permitted the amount of exercise he is capable of taking without becoming breathless or fatigued. Exercise, such as a brisk walk, swimming or playing golf, keeps a person in better physical health. Business executives who go to office in a car, sit at the desk during the day, and whose recreation consists of theatres or dinner parties, seldom remain physically fit. They are obese and become breathless on moderate exertion. It is argued that it requires several miles of walking to burn the energy supplied by one slice of bread, and that an average individual feels more hungry after exercise; the consequent excess food consumed more than offsets the benefits of exercise. The conclusions may be true for short-term observations. If we look around we seldom see obesity in persons taking regular exercise but when they stop doing so, they rapidly put on weight. There is no better method of keeping healthy than taking exercise in moderation.

Some cardiologists prohibit their patients even from sitting up in bed during an acute attack of coronary infarction. Nursing a coronary patient by *propping up in bed* is, however, advantageous as it does not affect the blood pressure but reduces pulmonary pressure and load on the right ventricle, as compared to lying down [43].

Diet

Dietary counselling is the first step in the management of patients with an abnormally high plasma cholesterol or triglyceride level. If diet alone does not bring about a satisfactory reduction, then lipid-lowering *drugs* should be added [13].

Fats. The *usual* dietary intake of fats (animal *and* vegetable), providing 28 per cent of total calories, shows a significant fall in serum cholesterol and mortality compared to that in those taking a higher amount of fat [44]. The patient is more likely to follow dietary instructions if advice is given merely to reduce the fat intake (this usually amounts to less than 28 per cent of total calories) rather than prescribing a long list of 'do's and don'ts'. Most people who usually consume a well-balanced diet have about 28 per cent fat. It is only among the affluent society that a higher amount of fat is consumed.

The *dietary* treatment for types III, IV and V hyperlipoproteinaemia consists of: (1) controlling weight; (2) restricting carbohydrates as they stimulate endogenous lipid synthesis. The carbohydrates permitted consist of up to 125 g, comprised of starches (potato, cereals) and excluding sugars and fruits; (3) restricting short- and medium-chain fatty acids, such as butter and coconut oil, as they are oxidized in the liver to two carbon precursors for the synthesis of cholesterol, triglycerides and lipoproteins; (4) avoiding *alcohol,* as it stimulates endogenous hyperlipidaemia by increasing calorie intake, and stimulates the liver to synthesize *beta-* lipoproteins [25].

Drugs

Clofibrate. Clofibrate (Chloro-phenoxy-iso-butrate : *Atromid-S*) interferes with cholesterol synthesis in the liver. In a daily dose of 25–30 mg/kg (1·5–2 G daily) in divided doses, it reduces serum cholesterol, but effect is more on triglycerides. The *side-effects* include mild anorexia and gastro-intestinal disturbances or occasional reduction in white cell count, hepatic enlargement and myositis. Clofibrate potentiates the effect of anticoagulants, whose dosage requires to be reduced. In primary biliary cirrhosis the high serum cholesterol rises further, despite clofibrate therapy [45].

D-Thyroxine (Dextrothyroxine). Thyroid accelerates cholesterol breakdown to bile acids. *D*-thyroxine concentrates in the liver and thus has a stronger hypolipidaemic effect than *L*-thyroxine. A prolonged trial with *D*-thyroxine with a gradually increasing dosage up to daily 5–7 mg reduces serum cholesterol. The effective dose may result in hyperthyroidism and aggravate angina, myocardial infarction, congestive cardiac failure or produce sudden death [46]. *D*-thyroxine therapy is useful in decreasing serum cholesterol particularly in those with preclinical hypothyroidism [47].

Nicotinic Acid. Nicotinic acid probably interferes with cholesterol and fatty acid synthesis from acetate, and probably decreases release of fatty acids from the adipose tissues. The dose is 0·3 G on the first day, which is increased to 3 G more in divided doses, by the tenth day. Maintaining this dose helps reduce serum cholesterol and total serum lipids. Nicotinic acid produces transient flushing due to cutaneous vasodilatation. However, the tendency to flushing subsides in about 7–10 days. Slow release aluminium nicotinate may require a lesser dose of 1·5–3 G a day, but produces nausea that may be relieved with unabsorbable antacids. Reduced carbohydrate tolerance, glycosuria and hepatic dysfunction may occur with nicotinic acid therapy [46]. Rarely bilateral amblyopia may occur.

Oestrogens and Testosterone

Women of reproductive age have lower cholesterol than men hence oestrogen has been tried as a hypocholesterolaemic agent. It reduces cholesterol in *men* with feminizing doses only and is likely to produce intravascular clotting. Testosterone is reported to reduce cholesterol and triglycerides.

CONCLUSIONS

Fashions in medical research and the conclusions drawn change rapidly, but that does not alter the basic laws of nature. A decade ago all the horrors of heart disease were ascribed to high blood cholesterol consequent to *ingestion* of cholesterol and saturated fats. However, the blood cholesterol is not necessarily related to the dietary cholesterol as its absorption is limited. The excess intake of cholesterol and saturated fats may have a role in the production of coronary heart disease in the United States, where on an average over 40 per cent of the calories are derived from fat. On the other hand the Masai tribe in East Africa consume 3000 *Calories,* 66 per cent of it being derived from fats, while the cholesterol intake is 500–2000 mg. This diet is comparable to that in the United States, yet the Masai have a paucity of atherosclerosis and have low serum cholesterol. Masai students fed with 2 g crystalline cholesterol when compared with those on a cholesterol-free diet, showed no significant difference in serum cholesterol, phospholipid, triglyceride levels or lipoprotein patterns [48]. It appears that feeding cholesterol reduces endogenous synthesis.

It should not be assumed that consuming only unsaturated fats is desirable. For excessive use of unsaturated fats may be a factor in the causation of the high incidence of carcinoma of the stomach among the Japanese and Swedes. In animals unsaturated fats accelerate the production of cirrhosis. If a moderate amount of fat is taken in both saturated and unsaturated form, so as to derive less than 28 per cent of the calories, then no ill effects need be feared. *High carbohydrate* intake is now found to be a factor in enhancing the body synthesis of lipids and raised plasma values. Soft drinking water and even the air we breathe, presumably contaminated with cadmium and sulphur, are also suspected to produce heart disease.

The answer to the elusive truth in the prevention of heart disease probably lies in observing the simple laws of nature: (1) Consuming only the adequate calories to maintain normal weight. (2) Taking three or four well balanced meals. (3) Avoiding mental tension as far as possible. (4) Avoiding smoking. (5) *Taking regular physical exercise. Physical exercise* in moderation is the most vital factor in the prevention of coronary heart disease. Many of the evils ascribed to diet are in reality due to lack of regular exercise. In short, following the habits of our forefathers may more effectively prevent heart disease, allowing us to survive until the day when the research scientists may inform us that the best way to avoid a heart disease is to follow the habits of our forefathers.

DIET IN PREVENTION AND TREATMENT OF HEART DISEASE

In the present state of our knowledge the following dietetic suggestions are useful for the prevention and treatment of coronary heart disease:

1. Restrict total calories to reduce the weight to the expected normal for the height, age and sex.
2. It is not desirable to restrict all forms of fats as severe restrictions result in mental and physical depression [49].
3. The total ingestion of fats should be less than 28 per cent of the total calories.
4. Fats should be consumed partly as unsaturated vegetable oils such as cotton-seed, groundnut, and olive oil.
5. Saturated fats, hydrogenated vegetable oil (*vanaspati*), margarine and animal fats, like butter, *ghee* and the fat of animal meat, should be taken in moderation.
6. Green vegetables, fruits, cereals, skimmed milk and lean meat should be the main items of diet.
7. Three or four smaller meals are preferable to two big meals. The evening meal should be about 2 hours before retiring.
8. Regular exercise is most useful but physical strain after a meal should be avoided.

REFERENCES

[1] Bor, I. (1969) Myocardial infarction and ischaemic heart disease in infants and children, *Arch. Dis. Childh.*, **44**, 268.
[2] Ho, K.J., and Taylor, C.B. (1970) Control mechanisms of cholesterol biosynthesis, *Arch. Path.*, **90**, 83.
[3] Kaplan, J.A., Cox, G.E., and Taylor, C.B. (1963) Cholesterol metabolism in man, *Arch. Path.*, **76**, 359.
[4] Wilson, J.D., and Lindsey, C.A. (1965) Studies on the influence of dietary cholesterol on cholesterol metabolism in the isotopic steady state in man, *J. clin. Invest.*, **44**, 1805.
[5] Fredrickson, D.S., Levy, R.I., and Lees, R.S. (1967) Fat transport in lipoproteins—an integrated approach to mechanisms and disorders, *New Engl. J. Med.*, **276**, 34, 94, 148, 215, 273.
[6] Lees, R.S., and Wilson, D.E. (1971) The treatment of hyperlipidemia, *New Engl. J. Med.*, **284**, 186.

[7] STOKER, D.J., and WYNN, V. (1966) Effect of posture on the plasma cholesterol level, *Brit. med. J.*, **1**, 336.

[8] OLIVER, M.F., GEIZEROVA, H., CUMMINGS, R.A., and HEADY, J.A. (1969) Serum-cholesterol and A B O and rhesus blood-groups, *Lancet*, **ii**, 605.

[9] HARVARD, C.W.H. (1966) Recovery after myocardial infarction, *Brit. med. J.*, **1**, 1525.

[10] Shah, V.V., SHAH, S.R., and PANSE, V.N. (1968) Nutritional and physical factors in coronary heart disease, *Geriatrics*, **23**, 99.

[11] LEVY, R.I., and GLUECK, C.J. (1969) Hypertriglyceridemia, diabetes mellitus, and coronary vessel disease, *Arch. intern. Med.*, **123**, 220.

[12] STOUT, R.W. (1968) Insulin-stimulated lipogenesis in arterial tissue in relation to diabetes and atheroma, *Lancet*, **ii**, 702.

[13] LEVY, R.I., and FREDRICKSON, D.S. (1970) The current status of hypolipidemic drugs, *Postgrad. Med.*, **47**, 130.

[14] KUO, P.T. (1970) Hyperlipidemia in atherosclerosis: dietary and drug treatment, *Med. Clin. N. Amer.*, **54**, 657.

[15] KUO, P.T. (1967) Hyperglyceridemia in coronary artery disease and its management, *J. Amer. med. Ass.*, **201**, 87.

[16] HEINLE, R.A., LEVY, R.I., FREDRICKSON, D.S., and GORLIN, R. (1969) Lipid and carbohydrate abnormalities in patients with angiographically documented coronary artery disease, *Amer. J. Cardiol.*, **24**, 178.

[17] MASAREI, J.R., et al. (1971) Lipoprotein electrophoretic patterns, serum lipids and coronary heart disease, *Brit. med. J.*, **1**, 78.

[18] DAYTON, S., et al. (1968) Controlled trial of a diet high in unsaturated fat for prevention of atherosclerotic complications, *Lancet*, **ii**, 1060.

[19] TURPEINEN, O., et al. (1968) Dietary prevention of coronary heart disease. Long term experiment, *Amer. J. clin. Nutr.*, **21**, 255.

[20] HARMAN, D. (1957) Atherosclerosis: possible ill-effects of the use of highly unsaturated fats to lower serum-cholesterol levels, *Lancet*, **ii**, 1116.

[21] GYORGY, P., GOLDBLATT, H., and GANZIN, M. (1959) Dietary fat and cirrhosis of the liver, *Gastroenterology*, **37**, 637.

[22] BENNETT, A.E., DOLL, R., and HOWELL, R.W. (1970) Sugar consumption and cigarette smoking, *Lancet*, **i**, 1011.

[23] MARUHAMA, Y. (1970) Conversion of ingested carbohydrate 14C into glycerol and fatty acids of serum triglyceride in patients with myocardial infarction, *Metabolism*, **19**, 1085.

[24] MANN, J.I., HENDRICKS, D.A., TRUSWELL, A.S., and MANNING, E. (1970) Effects on serum-lipids in normal men of reducing dietary sucrose or starch for five months. *Lancet*, **i**, 870.

[25] ISSELBACHER, K.J., and GREENBERGER, N.J. (1964) Metabolic effects of alcohol on the liver, *New Engl. J. Med.*, **270**, 351.

[26] SLOAN, J.M., Mackay, J.S., and SHERIDAN, B. (1970) Glucose tolerance and insulin response in atherosclerosis, *Brit. med. J.*, **4**, 586.

[27] SHAFFER, C.F. (1970) Ascorbic acid and atherosclerosis, *Amer. J. clin. Nutr.*, **23**, 27.

[28] ALLISON, S.P., CHAMBERLAIN, M.J., and HINTON, P. (1969) Intravenous glucose tolerance, insulin, glucose and free fatty acid levels after myocardial infarction, *Brit. med. J.*, **4**, 776.

[29] YACOWITZ, H., FLEISCHMAN, A.I., and BIERENBAUM, M.I. (1965) Effects of oral calcium upon serum lipids in man, *Brit. med. J.,* **1,** 1352.

[30] TILLER, J.R., Schilling, R.S.F., and MORRIS, J.N. (1968) Occupational toxic factor in mortality from coronary heart disease, *Brit. med. J.,* **4,** 407.

[31] CORROLL, R.E. (1966) The relationship of cadmium in the air to cardiovascular disease death rates, *J. Amer. med. Ass.,* **198,** 267.

[32] VOORS, A.W. (1969) Does lithium depletion cause atherosclerotic heart disease? *Lancet,* **ii,** 1337.

[33] CRAWFORD, M.D., and CRAWFORD, T. (1969) Lead content of bones in the soft and hard water area, *Lancet,* **i,** 699.

[34] CRAWFORD, M.D., GARDNER, M.J., and MORRIS, J.N. (1968) Mortality and hardness of local water-supplies, *Lancet,* **i,** 827.

[35] SELTZER, C.C. (1970) Effects of cigarette smoking on coronary heart disease. Where do we stand now?, *Arch. environm. Hlth,* **20,** 418.

[36] POZNER, H., and Billimoria, J.D. (1970) Effect of smoking on blood clotting and lipoprotein levels, *Lancet,* **i,** 1318.

[37] DOYLE, J.T., *et al.* (1962) Cigarette smoking and coronary heart disease; combined experience of the Albany and Framingham studies, *New Engl. J. Med.,* 266, 796.

[38] DOLL, R., and HILL, A.B. (1964) Mortality in relation to smoking, : ten years' observations of British doctors, *Brit. med. J.,* **1,** 1399, 1460.

[39] GRUNDY, S.M., and GRIFFIN, A.C. (1959) Relationship of periodic mental stress to serum lipoprotein and cholesterol levels, *J. Amer. med. Ass.,* **171,** 1794.

[40] COOPER, K.H., and ZECHNER, A. (1971) Physical fitness in United States and Austrian military personnel. A comparative study, *J. Amer. med. Ass.,* **215,** 931.

[41] FRANK, C.W., WAINBLATT, E., SHAPIRO, S., and SAGER, R.V. (1966) Physical inactivity as a lethal factor in myocardial infarction among men, *Circulation,* **34,** 1022.

[42] VARNAUSKAS, E., BERGYN, H., HOUK, P., and Bjorntorp, P. (1966) Haemodynamic effects of physical training in coronary patients, *Lancet,* **ii,** 8.

[43] EDDY, J.D., and SINGH, S.P. (1969) Nursing posture after acute myocardial infarction, *Lancet,* **ii,** 1378.

[44] BIERENBAUM, M.L., *et al.* (1967) Modified-fat dietary management of the young male with coronary disease, *J. Amer. med. Ass.,* **202,** 1119.

[45] SCHAFFNER, F. (1969) Paradoxical elevation of serum cholesterol by clofibrate in patients with primary biliary cirrhosis, *Gastroenterology,* **57,** 253.

[46] PARSONS, W.B. (1965) Chemotherapy of hyperlipidemia, *Mayo Clin. Proc.,* **40,** 822.

[47] CALAY R., *et al.* (1971) Dextrothyroxine therapy for disordered lipid metabolism in preclinical hypothyroidism, *Lancet,* **i,** 205.

[48] Biss, K. *et al.* (1971) Some unique biologic characteristics of the Masai of East Africa, *New Engl. J. Med.,* **284,** 694.

[49] VAN HANDEL, E., NEUMANN, H. and BLOEM, T. (1957) A diet restricted in refined cereals and saturated fats: Its effect on the serum-lipid level of atherosclerotic patients, *Lancet.* **1,** 245.

75. HIGH BLOOD PRESSURE

High blood pressure is a common disorder of civilization particularly amongst the middle and the old age groups. It may sometimes be secondary to diseases of kidneys or endocrine glands like ovaries, supra-renals or pituitary that may respond to treatment. However, the majority of the patients with high blood pressure are labelled 'essential hypertension' as no definite cause could be found.

The heart during systole pumps blood in the elastic arteries that stretch. The recoil of arteries exerts diastolic pressure that serves to maintain the blood flow during diastole. Pumping blood against a raised diastolic pressure strains the heart muscle.

Over 150 mm systolic or over 95 mm diastolic is considered high blood pressure. People living in primitive conditions have a lower range of normal blood pressure. The detection of high blood pressure and its pronouncement by the physician creates anxiety to a patient. A temporary increase of pressure may occur during mental stress. The systolic pressure may rise by 30 points or more during the evening on a busy day as compared to that recorded on a Sunday morning during rest. The auscultatory reading on a manometer may show more than 30 mm Hg above or below the intra-arterial pressure. These variations depend upon the circumference of the arm, the blood pressure reading being too high with a larger arm and too low with a smaller one [1]. It is a mistake on the part of a patient to insist on knowing his blood pressure reading because the normal fluctuations may cause unnecessary anxiety.

Only high systolic pressure without much elevation of the diastolic pressure (divergent hypertension) occurs with arteriosclerosis, anaemia, pregnancy, etc. The heart is not particularly strained and the extreme ill effects on the eyes and kidneys do not occur. Persistent elevation of both the systolic and diastolic pressure (convergent hypertension) could be troublesome. Marked persistent elevation of the diastolic pressure strains the heart, damages the kidneys and produces retinal artery changes.

Predisposing Factors

Though the cause of 'essential hypertension' is not known there are factors which predispose to it.

1. *Hereditary* predisposition to high blood pressure is recognized.
2. *Obesity* tends to increase while weight reduction tends to reduce high blood pressure.
3. The *stress* and *strain* of modern life undoubtedly plays a role. A villager leading a quiet life is less likely to develop hypertension than a city dweller working constantly under pressure. Marked elevation in blood pressure during mental strain, as worrying over a visit to a doctor's office, may also show high readings. Many patients find a remarkable improvement in blood pressure if the physician tries to understand the cause of stress, and succeeds in removing the same and in helping the patient to accept a situation without mental reaction.

KEMPNER'S RICE DIET [2]

Kempner has advocated a rigid rice-fruit-sugar diet for hypertension that gives impressive results even in severe cases. It provides about 2000 Calories, 5 g fat, 20 g protein, 200 mg chloride and 150 mg sodium. Boiled or steamed *rice,* 250–350 g (dry weight), is allowed daily. All *fruit juices* and *fruits* are permitted. Nuts, dates, avocados, dried or canned fruit and fruit derivatives to which substances other than white sugar have been added, are avoided. Not more than one banana is allowed daily. *Sugar* is permitted *ad libitum.* An average patient takes about 100 g daily but even 500 g may be used. Usually no water is given and the *fluid* intake is limited to 700–1000 ml of fruit juice per day. *Vitamin* supplements advised are, vitamin A 5000 Units, vitamin D 1000 Units, thiamine chloride 5 mg, riboflavine 5 mg, niacinamide 25 mg, calcium pantothenate 2 mg.

Some authorities point out that the improvement with the above diet is not due only to low protein, low fat and low sodium but also due to the weight loss and rest under hospital conditions.

DIETETIC MANAGEMENT

Calories

An obese patient must be reduced to normal body weight with a low calorie diet as recommended for obesity.

Proteins

A diet of 50 g protein is necessary to maintain proper nutrition. In

severe hypertension protein restriction to 20 g as advocated by Kempner [2] may be necessary as a temporary measure.

Fats

Atherosclerosis is not an unusual accompaniment of hypertension
hence it may be advisable to avoid a high intake of animal fats or
hydrogenated oils (*vegetable ghee; vanaspati;* margarine). About 40–50
g fats partly as vegetable oil is permitted.

Carbohydrates

Easily digestible carbohydrate is of great help in the dietetic management of hypertension.

Minerals

Sodium. Low sodium diet may be beneficial. Improvement on Kempner's rice diet is partly ascribed to the low sodium content. In a
resistant case the diet has to be very low in sodium [3] (not more than
0·5 g sodium chloride a day). Ingestion of foodstuffs or drugs with a
sodium retaining activity, e.g. liquorice, tends to produce hypertension [4]. In hypertensive patients the sweat sodium excretion is low [5].
It is difficult for an ambulatory patient to follow sodium-poor diet and
the beneficial effects of sodium restriction may be due to physical
and even mental rest in a hospital. If the sodium-poor diet of 0·2 g
sodium (0·5 g sodium chloride) does not produce beneficial effect then
further persistence is of no vlaue. Indeed, in some cases of chronic
renal disease with polyuria, severe restriction of sodium chloride may
be fatal [6].

With effective oral sodium-excreting diuretics now available, stringent
sodium restriction is not necessary.

Potassium. If diuretics are administered to a hypertensive patient,
supplements of fruit juice or potassium salts such as 2–4 g potassium
citrate three times a day are administered.

Low serum potassium values in a patient of high blood pressure
points to aldosterone-secreting suprarenal tumour (Conn's syndrome,
p. 167).

Fluids

With a free flow of urine, fluid restriction is not necessary. With oedema following cardiac failure the fluid requirement is regulated as described on p. 555.

Low Blood Pressure

Finding a blood pressure lower than the standard reading, and its pronouncement, creates *'physician-induced disease'* in the mind of the patient. Low blood pressure *without* shock or any other accompanying disease, that does not bother him, is best not mentioned to the patient. A well rested patient recovering from surgical operation exhibiting systolic pressure even as low as 80 mm Hg, with *normal pulse rate,* may indicate uneventful progress. It should not be treated with drugs, as is frequently done by enthusiastic but inexperienced doctors. During early sleep in normal individuals the systolic blood pressure may also be lower than 80 mm Hg.

HIGH BLOOD PRESSURE
SODIUM-POOR DIET

(Less than 0·2 g sodium or 0·5 g sodium chloride)

Foods	*Remarks*
Bread or *chappatis* of wheat, rice, maize, *jowar, bajra* or *ragi*	Permitted, unsalted
Breakfast cereal of wheat, rice, oatmeal or maize	Permitted, unsalted
Rice, cooked	Permitted
Pulses (*dal*) or beans	Permitted
Meat, fish or chicken	Excluded
Eggs	Excluded
Milk or milk products	2 tablespoons permitted for tea or coffee
Soup	Vegetable soups only
Vegetable salad	Permitted, exclude radish, beetroot, carrot and spinach
Vegetables, cooked	
Potato, sweet potato or yam	Permitted
Fat for cooking, or butter	Permitted, partly as vegetable oil; butter should be unsalted
Sugar or jaggery or honey	Permitted
Jam or *murabba*	Permitted
Pastry	Excluded

Foods	*Remarks*
Dessert	Permitted
Sweet or sweetmeat	Permitted
Fruit, fresh	Permitted
Fruit, dried	Permitted, exclude dried figs, raisins, sultanas
Nuts	Permitted unsalted, exclude coconut water
Condiments	Permitted, exclude ready-made curry powders
Papad, chutney, pickles	Excluded
Beverage	Permitted
Fluid	Total intake 1500 ml if oedema

No salt or baking soda to be used in cooking.

No salt permitted at the table.

If salt-free bread is not available then any cereal flour can be used to bake bread or *chappatis* at home.

No canned products permitted unless declared to be salt free.

SODIUM-POOR DIET
(Less than 0·2 g sodium)

(For vegetarians *and* non-vegetarians)

Breakfast

Tea with 1 tablespoon milk and sugar
Puffed rice with cream, 2 tablespoons, and sugar
Bread* or *chappatis* with honey or jam
Orange

11 a.m.

Orange juice, 1 cup

Lunch

Rice with tomato soup
Baked potato or *dal*
Cooked pumpkin
Bread* or *chappatis*
Grapes

4 p.m.

Tea with milk, 1 tablespoon, and sugar

Almonds* or cashew nuts*

Dinner

Rice with mixed vegetable soup and sour lime
Boiled potato or *dal*, 1 cup
French beans
Bread* or *chappatis*
Baked apple

*Unsalted
No salt or baking soda to be used in cooking.
No salt permitted at the table.
Sour lime or vinegar may be used to make food palatable.
If salt-free bread is not available then any cereal flour to be used to bake bread or *chappatis* at home.

LOW SODIUM DIET
(Less than 0·5 g sodium)

Foods	Remarks
Bread or *chappatis* of wheat, rice, *jowar, bajra* or *ragi*	Permitted, if unsalted
Breakfast cereal of wheat, rice, oatmeal or maize	Permitted, if unsalted
Rice, cooked	Permitted
Pulses (*dal*) or beans	Permitted
Meat, fish or chicken	Permitted, all salted meat to be excluded
Egg	One
Milk or milk products	One cup. 2 cups for vegetarians
Soup	Vegetable soups
Vegetables, cooked	Permitted, radish, beetroot, carrot or spinach only once a week
Potato, sweet potato or yam	Permitted
Cooking fat or butter	Permitted, partly as vegetable oil; butter should be unsalted
Sugar, jaggery or honey	Permitted
Jam or *murabba*	Permitted
Pastry	Excluded
Dessert	Permitted

Foods	Remarks
Sweet or sweetmeat	Permitted
Fruit, fresh	Permitted
Fruit, dried	Permitted, exclude figs, raisins, sultanas
Nuts	Permitted, unsalted
Condiments	Permitted, exclude ready-made curry powders
Papad, chutney, pickles	Excluded
Beverages	Permitted
Fluid	Permitted, total intake 1500 ml

No salt or baking soda to be used in cooking.

No salt permitted at the table.

If salt-free bread is not available any cereal flour can be used to bake bread or *chappatis* at home.

No canned products permitted unless declared to be salt free.

HIGH BLOOD PRESSURE
LOW SODIUM DIET

(Less than 0·5 g sodium)

Mixed	Vegetarian
Tea with milk, 2 tablespoons, and sugar	Tea with milk, 2 tablespoons, and sugar

Breakfast

Mixed	Vegetarian
Fruit juice	Puffed rice with milk, ½ cup, and sugar
Cornflakes with cream and sugar	
Egg, 1 poached	Bread* or *khakhra* with butter*, 2 teaspoons
Bread* with butter*, 2 teaspoons, and jelly	Sweet lime
Apple	

Mixed	Vegetarian

Lunch

Mixed	Vegetarian
Vegetable soup with sour lime	Vegetable soup with sour lime
Mutton chop with boiled peas and mashed potato	Potato, baked
Bread*	Rice with *dal*
	Cauliflower

Orange	Bread* or *chappatis*
	Banana

4 p.m.

Tea with milk, 2 tablespoons, and sugar	Tea with milk, 2 tablespoons, and sugar
Toast* with honey	Bread* or *chappatis* with jam
	Cashew nuts* or groundnuts*

Dinner

Tomato soup	Cooked brinjals
Roast chicken with boiled potato and french beans	Rice with *dal*
	Buttermilk, 1 cup
Bread*	Bread* or *chappatis*

*Unsalted

No salt or baking soda to be used in cooking.

No salt to be used at the table.

Sour lime or vinegar may be used to make food more palatable.

If salt-free bread is not available then any cereal flour to be used to bake *chappatis* at home.

REFERENCES

[1] RAGAN, C., and BORDLEY, J. III (1941) The accuracy of clinical measurements of arterial blood pressure, *Bull. Johns Hopk. Hosp.*, **69**, 504.

[2] KEMPNER, W. (1948) Treatment of hypertensive vascular disease with rice diet, *Amer. J. Med.*, 4, 545.

[3] GROLLMAN, A., *et al.* (1945) Sodium restriction in the diet for hypertension, *J. Amer. med. Ass.*, **129**, 533.

[4] CONN, J.W., ROVNER, D.R., and COHEN, E.L. (1968) Licorice-induced pseudo-aldosteronism, *J. Amer. med. Ass.*, **205**, 492.

[5] QUINTERO-ATENCIO, J., VASQUEL-LEON, H., and PINO-QUEINTERO, L.M. (1966) Association of sweat sodium with arterial blood pressure, *New Engl. J. Med.*, **274**, 1224.

[6] SCHROEDER, H.A. (1948) Low salt diets and arterial hypertension, *Amer. J. Med.*, **4**, 578.

76. CONGESTIVE CARDIAC FAILURE

The heart is considered to be in failure when it is unable to supply sufficient blood for the usual metabolic needs of the body. Cardiac failure may result from:

1. Damage to the heart *muscle* as a result of high blood pressure, myocarditis following diphtheria or rheumatic fever. 2. Damage to the heart *valves* from rheumatic disease, syphillis or atheroma. 3. *Pericarditis* producing cardiac tamponade. 4. Obstruction to the coronary *arteries* in coronary thrombosis. 5. Chronic *pulmonary* disease. 6. *Congenital* heart diseases.

Obesity

Obesity increases pericardial fat, abdominal fat that raises the diaphragm displacing the normal position of the heart, and adds kilometres of capillaries to the circulatory system, all of which increase the cardiac work load. Reducing the body weight of an obese patient with heart disease is an important therapeutic measure.

Constipation

Regular bowel movements are of great help to a patient with heart disease. Constipation produces abdominal distension and discomfort. Straining during defaecation to pass hard constipated stools increases the work on the heart. Adequate fluid intake aided by figs, *isphgul* (*Isogel*) may be tried for a regular bowel movement [see Chapter 54]. Mild laxatives like milk of magnesia may be indicated.

Flatulence

Excess abdominal gas is distressing and interferes with night sleep that is so important to a cardiac patient. Excess carbohydrate like glucose or fruit juice aggravates flatulence. Constipation aggravates protein putrefaction or carbohydrate fermentation by colonic bacteria. Regular bowel movements and avoiding excessive amount of milk, pulses or vegetables are helpful in making a cardiac patient comfortable.

DIETETIC MANAGEMENT

Calories

A person confined to bed requires about 24 Calories per kg body weight. For an obese subject less calories are given.

Proteins

About 1 g protein per kg body weight is adequate.

Fats

Fats are more difficult to digest and only 30 g fats per day should be given. Fried foods should be avoided.

Carbohydrates

After supplying the above-mentioned amount of proteins and fats the remaining calories are supplied by carbohydrates.

Vitamins

Supplements of vitamins may be necessary during a restricted diet.

Minerals

Sodium. With right-sided failure there may be oedema due to inadequate renal perfusion and sodium retention. Restriction of fluids does not cure the oedema unless the retained sodium is excreted. Salt is completely avoided in cooking. Foods rich in sodium are avoided [see p. 161]. Mercurial or thiazide diuretics are helpful in excreting retained sodium.

Potassium. During diuresis with digitalis and diuretics the body potassium is depleted. Fruit juice, vegetable soups or oral potassium salts as potassium citrate, 2–4 G three times a day, are given to supplement the potassium loss.

Fluids

The oedema in cardiac failure is secondary to retention of sodium. The sodium-poor diet contains about 1500 ml fluids. When the oedema does not respond to diuretics, a dilutional hyponatraemia due to water retention is a possibility. In such patients the total fluid and calorie intake is supplied by 600 ml of sodium-free milk containing 100 mEq of potassium. No other food or fluid is permitted [1].

Principles of Diet

Easily digestible frequent small feeds should be given to avoid abdominal discomfort and to correct obesity. The evening meal should be smaller and eaten at least 2 hours before retiring.

CONGESTIVE CARDIAC FAILURE
OR CORONARY INFARCTION

Foods	Remarks
Bread or *chappatis* of wheat, rice, maize, *bajra, jowar* or *ragi*	Permitted
Breakfast cereals of wheat, rice, oatmeal or maize	Permitted
Rice, cooked	Permitted
Pulses (*dal*) or beans	Permitted as thin *dal* only
Meat, fish or chicken	Permitted with minimum fat
Eggs	Permitted
Milk or milk products	Permitted as skimmed milk
Soup	Permitted
Vegetable salad	Permitted in a small quantity
Vegetables, cooked	Permitted
Potato, sweet potato or yam	Permitted
Cooking, fat or butter	Permitted, 2 tablespoons a day preferably as oil
Sugar, jaggery or honey	Permitted
Jam or *murabba*	Permitted
Pastries	Permitted as biscuits or light cake
Dessert	Permitted as light custard, jelly or ice cream
Sweet or sweetmeat	Permitted in small helpings
Fruits, fresh	Permitted
Fruits, dried	Permitted occasionally as small helping
Nuts	Permitted occasionally as small helping
Condiments and spices	Permitted in small quantity, pungent spices to be excluded
Papad, chutney or pickles	Excluded
Beverage	Permitted as light tea or coffee
Fluids	To be restricted to 5 cups a day during oedematous stage

N.B.—Salt not permitted during cooking or at the table during oedematous stage.

CONGESTIVE CARDIAC FAILURE
OR CORONARY INFARCTION
SAMPLE MENU

Mixed Diet		*Vegetarian Diet*	
Approximately		*Approximately*	
Proteins	50 g	Proteins	50 g
Fats	30 g	Fats	30 g
Carbohydrates	255 g	Carbohydrates	255 g
Calories	1500	Calories	1500

Morning

Cornflakes, ¾ cup with skimmed milk, ½ cup, and sugar, 2 teaspoons
Egg, 1 poached
Toast, 1
Papaya, (Paw-Paw)

Puffed rice, ¾ cup with skimmed milk, 1 cup, and sugar, 2 teaspoons
Toast, 1
Jam, 1 teaspoon
Orange

Mid-morning

Orange juice, ½ cup

Buttermilk, 1 cup

Lunch

Chicken soup
Minced meat, 2 tablespoons
Boiled lady's fingers (okra)
Toast, 1
Rice pudding, 3 tablespoons

Tomato soup, 1 cup
Cooked pumpkin
Rice, 2 tablespoons
Dal, ½ cup
Chappatis, 2
Banana

3.30 p.m.

Tea, 1 cup
Biscuits, 2

Tea, 1 cup
Biscuits, 2

5.30 p.m.

Banana, 1

Sweet lime juice, 1 cup

7.30 p.m.

Vegetable soup
Roast leg of chicken
Cooked french beans
Bread, 1 slice

Vegetable soup with lemon juice
Skimmed milk curd, 1 cup
Cooked carrot
Bread, 1 slice or *chappatis,* 2

| *Mixed Diet* | *Vegetarian Diet* |
| Stewed apple with 1 tablespoon sugar | Ice-cream, ½ cup |

Before retiring

Skimmed milk, 1 cup   Skimmed milk, 1 cup

REFERENCE

[1] FUISZ, R.E. (1963) Hyponatremia. *Medicine* (*Baltimore*), **42,** 149.

77. ACID AND ALKALINE FOODS

It is surprising that where the authorities on nutrition are reluctant to give opinions, the food faddists have definite ideas about the acidity or alkalinity of foods. When a food is claimed to be 'acid' or 'alkaline' it is seldom clarified whether it refers to: (1) the acid or base content of food; (2) reaction in the raw state; (3) the reaction when cooked; (4) the effect on gastric secretion; (5) the effect on blood; or (6) the reaction of urine on excretion. Unless it is specified which of the above factors is referred to, a mere statement that a food is acid or alkaline has no meaning. To take a simple example, sour lime contains citric acid, has an acid reaction and on combustion forms carbonic acid which on excretion combines with a base and tends to make the urine alkaline. However, the quantity of sour lime ingested is so little that it has neglible effect on the metabolism.

ASH

The mineral element left after the combustion of food is known as ash, which may be acid or alkaline. Sodium, potassium, calcium, magnesium are alkaline radicals. Chloride, phosphate and sulphate are acid radicals. The reaction of the ash is determined by the preponderance of the alkaline or acid radical. Thus vegetables are rich in potassium and yield an alkaline ash.

TABLE 33

ACID OR ALKALINE ASH FOODS [1, 2]

Acid	Alkaline
Bacon, beef, brain, cereals (except *ragi*), egg, fish, groundnut, ham, mutton, pork and walnut.	Almonds, beverages, chestnut, coconut, dried fruits, fresh fruits including citrus, milk, pulses and vegetables (except cauliflower, *knol-khol,* peas).

Acid or Alkaline Ash Diet

In Health. Healthy kidneys are highly efficient and keep the blood reaction constant by excreting acid or alkaline urine, according to the body requirement. In a healthy person an attempt to balance acid ash with alkaline ash diet is unnecessary. It is not possible to counteract a highly efficient chemical mechanism of the kidneys by diet alone.

Renal Damage. In severe kidney damage the alkali reserve of the blood may be disturbed and an acid or alkaline ash diet perhaps may have some value, provided repeated estimations of alkali reserve are made; otherwise there is a grave danger of producing acidosis or alkalosis.

Urinary Calculi. Precipitation of calcium oxalate crystals is not greatly influenced by changes in the reaction of urine but the associated calcium phosphate crystals are soluble in acid urine. It would appear that an acid ash diet could be beneficial for calcium stones. In practice this does not occur because: (1) with diet alone it is not possible to make the urine sufficiently acid; (2) to produce acid ash, a diet rich in protein but without vegetables, fruits and milk is required (such a diet is not feasible for a prolonged period); (3) with acid urine, kidneys tend to convert urea into ammonia thereby making the urine alkaline; (4) associated urinary infection with urea-splitting organisms may convert urea into ammonia and make the urine alkaline; (5) high protein diet, if persisted with, may precipitate other crystals such as uric acid.

A rigid acid or alkaline ash diet therefore has no practical value in the treatment of urinary calculi. However, foods rich in calcium, oxalate and uric acid should be restricted according to the nature of the stone [see CHAPTER 73].

Ketogenic Diet. High fat diet to produce ketosis was once advocated for the treatment of epilepsy and urinary infections. With the potent and efficient drugs now available the unpleasant and impracticable ketogenic diet has been abandoned by most physicians.

REFERENCES

[1] McCance, R.A., and Widdowson, E.A. (1960) The composition of foods, *Spec. Rep. Ser. med. Res. Coun. (Lond.)*, No. 297, London, H.M.S.O.

[2] Aykroyd, W.R. (1963) *The Nutritive Value of Indian Foods and the Planning of Satisfactory Diets*, 6th ed, rev. Gopalan, C., and Balasubramaniam, S.C., Indian Council of Medical Research, New Delhi.

78. TUBE FEEDING

Oral feeding is the best method for nourshing a patient. It is only when a patient is unable to take oral feeds that tube or parenteral feeding becomes necessary. Tube feeding can be performed through: (1) nasogastric tube; (2) stoma of gastrostomy or jejunostomy; (3) rectal tube.

NASOGASTRIC TUBE

A gastric tube passed through the nose is the next best alternative to feeding by mouth. It has various advantages: (1) the tube can be passed without any danger if ordinary precautions are taken; (2) the tube can be easily retained and nutrition can be maintained even when travelling under adverse conditions; (3) the tube can be inserted or taken out several times a day, if necessary; (4) there is no danger of overloading the circulation with fluids and electrolytes if ordinary care is taken; (5) sterilization of food is not necessary; (6) almost any easily digestible food which passes through the tube can be fed to the patient; and (7) drugs can be administered through the tube.

Indications

(1) Semiconsciousness or unconsciousness; (2) persistent anorexia, nausea and vomiting not due to pyloric or intestinal obstruction; (3) paralysis of muscles of deglutition in diphtheria and poliomyelitis;

(4) renal failure; (5) peptic ulcer resistant to routine treatment.

1. *A semiconscious or unconscious* patient is unable to swallow food properly and the food is liable to pass through the larynx into the lungs, resulting in aspiration pneumonia.

2. *For anorexia, nausea and vomiting* such as occurs in viral hepatitis, a nasogastric tube is of great help. A well nourished liver cell is able to withstand infection or toxin far better than a depleted one. In viral hepatitis, maintenance of nutrition should always be aimed at and if the patient with marked anorexia can be induced to retain the nasogastric tube then the necessity of intravenous drip can be avoided. In hysterical vomiting also nasogastric tube feeding is of great help.

3. *During paralysis of the muscles of deglutition* as in diphtheria or poliomyelitis, nasogastric tube feeding is a very important factor in recovery as it maintains nutrition and prevents aspiration of food into the lungs.

4. *In acute renal failure* enthusiastic but ill-understood intravenous fluid and electrolyte therapy may cause death. When expert medical and laboratory aid is not available then the best chance of recovery lies in feeding the patient with a solution of glucose or lactose, 15–20 per cent, through a nasogastric tube. One thousand ml fluid is supplied to replace the daily loss by evaporation.

5. When a peptic ulcer is resistant to ordinary treatment a continuous intragastric drip is advocated to supply milk even when the patient is asleep. The object of the drip is to neutralize the gastric contents, and to do this an antacid or alkali such as sodium bicarbonate is also added to milk. There is no evidence that a milk drip increases the rate of healing in gastric ulcer and the evidence in duodenal ulcer is at present scanty.

Method of Intubation

For prolonged nasogastric feeds a modified Penrose tubing, collapsible when empty, causes less nasal, throat and oesophageal irritation and allows competent functioning of the cardio-oesophageal sphincter [1]. Alternatively a small bore plastic tube is preferred. About 10 Fr or a less gauge tube is adequate for a liquid drip. The tip of the boiled gastric tube is dipped in a lubricant like paraffin and inserted into either nostril. A deviated nasal septum may make one side easier to pass the tube than the other. Some patients retch when the tube touches the pharynx and for them a local anaesthetic spray is useful. As the tube is being pushed down it can be seen, if necessary, in the oropharynx. If a conscious patient can swallow it helps the passage of the tube. When the tip of the tube has been passed 60–65 cm from the nostril the tube is secured to the nose with adhesive tape. Some prefer passing the tube up to 30 cm from the nostrils so that the tube lies above the cardia. This tends to prevent oesophagitis (and is also a good method for treating oesophagitis). A thin collapsible tube may be retained in the stomach for a week. A thicker tube should be withdrawn every 2 or 3 days, cleaned and reintroduced, if necessary, after a few hours. The feeds can be given intermittently with a funnel or a syringe or given as a continuous drip. It is essential in an unconscious patient to be sure that the tube is not in the trachea. Aspiration of gastric juice, acid to litmus, shows that the tube is in the stomach. If the tube is in the bronchi, cotton-wool held over the end of the tube moves with respiration. If the tube is in the trachea, respiratory sounds are audible when the end of the tube is held near the diaphragm of the stethoscope. There are two other 'dodges' for detecting where the tip of the tube is: (1) blow air down and listen for a bubbling noise over the stomach with a stethoscope; (2) inject a few ml of sterile water and see if the patient coughs, provided the cough reflex is still present.

There is considerable elasticity in tube feeding. It is possible to give as much fluid and as many calories as are needed.

Calories

An average patient requires about 1500–2000 Calories. After surgical operation, injury or burn there is increase in metabolic rate and a provision of even 3000 Calories may be necessary. If adequate calories are not supplied, progressive calorie deficit soon develops resulting in wasting and prolonged convalescence before the patient feels able to to return to work [1]. For feeding programme, see p. 565.

Protein

High protein intake without sufficient total calories will not lead to positive nitrogen balance. A high protein diet can even be harmful as it produces a diuresis due to increased urea production and in the absence of a high fluid intake this diuresis leads to loss of water [2]. About 60–75 g protein is adequate for an average patient but even up to 300 g protein may be necessary in a protein depleted person or with marked protein loss from a raw surface such as burns or colon in ulcerative colitis. High protein can be supplied as skimmed milk powder, *Casilan or Complan* (Glaxo).

Fat

Fat is supplied to provide calories. The total fat intake may be up to 50 per cent of the total calorie needs. On taking high fat feeds some patients may get diarrhoea but it passes off and the over-all effect of high fat diet may be constipation [2]. Fat in the form of homogenized milk or fat emulsion is better tolerated. *Medium chain triglycerides* are easily absorbed by those who have malabsorption of fats.

Carbohydrate

Compared with glucose or sucrose, lactose has the highest molecular weight, therefore, weight for weight it will have the lowest osmolarity. Its solubility factor on the other hand is less than that of the other two. Lactose, however, precipitates diarrhoea in those with intestinal deficiency of the enzyme lactase. According to the tolerance of the patient 60–250 g. sugar can be added to the feeds. *Dextrimaltose* or liquid glucose, which is gradually absorbed as a 10–15 per cent solution, is well tolerated.

Liquid Glucose. Commercial starch is hydrolysed to form glucose as well as several partial end products of starch digestion, and this *mixture* is known as liquid glucose or glucose syrup. The composition of liquid glucose can be varied to suit the particular requirements.

CARBOHYDRATE CONTENT OF LIQUID GLUCOSE*
(British Pharmaceutical Codex)

CARBOHYDRATE COMPONENT	grams/100 g carbohydrate
Glucose (dextrose)	19·3
Maltose including isomaltose	14·3
Trisaccharides	11·3
Tetrasaccharides	10·8
Pentasaccharides	8·4
Hexasaccharides	6·6
Heptasaccharides	5·6
Octa and high-saccharides	24·0
Total carbohydrate	100·0

* Allen, R.J.L., and Brook, M. (1967) Carbohydrate and the United Kingdom Food Manufacturer, *Amer. J. clin. Nutr.*, **20**, 163.

Electrolytes

Sodium as common salt can be easily supplied through the nasogastric tube. High concentration of sodium chloride may produce similar effect as saline purge [2]. Since the kidneys conserve sodium, daily 30–40 mEq sodium may be adequate [2]. With a low sodium intake there is a negative balance before regulatory mechanisms come into play.

Potassium requirement is about 60 mEq per day. If fruit juice, coconut water and vegetable soups are provided, then potassium supplement is not necessary. Potassium salts may be administered if necessary [see CHAPTER 21].

Vitamins

Vitamin preparations can be supplied through the nasogastric tube.

Fluid

The daily requirement of fluids of about 2500–3000 ml can be easily provided. It is always advisable to slightly under-replace rather than over-replace fluids particularly in elderly patients with heart and chronic lung disease.

Foods and beverages that can be supplied by tube feeding are water, barley water, buttermilk, coffee, *dal* water, egg flip, *kanjee,* milk, milk beverages prepared with cocoa, *Casilan, Complan, Horlicks, Ovaltine, Bournvita;* strained porridge, saline, soup, tea, water, vegetable juices or any other liquid preparation which can pass through the tube. TABLES 34 and 35 are helpful in designing tube feeds.

The most convenient nasogastric feeding is easily provided by *Complan* 100 g, glucose 100 g, methylcellulose 3 g, and water added to make 1 litre of solution [3] with the following composition for 1, 2 and 3 litre feeds [p. 565].

NASOGASTRIC TUBE FEEDING

Fluids	2500 ml
Calories	1500
Protein	60 g

6.00 a.m.	1 cup milk tea ($\frac{1}{2}$ cup milk, $\frac{1}{2}$ cup water)
8.00 a.m.	1 cup milk or egg flip
9.00 a.m.	1 cup coconut water or fruit juice
10.00 a.m.	1 cup strained porridge or arrowroot *kanjee*

FOOD VALUES FOR NASOGASTRIC FEEDS

Complan	Glucose or Dextrimaltose or Liquid glucose	Total mixture	Water	Calories	Protein	Fat	Carbohydrates	Na	K	Cl
G	G	ml	ml		G	G	G	mEq	mEq	mEq
100	100	1000	850	860	31	16	144	22	28	20
200	200	2000	1700	1720	62	32	288	44	56	40
300	300	3000	2550	2580	93	48	432	66	84	60

Every hour about 100–200 ml is administered through the nasogastric tube.

12.00 noon	1 cup tomato or meat soup
1.00 p.m.	1 cup barley water
2.00 p.m.	1 cup buttermilk
4.00 p.m.	1 cup milk tea
5.00 p.m.	1 cup coconut water or fruit juice
6.00 p.m.	1 cup buttermilk
8.00 p.m.	1 cup strained porridge or *kanjee*
10.00 p.m.	1 cup milk (with cocoa) or egg flip

From the above mixture adequate fluids, proteins, fats and carbohydrates are provided for a 70 kg man. By decreasing the amounts it could be made suitable for a smaller individual. Extra sodium chloride if required is made up by adding salt.

GASTROSTOMY, JEJUNOSTOMY, AND RECTAL FEEDING

Gastrostomy

It may be necessary to feed a patient with a stricture or carcinoma of the oesophagus through a gastrostomy. The feeds already described can be used.

Jejunostomy

Feeding through jejunostomy may be necessary with extensive inflammation or malignancy of the oesophagus and stomach or after oesophageal resection or total gastrectomy. For jejunal feeding the food must be easily digestible or predigested because salivary and gastric digestion are completely eliminated and pancreatic and intestinal digestion are reduced. Complications of jejunal feeding may be nausea, vomiting, distension, abdominal cramps, diarrhoea and enteritis. These symptoms can be reduced by giving the feed as a drip or by injecting about 100 ml of feed every 15 minutes and by using homogenized milk. A special formula consisting of cream with predigested proteins and carbohydrates together with vitamin and mineral supplement has also been recommended [4].

Rectal Feeding (Colonic Feeding)

Human *rectum* does not absorb sodium, chloride and water, while the rest of the colon does [5]. Potassium and bicarbonate are normally *secreted* by the colon for excretion. However, when the concentration of potassium and bicarbonate is higher than circulating blood, then they are *also* absorbed [6]. *Calcium* and *magnesium* are also absorbed from the normal colon [7].

TABLE 34**

2000 CALORIE FEED FOR FULL NOURISHMENT IN CHILDREN
OR PARTIAL NOURISHMENT IN ADULTS*

INGREDIENT	QUANTITY	PROTEIN (G)	FAT (G)	CARBO-HYDRATE (G)	CALORIES
Cow's milk	2000 ml	68	74	96	1,320
50 per cent fat emul-sion (*Prosparol*)	100 ml	—	50	—	465
Lactose	60 g	—	—	63*	236
Water	400 ml	—	—	—	—
Total	2500 ml	68	124	159	2,021

Weight of feed=2617 g. Volume of feed=2500 ml. Water content=2400 ml (approx.). Sodium content=50 mEq. Potassium content=80 mEq.
* Calculated as monosaccharide.
** Masterton, J.P., Dudley, H.A.F., and MacRae, S. (1963) Design of tube feeds for surgical patients, *Brit. med. J., 2,* 909.

Method. If the lower bowel is loaded with faeces it is evacuated by an enema. A rubber tube preferably with multiple holes is used so as to avoid blockage with faeces. The tube is lubricated with paraffin or vaseline and inserted 20–25 cm. The fluid is administered by connecting the other end of the tube to an enema can or bottle raised to a height of 25–30 cm above the bed. About 20 drops a minute are usually well tolerated. The following can be administered rectally: (1) water; (2) one teaspoon of common salt added to a litre of drinking water; (3) glucose, 5 teaspoons to half a litre of water.

With a rectal drip sterilization of the water is unnecessary. Drinking water is used. The usefulness of a rectal drip is limited as an adequate calorie intake cannot be provided but it is an excellent method for treating mild dehydration and sodium depletion where facilities for intravenous therapy are not available.

TABLE 35**

3000 CALORIE FEED FOR FULL NOURISHMENT

INGREDIENT	QUANTITY	PROTEIN (G)	FAT (G)	CARBO- HYDRATE (G)	CALORIES
Cow's milk	1000 ml	34	37	48	660
50 per cent fat emul- sion (*Prosparol*)	270 ml	—	135	—	1,256
Lactose	250 g	—	—	262*	983
Milk protein (*Casilan*)	35 g	35	—	—	144
Water	1700 ml	—	—	—	—
Total	2970 ml	69	172	310	3,043

Weight of feed=3273 g. Volume of feed=2970 ml. Water content=2800 ml (approx.). Sodium content=25 mEq. Potassium content=40 mEq. To increase protein intake to 100 g / day add 30 g milk protein. To increase protein intake to 200 g/day add 130 g milk protein. To increase protein intake to 300 g/day add 230 g milk protein.

* Calculated as monosaccharide.
** Masterton, J.P., Dudley, H.A.F., and MacRae, S. (1963) Design of tube feeds for surgical patients, *Brit. med. J.*, **2**, 909.

REFERENCES

[1] DAVIS, L.E., and HOFMANN, W. (1969) A long-term nasogastric feeding tube made from modified Penrose tubing, *J. Amer. med. Ass.*, **209**, 685.
[2] MASTERTON, J.P., DUDLEY, H.A.F., and MACRAE, S. (1963) Design of tube feeds for surgical patients, *Brit. med. J.*, **2**, 909.
[3] PEASTON, M.J.T., (1966) External metabolic balance studies during nasogastric feeding in serious illness requiring intensive care, *Brit. med. J.*, **2**, 1367.
[4] HOLLANDER, F., ROSENAK, S., and COLP, R. (1945) A synthetic predigested aliment for jejunostomy feeding, *Surgery*, **17**, 754.
[5] DEVROEDE, G.J., and PHILLIPS, S.F. (1970) Failure of human rectum to absorb

electrolytes and water, *Gut,* **11,** 438.

[6] DEVROEDE, G.J., and PHILLIPS, S.F. (1969) Conservation of sodium, chloride and water by the human colon, *Gastroenterology,* **56,** 101.

[7] GOOPTU, D., TRUELOVE, S.C., and WARNER, G.T. (1969) Absorption of electrolytes from the colon in cases of ulcerative colitis and in control subjects, *Gut,* **10,** 555.

79. INTRAVENOUS FEEDING

The human body can tolerate starvation for several weeks but dehydration is rapidly fatal. The immediate objective in intravenous feeding is to provide water and electrolytes for daily needs and to correct imbalances produced by starvation or loss. It is advisable to avoid drugs in intravenous infusions [1].

Intravenous Feeding [2]

For a majority of surgical procedures the nutrition of the patient before and after surgery is not a problem. The period of relative starvation is well tolerated.

The resting metabolic expenditure (RME) rises by 10–15 per cent after surgery. Peritonitis and severe infections raise the expenditure 20–45 per cent above normal. When a long-term operative management is necessary it may be difficult to maintain nutrition, due either to the disease or surgical procedure. Under such conditions intravenous proteins, carbohydrates and fats are required.

Indications for Intravenous Feeding

(1) *Obstructive lesions* of the gastro-intestinal tract and *massive bowel resection;* (2) *inflammatory bowel diseases:* (a) ulcerative colitis; (b) regional enteritis; (3) *intestinal fistulae;* (4) *hypermetabolic states,* burns, severe infections; (5) *hepatic failure;* (6) *neonatal infants* with congenital anomalies; (7) anorexia nervosa [3].

This intravenous alimentation is not confined merely to operated patients in surgical practice. It may also allow natural closure of enterocutaneous *fistula,* pancreatic fistula, etc. Due to associated skin infection, surgery in such patients is not desirable. Remissions also occur with intravenous hyperalimentation in the inflammatory bowel lesions of *ulcerative colitis, granulomatous colitis* or *regional enteritis* [4].

Techniques of Parenteral Feeding

1. *Peripheral venous infusion* is suitable for giving isotonic solutions of glucose, saline and other electrolytes for a short period. The needle should be inserted in the upper limb veins. Lower limb immobilization and irritations by the perfusing fluid is more likely to cause superficial or deep vein thrombosis and embolism.

2. *Infusion through a polythene tube* by threading a tube into the deep veins or superior or inferior vena cava is ideal for those requiring intravenous therapy for several days or when hypertonic solutions have to be given. With this procedure the limbs can be moved freely. Unless strict aseptic precautions are taken there is danger of infection.

Proteins

The minimal nitrogen loss in the urine and faeces is about 5·7 g, and for tissue building about twice the amount is replaced.

Blood. One litre of blood provides 180 g of protein including haemoglobin. However, this amount is not rapidly available to the body for protein synthesis. Blood is therefore best used to combat anaemia and circulatory failure.

Plasma and Human Albumin. One litre of plasma contains 60–70 g of protein but since the half-life of the proteins is between 14 and 26 days the amino acids are only slowly released for re-utilization. Plasma infusion is best given as a temporary measure to raise the serum protein level when albumin synthesis is poor.

Amino Acids

Amino acids can be administered as : (1) *hydrolysate* of protein (casein); or (2) *synthetic amino acids mixture*. *Acid hydrolysis* of proteins results in destruction of tryptophan, and the hydrolysate produces reactions during intravenous administration. *Enzymatic hydrolysate* has no adverse reactions and is well utilized.

Synthetic amino acids mixture is made up of *essential* amino acids mainly in the *Laevo* form (*Tryphosan, Intramin*), in a higher proportion than that advocated as the minimal essential requirement [pp. 15-16]. Non-essential amino acids are also added to provide additional nitrogen. Simultaneous administration of calories as carbohydrate (fructose, sorbitol or ethanol) prevents metabolism of amino acids for calorie requirement, and amino acids are thus spared for the utilization of protein synthesis. About 15 per cent of infused amino acids are lost in the urine.

Fats [5]

The chief advantage of fat emulsion for intravenous use is its calorie value of 9 per g. This reduces the volume of fluid to be administered and considerably helps to replenish the calories. The previously used cotton-seed emulsions were toxic. *Soya-bean* emulsions are well tolerated. The addition of egg phosphatide helps to stabilize fat emulsions. The commercial preparation *Intralipid* is available in 10 and 20 per cent emulsions. In 24 hours not more than 3 g per kg body weight, i.e. 1 litre of 20 per cent emulsion in 70 kg man, should be administered. Infused fat takes about 18 hours to clear from the plasma. Administration of 5000 Units of heparin for each 500 ml 20 per cent *Intralipid* is advocated for activating lipoprotein lipase, which helps to clear the plasma of infused fat.

Toxic reactions immediately produced on fat infusion are: dyspnoea, cyanosis, fever, urticaria, tachycardia, flushing, nausea, vomiting and muscle pain. Prior to starting fat infusion each day, the plasma should be inspected for milkiness and further fat infusions are not administered until the plasma is clear. Persistent lipaemia results in fatty liver, disordered liver function, hypoprothrombinaemia and thrombocytopenia. *Nothing should be added to the fat emulsion* as it is likely to crack. The emulsion is preserved in a refrigerator.

Carbohydrates

For short-term therapy the minimum daily requirement of 600 calories is met with 5 per cent *glucose*, in 3 litres, that is excessive fluid. A higher concentration of glucose is likely to result in thrombophlebitis of the infused vein. *Fructose* is preferable to glucose because: (1) solutions of 10–15 per cent do not cause thrombophlebitis; (2) in equal concentration, less is excreted through the kidneys and less diuresis results; (3) the metabolism is rapid and is less dependent on insulin; (4) when administered with amino acids, fructose causes more rapid protein synthesis than glucose.

Sorbitol [p. 463] is less irritant to veins and even up to 30 per cent solution is advocated for intravenous use in surgical practice [6]. When mixed with protein hydrolysates or amino acid mixture, sorbitol is sometimes preferred to glucose or fructose which caramelizes during the autoclaving of amino acids and produces reactions.

Alcohol

Intravenous alcohol can be given at a rate of up to 10 g per hour as 3 per cent solution. A higher concentration produces venous thrombosis. Alcohol provides 7 Calories per g. Fructose enhances alcohol metabolism, hence intravenous nutrition of fructose and alcohol is best suited. As long as the rate of administration does not exceed 10 g per hour (320 ml of 3 per cent solution) there is no danger of alcohol intoxication.

Vitamins

With parenteral feeding as the only source of nutriment, an ampoule of a mixture of thiamine 5 mg, riboflavine 5 mg, nicotinamide 20 mg, pyridoxine 2 mg, and pantothenic acid 5 mg, with 100 mg of vitamin C should be added to the infusion.

Electrolytes

Sodium. In the absence of deficiency about ½ to 1 litre of isotonic saline (0·85 per cent sodium chloride) is usually sufficient to meet the daily requirements. Sodium deficiency due to diminished intake and loss from intestinal aspiration or fistulae has to be made up. (1) *Mild* deficiency, which may produce nausea, occurs if a patient is not fed orally for a day or two. About 1–2 litres of isotonic saline is required to correct this mild deficiency. (2) *Moderate* deficiency may be suspected when, in addition to the history of poor intake or loss, there is associated giddiness and hypotension. About 2–3 litres of isotonic saline are required to correct the deficiency. (3) *Severe* deficiency should be suspected with circulatory failure and a systolic blood pressure of less than 90 mm Hg, inelastic skin and flaccid eye-balls. There is no thirst in pure sodium deficiency. About 4–6 litres of isotonic saline or more concentrated saline may be necessary. For further information see CHAPTER 20.

Sodium Chloride. Sodium chloride has a higher proportion of chloride to sodium ion than in the body and the correction of large deficits of sodium with saline causes 'dilutional acidosis'. This can be prevented by administering 1 litre of $\frac{1}{6}$ molar lactate for every 4 litres of isotonic saline.

Sodium During Amino Acid Therapy. The casein hydrolysate *Aminosol* 10 per cent solution is rich in sodium, 160 mEq per litre, and care is therefore necessary in the elderly or those with cardiovascular disease. *Amigen* in glucose or *Amigen* 800 has a sodium content of 35 mEq per litre, while synthetic amino acids (*Tryphosan*) have sodium 6 mEq/l [5].

Potassium. Potassium deficiency occurs with starvation or loss of intestinal secretion due to diarrhoea, intestinal aspiration or fistulae. Potassium is required not only to maintain the body function but also for tissue formation. Intravenous potassium is best avoided unless there is marked deficiency. Not more than 3 g of potassium chloride is added to each litre of fluid and given by slow intravenous drip. In dehydrated patients with marked oliguria the urine output is first restored by saline infusions before intravenous potassium is given.

The amino acid solution and fat emulsions are poor in potassium and supplement may be necessary. The usual required daily total amount of potassium may be 60 mEq. Potassium chloride ampoules are prepared in quantities of 1·5 g (20 mEq) or 2 g (26 mEq). One ampoule is added to each 500 ml of amino acid mixture to provide a total of 4·5–6 g potassium chloride. Potassium is not added to fat emulsion for fear of cracking the same.

Water

The daily minimum water requirement is about 1·5 litres which can be supplied as 5 per cent glucose or with the required amount of electrolytes. To this should be added an amount of water equal to the volume of urine voided during the previous 24 hours.

Additional water as glucose or saline may have to be given to correct any deficit that may have occurred before the start of therapy. This deficit may clinically manifest as: (1) *mild symptoms* of thirst and oliguria which denotes a deficiency of about 2 per cent of body weight (1·2 litres in a 60 kg man); (2) *moderate symptoms* of thirst, oliguria and mental confusion denoting about 6 per cent water deficiency (3·5 litres in a 60 kg man); (3) *severe symptoms* of great prostration, severe oliguria with a history of a long period of dehydration denoting water deficiency of about 7–14 per cent (4–9 litres in a 60 kg man). The deficiency should be made up in about 24 hours with the aim of restoring the urine output to about 300–400 ml every 8 hours.

In routine practice, intravenous feeding consists of administering solutions of glucose or saline. For more intensive intravenous feeding the following solutions are advocated in the United Kingdom and European continent.

Aminosol-Fructose-Ethanol-Potassium Chloride Mixture

Aminosol	3·3 %
Fructose	15·0 %
Ethanol	2·5 %
Potassium chloride	2·0 g (26 mEq)

A	B
1. 500 ml *Aminosol*-fructose-ethanol-potassium chloride mixture	500 ml *Intralipid* 20 % Heparin 5000 Units
2. 500 ml *Aminosol*-fructose-ethanol-potassium mixture	500 ml *Aminosol* 10 %
3. 500 ml *Aminosol*-fructose-ethanol-potassium chloride mixture	500 ml *Intralipid* 20 % Heparin 5000 Units

The amino acids irritate the veins while fat emulsions do not do so; but addition of any substance to the emulsion may result in cracking and the consequent danger of fat embolism. The above pairs A and B are in two separate bottles running simultaneously and are connected by a Y-tube just before opening in the veins.

Each pair is infused over an 8 hour period. The above infusions provide the following in 24 hours:

Fluid	3000 ml
Calories	3500
Sodium	161 mEq
Potassium	78 mEq
Nitrogen	12·75 g

In order to reduce calorie intake, *Intralipid* 10 per cent solutions are used instead of 20 per cent.

North America fat emulsions are not in vogue, therefore the

caloric requirement is made up with 20 per cent glucose. The concentrated glucose administration may produce about 2 per cent glycosuria. The normal pancreas responds to high glucose intake with increased endogenous insulin output. In diabetics, insulin replacement is necessary. Sudden stoppage of hyperalimentation may produce hypoglycaemia so the patient should be gradually weaned.

The intravenous feeds recommended in North America are given in TABLE 36. They are recommended to be given through the *subclavian vein*.

The high concentration of glucose in the deep veins during prolonged intravenous hyperalimentation predisposes to fungal septicaemia [7]. This may possibly be prevented by external arteriovenous shunts in the arm or leg [8]. Air embolism is also a likely complication.

TABLE 36

INTRAVENOUS HYPERALIMENTATION [2]:

COMPOSITION OF DAILY INTRAVENOUS NUTRIENT RATION IN THE AVERAGE ADULT

Water	2,500—3,500 ml	Vitamin A	5,000 — 10,000 USP Units
Protein hydrolysates (amino acids)	100— 140 gm	Vitamin D	500 — 1,000 USP Units
Nitrogen	12·20 g	Vitamin E	2·5 — 5·0 IU
Carbohydrate (dextrose)	525— 750 gm	Vitamin C	250 — 500 mg
Calories	2,500—3,500 Cal	Thiamine	25 — 50 mg
Sodium	125— 150 mEq	Riboflavine	5 — 10 mg
Potassium	75— 120 mEq	Pyridoxine	7·5 — 15 mg
Magnesium	4— 8 mEq	Niacin	50 — 100 mg
		Pantothenic acid	12·5 — 25 mg

COMPOSITION OF 100 ml ESSENTIAL AMINO ACID SOLUTION

ESSENTIAL AMINO ACIDS	MINIMAL DAILY REQUIREMENTS (gm)
L-isoleucine	0·70
L-leucine	1·10
L-lysine	0·80
L-methionine	1·10

Table 36 cotd.

ESSENTIAL AMINO ACIDS	MINIMAL DAILY REQUIREMENTS (gm)
L-phenylalanine	1·10
L-threonine	0·50
L-tryptophan	0·25
L-valine	0·80
Total	6·35 gm/100 ml

REFERENCES

[1] LANCET (1970) Adding drugs to intravenous infusions, *Lancet, ii,* 556.
[2] DUDRICK, S.J., LONG, J.M., STEIGER, E., and RHOADS, J.E. (1970) Intravenous hyperalimentation, *Med. Clin. N. Amer.,* **54,** 577.
[3] DUDRICK, S.J., WILMORE, D.W., VARS, H.M., and RHOADS, J.E. (1968) Long term total parenteral nutrition with growth, development and positive nitrogen balance, *Surgery,* **64,** 134.
[4] DURICK, S.J., and RHOADS, J.E. (1971) New horizons for intravenous feeding, *J. Amer. med. Ass.,* **215,** 939.
[5] BRITISH MEDICAL JOURNAL (1970) Solutions for intravenous feeding, *Brit. med. J.,* **1,** 352.
[6] BYE, P.A. (1969) The utilization and metabolism of intravenous sorbitol, *Brit. J. Surg.,* **56,** 653.
[7] CURRY, C.R., and QUIE, P.G. (1971) Fungal septicemia in patients receiving parenteral hyperalimentation, *New Engl. J. Med.,* **285,** 1221.
[8] SCRIBNER, B.H., *et al.* (1970) Long-term total parenteral nutrition, *J. Amer. med. Ass.,* **212,** 457.

80. PREGNANCY AND LACTATION

Pregnancy is a most remarkable anabolic process whereby out of food, vitamins, minerals and hormones, a seven-pound baby is born within 9 months. The foetus is in a sense a parasite to the mother and draws its nourishment from her diet. If the nutrition of the mother is inadequate then her body reserves are drawn upon and depleted. The incidence of prematurity rises with a decrease in the nutritional status of pregnant women. Low birth weights, low vitality and a large number of early deaths occur among infants born to poorly nourished mothers. Improving the nutrition of the mother, even in the third trimester of pregnancy, improves the status of the infants.

IDEAL WEIGHT

After conception, restriction of calories for weight reduction is not desirable. However, an optimum weight before conception is most desirable for normal pregnancy and delivery. In obese mothers toxaemias of pregnancy are more frequent, the foetus is likely to be bigger and the delivery more difficult and dangerous. If the mother is underweight the chances of premature birth are increased.

The optimum weight gain for a mother during pregnancy is about 1·5 kg in the first three months. In each subsequent month the average gain should be 1·5 kg, being a little more in the last 2 or 3 months. At full term the total gain is about 10–12 kg. With excessive vomiting in early pregnancy slight loss of weight may occur. Sudden changes in weight, either gain or loss, may be harmful.

Dyspepsia in Pregnancy

Morning nausea and vomiting are common in early pregnancy and may continue during the later months. The aetiology of these symptoms is obscure but they are aggravated by mental stress. A well adjusted and emotionally mature person can succeed in overcoming them to an appreciable extent. The hydrochloric acid secretion is decreased during pregnancy. Heartburn in later pregnancy is due to the upward displacement of the digestive organs and regurgitation of gastric contents into the lower oesophagus. Constipation aggravates flatulence and heartburn. Frequent, small and easily digestible feeds, adequate fluids and dried fruits like prunes, figs, and apricots, help to combat the constipation [see CHAPTER 54]. Repeated purgation is not desirable.

NUTRITION IN PREGNANCY

A 3·2 kg full term infant is born with about 300 ml blood, 500 g proteins, 30 g calcium, 15 g phosphorus and about 300–400 mg iron. All these are drawn from the mother. Additional dietary demands on the mother are: (1) a 20–25 per cent increase in basal metabolism in the later stages of pregnancy; (2) formation of the placenta; and (3) blood loss during parturition. The diet of the mother should be adequate to supply the above requirements.

Calories

About 2000 Calories a day are recommended for a mother of 45 kg (100 lb). The calorie requirement is greater for mothers of larger build.

Lactating women produce 850–1000 ml milk, that is, the equivalent of 600 calories. British lactating women were found to consume approximately 600 Calories more than those not lactating [1].

Proteins

During pregnancy additional protein laid down for the foetus, placenta, etc., is about 950 g, roughly estimated as daily 0·5, 3·0, 4·5 and 5·7 g during each successive 10 week period. In order to convert this amount of tissue protein, an additional 10–12 g of mixed protein allowance for the mother is recommended daily.

During lactation daily milk produced is 850–1000 ml. Assuming 1 per cent protein in human milk, the daily excretion is 10 g. Therefore, about 25 g extra daily protein for the mother is recommended. Amongst vegetarians, a daily supplement of 2–3 cups of milk and milk products should supply the daily need for protein. Non-vegetarians are advised, besides about 2 cups of milk, to take one average helping of meat, fish, chicken or eggs at *each* meal. If the mother can take only a small quantity of food, due to vomiting or any other cause, then carbohydrates and fats may be curtailed but the intake of protein-rich foods should be maintained.

Carbohydrates and Fats

Carbohydrates and fats should be supplied as in an ordinary diet to provide the necessary calories.

Glycosuria and Diabetes

The presence of sugar in the urine during pregnancy may not be due to diabetes but may be a temporary alteration in the carbohydrate metabolism that reverts to normal after the termination of pregnancy. The carbohydrate metabolism may be altered due to high blood sugar, increased glomerular filtration, or diminished tubular reabsorption of glucose. On overnight fasting state, the first urine is discarded but subsequent urine (without food) showing sugar with glucose oxidase method (*Clinistix*) is likely to be due to diabetes and requires a glucose tolerance curve [2].

The oral glucose tolerance during pregnancy shows gross variations in the same individual, and in the absence of gross abnormality no result should be labelled abnormal without at least one confirmatory test. The British Diabetic Association recommends that blood glucose is considered abnormal when by to glucose oxidase method the capillary blood glucose level is over 120 mg per 100 ml at 2 hours of glucose tolerance test and over 180 mg per 100 ml at any time during the test [3]. This approximately corresponds to 110 mg and 160 mg respectively of venous blood.

Vitamins and Minerals

So that the infant is born with adequate stores, vitamin deficiency should not be allowed to occur during pregnancy. There are no definite experimental observations nor general opinions about the exact requirements, but the recommendations in TABLE 37 are considered to be reasonable. Ideally, the diet should supply all these vitamins but this is not feasible and one tablet of a multivitamin preparation should be administered daily.

TABLE 37

REQUIREMENTS DURING PREGNANCY AND LACTATION

Calories	2000–2500
Proteins	70–90 g
Vitamin A	6000 Units
Thiamine	1·5 mg
Riboflavine	2·0 mg
Nicotinic acid	15 mg
Folic acid	5–10 mg
Vitamin C	45 mg
Vitamin D	400 Units
Calcium	1·5 g
Iron	15 mg

Calcium

The calcium requirement increases particularly during the last 3 months of pregnancy when the bones of the foetus are ossifying. About 25 mg of calcium is required daily for the foetus at the third month and the demand gradually increases till 300 mg daily is necessary in the ninth month. If the extra supply of calcium is not available from the diet then the calcium stores in the bones of the mother are depleted. In extreme cases this leads to osteomalacia. Only about one-third of dietary calcium is utilized and so a liberal calcium intake is necessary. Unless the diet is adequate in milk and milk products, it does not supply the necessary calcium and a commercial calcium supplement should be given. The total daily intake of calcium should be 1·5 g. Absorption of calcium is increased during pregnancy [4].

The intake of calories, protein, vitamins and minerals should be gradually increased so as to reach the maximum recommended during the last 3 months of pregnancy.

Smoking

Mothers who smoke during pregnancy have smaller babies than non-smokers. This effect may be due to reduced blood flow to the placenta. The growth of the foetus is not affected if the mother had smoked prior to pregnancy or had stopped early in the pregnancy. The incidence of abortion, stillbirth and perinatal death is higher among smokers [5]. Surprisingly enough, the smokers have comparatively lower blood pressure [5] and a lower incidence of pre-eclamptic toxaemia ([6].

PRINCIPLES OF DIETETICS

Frequent small feeds during first 3 months if there is vomiting.

TABLE 38 suggests satisfactory intake of certain foods during pregnancy and lactation. The diet requires to be gradually increased as pregnancy proceeds.

ANAEMIAS IN PREGNANCY

Physiological changes in the blood occur progressively during normal pregnancy. The plasma volume rises by 30 per cent. The whole blood volume increases by 45 per cent, and there is a 40 per cent rise in the circulating red cells. The total haemoglobin mass increases from 550 g at the beginning of pregnancy to 725 g in the seventh month of pregnancy. The haemoglobin concentration thus drops from 13·4 to 11·6 g per 100 ml.

A pregnant woman is labelled anaemic if from the 28th week onwards the haemoglobin is less than 10 g per 100 ml (70 per cent) of blood. Anaemia during pregnancy is common in Western countries and is more frequent still in the tropics with poor nutrition and repeated pregnancies, worm infestation and sometimes associated haemoglobinopathies [7].

TABLE 38

SUGGESTED DAILY INTAKE OF CERTAIN NUTRITIVE
FOODS DURING PREGNANCY AND LACTATION

	Mixed Diet	Vegetarian Diet
Milk	2 cups	3 cups
Cereals	As required	As required
Pulses	—	2 cups cooked dal
Eggs	2	—
Meat, fish or poultry	2 average helpings	—
Leafy vegetables	2 helpings	2 helpings
Potato, medium	1–2	1–2
Fruits	1–2 helpings	1–2 helpings

Iron Deficiency

In pregnancy 550 mg of iron is required for the formation of foetus (400 mg in foetus, 100 mg in placenta, and 50 mg in uterine muscles), 175 mg is lost during parturition and 180 mg is excreted in the milk during lactation. An additional 500 mg is utilized in the formation of the increased haemoglobin mass, which, however, is not lost to the mother. On the other hand, there is also a saving of about 225 mg of iron which would have been lost during nine menstrual cycles. Thus the total loss of iron to the mother during each pregnancy is about

680 mg if the infant is breast fed and 500 mg if it is not breast fed.

The predominantly cereal diet in the tropics should be able to provide 40 mg iron per day [8]. The iron intake of pregnant British women is 14·2 mg per day [9].

The ability to absorb iron is increased during pregnancy and the maximum absorption occurs during the last trimester. In pregnant women with a urinary infection the incidence of iron deficiency anaemia is increased. Therapeutic administration of iron can produce a rise in the haemoglobin level even of non-anaemic pregnant women. It is justifiable to prescribe iron for all pregnant women particularly in those with haemoglobin level below 12 g per 100 ml blood because the iron stores are like to be deficient. However, the intolerance to oral iron is usually due to high dosage. The rate of haemoglobin formation does not differ whether iron is administered orally or parenterally. Administration of 30 mg elemental iron per day after the first trimester of pregnancy prevents fall in haemoglobin level [10]. About 32 per cent of pregnant women fail to take the prescribed iron tablets and this may account for lack of response to prophylactic therapy [11].

Parenteral iron therapy is indicated when: (1) the patient is not relied upon to take oral iron; (2) malabsorption states occur; (3) haemoglobin is less than 6 g per 100 ml after 30th week of pregnancy. Iron-destran complex (*Imferon*) or iron-sorbitol complex (*Jectofer*), 100 mg intramuscularly daily or on alternate days, may then be given. Enthusiasm to give an *intravenous total dose* of iron-dextran as a single large dose of up to 2 G in 500 ml dextrose or normal saline should be curbed. Only an experienced person who is prepared to give the injection under his direct supervision may attempt it, since anaphylactic shock and even death may occur.

Folic Acid

The demand for folate is increased because of increased cellular proliferation. The low folate levels are not due to deficient absorption as was previously believed but to deficient intake.

Premature infants are sometimes reported as being born to folate-deficient mothers of the poorer class, but the incidence is reduced with folic acid supplements [12]. On the other hand, even when folic acid deficiency was severe enough to produce megaloblastic anaemia in mothers, the incidence of perinatal mortality, foetal malformation, prematurity, low weight and neonatal haemoglobin concentration was not different from that in the general population [13]. Though premature separation of placenta has been repeatedly blamed on folic acid deficiency, this claim has not been substantiated [14].

The *requirement* of 'free folate' (in absorbable form and not requiring intestinal conjugase digestion) is 300 micrograms during pregnancy and 400 micrograms during lactation. In practice, 5 mg folic acid supplement ensures adequate supply. The fear of this prophylactic therapy precipitating subacute combined degeneration in patients with pernicious anaemia is not quite justified, as chances of such an occurrence are very remote compared to the benefit. Folates are easily destroyed by cooking, hence fresh vegetables such as *lettuce, cabbage* and *cucumber* are recommended as preventive measures.

Vitamin B_{12}

Anaemia due to vitamin B_{12} deficiency in pregnancy is comparatively uncommon but has been noted [15]. The mean vitamin B_{12} level in the serum of the mother at parturition was 190 micromicrograms per ml, while it was 390 micromicrograms per ml in the infant's serum, in one series [16]. A single injection of 40 micrograms of vitamin B_{12} is enough to produce a maximum response in 10 days in mothers who are deficient in it, but usually larger therapeutic doses are given. [15].

REFERENCES

[1] THOMSON, A.M., HYTTEN, F.E., and BILLEWICZ, W.Z. (1970)The energy cost of human lactation, *Brit. J. Nutr.*, **24**, 565.

[2] SUTHERLAND, H.W., STOWERS, J.M., and MCKENZIE, C. (1970) Simplifying the clinical problem of glycosuria in pregnancy, *Lancet*, **i**, 1069.

[3] FITZGERALD, M.G., and KEEN, H. (1964) Diagnostic classification of diabetes, *Brit. med. J.*, **1**, 1568.

[4] SHENOLIKAR, I.S. (1970) Absorption of dietary calcium in pregnancy, *Amer. J. clin. Nutr.*, **23**, 63.

[5] RUSSELL, C.S., TAYLOR, R., and LAW, C.E. (1968) Smoking in pregnancy, maternal blood pressure, pregnancy outcome, baby weight and growth and other related factors, *Brit. J. prev. soc. Med.*, **22**, 119.

[6] DUFFUS, G.M., and MACGILLIVNA, I. (1968) The incidence of pre-eclamptic toxaemia in smokers and non-smokers, *Lancet*, **i**, 994.

[7] MEHTA, B.C., JHAVERI, K., and PATEL, J.C. (1971) Anaemia in pregnancy, *Indian J. med. Sci.*, **25**, 301.

[8] APTE, S.V., and IYENGAR, L. (1970) Absorption of dietary iron in pregnancy, *Amer. J. clin. Nutr.*, **23**, 7.

[9] CHANARIN, I., ROTHMAN, D., PERRY, J., and STRATFULL, D. (1968) Normal dietary folate, iron and protein intake, with particular reference to pregnancy, *Brit. med. J.*, **2**, 394.

[10] IYENGAR, L., and APTE, S.V. (1970) Prophylaxis of anaemia in pregnancy, *Amer. J. clin. Nutr.*, **23**, 725.

[11] BONNAR, J., GOLDBERG, A., and SMITH, J.A. (1969) Do pregnant women take their iron?, *Lancet*, **i**, 457.

[12] BAUMSLAG, N., EDELSTEIN, T., and METZ., J. (1970) Reduction of incidence of prematurity by folic acid supplementation in pregnancy, *Brit. med. J.* **1**, 16.

[13] PRITCHARD, J.A., SCOTT, D.E., WHALLEY, P.J., and HALING, R.F. (1970) Infants of mothers with megaloblastic anaemia due to folate deficientcy, *J. Amer. med. Ass.*, **211**, 1982.

[14] ALPERIN, J.B., HAGGARD, M.E., and MCGANITY, W.J. (1969) Folic acid, pregnancy and abruptio placentae, *Amer. J. clin. Nutr.*, **22**, 1354.

[15] PATEL, J.C., and KOCHER, B.R. (1950) Vitamin B_{12} in macrocytic anaemia of pregnancy and the puerperium, *Brit. med. J.*, **1**, 924.

[16] BAKER, H., ZIFFER, H., PASHER, I., and SOBOTKA, H. (1958) A comparison of maternal and foetal folic acid and vitamin B_{12} at parturition, *Brit. med. J.*, **1**, 978.

81. BOWEL TRAINING AND COMMON DIGESTIVE AILMENTS IN INFANCY

Bowel Training

A vigilant mother anticipates when her child is about to pass urine or stool. An infant is likely to empty the bladder or pass a stool on awakening from sleep or after a feed. If the baby is held over a pot as soon as he wakes up or after each feed, he can be trained to open his bowels and pass urine regularly. This procedure helps by reducing the number of dirty napkins thus saving the mother trouble and by avoiding napkin rash due to irritation of the skin by the excreta.

COMMON DIGESTIVE AILMENTS OF INFANCY

The common digestive ailments in infancy are: (1) constipation; (2) diarrhoea; (3) vomiting; and (4) colic.

CONSTIPATION

Constipation is one of the commonest variations in the infant's bowel habit that disturbs the mother. If the infant does not move his bowels every day, but passes a well formed semi-solid stool every other day and is happy and contented, this should not be considered as constipation and purgatives are not needed. It is only when the infant is distressed during the passage of dry, hard stools that the bowels require attention.

Aetiology

1 *Insufficient fluid intake* is the most common cause of constipation in the tropics

2. *Underfeeding* constitutes an important cause of constipation in infants in the lower economic group. Underfeeding in a breast fed infant can be diagnosed only by test weighing. In an artificially fed infant the amount and quality of the feeds can be easily determined.

3. *Artificial feeding* may produce constipation. Usually breast fed infants pass greenish unformed stools because of the relatively high content of lactose in mother's milk. Artificially fed infants tend to pass hard light coloured stools because, compared to human milk, animal milk contains: (a) more casein, which is liable to form larger and harder curds; (b) less sugar, which diminishes intestinal fermentation; and (c) more calcium, which combines with fatty acids to form insoluble soaps.

4. A *diet* wholly of milk, when additional foods ought to have been added, may produce constipation in an infant.

5. *Purgatives* administered injudiciously may cause irregularity of the natural bowel movement and a laxative habit may be started which sometimes persists throughout our life.

6. *Acute anal fissure* is sometimes a cause of constipation in children— the child being reluctant to have his bowels opened due to pain.

7. *Congenital anomalies* like pyloric stenosis and megacolon are rare causes of constipation in infancy.

Treatment

If an infant does not pass a stool each day, the mother should not rush for a bottle of laxative. This will not cure constipation but perpetuate it. The diet should be readjusted first and a laxative should only be given as a last resort.

1. At least 150 ml of *fluid* per kg ($2\frac{1}{2}$ oz per lb) of body weight per day, and more during the hot season, must be given to a baby. Most of the fluid is supplied by milk but some water is also needed. It is best to give water to the infant two hours after each feed.

2. *Test weighing* of a breast fed infant may show that the *milk intake*
is insufficient and, if so supplementary or complementary feeds should
be given.

3. If the hard *casein curds* of animal milk are responsible for bowel
irregularity then boiling the milk for 5 minutes before making a feed
may help.

4. *Carbohydrates* such as ripe banana, prune juice or syrup of figs
help in passing a natural stool. The addition of 1 or 2 teaspoons of
sugar or extract of malt to feeds also promotes bowel movement.

If, despite these measures, constipation persists, 1 or 2 teaspoons
of milk of magnesia may be given. This medicine should be resorted
to only occasionally as its regular use is liable to lead to habit formation.
Occasionally, for quick relief, a soap stick or glycerin suppository
may be inserted into the rectum.

DIARRHOEA

Aetiology

1. *Infection* of the intestinal tract due to faulty sterilization of utensils,
milk, water or food, or uncleanlines in the management of the infant,
predispose to diarrhoea. Respiratory or other systemic infections in
the infant may be accompanied by diarrhoea. Organisms thrive in
the warm climate of the tropics and food that is not properly boiled
or preserved may produce gastro-enteritis. Not infrequently, tonsillitis,
otitis media, pyelitis or other infection may manifest itself as diarrhoea
and a search for the primary cause should always be made.

2. *Excess of carbohydrates or of fats* may produce diarrhoea. Excess
of carbohydrates leads to acid fermentation and frequent loose stools.
Excess of fat, if not split, produces fatty diarrhoea.

3. *Underfeeding* may also produce frequent small stools. This is
often referred to as hunger diarrhoea.

Treatment

Prevention of diarrhoea, which should be the aim, is best achieved
by giving feeds of the correct composition and amount by carefully
sterilizing utensils and feeds, and by protecting the infant from systemic
infections.

The precise treatment of diarrhoea depends on its cause and severity.
Every case of diarrhoea requires fluid and electrolyte management to

forestall the disastrous complication of dehydration and electrolyte loss [see CHAPTERS 20, 21 and 32.]. Careful nursing may prevent deterioration in the infant's condition and avoid any necessity for parenteral fluid and electrolyte therapy.

Infants are very sensitive to loss of fluid such as occurs with diarrhoea. Water should be given freely. Regular feeds should be stopped, but, to prevent dehydration, 0·45 per cent saline ($\frac{1}{4}$ teaspoon of common salt dissolved in a glass of water) should be given frequently. Sugar is also added to supply calories and to prevent ketosis which quickly develops if an infant is starved. Potassium is supplied by giving fruit juice. In severe diarrhoea, potassium citrate, $\frac{1}{4}$ teaspoon daily, may be given. A practical way of administering fluids and electrolytes during acute diarrhoea is to give the following 'elixir.':

Sugar or dextrose	2 tablespoons
Common salt (sodium chloride)	$\frac{1}{4}$ teaspoon
Juice of fresh fruit in season (orange, etc.)	100–150 ml
Water (boiled and cooled) add to 1 glass (300 ml)	

Two to four tablespoons of this 'elixir' should be given every hour.

Lime-whey. In both breast fed and artificially fed infants, a useful household preparation that may be given with advantage before restarting milk feeds is lime-whey. This is prepared by bringing milk to the boil and adding sour lime drop by drop until suddenly the milk 'breaks', i.e., solids form into masses and float in a clear yellowish liquid. The fluid is strained through a clean muslin cloth, sugar is added, and when cool enough, it is given to the baby. Lime-whey is virtually free from fat and casein, but contains the lactalbumin, sugar and minerals of natural milk. Its potassium content is sufficiently high to prevent the deficiency which is sometimes a feature of severe diarrhoea with dehydration.

Milk Feeds. In severe diarrhoea, milk should be stopped. When the diarrhoea has been controlled, the infant is started on his feeds by diluting one part of milk with three parts of water. The concentration of milk is gradually increased until the normal for his age is reached.

VOMITING

A small amount of milk is usually vomited by infants who have taken too much at a feed. As long as the infant is otherwise thriving, and gaining weight normally, such vomiting should be ignored and the mother reassured.

Aetiology

The commonest causes of vomiting in infancy are: (1) air swallowing; (2) over-feeding; (3) large casein curds; (4) nervousness; (5) acute infections, especially upper respiratory infections; and (6) stenosis of the pylorus or oesophagus.

1. *Air swallowing* (aerophagy) occurs in every infant during feeds. It is more likely if : (a) the infant is excessively hungry and gulps milk rapidly; (b) there is not enough milk in the breasts and he is left to feed too long so that he sucks vigorously on an empty breast; (c) the hole in the teat of the feeding bottle is too small. When the baby is put on his back after a feed the swallowed air cannot escape through the oesophagus. The stomach is distended and expels some air and milk which is interpreted as vomiting. This regurgitation can be prevented by holding the child upright after a feed and rubbing his back gently until air is expelled by 'burping'. The baby should also be encouraged to burp when he is changed from one breast to the other. A bottle fed infant should be allowed to burp once or twice, half way through the feed. Feeding should be so regulated that the infant does not become excessively hungry.

2. *Over-feeding* is sometimes a cause of vomiting during infancy amongst wealthy families. The amount and concentration of the feeds needs to be adjusted appropriately.

3. *Large casein curds* form in the stomach when animal milk is fed. This can be corrected by boiling the milk for 5 minutes before preparing the feed.

4. *Nervous* vomiting is likely to occur when foods other than milk are being introduced. Allowing the baby to taste each new food before feeding may help.

5. *Upper respiratory infections* sometimes start with vomiting. Every infant brought because of vomiting should be examined carefully for evidence of infection.

6. *Stenosis of the pylorus or oesophagus* is not frequent but when present may require surgical management.

Treatment
The treatment of vomiting involves correction of the primary cause rather than the administration of drugs.

COLIC

Colic is an acute intermittent abdominal pain, often associated in infants with the passage of gas; the infant cries with pain during an attack of colic. Common causes of colic are air swallowing (aerophagy), due for example, to thumb sucking, and an excess of carbohydrate and fruit juice causing intestinal fermentation and gas production. Some infants appear to be particularly prone to colic during the second and third months.

Treatment
Feeding at proper intervals avoids thumb-sucking. In an infant prone to colic, the quantity of sugar and fruit juice should be reduced. An acute attack of colic often responds to atropine methonitrate (*Eumydrin*).

82. DIET FOR CHILDREN

A child needs a balanced and adequate diet to supply the materials and energy needed for growth.

REQUIREMENTS

Calories
A child requires more calories per kilogram body weight than an adult because: (1) basal metabolism is highest during infancy and then steadly declines throughout life except for a small rise during adolescence; (2) physical activity of the child far exceeds that of an adult; and (3) extra calories are needed for growth.

Proteins
A child requires relatively more protein than an adult because it is

needed not only for tissue repair but also for growth. About 14 per cent of the calories should be supplied as protein.

The main sources of protein are milk and milk products, meat, fish, fowl, eggs, nuts, cereals and pulses.

Carbohydrates and Fats

Carbohydrates and fats are supplied mainly for their caloric value. Care should be taken that sweets are not sucked constantly as they ferment in the mouth and damage the teeth. Liberal helpings of raw and cooked vegetables and fruits should be allowed at each meal.

Vitamins and Minerals

If the diet is well balanced, supplements of vitamins and minerals are not necessary.

Fluids

Fluid intake should be sufficient to ensure a free flow of urine. Childern who run about and sweat profusely need extra fluids.

FOOD HABITS

It is preferable to give feeds at the intervals suggested below:

8.00 a.m.	Breakfast
10.30 a.m.	Fruit juice, biscuits or *puris,* milk, 1 cup
12.30 p.m.	Lunch
4.00 p.m.	Biscuits, cakes or *puris,* milk, 1 cup
7.00 p.m.	Dinner

The meal hours should be regular and nibbling between meals should be discouraged. At meal time there should be no comments about likes and dislikes regarding food. If a child does not eat, the parent should not feed forcibly or scold as this only makes a child obstinate. If after a mild persuasion the child refuses to eat then no further attempt should be made to feed him at that meal. If the parent's sole complaint is that a child is indifferent towards food, despite being healthy, physically fit and happily playing about, it is the parent who requires instruction. A child should never be made conscious that he obliges his parent by eating. No 'tonics', digestives or injections have ever produced an appetite in a child who refused to eat.

Frequently the child refuses to eat because of lack of ingenuity on the part of the mother in serving food. Milk and eggs in particular are refused because they are served in a monotonous way day after day. Milk can easily be made appetizing by the addition of various kinds of flavouring agents and syrups which increase calories and impart attractive colours. Milk and eggs can be served as custard, pudding or ice-cream. Confectionary can also be made into various appealing shapes and shades. An occasional lunch or dinner served in the back-yard or garden with friends may create a ravenous appetite. Thus a little imagination in the preparation and serving of a meal can be richly rewarded.

DIET FOR SCHOOL CHILDREN

School children usually have a good appetite but their food should be judiciously selected. Their liking for sweets makes the diet adequate in calories but deficient in proteins. Roasted groundnuts and Bengal gram are good sources of inexpensive protein relished by children.

Children who are reluctant to go to bed early have difficulty in waking up in the morning and may rush their breakfast before going to school. School lunch may also be hurried so as to get more time for play during the lunch interval. In the evening, when they return from school, children are usually thirsty and may gulp down a lot of liquid which dulls their appetite. If good nutrition is to be assured these bad habits should be corrected.

If it is not possible to send a hot lunch to school, a nutritious dry lunch can be prepared as advised below:

Diet for School Children

Breakfast:	Cereal with a cup of milk
	One egg (any preparation)
	Toast with butter and jam or *chappatis* with ghee and sugar or honey
Mid-morning	Biscuits or *puris*
Lunch (dry)	Mutton or cottage cheese sandwiches
	Boiled egg or potato chips
	Fruit in season like banana, orange, apple or mango
	Roasted groundnuts or Bengal gram about 30–60 g
4.00 p.m.	Milk, 1 cup
	Cakes, biscuits or *puris*

Dinner	Meat, fish, chicken or curd
	Cooked *dal* or butter-milk
	Cooked vegetables
	Potato, baked or boiled
	Bread or *chappatis*
	Custard pudding or home-made sweets
Before retiring	A cup of milk

83. DIET IN OLD AGE

With advances in medicine, more people are reaching a ripe old age. The factors in increasing longevity have been hygiene, nutrition, preventive medicine and (possibly) antibiotics. Diseases of old age like diabetes are better managed. The recognition of the dangers of obesity, made evident by statistics from life insurance companies, have induced many to regulate their weight, resulting in a reduced death rate.

Mental faculty is depressed not only due to arteriosclerosis but also by poor nutrition of vitamins and minerals.

The management of older people has become a problem in modern society. With a joint family system the elderly were well looked after. They stayed mostly in the villages in healthy surroundings and had good wholesome food. With the exodus of younger people from the countryside into congested cities accommodation and care for the aged has become a problem.

A diet for old people should be such as to help them maintain good health. If they are living alone, their diet tends to become unbalanced as they are reluctant to cook and, to avoid the trouble of going to a restaurant, they skip meals and frequently subsist on tea and snacks. Their food intake may be further limited by exclusion of certain foods for high blood pressure, diabetes, heart failure and kidney diseases. Their appetite may be reduced due to restriction of physical activity by arthritis, worries about their own failing health and constipation. Digestion may be impaired by improper mastication with artificial teeth.

The bones show osteoporotic changes in old age because of deficiency of calcium, protein, vitamins, minerals and hormones.

DIETETIC MANAGEMENT

Calories

The lowered metabolic rate in the elderly reduces the calorie requirement. A retired life, arthritis and angina reduce physical activities to a minimum. The calories should be restricted to combat any tendency to obesity. If there is loss of weight and emaciation, adequate calories should be supplied to regain normal weight. The total calorie requirement is an individual problem which is best judged by observing the weight of the patient.

Proteins

Deficiency of protein is common in the elderly and is one of the factors producing oedema, anaemia and lowered resistance to infections. Protein-rich foods like meat and fish are expensive, require cooking, and may be difficult to chew without teeth. Amongst the vegetarians, pulses provide an appreciable amount of protein, though in old age such food-stuffs increase flatulence. The protein intake should be about 70 g. If this amount cannot be provided with regular meals then commercial protein preparations or skimmed milk powder should be given as a supplement.

If mastication is a problem then minced meat, half-boiled eggs, and milk products, like curds. buttermilk, custard and puddings are useful.

Fats

With advancing age fats become difficult to digest. Older people tend to have a high blood cholesterol level. Ingestion of unsaturated fats, like vegetable oils (except coconut and palm), reduce blood cholesterol and part of the fat intake may with advantage be given in this form. About 40–50 g of fat daily should be advised.

Carbohydrates

Old people tend to take much carbohydrate and little protein. Bread, biscuits, cakes and pastry are cheap, readily available, do not require cooking and can be stored, hence they form the bulk of the diet. Such a diet produces protein deficiency, anaemia and constipation due to lack of roughage. Anaemia and constipation in turn reduce appetite and enhance malnutrition.

Vitamins and Minerals

Vitamin deficiency, particularly of the vitamin B complex, is common with unbalanced diet and daily supplement with a *multivitamin* tablet is advisable.

The blood pressure, particularly the systolic pressure, rises with old age but the intake of sodium should not be drastically reduced. A sodium-poor diet is also deficient in protein [see pp. 549 and 551].

Osteoporosis is common in old age. The exact reason for it is not determined but it may be partly due to diminished intake and absorption of calcium and partly to a deficiency of sex hormones leading to loss of protein. A combination of androgen and oestrogen has been recommended for senile osteoporosis. Senile *osteomalacia* is common, particularly in women confined indoors and taking less than 70 IU vitamin D. Lactase-deficient people avoid milk, which leads to diminished calcium and vitamin D intake resulting in osteoporosis and osteomalacia. Half a litre of milk and 2–3 eggs daily may substantially aid in ensuring an adequate supply of calcium and protein.

Anaemia is common in the elderly. Salicylates taken over a prolonged period for chronic arthritis tend to produce alimentary blood loss and anaemia. Iron deficiency is common. Hypofunction of the thyroid, diminished activity of the bone marrow and diminished protein intake are other possible factors contributing to anaemia in the aged. Anaemia in the elderly should be investigated to exclude carcinoma. Vitamin B and folic acid deficiency are also common [1].

Potassium deficiency occurs with less than 50 mEq intake per day. The patients exhibit muscle weakness, apathy and faecal impaction. Constipation leads to anorexia and further restriction in food intake.

Fluids

An adequate fluid intake should be ensured. The intake may be varied according to the diet and the season. The excretion of over 1200 ml of urine indicates proper fluid balance. Many old people are reluctant to drink liquids as they have to urinate frequently, particularly with diseases like diabetes, chronic nephritis and prostatic enlargement. They should be induced to take sufficient liquids during the day and refrain from drinking at night so that their sleep is not disturbed. They should not drink water before, during, or immediately after meals, as they may feel bloated which restricts adequate food intake.

Meal Pattern

The elderly should be given small frequent feeds and an early evening dinner. This prevents disturbed sleep due to gaseous distension. Old people not infrequently have a poor coronary circulation, and so physical exertion, particularly climbing stairs, immediately after a meal should be avoided.

OLD AGE

Mixed Diet	*Vegetarian Diet*
On rising	
A glass of warm water	A glass of warm water
Tea or coffee	Tea or coffee
Breakfast	
Eggs, 2, half boiled or scrambled	Porridge with milk and sugar
Toast, butter, jam	Toast or *chappatis,* butter, jam
Banana	Banana
11 a.m.	
Fruit juice, 1 cup	Fruit juice, 1 cup
Lunch	
Meat or fish	Curd, 1 cup
average helping with baked	*Dal,* 1 cup
potato and french beans	Cooked vegetables
Bread or *chappatis*	Potato, mashed
	Bread or *chappatis*
4 p.m.	
Tea	Tea
Biscuits	Biscuits
Dinner	
Chicken, roast with pumpkin	Curd, 1 cup
Bread or *chappatis*	Cooked vegetables
Custard, ½ cup	Bread or *chappatis*
	Ice cream, ½ cup

REFERENCE

[1] READ, A.E., GOUGH, K.R., PARDOE, J.L., and NICHOLAS, A. (1965) Nutritional studies on the entrants to an old peoples home, with particular reference to folic acid deficiency, *Brit. med. J.,* **2**, 843.

PART IV

TABLES OF FOOD VALUES, ETC.

In the following tables values are given for proteins, fats, carbo-hydrates, calories, vitamins and minerals for the *cooked* average portion served. Values of raw food are given where data for cooked food are not available.

The food values are mainly derived from the following sources:

REFERENCES

[1] *Bowes and Church's Food Values of Portions Commonly Used* (1963) 9th ed., rev. Church, C.F., and Church, H.N., Philadelphia.

[2] McCANCE, R.A., and WIDDOWSON, E.M. (1960) The composition of foods, *Spec. Rep. Ser. med. Res. Coun. (Lond.)*, No. 297, London, H.M.S.O.

[3] AYKROYD, W.R. (1963) *The Nutritive Value of Indian Foods and Planning of Satisfactory Diets,* 6th ed. rev. Gopalan, C., and Balasubramanian, S.C., Indian Council of Medical Research, New Delhi.

TABLE 39A

CALORIE VALUE OF ALCOHOLIC BEVERAGES

ALOCOHOLIC BEVERAGES	AVERAGE PORTION	ML	CALORIES
Beer	1 glass	240	98
Benedictine	1 measure	20	69
Brandy, cognac	1 oz	30	73
Cider	1 small glass	180	71
Gin	1 measure	43	105
Rum	1 measure	43	105
Sherry	1 measure	100	120
Toddy, fermented	1 glass	240	24
Toddy, sweet	1 glass	240	144
Whisky, Scotch	1 measure	43	119

TABLE 39B

PROTEIN, FAT, CARBOHYDRATE AND CALORIE VALUES OF AVERAGE PORTIONS *served*

NAME	AVERAGE PORTION	WEIGHT G	PROTEIN G	FAT G	CARBO-HYDRATE G	CALORIES
BEVERAGES						
Bournvita, 2 tablespoons, cow's milk, 1 cup	1 cup	230	10·2	11·1	28·8	265
Bovril	1 tablespoon	15	2·5	0·1	—	11
Coca Cola	1 bottle	170	—	—	20·4	78
Cocoa powder	2 tablespoons	30	5·8	6·6	9·9	128
Cocoa, 1 tablespoon, cow's milk, 1 cup	1 cup	215	9·9	12·3	14·5	224
Coffee, cow's milk, 2 tablespoons, sugar, 2 teaspoons	1 cup	200	0·9	1·1	11·4	60
Horlicks	2 tablespoons	30	4·1	2·3	20·1	113
Lemonade, fresh lemon juice, 2 tablespoons, sugar, 3 teaspoons	1 glass	240	—	—	17·4	73
Ovaltine	2 tablespoons	30	3·8	1·8	20·6	109
Ovaltine, 1 tablespoon, cow's milk, 1 cup	1 cup	215	9·0	10·0	20·0	215
Tea, cow's milk, 2 tablespoons, sugar, 2 teaspoons	1 cup	200	0·9	1·1	11·4	60
CEREALS AND CEREAL FOODS						
Arrowroot	1 tablespoon	8	—	—	7·0	29
Bajra (*Pennisetum typhoideum*), 30 g flour	1 small *chappati*	45	3·5	1·5	20·1	108
Barley, pearled (2 tablespoons, dry)		30	2·3	0·3	22·3	99

TABLE 39B—(Continued)

PROTEIN, FAT, CARBOHYDRATE AND CALORIE VALUES
OF AVERAGE PORTIONS *served*

NAME	AVERAGE PORTION	WEIGHT G	PROTEIN G	FAT G	CARBO-HYDRATE G	CALORIES
CEREALS AND CEREAL FOODS (*Contd.*)						
Cornflakes	1 cup	25	2·1	0·1	21·0	95
Corn flour	¼ cup	25	2·1	0·1	21·0	95
Farex	2 tablespoons	30	3·7	0·7	20·7	97
Grape nuts	¼ cup	30	2·8	0·2	24·0	110
Jowar (*Sorghum vulgare, cholam*), 30 g flour	1 small *chappati*	45	3·1	0·6	22·2	106
Macaroni, cooked	⅔ cup	—	3·6	0·1	21·7	107
Maize (30 g flour)	1 *chappati*	45	3·3	1·1	19·8	102
Maize cake (*tortilla*)	1 cake	10	0·5	0·2	4·5	21
Oat meal, porridge cooked	1 cup	236	5·4	2·8	26·0	148
Ragi (*Elusine coracana*), 30 g flour	1 *chappati*	45	2·1	0·4	21·6	98
Rice, milled, boiled (3 tablespoons, dry)	1 cup	—	2·9	0·1	30·2	138
Rice, puffed	1 cup	13	0·8	0·1	11·5	51
Spaghetti plain, cooked	1 cup	146	7·4	0·9	44·1	218
Spaghetti, with tomato sauce	1 cup	220	7·0	1·5	34·3	179
Wheat, All Bran, Kellog's	½ cup	28	3·1	0·7	21·4	95
Wheat bread	1 slice	30	2·3	0·5	15·0	75
Wheat bread, butter, 1 teaspoon, and jam, 1 teaspoon	1 slice	40	2·6	4·6	19·7	130
Wheat bun	1 average	35	2·6	3·2	20·0	120

TABLE 39B—(Continued)

PROTEIN, FAT, CARBOHYDRATE AND CALORIE VALUES OF AVERAGE PORTIONS *served*

NAME	AVERAGE PORTION	WEIGHT G	PROTEIN G	FAT G	CARBO-HYDRATE G	CALORIES
CEREALS AND CEREAL FOODS (*Contd.*)						
Wheat *chappati* (15 g flour)	1 thin		1·2	0·1	8·0	40
Wheat coffee cake, iced	1	70	3·9	6·1	31·6	196
Wheat doughnut	1	32	2·2	6·5	17·5	135
Wheat *khakhra* (15 g flour)	1		1·2	0·1	8·0	40
Wheat *parotha* (atta, 60 g and fat, 2 tea-spoons)	1		4·8	10·4	36·0	256
Wheat shredded	1 biscuit	22	2·2	0·5	18·3	84
DESSERTS						
Blancmange	½ cup	125	4·2	4·7	23·8	152
Cake, angel	1 piece	45	3·4	0·1	33·0	145
Cake, plain	1 piece	75	3·5	8·3	32·3	218
Cake, plain with chocolate icing	1 piece	87	3·9	10·4	48·1	302
Cake, chocolate	1 piece	45	2·2	7·6	35·5	185
Cake, sponge	1 piece	50	3·4	2·4	29·5	153
Custard, baked	1 helping	157	8·8	9·1	22·8	205
Custard, boiled	½ cup	130	7·1	7·3	18·2	164
Jello-plain	1 serving	65	1·6	—	15·1	65

TABLE 39B—(Continued)

PROTEIN, FAT, CARBOHYDRATE AND CALORIE VALUES
OF AVERAGE PORTIONS *served*

NAME	AVERAGE PORTION	WEIGHT G	PROTEIN G	FAT G	CARBO-HYDRATE G	CALORIES
DESSERTS (*Contd.*)						
Pie	Average helping					
Apple, blackberry, chocolate cream, pineapple, lemon-meringue, strawberry		160	3·8	14·3	60·2	377
Pudding, bread, with raisins	½ cup	110	5·9	6·6	32·0	210
Pudding, rice, with raisins	½ cup	100	4·6	4·3	28·2	166
Shortcake, peach, strawberry, raspberry, blackberry	1 piece	150	3·2	6·3	42·4	266
EGGS, MEAT, POULTRY						
Bacon, cooked (30 g raw)	1 slice	7	1·8	4·4	—	48
Beef, corned, tinned	1 slice	28	7·1	3·4	—	60
Beef hamburger (100 g raw)	1	75	19·0	13·2	—	195
Beef steak, porterhouse, broiled (240 g raw)		100	25·4	14·7	—	242
Beef steak, sirloin, broiled (240 g raw)		125	31·9	13·8	—	260
Beef steak, tenderloin, broiled (120 g raw)		66	17·2	8·3	—	148
Beef stew (90 g beef, 2 small potatoes, 1 carrot, 1 onion)		485	28·1	19·6	56·1	529

TABLE 39B—(Continued)

PROTEIN, FAT, CARBOHYDRATE AND CALORIE VALUES OF AVERAGE PORTIONS served

NAME	AVERAGE PORTION	WEIGHT G	PROTEIN G	FAT G	CARBO-HYDRATE G	CALORIES
EGGS, MEAT, POULTRY (Contd.)						
Brain	1 serving	100	12·0	5·8	—	103
Chicken, boiled (weighed with bone)	1 serving	100	17·0	6·7	—	132
Chicken, roast	1 serving	100	29·6	7·3	—	189
Chicken soup	1 cup	200	4·0	2·0	—	34
Duck, roast	1 serving	100	22·8	23·6	—	310
Egg, small, boiled	1	30	4·0	4·0	0·2	52
Egg, medium, boiled	1	48	6·1	5·5	0·3	77
Egg, medium, fried	1	52	6·1	9·2	0·3	120
Egg, 1 medium omelette	1	62	6·6	9·8	0·3	120
Egg, 1 medium scrambled with milk and fat		62	6·6	9·8	1·0	120
Goose, roast	3 slices	100	28·1	22·4	—	322
Ham, fresh cooked (100 g raw)	1 slice	50	18·5	4·5	—	118
Heart, roast		100	20·0	4·3	0·8	125
Kidney, fried		50	14·0	4·5	—	100
Liver, sliced, fried after rolling in flour	1 serving	50	14·7	8·0	2·0	142
Luncheon meat	1 slice	30	4·6	6·8	0·5	80
Meat paste	1 teaspoon	5	1·0	0·6	0·2	10

TABLE 39B—(Continued)

PROTEIN, FAT, CARBOHYDRATE AND CALORIE VALUES
OF AVERAGE PORTIONS *served*

NAME	AVERAGE PORTION	WEIGHT G	PROTEIN G	FAT G	CARBO-HYDRATE G	CALORIES
EGGS, MEAT, POULTRY (*Contd.*)						
Mutton chop, covered with egg and bread crumbs and fried		50	11·4	12·6	2·3	170
Mutton, lean only	1 slice	30	8·8	1·8	—	53
Mutton, leg with fat, roast	1 serving	100	20·6	14·5	—	220
Mutton soup, thin	1 cup	200	4·0	2·0	—	34
Pork, leg, roast	1 serving	100	24·6	23·2	—	317
Sausage, cooked	1 serving	20	3·5	8·8	—	94
Turkey, roast (flesh only)	1 slice	40	12·4	3·0	—	80
Veal, cutlet	1	100	33·2	15·0	—	277
Venison, roast	1 serving	100	33·5	6·4	—	197
FATS AND OILS						
Butter	1 teaspoon	5	—	4·0	—	36
Ghee (clarified butter)	1 teaspoon	5	—	5·0	—	45
Lard	1 tablespoon	14	—	14·0	—	126
Margarine	1 tablespoon	14	Tr.	11·3	—	100
Oil, corn	1 tablespoon	14	—	14·0	—	126
Oil, groundnut	1 tablespoon	14	—	14·0	—	126

TABLE 39B—(Continued)

PROTEIN, FAT, CARBOHYDRATE AND CALORIE VALUES
OF AVERAGE PORTIONS *served*

NAME	AVERAGE PORTION	WEIGHT G	PROTEIN G	FAT G	CARBO-HYDRATE G	CALORIES
FATS AND OILS (*Contd.*)						
Oil, olive	1 tablespoon	14	—	14·0	—	126
Oil, *til*	1 tablespoon	14	—	14·0	—	126
FISH						
Caviare, canned	1 round teaspoon	10	3·4	1·7	—	30
Crab, boiled without shell		100	19·2	5·2	—	127
Herring, smoked, kippered	½ large	100	22·2	12·9	—	211
Herring roe, rolled in flour and fried		100	23·4	15·8	4·7	260
Lobster, boiled (¾ lb, 2 teaspoons butter)	1 average	334	20·0	24·9	0·8	308
Mackerel, fried, weighed with skin and bone	1 serving	100	14·6	8·3	—	136
Oysters, fried	6 oysters	135	15·1	29·6	18·2	412
Plaice, covered with crumbs and fried	1 serving	100	18·0	14·4	7·0	234
Pomfret, fried	1 serving	100	22·0	13·0	—	205
Prawns, cooked without shell		100	21·2	1·8	—	104
Salmon, steamed		100	19·1	13·0	—	199
Salmon, canned	½ cup	100	19·7	6·0	—	137
Sole, baked		102	16·9	20·0	—	204
Sardines, canned, after draining oil		100	20·4	22·6	—	294

TABLE 39B—(Continued)

PROTEIN, FAT, CARBOHYDRATE AND CALORIE VALUES OF AVERAGE PORTIONS *served*

NAME	AVERAGE PORTION	WEIGHT G	PROTEIN G	FAT G	CARBO-HYDRATE G	CALORIES
FISH (*Contd.*)						
Shrimps, boiled, weighed without shell		100	22·3	2·4	—	114
Shrimps, fried		75	15·3	9·3	8·3	180
Trout (4 oz raw)		90	21·9	13·7	—	216
Tuna, canned	⅝ cup	100	29·0	8·2	—	198
FRUITS						
Apple	1 medium	150	0·3	0·2	16·5	66
Apple juice, canned	½ cup	100	0·1	—	12·5	50
Apricots	2–3 medium	100	1·0	0·1	9·8	51
Avocado pear	½	108	2·0	18·0	6·0	185
Banana	1	150	1·8	0·3	34·5	132
Bullock heart (*Anona reticulata*) *ramphal*		100	1·4	0·2	15·7	70
Blackberries, raw	⅝ cup	100	1·2	1·0	12·5	57
Cashew fruit		100	0·2	0·1	11·6	48
Figs, fresh	3 small	100	2·1	—	18·1	77
Fruit cocktail, canned	½ cup	100	1·4	0·4	19·6	79
Grape-fruit	½ medium	115	0·4	0·3	21·4	81
		180	0·9	0·4	18·2	72

TABLE 39B—(Continued)

PROTEIN, FAT, CARBOHYDRATE AND CALORIE VALUES
OF AVERAGE PORTIONS *served*

NAME	AVERAGE PORTION	WEIGHT G	PROTEIN G	FAT G	CARBO-HYDRATE G	CALORIES
FRUITS (*Contd.*)						
Grapes	22–24	100	1·4	1·4	14·9	70
Guava	1 medium	100	0·9	0·3	11·2	51
Jack fruit		100	1·9	0·1	19·8	88
Jambu (*Syzigium cumini*)		100	0·7	0·3	14·0	63
Lemon, sour		100	0·6	0·7	8·2	42
Lime, sweet (*musambi*)	1 average	150	1·2	0·5	13·8	63
Mango, Alphonso, Bulsar	1	150	0·6	1·2	27·0	122
Mango, Alphonso, Ratnagiri	1	150	0·6	1·3	24·5	111
Melon	½ medium	150	0·9	0·2	8·1	37
Orange	1 medium	150	1·4	0·3	16·8	68
Orange juice	1 cup	200	1·6	1·0	21·0	96
Papaya	⅓ medium	100	0·6	0·1	7·2	32
Peach, fresh	1 medium	100	1·2	0·3	10·5	50
Pears	1	150	1·3	0·3	19·4	84
Pineapple	1 slice	84	0·3	0·2	11·5	44
Pineapple juice	1 cup	200	0·8	0·2	26·8	106
Plums	1	60	0·7	0·1	7·7	30
Pomegranate		100	1·5	1·2	20·9	90
Raspberries	⅔ cup	100	1·2	0·4	13·8	57

TABLE 39B—(Continued)

PROTEIN, FAT, CARBOHYDRATE AND CALORIE VALUES OF AVERAGE PORTIONS served

NAME	AVERAGE PORTION	WEIGHT G	PROTEIN G	FAT G	CARBO-HYDRATE G	CALORIES
FRUITS (Contd.)						
Strawberries	10 large	100	0·8	0·5	8·2	37
Tangerines	1 large	150	1·2	0·4	16·3	66
Watermelon cubes	—	100	0·5	0·2	6·9	28
FRUITS DRIED						
Currants	½ cup	100	2·3	0·5	71·2	268
Dates, seeds removed	3 to 4	30	0·6	0·2	22·6	85
Figs, dried	2 small	30	1·2	0·4	20·5	81
Peaches, dried	½ cup	80	2·4	0·5	55·5	212
Prunes, dried	6 medium	50	1·1	0·3	35·5	134
Raisins, seedless	1 tablespoon	10	0·2	0·1	7·1	27
MILK AND MILK PRODUCTS						
Butter	1 teaspoon	5	—	4·0	—	36
Buttermilk, buffalo's (curd, 1 cup making 3 cups of buttermilk)	1 cup	200	2·7	4·6	2·1	62
Buttermilk, cow's (curd, 1 cup making 3 cups of buttermilk)	1 cup	200	2·3	3·0	2·1	45
Cheese, Cheddar	1 piece	28	7·0	9·0	0·6	111

TABLE 39B—(*Continued*)

PROTEIN, FAT, CARBOHYDRATE AND CALORIE VALUES
OF AVERAGE PORTIONS *served*

NAME	AVERAGE PORTION	WEIGHT G	PROTEIN G	FAT G	CARBO-HYDRATE G	CALORIES
MILK AND MILK PRODUCTS (*Contd.*)						
Cheese, cottage	1 round table-spoon	28	5·5	0·1	0·6	27
Cream, light	2 tablespoons	30	0·8	5·4	1·2	56
Curds, buffalo milk	1 cup	200	8·0	14·0	6·3	182
Curds, skimmed milk, buffalo's or cow's	1 cup	200	8·4	0·2	6·3	69
Ghee (clarified butter)	1 teaspoon	5	—	5·0	—	45
Ice cream	1 helping	100	4·1	11·3	19·8	196
Milk, buffalo's	1 cup	200	8·0	14·0	10·4	206
Milk, buffalo's skimmed	1 cup	200	8·4	0·2	10·8	78
Milk, cow's	1 cup	200	7·0	9·0	9·6	160
Milk, cow's, skimmed	1 cup	200	7·2	0·2	10·0	70
Milk, condensed, sweetened	1 tablespoon	20	1·5	1·7	10·1	62
Milk, goat's	½ cup	100	3·3	4·1	4·7	75
Milk, whole, powdered	1 tablespoon	7	1·9	1·9	2·7	35
Milk, skimmed, powdered	1 tablespoon	7	2·6	Tr.	3·7	26
NUTS						
Almonds	12-15	15	2·8	8·1	2·9	90
Brazil nuts, shelled	4 medium	15	2·2	9·9	1·7	97

TABLE 39B—(Continued)

PROTEIN, FAT, CARBOHYDRATE AND CALORIE VALUES
OF AVERAGE PORTIONS *served*

NAME	AVERAGE PORTION	WEIGHT G	PROTEIN G	FAT G	CARBO-HYDRATE G	CALORIES
NUTS (Contd.)						
Butter nuts	4–5	15	3·6	9·2	1·3	96
Cashew nuts	6–8	15	2·8	7·2	4·1	88
Chestnuts, fresh	3 small	15	0·4	0·2	6·2	29
Coconut, fresh	1 piece	15	0·5	5·2	2·1	54
Coconut water	1 glass	240	0·2	0·2	10·8	46
Hazel nuts	10–12	15	1·6	9·5	3·0	97
Hickory nuts	15 small	15	2·1	10·1	2·0	101
Peanuts (groundnuts), roasted	1 tablespoon	15	4·0	7·0	3·3	86
Peanut butter	1 tablespoon	15	3·9	7·2	3·2	86
Pistachio nuts	30	15	2·9	8·0	2·8	88
Walnuts	8 halves	20	3·2	12·8	3·2	128
PULSES, DRIED PEAS AND BEANS						
Bengal gram (*chana dal*)	1 cup cooked thin *dal*	200	7·0	2·3	14·0	105
Bengal gram (*bhuna chana : futana*), roasted	—	100	22·5	5·2	58·1	369

TABLE 39B—(Continued)

PROTEIN, FAT, CARBOHYDRATE AND CALORIE VALUES
OF AVERAGE PORTIONS served

NAME	AVERAGE PORTION	WEIGHT G	PROTEIN G	FAT G	CARBO-HYDRATE G	CALORIES
PULSES, DRIED PEAS AND BEANS (Contd.)						
Black gram (urd dal)	⎫					
Green gram (mung dal)	⎬ 1 cup cooked					
Field bean (val dal)	⎭ thin dal	200	7·0	2·3	14·0	105
Lentil (masur dal)						
Peas, dried (vatana dal)						
Red gram (tur dal)						
Beans, baked	½ cup	100	6·0	0·4	17·3	92
Peas, roasted	—	100	22·9	11·4	58·1	340
SUGAR, JAM, CHOCOLATE, ETC.						
Chocolate, milk-shake one glass (8 oz), 60 g ice-cream, 45 g chocolate syrup	1 glass	345	11·2	17·8	58·0	421
Chocolate, nut	1 piece	28	2·4	7·9	16·9	142
Chocolate, milk	1 piece	28	2·4	9·5	15·9	152
Glucose	1 tablespoon	12	—	—	11·0	45
Honey	1 tablespoon	21	0·1	—	16·4	64
Jams, assorted	1 tablespoon	20	0·1	0·1	14·2	55
Jaggery	1 tablespoon	15	0·2	0·1	14·0	56

TABLE 39B—(Continued)

PROTEIN, FAT, CARBOHYDRATE AND CALORIE VALUES OF AVERAGE PORTIONS *served*

NAME	AVERAGE PORTION	WEIGHT G	PROTEIN G	FAT G	CARBO-HYDRATE G	CALORIES
SUGAR, JAM, CHOCOLATE, ETC. (Contd.)						
Marmalade, orange	1 tablespoon	20	0·2	0·1	14·0	56
Molasses	1 tablespoon	20	—	—	13·0	50
Sugar, white granular	1 teaspoon level	5	—	—	5·0	20
Sugar, white granular	1 teaspoon rounded	8	—	—	8·0	32
Sugar, cube	1 piece	6	—	—	6·0	24
Syrup, golden	1 tablespoon	20	—	—	14·8	59
VEGETABLES						
Amaranth (Chinese spinach:*rajgira*), cooked	½ cup	100	2·8	0·4	6·8	42
Artichoke, cooked	½ large	100	2·7	0·2	5·9	29
Asparagus, canned	6 medium	115	2·2	0·4	3·4	20
Bamboo, tender shoots	¾ cup	100	2·3	0·2	6·1	29
Bengal gram leaves, raw		100	7·0	1·4	14·9	97
Brinjal (egg plant), raw		100	1·4	0·3	4·0	24
Broad beans, raw		100	4·5	0·1	7·2	48
Beetroot, cooked	½ cup	83	0·8	0·1	8·1	34
Broccoli, cooked	¾ cup	100	3·3	0·2	5·5	29
Brussels sprouts, cooked	5–6	70	3·1	0·4	6·2	33

TABLE 39B—*(Continued)*

PROTEIN, FAT, CARBOHYDRATE AND CALORIE VALUES
OF AVERAGE PORTIONS *served*

NAME	AVERAGE PORTION	WEIGHT G	PROTEIN G	FAT G	CARBO-HYDRATE G	CALORIES
VEGETABLES (*Contd.*)						
Cabbage, shredded, raw	½ cup	50	0·7	0·1	2·7	12
Cabbage, cooked	½ cup	85	1·2	0·2	4·5	20
Carrot, cooked	½ cup	75	0·5	0·4	4·8	23
Carrot, raw	1 large	100	1·2	0·3	9·3	42
Carrot leaves, raw		100	5·1	0·5	13·1	77
Cauliflower, cooked	½ cup	60	1·5	0·1	3·0	15
Celery, raw	3 inner stalks	50	0·6	0·1	0·8	9
Cluster beans (*guarphalli*), raw		100	3·2	0·4	11·0	59
Colocasia, green (*alu*)		100	3·9	1·5	6·8	56
Coriander leaves (*kothmir*), raw		100	3·3	0·6	7·5	48
Corn (maize), tender, boiled	1	140	2·7	0·7	20·0	84
Cucumber, raw	½ medium	50	0·4	—	1·4	6
Curry leaves		100	6·1	1·0	18·7	108
Double beans, raw		100	8·3	0·3	12·3	85
Drumstick (*Moringa oleifora*), raw		100	2·5	0·1	3·7	26
Drumstick leaves, raw		100	6·7	1·7	12·5	92
Fenugreek (*methi sag*) leaves, raw		100	4·4	0·9	6·0	49
French beans, raw		100	1·7	0·1	4·5	26
Knol-khol, raw		100	1·1	0·2	3·8	27

TABLE 39B—(Continued)

PROTEIN, FAT, CARBOHYDRATE AND CALORIE VALUES
OF AVERAGE PORTIONS *served*

NAME	AVERAGE PORTION	WEIGHT G	PROTEIN G	FAT G	CARBO-HYDRATE G	CALORIES
VEGETABLES *(Contd.)*						
Lady's fingers (okra; *bhendi*)	8 or 9 pods	85	1·5	0·2	6·3	28
Lettuce	3 small leaves	30	0·4	0·1	0·9	5
Mango, green, without seed		100	0·7	0·1	10·1	44
Mushrooms, fried	7 small	70	1·7	7·4	2·8	78
Onion, mature, raw	1 average	100	1·4	0·2	10·3	45
Onion stalks		100	0·9	0·2	8·9	41
Parsley, raw	10 small twigs	10	0·4	0·1	0·9	5
Parsnips, cooked	½ cup	78	0·8	0·4	10·7	47
Peas, green, cooked	½ cup	80	3·8	0·3	9·7	56
Peas (dried 30 g), cooked	½ cup	—	7·1	0·4	18·1	102
Peas, fresh, raw, shelled	¾ cup	100	6·7	0·4	17·7	98
Pepper, green, leaked, without stuffing	1 average	65	0·8	0·1	3·9	17
Potato, baked	1 medium	100	2·4	0·1	22·5	98
Potato, boiled	1 medium	100	2·0	0·1	19·1	83
Potato, chips	10 pieces	20	1·3	7·4	9·8	108
Potato, french fried	10 pieces	50	2·7	9·6	26·0	197
Potato, mashed with butter and milk	½ cup	100	2·1	15·9	6·0	123
Pumpkin, cooked	½ cup	100	1·0	0·3	7·9	33
Pumpkin leaves, raw		100	4·6	0·8	7·7	56
Radish, red, raw	1 small	10	0·1	Tr.	0·4	2

TABLE 39B—(Continued)

PROTEIN, FAT, CARBOHYDRATE AND CALORIE VALUES
OF AVERAGE PORTIONS served

NAME	AVERAGE PORTION	WEIGHT G	PROTEIN G	FAT G	CARBO-HYDRATE G	CALORIES
VEGETABLES (Contd.)						
Radish, white	1 large	100	0.7	0.1	4.2	21
Rhubarb stalk, raw		100	1.1	0.5	3.7	24
Ridge gourd (turiya), raw		100	0.5	0.1	3.4	17
Spinach, cooked	½ cup	90	2.8	0.6	3.3	23
Squash, cooked	½ cup	100	0.6	0.1	3.9	16
Snake gourd (padwal), raw		100	0.5	0.3	3.3	18
Sweet potato, baked	1 medium	120	2.6	1.1	41.3	183
Tinda (giloda), raw		100	1.4	0.2	3.4	21
Tomato, raw	1 medium	100	1.0	0.3	4.0	20
Tomato, canned	½ cup	100	1.0	0.2	3.9	19
Tomato, catchup	1 tablespoon	17	0.3	0.1	4.2	17
Tomato juice, canned	½ cup	100	1.0	0.3	4.6	22
Tomato soup, canned	1 cup	200	1.6	2.0	12.1	73
Turnip, cooked	½ cup	73	2.1	0.3	3.9	22
Vegetable juices	½ cup	100	0.9	0.1	4.3	18
Vegetable marrow, cooked	½ cup	100	0.6	0.1	3.9	16
Water chestnut (singhara)	4	25	0.4	—	4.5	18
Watercress, raw	10 medium sprigs	10	0.2	—	0.3	2
Yam, cooked	½ cup	100	2.4	0.2	24.1	105

TABLE 40

THIAMINE, RIBOFLAVINE, NICOTINIC ACID EQUIVALENT OF FOODS AS *served*

NAME	AVERAGE PORTION	WEIGHT G	THIAMINE MICROGRAMS	RIBOFLAVINE MICROGRAMS	NICOTINIC ACID EQUIVALENT* MG
CEREALS AND CEREAL FOODS					
Bajra (*Pennisetum typhoideum*) (30 g flour)	1 small *chappati*	45	70	50	2·0
Cornflakes	1 cup	25	100	20	0·7
Grape nuts	¼ cup	28	100	–	1·5
Jowar (*Sorghum vulgare : cholam*) (30 g flour)	1 small *chappati*	45	97	80	1·0
Oatmeal porridge	1 cup	236	220	50	1·6
Ragi (*Eleusine coracana*) (30 g flour)	1 *chappati*	45	107	50	0·7
Rice, milled, boiled (3 tablespoons, dry)	1 cup	–	27	11	1·0
Spaghetti with tomato sauce	1 serving	220	308	242	4·7
Wheat, All Bran, Kellog's	½ cup	28	110	90	5·0
Wheat bun	1 average	35	82	79	1·1
Wheat *chappati* (15 g flour)	1 thin	–	45	45	0·9
Wheat coffee cake, iced	1	70	103	105	1·5
Wheat, shredded	1 biscuit	22	65	23	1·3
EGGS, MEAT, POULTRY					
Bacon, cooked (30 g raw)	1 strip	7	40	22	0·6
Beef, corned, canned	1 slice	30	6	67	2·2
Beef, hamburger (100 g raw)	1 serving	75	120	135	7·6

*Nicotinic acid equivalent=Nicotinic acid in mg plus trytophan content.
60mg tryptophan=1 mg nicotinic acid.

TABLE 40—(*Continued*)

THIAMINE, RIBOFLAVINE, NICOTINIC ACID

EQUIVALENT OF FOODS AS *served*

NAME	AVERAGE PORTION	WEIGHT G	THIAMINE MICROGRAMS	RIBOFLAVINE MICROGRAMS	NICOTINIC ACID EQUIVALENT† MG
EGGS, MEAT, POULTRY (*Contd.*)					
Beef steak, porterhouse, broiled (240 g raw)		100	100	120	11·1
Beef steak, sirloin, broiled (240 g raw)		125	125	575	10·3
Beef steak, tenderloin, broiled (120 g raw)		66	66	304	5·5
Beef stew (90 g beef, 2 small potatoes, 1 carrot, 1 onion)	1 serving	485	255	280	9·9
Chicken, roast	1 serving	100	80	180	13·0
Egg, small, boiled	1	30	30	94	1·2
Egg, medium, boiled	1	48	40	130	1·6
Egg, medium, fried	1	52	40	130	1·6
Ham, fresh, cooked (100 g raw)	1 slice	50	325	150	6·6
Heart, roast	1 serving	100	270	680	9·2
Kidney, fried	1 serving	50	150	1000	4·3
Liver, sliced, fried after rolling in flour	1 serving	50	120	1700	9·7
Mutton, lean only	1 slice	30	70	95	4·2
Mutton, leg with fat, roast	1 serving	100	166	223	9·5
Sausage, cooked	1 average	20	98	48	0·6†
Turkey, roast (flesh only)	1 slice	40	32	69	2·9†
Veal, cutlet	1	100	122	322	13·6

†Tryptophan values not added.

TABLE 40—(Continued)

THIAMINE, RIBOFLAVINE, NICOTINIC ACID OF AVERAGE PORTIONS *served*

NAME	AVERAGE PORTION	WEIGHT G	THIAMINE MICROGRAMS	RIBOFLAVINE MICROGRAMS	NICOTINIC ACID EQUIVALENT MG
FISH					
Crab, boiled without shell	1 average	100	100	150	5·2
Lobster, boiled (¾lb, 2 teaspoons butter)		334	111	61	3·0
Oysters, fried	6 oysters	135	134	274	1·2†
Sole, baked		100	49	54	4·3
Tuna, canned	⅝ cup	100	50	120	18·6
MILK AND MILK PRODUCTS					
Cheese, Cheddar	1 piece	28	6	118	1·5
Milk, buffalo's	1 cup	200	80	280	2·3
Milk, cow's	1 cup	200	100	360	2·3
NUTS					
Almonds	12–15	15	38	100	0·9
Cashew nuts	6–8	15	95	29	1·5
Peanuts (goundnuts), roasted	1 tablespoon	15	38	39	3·3
Walnuts	8 halves	20	96	120	0·8

†Tryptophan values not added.

TABLE 40—(Continued)

THIAMINE, RIBOFLAVINE, NICOTINIC ACID OF AVERAGE PORTIONS served

NAME	AVERAGE PORTION	WEIGHT G	THIAMINE MICROGRAMS	RIBOFLAVINE MICROGRAMS	NICOTINIC ACID EQUIVALENT MG
PULSES AND BEANS					
Bengal gram (*chana dal*)	1 cup thin *dal*	200	87	127	1·1
Black gram (*urd dal*)	1 cup thin *dal*	200	76	92	1·5
Green gram (*mung dal*)	1 cup thin *dal*	200	130	38	—
Field bean (*val dal*)	1 cup thin *dal*	200	94	40	—
Lentil (*masur dal*)	1 cup thin *dal*	200	81	125	1·0
Red gram (*tur dal*)	1 cup thin *dal*	200	—	127	—
Peas, dried (*vatana dal*)	1 cup thin *dal*	100	81	92	—
VEGETABLES					
Asparagus, canned	6 medium	115	90	110	1·0
Brussels sprouts, cooked	5–6	70	28	84	—
Cabbage, shredded, raw	½ cup	50	30	25	—
Cabbage, cooked	½ cup	85	40	40	—
Carrot, cooked	½ cup	75	38	38	—
Carrot, raw	1 large	100	60	60	—
Peas, green, cooked	½ cup	80	200	110	—
Peas, fresh, raw, shelled	¾ cup	100	340	160	—
Turnip, cooked	½ cup	73	45	300	—

TABLE 41
VITAMIN C
CONTENT OF FOODS

NAME	AVERAGE PORTION	WEIGHT G	VITAMIN C MG
FRUITS			
Apple	1 medium	150	7
Avocado pear	½	108	17
Banana	1 medium	150	15
Blackberries, raw	⅝ cup	100	21
Grape-fruit	½ medium	180	72
Grapes	22–24	100	4
Guava	1 medium	100	300
Jack fruit	1 medium	100	7
Jambu (*Syzigium cumini*)		100	18
Lime, sour		100	26
Lime, sweet (*musambi*)	1 average	150	66
Mango, Alphonso, Bulsar	1	150	54
Mango, Alphonso, Ratnagiri	1	150	37
Melon	½ medium	150	48
Orange	1 medium	150	74
Orange juice	1 cup	200	96
Papaya	⅓ medium	100	57
Peach, fresh	1 medium	100	6
Pineapple	1 slice	84	20
Plums	1	60	3
Raspberries	⅔ cup	100	24
Strawberries	15 average	100	60
Tangerines	1 large	150	48
FRUITS, DRIED			
Currants, black, raw		100	200
Prunes, dried	6 medium	50	1·5
MILK AND MILK PRODUCTS			
Milk, buffalo's	1 cup	200	6
Milk, cow's	1 cup	200	4
VEGETABLES			
Amaranth (Chinese spinach: *rajgira*), cooked	½ cup	100	3
Asparagus, canned	6 medium	115	17
Beetroot, cooked	½ cut	83	6
Broccoli, cooked	¾ cup	100	74
Brussels sprouts, cooked	5–6	70	33
Cabbage, shredded, raw	½ cup	50	39
Cabbage, cooked	½ cup	85	58
Carrot, cooked	½ cup	75	3

TABLE 41—(*Continued*)
VITAMIN C
CONTENT OF FOODS

NAME	AVERAGE PORTION	WEIGHT G	VITAMIN C MG
VEGETABLES (*Contd.*)			
Carrot leaves, raw		100	79
Cauliflower, cooked	½ cup	60	17
Coriander leaves (*kothmir*), raw		100	135
Drumstick (*Moringa oleifera*), raw		100	120
Drumstick leaves, raw		100	220
Fenugreek leaves (*methi sag*). raw		100	54
French beans, raw		100	14
Mango, green, without seed		100	3
Onion, mature, raw	1 average	100	9
Onion stalks		100	17
Parsley, raw	10 small twigs	10	19
Parsnips, cooked	½ cup	78	10
Peas, green, cooked	½ cup	80	12
Peas, fresh, raw, shelled	¾ cup	100	26
Potato, baked	1 medium	100	17
Potato, boiled	1 medium	100	14
Potato, mashed with butter and milk	½ cup	100	7
Radish, red, raw	1 small	10	8
Spinach, cooked	½ cup	90	27
Squash, cooked	½ cup	100	11
Sweet potato, baked	1 medium	120	28
Tomato, raw	1	100	23
Tomato, canned	½ cup	100	16
Tomato juice, canned	½ cup	100	16
Turnip, cooked	½ cup	73	44
Vegetable juices	½ cup	100	5
Vegetable marrow, cooked	½ cup	100	11
Watercress, raw	10 medium sprigs	10	8

TABLE 42A

VITAMIN A
CONTENT OF FOODS

NAME	AVERAGE PORTION	WEIGHT G	VITAMIN A IU	RETINOL MICROGRAM
EGGS, MEAT, POULTRY				
Egg, small, boiled	1	30	410	123
Egg, medium, boiled	1	48	550	165
Kidney, fried	1 serving	50	650	195
Liver, sliced fried after rolling in flour	1 serving	50	24600	7380
FISH				
Lobster, boiled 3/4 lb, 2 teaspoons butter	1 average	334	920	276
Oysters, fried	6 oysters	135	1539	462
Cod-liver oil	1 teaspoon	5	1000–2000	333–666
Halibut-liver oil	1 drop		600–2000	180–666
Shark-liver oil	1 teaspoon	5	1000	333
MILK and MILK PRODUCTS				
Butter	1 teaspoon	5	165	50
Cheese, Cheddar	1 piece	28	392	118
Cream, light	2 tablespoons	30	226	68
Ghee (clarified butter)	1 teaspoon	5	165	50
Milk, buffalo's	1 cup	200	480	144
Milk, cow's	1 cup	200	300	90
Milk, goat's	½ cup	100	182	55
Milk, human (early lactation)		100	46	14
Milk, human (late lactation)		100	30	9

TABLE 42 B
CAROTENE CONTENT OF FOODS

FOOD	AVERAGE PORTION	WEIGHT G	CAROTENE IU
CEREALS AND CEREAL FOODS			
Spaghetti with tomato sauce	1 serving	220	807
Wheat coffee cake, iced	1	70	214
FRUITS			
Apricots	2 or 3 medium	100	2030
Mango, Alphonso, Bulsar	1	150	16130
Mango, Alphonso, Ratnagiri	1	150	22500
Melon	$\frac{1}{2}$ medium	150	670
Papaya	$\frac{1}{3}$ medium	100	1110
FRUITS, DRIED			
Peaches	$\frac{1}{2}$ cup	80	2600
Prunes	6 medium	50	945
VEGETABLES			
Amaranth (Chinese spinach: rajgira), cooked	$\frac{1}{2}$ cup	100	11500
Asparagus, canned	6 medium	115	690
Broccoli, cooked	$\frac{3}{4}$ cup	100	3400
Brussels sprouts, cooked	5–6	70	280
Carrot, cooked long time in much water	$\frac{1}{2}$ cup	75	9375
Carrot, raw	1 large	100	12000
Carrot leaves, raw		100	9500
Coriander leaves (kothmir), raw		100	11530
Drumstick leaves, raw		100	11300
Fenugreek leaves (methi sag), raw		100	6450
French beans, raw		100	221
Lettuce	3 small leaves	30	162
Mango, green, without seed		100	150
Onion, mature, raw	1 average	100	50
Onion stalks		100	993
Parsley, fresh	10 small twigs	10	823
Peas, green, cooked	$\frac{1}{2}$ cup	80	575
Peas, fresh, raw, shelled	$\frac{3}{4}$ cup	100	680
Pumpkin, cooked	$\frac{1}{2}$ cup	100	3400
Spinach, cooked	$\frac{1}{2}$ cup	90	10600
Sweet potato, baked	1 medium	120	11410
Tomato, raw	1 medium	100	1200
Tomato, canned	$\frac{1}{2}$ cup	100	1050
Tomato juice, canned	$\frac{1}{2}$ cup	100	1050
Turnip, cooked	$\frac{1}{2}$ cup	73	7685
Vegetable juice	$\frac{1}{2}$ cup	100	882
Watercress, raw	10 medium sprigs	10	472
Yam, cooked	$\frac{1}{2}$ cup	100	3000

TABLE 43

VITAMIN D

CONTENT OF FOODS

NAME	AVERAGE PORTION	WEIGHT G	VITAMIN D IU
Butter	1 teaspoon	5	2
Cream	1 tablespoon	14	2
Milk, buffalo's, whole	1 cup	200	14
Milk, cow's, whole	1 cup	200	8
Ghee (clarified butter)	1 tablespoon	14	14
Egg	1 medium	48	27
Cod-liver oil	1 teaspoon	5	350
Halibut-liver oil	1–2 drops	–	400
Shark-liver oil	1 teaspoon	5	100

TABLE 44

MINERAL CONTENT OF FOODS

NAME	AVERAGE PORTION	WEIGHT G	CALCIUM MG	IRON MG	MAGNE-SIUM MG	PHOS-PHORUS MG	SODIUM MG	POTAS-SIUM MG
CEREALS AND CEREAL FOODS								
Bajra (Pennisetum typhoideum)								
30 g flour	1 *chappati*	45	13	4·3	37	80	3	9
Cornflakes	1 cup	25	6	0·5	–	16	165	40
Farex	2 tablespoons	30	251	6·9	24	167	78	84
Jowar (Sorghum vulgare)								
30 g flour	1 *chappati*	45	7	1·6	42	66	2	39
Maize, 30 g flour	1 *chappati*	45	3	0·6	86	105	5	86
Oatmeal porridge	1 cup	236	21	1·7	–	158	1	130
Ragi (Eleusine coracona)								
30 g flour	1 *chappati*	45	102	5·1	57	84	3	124
Rice, milled, boiled (3 tablespoons dry)	1 cup	–	9	0·3	–	52	1	49
Wheat, All Bran, Kellog's	½ cup	28	24	2·9	119	350	370	271
EGGS, MEAT, POULTRY								
Bacon	1 rasher	7	1	0·2	2	22	76	17
Beef, corned, canned	1 slice	28	6	1·2	–	30	268	17
Beef hamburger (100 g raw)	1	75	5	–	15	165	35	335

TABLE 44—(Continued)

MINERAL CONTENT OF FOODS

NAME	AVERAGE PORTION	WEIGHT G	CALCIUM MG	IRON MG	MAGNESIUM MG	PHOSPHORUS MG	SODIUM MG	POTASSIUM MG
EGGS, MEAT, POULTRY (Contd.)								
Beef steak, porterhouse, broiled (240 g raw)		100	11	—	20	183	52	398
Beef steak, sirloin, broiled (240 g raw)		100	18	4·8	26	282	57	545
Brain, boiled		100	16	2·0	13	355	147	270
Chicken, boiled (weighed with bone)		100	7	1·4	17	175	64	248
Chicken, roast		100	14	2·6	23	271	80	355
Duck, roast	1	100	19	5·8	24	231	195	319
Egg, hen's, small, boiled	1	30	20	0·7	—	—	30	36
Egg, hen's, medium, boiled	1	48	26	1·1	—	101	39	48
Goose, roast	3 slices	100	10	4·6	31	265	145	406
Ham, fresh, cooked	1 slice	50	4	1·2	15	140	35	245
Kidney, fried		50	8	7·2	13	216	130	150
Liver, sliced, fried		50	4	10·3	13	225	46	193
Mutton, chop, fried	1 slice	50	8	1·5	13	111	58	175
Mutton, lean	1 slice	30	2	1·0	7	67	26	156
Mutton, roast, leg with fat		100	6	3·1	22	199	61	369
Pork, leg, roast		100	5	1·7	22	363	66	308
Turkey, roast	1 slice	40	12	1·5	12	128	52	146
Veal, cutlet	1	100	10	4·2	23	288	54	527

TABLE 44—(Continued)

MINERAL CONTENT OF FOODS

NAME	AVERAGE PORTION	WEIGHT G	CALCIUM MG	IRON MG	MAGNESIUM MG	PHOSPHORUS MG	SODIUM MG	POTASSIUM MG
FISH								
Crab, boiled		100	29	1·3	48	350	366	271
Lobster, boiled (350 g with butter, 2 teaspoons)	1 average	334	80	0·7	–	229	210	180
Mackerel, fried, weighed with skin and bone		100	21	0·9	25	204	112	305
Plaice, covered with crumbs and fried		100	45	0·8	24	251	124	219
Prawns, cooked without shell		100	145	1·1	42	349	–	260
Salmon, steamed		100	29	0·8	29	302	107	333
Salmon, canned		100	66	1·3	30	235	538	320
Sardines, canned with bones after draining oil		100	409	4·0	41	683	785	433
FRUITS								
Apple	1 medium	150	5	0·5	4	6	14	68
Apricots	2–3 medium	100	11	1·1	11	23	5	276
Banana	1 medium	150	12	0·9	–	42	1	630
Custard apple		100	12	0·5	24	51	14	578
Guava	1 medium	100	10	1·4	8	28	5	91
Lime, sweet (musambi)	1 medium	150	60	1·0	–	45	Tr	735

TABLE 44—(Continued)

MINERAL CONTENT OF FOODS

NAME	AVERAGE PORTION	WEIGHT G	CALCIUM MG	IRON MG	MAGNESIUM MG	PHOSPHORUS MG	SODIUM MG	POTASSIUM MG
FRUITS (Contd.)								
Orange	1 medium	150	50	0·6	–	35	Tr	360
Papaya	1/6 medium	100	17	0·5	11	13	6	69
Peach	1 medium	100	15	2·4	21	41	2	453
FRUITS, DRIED								
Currants	1/2 cup	100	75	2·7	–	138	22	730
Peach	1/2 cup	100	35	5·5	–	101	12	1100
Raisins, seedless	1 tablespoon	10	8	0·3	–	13	2	73
MILK AND MILK PRODUCTS								
Cheese, Cheddar	1 piece	28	203	0·3	–	139	190	–
Cheese, cottage	1 piece	28	27	0·1	–	53	81	–
Milk, buffalo's	1 cup	200	300	0·2	–	260	38	180
Milk, cow's	1 cup	200	244	0·2	–	192	32	280
Milk, skimmed, powder	1 tablespoon	7	96	–	8	75	42	94
NUTS								
Almonds	12–15	15	38	0·7	–	71	Tr	104
Brazil nuts, shelled	4 medium	15	28	0·5	–	104	Tr	100
Cashew nuts, roasted	6–8	15	7	0·8	–	64	2	84
Coconut, fresh	1 piece	15	3	0·3	–	15	2	116

Tr = trace

TABLE 44—(Continued)

MINERAL CONTENT OF FOODS

NAME	AVERAGE PORTION	WEIGHT G	CALCIUM MG	IRON MG	MAGNES-IUM MG	PHOS-PHORUS MG	SODIUM MG	POTASS-IUM MG
PULSES AND BEANS								
Bengal gram (*chana dal*) 30 g dry	1 cup thin *dal*	200	16	2·7	41	99	22	216
Black gram (*urd dal*) 30 g dry	1 cup thin *dal*	200	45	2·7	55	115	12	240
Field bean (*val dal*) 30 g dry	1 cup thin *dal*	200	18	0·8	–	130	–	–
Green gram (*mung dal*) 30 g	1 cup thin *dal*	200	22	2·5	57	100	8	345
Lentil (*masur dal*) 30 g dry	1 cup thin *dal*	200	20	1·4	28	88	12	188
Red gram (*tur dal*) 30 g dry	1 cup thin *dal*	200	22	1·6	40	90	9	330
Beans, baked		100	62	2·0	37	184	591	344
Peas, roasted		100	81	6·4	122	345	15	750
VEGETABLES								
Amaranth leaves (Chinese spinach: *rajgirah*), raw		100	397	25·5	247	83	230	341
Artichoke, cooked	½ large	100	44	0·8	–	58	43	430
Brussels sprouts, boiled		100	27	0·6	11	44	8	247
Cabbage, boiled		100	30	0·5	6	32	12	108

TABLE 44—(Continued)

MINERAL CONTENT OF FOODS

NAME	AVERAGE PORTION	WEIGHT G	CALCIUM MG	IRON MG	MAGNESIUM MG	PHOSPHORUS MG	SODIUM MG	POTASSIUM MG
VEGETABLES (Contd.)								
Cabbage, raw	½ cup	50	23	0·3	–	16	5	230
Carrot, boiled	1 large	100	29	0·4	8	30	22	237
Carrot, raw	1 large	100	39	0·8	–	37	31	410
Carrot leaves		100	340	8·8	–	110	–	–
Cauliflower, boiled		100	23	0·5	7	33	11	152
Cauliflower, green leaves		100	626	40·0	–	107	–	–
Cauliflower, raw		100	18	0·6	–	75	10	408
Cluster beans, raw (guar-phalli)		100	111	4·5	–	57	–	–
Coriander leaves, raw		100	184	18·5	64	62	58	256
Drumstick, raw		100	30	5·3	24	110	–	259
Fenugreek leaves (methi sag), raw		100	360	17·2	67	51	76	31
French beans, raw		100	50	1·7	29	28	4	120
Lady's-fingers, raw		100	66	1·5	43	56	7	103
Onion, boiled		100	24	0·2	5	16	7	78
Onion, mature, raw		100	180	0·7	–	50	10	137
Peas, green, boiled		100	13	1·2	21	83	–	174
Peas, green, raw		100	20	1·5	34	139	8	79
Potato, old, boiled	1 average	100	4	0·5	15	29	3	325
Spinach, boiled		100	595	4·0	59	93	123	490

TABLE 45

FOOD VALUES OF CEREALS (UNCOOKED) PER 100 G*

NAME	PRO-TEIN G	FAT G	CAR-BOHY-DRATE G	CALO-RIES	THIA-MINE MICRO-GRAMS	RIBO-FLA-VINE MICRO-GRAMS	NICO-TINIC ACID MG	CAL-CIUM MG	IRON MG	MAG-NES-IUM MG	PHOS-PHO-RUS MG	SOD-IUM MG	POT-ASS-IUM MG
BAJRA (Pennisetum typhoideum: cambu)	11·6	5·0	67·5	356	330	160	3·2	42	14·3	125	269	11	30
BARLEY (Hordeum vulgare: juv)	11·5	1·3	69·6	336	470	200	5·4	26	3·4	127	215	16	253
JOWAR (Sorghum vulgare: cholam)	10·4	1·9	72·6	349	370	280	1·8	25	5·8	140	222	7	131
MAIZE, tender (Zea maya: makai)	4·7	0·9	24·6	125	110	170	0·6	9	1·1	40	121	52	151
MAIZE, dry (Zea maya: makai)	11·1	3·6	66·2	342	420	10	1·4	10	2·0	144	348	16	286
OATMEAL (Avena sterilis)	13·6	7·6	62·8	374	540	120	1·1	50	3·8	-	380	-	-
RAGI (Eleusine coracana: nachni)	7·3	1·3	72·0	328	420	100	1·1	344	17·4	191	283	11	408
RICE, raw, home pounded	7·5	1·0	84·2	345	210	160	3·9	12	2·9	-	175	-	-
RICE, raw, milled	6·8	0·5	78·2	345	90	30	1·9	10	3·1	48	160	8	70
RICE, parboiled, home pounded	8·5	0·6	77·4	349	270	120	4·0	10	2·8	-	280	-	-

TABLE 45—(Continued)

FOOD VALUES OF CEREALS (UNCOOKED) PER 100 G*

NAME	PRO-TEIN G	FAT G	CAR-BOHY-DRATE G	CALO-RIES	THIA-MINE MICRO-GRAMS	RIBO-FLA-VINE MICRO-GRAMS	NICO-TINIC ACID MG	CAL-CIUM MG	IRON MG	MAG-NES-IUM MG	PHOS-PHO-RUS MG	SOD-IUM MG	POT-ASS-IUM MG
RICE, parboiled, milled	6·4	0·4	79·0	348	210	90	3·8	9	4·0	38	143	10	117
RICE, bran	13·5	16·2	48·4	393	2700	480	–	67	35·0	–	1410	–	–
WHEAT													
INDIAN													
Wheat, whole	11·8	1·5	71·2	346	450	120	5·0	41	4·9	139	306	17	284
Wheat flour, whole (atta)	12·1	1·7	69·4	341	490	290	4·3	48	11·5	55	423	20	315
Wheat flour, refined (maida)	11·0	0·9	73·9	348	120	70	0·9	23	2·5	42	121	9	130
ENGLISH													
Wheat, whole	8·9	2·2	73·4	333	290	170	4·8	36	3·0	106	340	3	361
Wheat, 80% extraction	8·2	1·3	80·8	348	180	80	0·9	22	1·6	24	118	2	151
Wheat, 70% extraction	7·9	1·0	81·9	349	90	60	0·8	19	1·4	14	84	2	111
MANITOBA													
Wheat, whole	13·6	2·5	69·0	339	360	170	5·5	28	3·8	141	350	3	312
Wheat, 80% extraction	13·2	1·4	75·5	350	200	80	1·1	15	2·5	45	139	3	112
Wheat, 70% extraction	12·8	1·2	76·9	352	70	70	1·0	13	2·2	27	97	2	82

*1. Aykroyd, W.R. (1963) *The Nutritive Value of Indian Foods and the Planning of Satisfactory Diets*, 6th ed., rev. Gopalan, C., and Balasubramanian, S.C., Indian Council of Medical Research, New Delhi.
2. McCance, R.A., and Widdowson, E.M. (1960) The composition of foods, *Spec. Rep. Ser. med. Res. Coun. (Lond.)*, No. 297, London, H.M.S.O.

TABLE 46

FOOD VALUES OF PULSES, DRIED PEAS AND BEANS (UNCOOKED) PER 100 G*

NAME	PRO-TEIN G	FAT G	CAR-BOHY-DRATE G	CALO-RIES	THIA-MINE MICRO-GRAMS	RIBO-FLA-VINE MICRO-GRAMS	NICO-TINIC ACID MG	CAL-CIUM MG	IRON MG	MAG-NES-IUM MG	PHOS-PHO-RUS MG	SOD-IUM MG	POT-ASS-IUM MG
BENGAL GRAM, whole (Cicer arietinum: chana hurbara)	17·1	5·3	60·9	360	300	510	2·1	202	10·2	168	312	37	808
BENGAL GRAM, dal (Cicer aerietinum: chana ki dal)	20·8	5·6	59·8	372	480	180	2·4	56	9·1	138	331	73	720
BLACK GRAM, dal (Phaseolus mungo: urd dal)	24·0	1·4	59·6	347	420	370	2·0	154	9·1	185	385	40	800
FIELD BEAN, dal (Dolichos lablab: val dal, kadwal)	24·9	0·9	60·1	347	520	160	1·8	60	2·7	–	433	–	–
GREEN GRAM, dal (Phaseolus aureus: mung dal)	24·5	1·2	59·9	351	720	150	2·4	75	8·5	189	405	27	1150

* Aykroyd, W.R. (1963) *The Nutritive Value of Indian Foods and Planning of Satisfactory Diets*, 6th ed., rev. Gopalan, C., and Balasubramaniam, S.C., Indian Council of Medical Research, New Delhi.

TABLE 46—(Continued)

FOOD VALUES OF PULSES, DRIED PEAS AND BEANS (UNCOOKED) PER 100 G*

NAME	PRO-TEIN G	FAT G	CAR-BOHY-DRATE G	CALO-RIES	THIA-MINE MICRO-GRAMS	RIBO-FLA-VINE MICRO-GRAMS	NICO-TINIC ACID MG	CAL-CIUM MG	IRON MG	MAG-NES-IUM MG	PHOS-PHO-RUS MG	SOD-IUM MG	POT-ASS-IUM MG
KHESARI, dal (*Lathyrus sativus*)	28·2	0·6	56·6	351	390	410	2·2	90	6·3	92	317	38	644
LENTIL (*Lens culinaris medic: masur dal*)	25·1	0·7	59·0	343	450	490	1·5	69	4·8	94	293	40	629
PEAS, DRIED (*Pisum sativum*)	19·7	1·1	56·5	315	470	380	1·9	75	5·1	124	298	20	725
RED GRAM (*Cajanus ajan: tur dal*)	22·3	1·7	57·6	355	450	510	2·6	73	5·8	133	304	29	1104
SOYA BEAN (*Glycine max*)	43·2	19·5	20·9	432	730	760	2·4	240	11·5	-	690	-	-

* Aykroyd, W.R. (1963) *The Nutritive Value of Indian Foods and the Planning of Satisfactory Diets*, 6th ed., rev. Gopalan, C., and Balasubramanian, S.C., Indian Council of Medical Research, New Delhi.

TABLE 47

FOOD VALUES OF SPICES PER 100 G *

NAME	PRO-TEIN G	FAT G	CAR-BOHY-DRATE G	CALO-RIES	THIA-MINE MICRO-GRAMS	RIBO-FLA-VINE MICRO-GRAMS	NICO-TINIC ACID MG	CAL-CIUM MG	IRON MG	MAG-NES-IUM MG	PHOS-PHO-RUS MG	SOD-IUM MG	POT-ASS-IUM MG
Asafoetida	4·4	1·1	67·5	297	–	40	0·3	690	22·2	–	50	–	:
Cardamom	10·2	2·2	42·1	229	220	170	0·8	130	5·0	–	160	–	–
Chillies, green	2·9	0·6	3·0	29	190	390	0·9	30	1·2	24	80	7	217
Chillies, dry	15·9	6·2	31·6	246	930	430	9·5	160	2·3	–	370	14	530
Cloves, dry	5·2	8·9	46·0	285	80	130	–	740	4·9	–	100	–	–
Coriander seeds	14·1	16·1	21·6	288	220	350	1·1	630	17·9	–	393	32	990
Cumin seeds	18·7	15·0	36·6	356	550	360	2·6	1080	31·0	–	511	126	980
Fenugreek seeds	26·2	5·8	44·1	333	340	290	1·1	160	14·1	–	370	19	530
Garlic, dry	6·3	0·1	29·0	142	160	230	0·4	30	1·3	–	310	–	–
Ginger, fresh	2·3	0·9	12·3	67	60	30	0·6	20	2·6	–	60	–	–
Nutmeg	7·5	36·4	28·5	472	330	10	1·4	120	4·6	–	240	–	–
Pepper, dry	11·5	6·8	49·5	305	90	140	1·4	460	16·8	–	198	–	–
Tamarind pulp	3·1	0·1	67·4	283	–	70	0·7	170	10·9	–	110	–	–
Turmeric	6·3	5·1	69·4	349	30	–	2·3	150	18·6	–	282	25	3300

*Aykroyd, W.R. (1963) *The Nutritive Value of Indian Foods and the Planning of Satisfactory Diets*, 6th ed., rev. Gopalan, C., and Balasubramanian, S. C., Indian Council of Medical Research, New Delhi

AGE** From— upto	WEIGHT	HEIGHT	CAL-ORIES	PRO-TEIN	VITAMIN A ACTI-VITY	VITAMIN D	VITA-MIN E ACTI-VITY	AS-COR-BIC ACID
				INFANTS				
Years	KG(LB)	CM(IN)	GM	GM	IU	IU	IU	MG
Birth–1/6	4(9)	55(22)	kg x 120‡	kg x 2.2	1500	400	5	35
1/6–1/2	7(15)	63(25)	kg x 110‡	kg x 2.0	1500	400	5	35
1/2–1	9(20)	72(28)	kg x 100‡	kg x 1.8	1500	400	5	35
				CHILDREN				
1– 2	12(26)	81(32)	1100	25	2000	400	10	40
2– 3	14(31)	91(36)	1250	25	2000	400	10	40
3– 4	16(35)	100(39)	1400	30	2500	400	10	40
4– 6	19(42)	110(43)	1600	30	2500	400	10	40
6– 8	23(51)	121(48)	2000	35	3500	400	15	40
8–10	28(62)	131(52)	2200	40	3500	400	15	40
				MALES				
10–12	35(77)	140(55)	2500	45	4500	400	20	40
12–14	43(95)	151(59)	2700	50	5000	400	20	45
14–18	59(130)	170(67)	3000	60	5000	400	25	55
18–22	67(147)	175(69)	2800	60	5000	400	30	60
22–35	70(154)	175(69)	2800	65	5000	—	30	60
35–55	70(154)	173(68)	2600	65	5000	—	30	60
55–75＋	70(154)	171(67)	2400	65	5000	—	30	60
				FEMALES				
10–12	35(77)	142(56)	2250	50	4500	400	20	40
12–14	44(97)	154(61)	2300	50	5000	400	20	45
14–16	52(114)	157(62)	2400	55	5000	400	25	50
16–18	54(119)	160(63)	2300	55	5000	400	25	50
18–22	58(128)	163(64)	2000	55	5000	400	25	55
22–35	58(128)	163(64)	2000	55	5000	—	25	55
35–55	58(128)	160(63)	1850	55	5000	—	25	55
55–75＋	58(128)	157(62)	1700	55	5000	—	25	55
PREGNANCY			＋ 200	65	6000	400	30	60
LACTATION			＋1000	75	8000	400	30	60

* The allowance levels are intended to cover individual variations among most stresses. The recommended allowances can be attained with a variety of have been less well defined.

** Entries on lines for age range 22–35 years represent the reference man and the specified age range.

† The folacin allowances refer to dietary sources as determined by *Lactobacillus* the RDA.

*** Niacin equivalents include dietary sources of the vitamin itself plus 1 mg

‡ Assumes protein equivalent to human milk. For proteins not 100 per cent

48

OF SCIENCES—NATIONAL RESEARCH COUNCIL
DIETARY ALLOWANCES* (*Revised* 1968)

FOLA-CIN†	NIA-CIN	RIBO-FLA-VINE	THIA-MINE	VITA-MIN B_6	VITA-MIN B_{12}	CAL-CIUM	PHOS-PHO-RUS	IO-DINE	IRON	MAG-NE-SIUM
				INFANTS						
MG	MG equiv	MG ***	MG	MG	μG	MG	MG	μG	MG	MG
0·05	5	0·4	0·2	0·2	1·0	0·4	0·2	25	6	40
0·05	7	0·5	0·4	0·3	1·5	0·5	0·4	40	10	60
0·1	8	0·6	0·5	0·4	2·0	0·6	0·5	45	15	70
				CHILDREN						
0·1	8	0·6	0·6	0·5	2·0	0·7	0·7	55	15	100
0·2	8	0·7	0·6	0·6	2·5	0·8	0·8	60	15	150
0·2	9	0·8	0·7	0·7	3	0·8	0·8	70	10	200
0·2	11	0·9	0·8	0·9	4	0·8	0·8	80	10	200
0·2	13	1·1	1·0	1·0	4	0·9	0·9	100	10	250
0·3	15	1·2	1·1	1·2	5	1·0	1·0	110	10	250
				MALES						
0·4	17	1·3	1·3	1·4	5	1·2	1·2	125	10	300
0·4	18	1·4	1·4	1·6	5	1·4	1·4	135	18	350
0·4	20	1·5	1·5	1·8	5	1·4	1·4	150	18	400
0·4	18	1·6	1·4	2·0	5	0·8	0·8	140	10	400
0·4	18	1·7	1·4	2·0	5	0·8	0·8	140	10	350
0·4	17	1·7	1·3	2·0	5	0·8	0·8	125	10	350
0·4	14	1·7	1·2	2·0	6	0·8	0·8	110	10	350
				FEMALES						
0·4	15	1·3	1·1	1·4	5	1·2	1·2	110	18	300
0·4	15	1·4	1·2	1·6	5	1·3	1·3	115	18	350
0·4	16	1·4	1·2	1·8	5	1·3	1·3	120	18	350
0·4	15	1·5	1·2	2·0	5	1·3	1·3	115	18	350
0·4	13	1·5	1·0	2·0	5	0·8	0·8	100	18	350
0·4	13	1·5	1·0	2·0	5	0·8	0·8	100	18	350
0·4	13	1·5	1·0	2·0	5	0·8	0·8	90	18	300
0·4	13	1·5	1·0	2·0	6	0·8	0·8	80	10	300
0·8	15	1·8	+0·1	2·5	8	+0·4	+0·4	125	18	450
0·5	20	2·0	+0·5	2·5	6	+0·5	+0·5	150	18	450

normal persons as they live in the United States under the usual environmental
common foods providing other nutrients for which human requirements

woman at age 22. All other entries represent allowances for the midpoint of

casei assay. Pure forms of folacin may be effective in doses less than 1/4 of

equivalent for each 60 mg of dietary tryptophan.
utilized, factors should be increased proportionately.

TABLE 49

DAILY DIETARY ALLOWANCES RECOMMENDED BY THE COMMITTEE OF
THE BRITISH MEDICAL ASSOCIATION (1950)

AGE AND SEX	REQUIREMENT	CALORIES	PROTEIN G	IRON G	CALCIUM G	VITAMIN A AND CAROTENE IU	VITAMIN D IU	THIAMINE MG	NIACIN MG	RIBOFLAVINE MG	VITAMIN C MG
Both 0-1		1000	37	6·5	1·0	3000	800	0·4	4	0·6	10
2-6		1500	56	7·5	1·0	3000	400	0·6	6	0·9	15
7-10		2000	74	10·5	1·0	3000	400	0·8	8	1·2	20
Males 11-14		2750	102	13·5	1·3	3000	400	1·1	11	1·6	30
15-19		3500	130	15·0	1·4	5000	400	1·4	14	2·1	30
20+	No work, almost basal	1750	51	12·0	0·8	5000		0·7	7	1·0	20
	Sedentary work and little travelling	2250	66	12·0	0·8	5000		0·9	9	1·4	20
	Light work and travelling	2750	80	12·0	0·8	5000		1·1	11	1·6	20
	Medium work and travelling	3000	87	12·0	0·8	5000		1·2	12	1·8	20
	Heavy work and travelling	3500	102	12·0	0·8	5000		1·4	14	2·1	20
	Very heavy work and travelling	4250	124	12·0	0·8	5000		1·7	17	2·6	20
	Extremely heavy work and travelling	5000	146	12·0	0·8	5000		2·0	20	3·0	20
Females 11-14		2750	102	13·5	1·2	3000	400	1·1	11	1·6	30
15-19		2500	93	15·0	1·1	5000	400	1·0	10	1·5	30
20+	No work, almost basal	1500	44	12·0	0·8	5000		0·6	6	0·9	20
	Sedentary work and little travelling	2000	58	12·0	0·8	5000		0·8	8	1·2	20
	Light work and travelling	2250	66	12·0	0·8	5000		0·9	9	1·4	20
	Medium work and travelling	2500	73	12·0	0·8	5000		1·0	10	1·5	20
	Heavy work and travelling	3000	87	12·0	0·8	5000		1·2	12	1·8	20
	Very heavy work and travelling	3750	109	12·0	0·8	5000		1·5	15	2·2	20
Pregnancy	First half	2500	93	12·0	0·8	6000	400	1·0	10	1·5	40
	Second half	2750	102	15·0	1·5	6000	600	1·1	11	1·6	40
Lactation		3000	111	15·0	2·0	8000	800	1·4	14	2·1	50

The height and weight of Indians show considerable variations in the different provinces and communities. The following Tables 50A, 50B, 50C, 50D are the average values for Indians derived from the exhaustive data prepared by Dr. J. J. Cursetji of Oriental Life Insurance Co.

TABLE 50A
HEIGHT (INCHES), WEIGHT (POUNDS)

FOR

INDIAN MALES

HEIGHT		AGE IN YEARS						
		20	25	30	35	40	45	50
FEET	INCHES	LB	LB	LB	LB	LB	LB	LB
4	10	93	97	101	104	107	109	111
4	11	96	99	104	107	110	112	114
5	0	99	103	107	110	113	115	117
5	1	102	106	110	114	116	118	120
5	2	106	109	114	117	119	122	123
5	3	110	113	117	121	123	125	127
5	4	112	115	121	124	127	129	131
5	5	117	121	126	129	132	134	135
5	6	120	124	129	133	136	138	140
5	7	125	129	133	137	141	143	145
5	8	128	133	137	141	145	148	151
5	9	133	137	142	146	150	154	157
5	10	137	141	146	151	156	159	160
5	11	141	146	151	157	162	164	166
6	0	146	151	157	162	167	170	172

TABLE 50B
HEIGHT (CENTIMETRES), WEIGHT (KILOGRAMS)
FOR
INDIAN MALES

HEIGHT	AGE IN YEARS						
	20	25	30	35	40	45	50
CM	KG	KG	KG	KG	KG	KG	KG
148	42·7	44·2	46·2	47·6	48·8	50·0	50·9
150	43·6	44·9	46·9	48·5	49·7	50·8	51·5
153	45·4	47·0	49·0	50·4	51·7	52·3	53·5
155	46·3	48·1	49·9	51·5	52·7	53·5	54·2
158	48·6	50·0	52·0	53·5	54·5	55·7	56·3
160	49·7	51·1	53·1	54·7	55·6	56·7	57·4
163	51·1	52·7	54·9	56·3	57·6	58·5	59·4
165	53·1	54·7	56·9	58·5	59·7	60·6	62·0
168	54·0	56·3	58·1	60·1	61·5	62·4	63·7
170	56·5	57·9	60·3	62·2	63·7	64·7	65·8
173	58·1	60·1	62·2	64·0	65·8	67·0	68·3
175	60·1	62·2	64·2	66·0	68·1	69·7	71·0
178	61·9	64·0	66·3	68·5	70·6	71·9	72·4
180	64·0	66·2	68·5	71·0	73·3	74·4	75·1
183	66·0	68·5	71·0	73·3	75·6	77·1	77·8

TABLE 50C
HEIGHT (INCHES), WEIGHT (POUNDS)
FOR
INDIAN FEMALES

HEIGHT		AGE IN YEARS						
		20	25	30	35	40	45	50
FEET	INCHES	LB	LB	LB	LB	LB	LB	LB
4	10	86	90	93	96	99	101	103
4	11	89	92	96	99	102	104	105
5	0	92	95	99	102	105	106	108
5	1	94	98	102	105	107	109	111
5	2	98	101	105	108	110	113	114
5	3	102	105	108	112	114	116	118
5	4	104	106	112	115	117	119	121
5	5	108	112	117	119	122	124	125
5	6	110	114	119	123	126	128	130

TABLE 50D
HEIGHT (CENTIMETRES), WEIGHT (KILOGRAMS)
FOR
INDIAN FEMALES

HEIGHT	AGE IN YEARS						
	20	25	30	35	40	45	50
CM	KG	KG	KG	KG	KG	KG	KG
148	38·6	41·0	42·6	44·0	45·1	46·3	47·1
150	40·3	41·6	43·5	44·8	46·0	47·0	47·7
153	41·9	43·5	45·3	46·6	47·9	48·4	49·5
155	42·8	44·3	46·2	47·7	48·8	49·5	50·1
158	44·9	46·3	48·1	49·5	50·4	51·6	52·1
160	46·0	47·3	49·1	50·6	51·5	52·4	53·0
163	47·3	48·8	50·8	52·1	52·2	54·1	54·9
165	49·1	50·6	52·6	54·1	55·3	56·0	57·3
168	50·0	52·1	53·8	55·6	56·8	57·7	59·0

TABLE 51A
DESIRABLE WEIGHTS FOR
MEN OF AGES 25 AND OVER *
in Pounds according to Frame
(in Indoor Clothing)

HEIGHT (WITH SHOES ON) 1-INCH HEELS		SMALL FRAME	MEDIUM FRAME	LARGE FRAME
FEET	INCHES			
5	2	112–120	118–129	126–141
5	3	115–123	121–133	129–144
5	4	118–126	124–136	132–148
5	5	121–129	127–139	135–152
5	6	124–133	130–143	138–156
5	7	128–137	134–147	142–161
5	8	132–141	138–152	147–166
5	9	136–145	142–156	151–170
5	10	140–150	146–160	155–174
5	11	144–154	150–165	159–179
6	0	148–158	154–170	164–184
6	1	152–162	158–175	168–189
6	2	156–167	162–180	173–194
6	3	160–171	167–185	178–199
6	4	164–175	172–190	182–204

TABLE 51B
DESIRABLE WEIGHTS FOR
WOMEN OF AGES 25 AND OVER *
Weight in Pounds according to Frame
(in Indoor Clothing)

HEIGHT (WITH SHOES ON) 2-INCH HEELS		SMALL FRAME	MEDIUM FRAME	LARGE FRAME
FEET	INCHES			
4	10	92–98	96–107	104–119
4	11	94–101	98–110	106–122
5	0	96–104	101–113	109–125
5	1	99–107	104–116	112–128
5	2	102–110	107–119	115–131
5	3	105–113	110–122	118–134
5	4	108–116	113–126	121–138
5	5	111–119	116–130	125 142
5	6	114–123	120–135	129–146
5	7	118–127	124–139	133–150
5	8	122–131	128–143	137–154
5	9	126–135	132–147	141–158
5	10	130–140	136–151	145–163
5	11	134–144	140–155	149–168
6	0	138–148	144–159	153–173

* Information supplied through courtesy of Metropolitan Life Insurance Company, U.S.A.

INDEX